HIGH ALTITUDE MEDICINE
AND PHYSIOLOGY

HIGH ALTITUDE MEDICINE AND PHYSIOLOGY

Fifth edition

John B West MD PhD DSc FRCP FRACP
Professor of Medicine & Physiology, School of Medicine,
University of California, San Diego, USA

Robert B Schoene MD
Clinical Professor of Medicine, Division of Pulmonary and Critical Care
Medicine, University of Washington School of Medicine, Seattle, USA

Andrew Luks MD
Associate Professor, Division Pulmonary and Critical Care Medicine,
Harborview Medical Center and University of Washington, Seattle,
Washington, USA

James S Milledge MBChB MD FRCP
Hon Professor, University College London, and formerly Consultant
Respiratory Physician and Medical Director, Northwick Park Hospital,
Harrow, UK

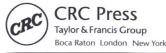

CRC Press
Taylor & Francis Group
Boca Raton London New York

CRC Press is an imprint of the
Taylor & Francis Group, an **informa** business

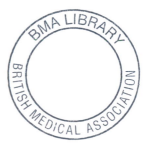

Preface

New advances in the areas of high altitude medicine and physiology continue to be made at a rapid pace. For example, since the last edition of this book in 2007, there have been dramatic advances in the area of genetics of high altitude. One of the most important discoveries has been the genetic differences between Tibetans and Han Chinese with the expectation that this will go a long way in explaining the remarkable adaptation of Tibetans to their environment. Additional important advances have been made on the functions of hypoxia-inducible factors which we now realize orchestrate many of the body's responses to hypoxia. Added to this has been a better understanding of the phenotypic differences between Andeans and Tibetans which are the two principal populations of the world that have so successfully adapted to high altitude. All this new work has justified a new chapter on genetics at altitude and this is written in a way that should make this somewhat technical topic accessible to those of us who do not have a strong background in the area.

Additional important advances have been made in the management of high altitude diseases. For example, the value of the different medications available for acute mountain sickness is addressed, together with new information on strategies for acclimatization. Advances in our understanding of the mechanism of high altitude pulmonary edema are discussed together with their therapeutic implications. Extensive additions have been made to the chapter on other high altitude related medical conditions. In addition, the chapter on pre-existing medical conditions has been extensively revised.

Another burgeoning area is the challenge presented to people who need to go to high altitude to work. Mines are being developed at increasingly high altitudes, particularly in South America. There are now very large telescopes located as high as 5000 m in north Chile and effective work at those altitudes is only possible using oxygen enrichment of room air. A striking technological advance is the new Chinese train to Lhasa which passes through an altitude over 5000 m. The ingenious solution has been to increase the oxygen concentration in every passenger car on the train. A sadder event is the continuing dispute between India and Pakistan in the region of the Siachen Glacier where troops are operating at over 6000 m with a correspondingly high morbidity.

For this new edition, all sections of the book have been carefully updated, but great pains have been taken to maintain a reasonable length. There are a number of new illustrations. The references have been brought up to date with some of them so recent that they have been completed in the proof stage.

A welcome addition to the group of editors is Andrew Luks MD from the University of Washington in Seattle. He is an avid mountaineer and has a particular interest in the clinical aspects of high altitude diseases. He has been responsible for updating several of the chapters in this area.

Mountains continue to attract increasing numbers of people for skiing, trekking or climbing. In addition, commercial activities at high altitude are increasing at a rapid rate. Happily, there has been a large increase in research on the diseases that affect permanent dwellers at high altitude, an area that has traditionally received less attention than should have been the case. Our hope is that this new edition will continue to improve the health and safety of all people who live, visit or work at high altitude. It is a pleasure to acknowledge the continuing support of Joanna Koster and her colleagues at Hodder Arnold.

John B West
Robert B Schoene
Andrew Luks
James S Milledge

Acknowledgements

We acknowledge help from many friends and colleagues who have read and provided comments on parts of the text. Tatum Simonson PhD gave advice in the chapter on Genetics and High Altitude, and Keith Lander provided general editorial assistance. Andrew Luks is grateful to Erik Swenson for support and mentorship through his career. Pat Howell read and corrected the chapters by Jim Milledge.

We would also like to thank all those who contributed to the original work on which much of this book is based. These include Sherpas, porters, climbers, scientists and other supporters who made the projects possible. We remember too, with gratitude, all those who share the adventure of science with colleagues in the high places of the world.

Conversion tables

Table F.1 Conversion of pressure units mmHg (millimeters of mercury) to kPa (kilopascals)

mmHg	kPa
1	0.133
10	1.33
20	2.67
30	4.00
40	5.33
50	6.67
60	8.00
80	10.7
100	13.3
200	26.7
300	40.0
500	66.7
700	93.3
760	101.3

1 torr = 1mmHg

Table F.2 Conversion of height units and barometric pressure according to the ICAO Standard Atmosphere and the actual pressure on most high mountains at low latitudes (see Table 2.1)

Altitude		Pressure mmHg	
m	ft	Standard	Actual
0	0	760	760
1 000	3 281	674	679
2 000	6 562	596	604
3 000	9 843	526	537
4 000	13 123	462	475
5 000	16 404	405	420
6 000	19 685	354	369
7 000	22 966	308	324
8 000	26 247	267	284
9 000	29 258	231	247

1 Watt = 6.12 kg. m min^{-1}

Table F.3 Conversion of temperature units, °C (degrees Celsius) to °F (degrees Fahrenheit)

°C	°F
−40	−40
−30	−20
−25	−13
−20	−4
−15	5
−10	14
−5	23
0	32
5	41
10	50
15	59
20	68
25	77
50	86
35	95
40	104

1 Watt = 6.12 kg. m min^{-1}

Table F.4 Conversion of energy units, kcal (kilocalories) to kJ (kilojoules)

kcal	kJ
50	209.4
100	418.8
250	1 047
500	2 094
1 000	4 188
2 000	8 375
3 000	12 563
4 000	16 750
5 000	20 938
6 000	25 126

1 Watt = 6.12 kg. m min^{-1}

List of abbreviations

ACE	angiotensin converting enzyme		CXEE	Caudwell Xtreme Everest Expedition
ACTH	adrenocorticotropic hormone		DLCO	diffusing capacity or carbon monoxide
ADH	aldosterone		E	estrogen
ADH	anti-diuretic hormone		E+P	estrogen plus progesterone
AFC	alveolar fluid clearance		ECF	extracellular fluid
AH	acute hypoxia		ECG	electrocardiogram
Aldo	aldosterone		ECMO	extra-corporeal membrane oxygenation
ALMA	atacama large millimeter/sub-millimeter array		EEG	electroencephalogram
			EMG	electromyography
AM	adrenomedullin		eNOS	endothelial nitric oxide synthase
AMREE	American Medical Research Expedition to Everest		EPO	erythropoietin
			ERB	endothelin receptor blocker
AMS	acute mountain sickness		ERPF	effective renal plasma flow
ANP	atrial natriuretic peptide		ESQ	environmental symptom questionnaire
ASHRAE	American Society of Heating, Refrigeration and Air-Conditioning Engineers		ET	endothelin
			ET-1	endothelin-1
ATP	adenosine triphosphate		FSH	follicle-stimulating hormone
AVP	arginine vasopressin		FVC	forced vital capacity
BAL	bronchoalveolar lavage		GABA	gamma aminobutyric acid
BBB	blood–brain barrier		HACE	high altitude cerebral edema
BCAA	branched-chain amino acid		HAPE	high altitude pulmonary edema
bFGF	basic fibroblast growth factor		HAPH	high altitude pulmonary hypertension
BMEME	British Mount Everest Medical Expedition		HAR	high altitude retinopathy
BMR	basal metabolic rate		Hb	hemoglobin
BNP	brain natriuretic peptide		[Hb]	hemoglobin concentration
BP	blood pressure		Hct	hematocrit
BTPS	body temperature and pressure saturated		HCVR	hypercapnic ventilatory response
CAD	coronary artery disease		HIF	hydroxia-inducible factor
CBF	cerebral blood flow		HIF-1	hypoxia-inducible factor 1
CF	cystic fibrosis		HIF-1α	hypoxia-inducible factor-1 alpha
CH	chronic hypoxia		HPVR	hypoxic pulmonary vascular response
CKD	chronic kidney disease		HRE	hypoxia response element
CMS	chronic mountain sickness		HVD	hypoxic ventilatory decline
CNS	central nervous system		HVR	hypercapnic ventilatory response
COLD	chronic obstructive lung disorder		I/D	insertion/deletion
COPD	chronic obstructive pulmonary disease		ICD	implantable cardiac defibrillator
CPAP	continuous positive airway pressure		ICP	intracranial pressure
CSF	cerebrospinal fluid		IH	intermittent hypoxia
CT	computed tomography		IHE	intermittent hypoxic exposure
CTS	comet-tail scores		iNOS	inducible nitric oxide synthase

INR	international normalized ratio
IOP	intraocular pressure
ISMM	International Society for Mountain Medicine
IT	interval training
IUGR	intra-uterine growth retardation
LASIK	laser-assisted in situ keratomeliusis
LH	luteinizing hormone
LHTL	live high, train low
LLS	Lake Louise Score
LLSS	Lake Louise Scoring System
LLTH	live low, train high
LLTL	live low, train low
LT	lactate threshold
LVF	left ventricular failure
MFNS	magnetic femoral nerve stimulation
MIGET	multiple inert gas elimination technique
MR	magnetic resonance
MRI	magnetic resonance imaging
MVV	maximal voluntary ventilation
NESP	novel erythropoiesis stimulating protein
NFPA	National Fire Protection Association
NHE1	sodium/hydrogen ion exchanger isoform 1
NIPPV	non-invasive positive pressure ventilation
NK	natural killer
NO	nitric oxide
NOx	no metabolites
NPY	neuropeptide y
NREM	non-rapid eye movement
NSAIDs	non-steroidal anti-inflammatory drugs
OHD	oxygen–hemoglobin dissociation
ONSD	optic nerve sheath diameter
OPS	orthogonal polarization spectral
PAC	plasma aldosterone concentration
PAL	physical activity level
PAP	pulmonary artery pressure
PASP	pulmonary artery systolic pressure
PCr	phosphocreatine
PCV	packed cell volume
PDE-5	phosphodiesterase type-5
PDGF	platelet-derived growth factor
PFO	patent foramen ovales
PHD	prolyl hydroxylase domain
PRA	plasma renin activity
PRK	photorefractive keratectomy
PV	plasma volume
PVR	pulmonary vascular resistance
RAS	renin–angiotensin system
RBC	red blood cells
RCM	red cell mass
RDBPC	randomized, double-blind, placebo-controlled
REDST	redox state
REM	rapid eye movement
rhEPO	recombinant human epo
RK	radial keratotomy
ROS	oxygen free radicals
ROS	reactive oxygen species
RQ	respiratory quotient
SAH	subarachnoid hemorrhage
SBP	systolic blood pressure
SDF	sidestream dark-field
17-OHCSs	17-hydroxycorticosteroids
SIDS	sudden infant death syndrome
SiEp	serum immunoreactive epo concentration
SL	sea level
SNP	single nucleotide polymorphism
STPD	standard temperature and pressure, dry gas
SWS	slow wave sleep
TBG	thyroxine-binding globulin
TBW	total body water
TEG	thromboelastography
TGF	transforming growth factor
TIA	transient ischemic attacks
TLC	total lung capacity
TRPC	transient receptor potential
TSH	thyroid-stimulating hormone
TT	time trial
2,3-DPG	2,3-diphosphoglycerate
UA	uterine arteries
Ub	ubiquitin
UKIRT	United Kingdom Infrared Telescope
V/Q	ventilation/perfusion
VAS	visual analog scale
VDH	ventilatory deacclimatization from hypoxia
VEGF	vascular endothelial growth factor
VHL	von Hippel–Lindau
WBC	white blood cells

History

SUMMARY

The history of high altitude medicine and physiology is one of the most colorful in the whole of the life sciences. Although there were a few anecdotal references to medical problems at high altitude before 1600, Joseph de Acosta's description of acute mountain sickness, originally published in 1590, is a watershed. Shortly after this the mercury barometer was invented by Evangelista Torricelli in 1644, and very quickly it was recognized that barometric pressure declined with altitude. Robert Boyle and Robert Hooke constructed the first air pump for physiological measurements in 1660 and Boyle then proposed his famous law. During the seventeenth and eighteenth centuries the nature of respiration was elucidated and the respiratory gases were first clearly described by Lavoisier in 1777. Soon the effects of acute ascent to high altitude were dramatically shown by the early balloonists including several fatalities from the severe hypoxia. The French physiologist, Paul Bert, was the first to clearly identify the low partial pressure of oxygen as responsible for high altitude illness with his landmark publication *La Pression Barométrique* in 1878.

When climbing became popular in the European Alps in the mid-nineteenth century many instances of acute mountain sickness were described. The construction of the Observatoire Vallot in France and the Capanna Margherita in Italy facilitated early medical and physiological studies of high altitude. The early twentieth century saw the beginning of special expeditions to high altitude to make medical and physiological measurements including the important Pikes Peak Expedition of 1911. A lively topic at this time was the possibility of oxygen secretion by the lung and this was finally resolved in favor of passive diffusion. Attempts to climb the highest mountain in the world, Mount Everest, comprise a great saga culminating in the first ascent in 1953 when supplemental oxygen was used, and the first ascent without bottled oxygen in 1978.

More recently, there have been several dedicated expeditions to explore the physiology of extreme altitude and generally an enormous increase in high altitude life sciences research. An important area has been the medical and physiological features of permanent residents of high altitude. A recent major advance was the discovery of genetic differences in Tibetans compared with Han Chinese. Another area of study is ways of improving the quality of life for people who are required to work at high altitude.

1.1 INTRODUCTION

This chapter provides an overall view of the history of high altitude medicine and physiology. More information about specific events is given at the beginning of subsequent chapters. Readers who desire more details can find these in West (1998). Table 1.1 shows a chronology of some of the principal events in the development of high altitude medicine and physiology.

1.2 CLASSICAL GREECE AND ROME

It is perhaps surprising that there are so few references to the ill effects of high altitude in the extensive writings of classical Greece and Rome. The Greek epics and myths, in particular, are so rich in the accounts of travels and the foibles of human nature that one might expect there to be a reference to the deleterious effects of high altitude but this is generally not the case. However, seventeenth century writers believed that the ancient Greeks were aware of the thinness of the air at high altitude. For example, Robert Boyle (1627–91) claimed that Aristotle (384–322 BC) held this view when he wrote:

Table 1.1   Chronology of some principal events in the development of high altitude medicine and physiology

Year	Event
c. 30 BC	Reference to the Great Headache Mountain and Little Headache Mountain in the *Ch'ien Han Shu* (classical Chinese history)
1590	Publication of the first edition (Spanish) of *Historia Natural y Moral de las Indias* by Joseph de Acosta with an account of mountain sickness
1644	First description of the mercury barometer by Torricelli
1648	Demonstration of the fall in barometric pressure at high altitude in an experiment devised by Pascal
1777	Clear description of oxygen and the other respiratory gases by Lavoisier
1783	Montgolfier brothers initiate balloon ascents
1786	First ascent of Mont Blanc (4807 m) by Balmat and Paccard
1878	Publication of *La Pression Barométrique* by Paul Bert
1890	Viault describes high altitude polycythemia
1890	Joseph Vallot builds a high altitude laboratory at 4350 m on Mont Blanc
1891	Christian Bohr publishes *Uber die Lungenathmung*, giving evidence for the secretion of both oxygen and carbon dioxide by the lung
1893	High altitude station, Capanna Regina Margherita, is built on a summit of Monte Rosa at 4559 m
1906	Publication of *Hohenklima und Bergwanderungen* by Zuntz *et al.*
1909	The Duke of the Abruzzi reaches 7500 m in the Karakoram without supplementary oxygen
1910	Zuntz organizes an international high altitude expedition to Tenerife
1910	August Krogh publishes *On the Mechanism of Gas-Exchange in the Lungs*, disproving the secretion theory of gas exchange

1911	Anglo-American Pikes Peak expedition (4300 m); participants C.G. Douglas, J.S. Haldane, Y. Henderson and E.C. Schneider
1913	T.H. Ravenhill publishes *Some Experiences of Mountain Sickness in the Andes*, describing *puna* of the normal, cardiac and nervous types
1920	Barcroft *et al.* publish the results of the experiment carried out in a glass chamber in which Barcroft lived in a hypoxic atmosphere for 6 days
1921	A.M. Kellas finishes his manuscript on 'A consideration of the possibility of ascending Mt Everest' which remained unpublished until 2001
1921–22	International High Altitude Expedition to Cerro de Pasco, Peru, led by Joseph Barcroft
1924	E.F. Norton ascends to 8500 m on Mount Everest without supplementary oxygen
1925	Barcroft publishes *The Respiratory Function of the Blood*. Part 1. *Lessons from High Altitude*
1935	International High Altitude Expedition to Chile, scientific leader D.B. Dill
1946	Operation Everest I carried out by C.S. Houston and R.L. Riley
1948	Carlos Monge M. publishes *Acclimatization in the Andes*, about the permanent residents of the Peruvian Andes
1949	H. Rahn and A.B. Otis publish *Man's Respiratory Response During and After Acclimatization to High Altitude*
1952	L.G.C.E. Pugh and colleagues carry out experiments on Cho Oyu near Mount Everest in preparation for the 1953 expedition
1953	First ascent of Mount Everest by Hillary and Tenzing (with supplementary oxygen)
1960–61	Himalayan Scientific and Mountaineering Expedition in the Everest region, scientific leader L.G.C.E. Pugh. Silver Hut laboratory at 5800 m, measurements up to 7440 m
1968–79	High altitude studies on Mount Logan (5334 m), scientific director C.S. Houston
1973	Italian Mount Everest Expedition with laboratory at 5350 m, scientific leader P. Cerretelli
1978	First ascent of Everest without supplementary oxygen by Reinhold Messner and Peter Habeler
1981	American Medical Research Expedition to Everest, scientific leader J.B. West
1985	Operation Everest II, scientific leaders C.S. Houston and J.R. Sutton
1983 to present	Research at Capanna Regina Margherita (4559 m) by O. Oelz, P. Bärtsch and co-workers from Zurich, Bern and Heidelberg
1984 to present	Studies at Observatoire Vallot (4350 m) on Mont Blanc by J.-P. Richalet and co-workers
1985	Studies on Mt McKinley (Denali) at 4400 m, leader P. Hackett
1990 to present	Research at Pyramid Laboratory, Lobuje, Nepal by P. Cerretelli and co-workers
1991	Expedition to Mt Sajama, 6542 m, leader J.-P. Richalet
1994	British Mount Everest Medical Research Expedition, leaders S. Currin, A. Pollard and D. Collier
1997	Operation Everest III (COMEX '97), leader J.-P. Richalet
1998	Medical Research Expedition to Kangchenjunga, leaders S. Currin, D. Collier and J. Milledge
1998	Expedition to Chacaltaya, 5200 m, leader B. Saltin
2007	Caudwell Xtreme Everest Expedition, leader M. Grocott
2010	Reports by several groups of genetic changes in Tibetans compared with Han Chinese

That which some of those that treat of the height of Mountains, relate out of Aristotle, namely, That those that ascend to the top of the Mountain Olympus, could not keep themselves alive, without carrying with them wet Spunges, by whose assistance they could respire in that Air, otherwise too thin for Respiration: . . .

(Boyle 1660, p. 357)

However, modern historians have not been able to find this statement in Aristotle's extensive writings. Similar attributions to Aristotle can be found in the writings of Francis Bacon (1561–1626) and St Augustine of Hippo (354–430). See West (1998) for additional information.

1.3 CHINESE HEADACHE MOUNTAINS

There is a tantalizing reference to what may have been acute mountain sickness in the classical Chinese history, the *Ch'ien Han Shu*, which dates from about 30 BC. One of the Chinese officials was warning about the dangers of traveling to the western regions, probably part of present day Afghanistan, when he stated that travelers would not only be exposed to attacks from robbers but they would also become ill. One of the translations reads:

> Again, on passing the Great Headache Mountain, the Little Headache Mountain, the Red Land, and the Fever Slope, men's bodies become feverish, they lose colour, and are attacked with headache and vomiting; the asses and cattle being all in like condition. . . .

Several people have tried to identify the site of the Headache Mountains, suggesting for instance that it is the Kilik Pass (4827 m) in the Karakoram Range on the route from Kashgar to Gilgit (Gilbert 1983). However, there is not universal agreement on this.

1.4 POSSIBLE EARLY REFERENCE TO HIGH ALTITUDE PULMONARY EDEMA

Fâ-Hien was a Chinese Buddhist monk who made a remarkable journey through China and adjoining countries in about AD 400. He related that when crossing the 'Little Snowy Mountains' (probably in Afghanistan) his companion became ill, 'a white froth came from his mouth' and he died. It is tempting to identify this as the first description of high altitude pulmonary edema.

1.5 JOSEPH DE ACOSTA'S DESCRIPTION OF MOUNTAIN SICKNESS

Joseph de Acosta (1540–1600) was a Jesuit priest who traveled to Peru in about 1570. While he was there he ascended the Andes and gave a very colorful account of illness associated with high altitude. This was first published in 1590 in Spanish (Acosta 1590) (Fig. 1.1), and an English translation entitled *The Naturall and Morall Historie of the East and West Indies* appeared in 1604 (Acosta 1604). Here are some passages from his account when the party were near the top of Mount Pariacaca.

> I was suddenly surprized with so mortall and strange a pang, that I was ready to fall from the top to the ground. . . .

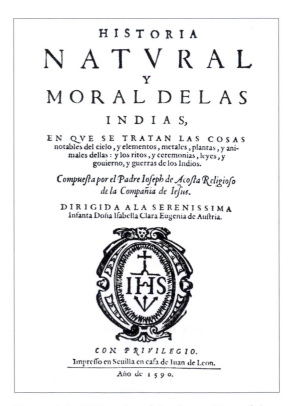

Figure 1.1 Title page of the first edition of the book by Joseph de Acosta published in Seville in 1590.

He then went on to add:

> I was surprized with such pangs of straining
> & casting, as I thought to cast up my heart
> too; for having cast up meate, fleugme &
> choller, both yellow and greene; in the
> end I cast up blood, with the straining
> of my stomacke. To conclude, if this had
> continued, I should undoubtedly have
> died. . . .

This is followed by an often-quoted passage:

> I therefore perswade my selfe that the
> element of the aire is there so subtile and
> delicate, as it is not proportionable with the
> breathing of man, which requires a more
> grosse and temperate aire, and I beleeve
> it is the cause that doth so much alter the
> stomacke, & trouble all the disposition.

It should be noted that this is not a typical account
of acute mountain sickness which usually comes
on gradually and is not associated with severe
vomiting. The description sounds more like a
gastrointestinal upset.

Acosta's book was widely read and, for example,
Robert Boyle was familiar with his description
of mountain sickness. Various people including
Gilbert (1991) have attempted to identify the site
of Pariacaca but there is some disagreement over
this.

1.6 INVENTION OF THE BAROMETER

A key advance in high altitude science was the
recognition that barometric pressure falls with
increasing altitude. In 1644 Evangelista Torricelli
(1608–47) wrote a letter to his friend Michelangelo
Ricci in which he described how he had filled a
glass tube with mercury and inverted it so that
one end was immersed in a dish of the same liquid
(Torricelli 1644) (Fig. 1.2). The mercury descended
to form a column about 76 cm high, and Torricelli
argued that the mercury was supported by the
weight of the atmosphere acting on the dish. His
letter included the striking sentence: 'We live

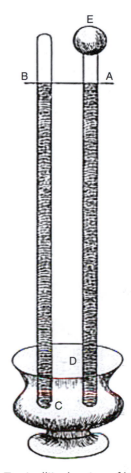

Figure 1.2 Torricelli's drawing of his
first mercury barometer, from his letter to
Michelangelo Ricci of 1644.

submerged at the bottom of an ocean of the
element air, which by unquestioned experiments is
known to have weight. . . .' This was a conceptual
breakthrough. Torricelli also speculated that on the
tops of high mountains the pressure might be less
because the air is 'distinctly rare'.

However, it was left to Blaise Pascal (1623–62) to
prove that barometric pressure falls with increasing
altitude. In 1648 he persuaded his brother-in-law,
Florin Perier, to carry a mercury barometer up
the Puy-de-Dôme in central France. This was an
elaborate experiment with careful controls and he
was successful in showing that on the summit the
pressure had fallen by approximately 12% of its
value in the village of Clermont.

1.7 INVENTION OF THE AIR PUMP

The first effective air pump was constructed by Otto von Guericke (1602–86) who was mayor of the city of Magdeburg in central Germany. In a famous experiment he constructed two metal hemispheres which fitted together accurately when the air within them was pumped out. Two teams of horses were then unable to separate the two hemispheres, graphically demonstrating the enormous force that could be developed by the air pressure.

However, Guericke's pump was cumbersome to operate and it was impossible to place objects in the hemispheres to study the effects of the reduced air pressure. This was first done by Robert Boyle (1627–91) and his colleague Robert Hooke (1635–1703). Hooke was a mechanical genius who designed an air pump consisting of a piston inside a brass cylinder. Above this was a large glass receiver into which various objects and small animals could be placed (Fig. 1.3). In his groundbreaking book *New Experiments Physico-Mechanicall, Touching the Spring of the Air, and its Effects. . .* (Boyle 1660), he demonstrated the effects of a reduced atmospheric pressure in a variety of experiments. In one of these a lark was placed in the receiver and Boyle wrote:

> the Lark was very lively, and did, being put into the Receiver, divers times spring

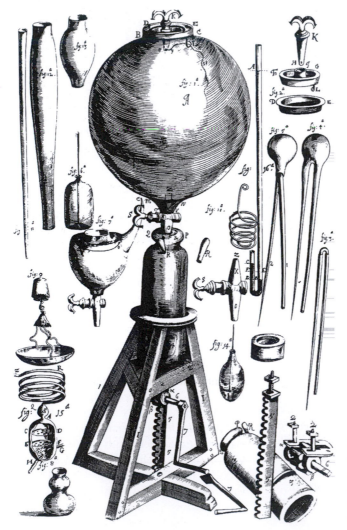

Figure 1.3 Air pump constructed by Robert Boyle and Robert Hooke. This enabled them to carry out the first experiments on hypobaric hypoxia. From Boyle (1660).

up in it to a good height. The Vessel being hastily, but carefully clos'd, the Pump was diligently ply'd, and the Bird for a while appear'd lively enough; but upon a greater Exsuction of the Air, she began manifestly to droop and appear sick, and very soon after was taken with as violent and irregular Convulsions, as are wont to be observ'd in Poultry, when their heads are wrung off. . . .

Following these experiments Hooke made a chamber large enough for a man to sit in it while it was partially evacuated and he reported to the young Royal Society:

that himself had been in it, and by the contrivance of bellows and valves blown out of it one tenth part of the air (which he found by a gage suspended within the vessel) and had felt no inconvenience but that of some pain in his ears at the breaking out of the air included in them, and the like pain upon the readmission of the air pressing the ear inwards.

1.8 DISCOVERY OF OXYGEN

Progress in the remainder of the seventeenth century and most of the eighteenth century was largely stymied until the nature of the respiratory gases was characterized. There is not space here to follow the interesting story of the work of Boyle, Hooke, Lower and Mayow in the seventeenth century and the discovery of oxygen by Joseph Priestley (1733–1804), Carl Scheele (1742–86) and Antoine Lavoisier (1743–94). John Mayow (1641–79) was aware in 1674 of what he called 'nitro-aerial spirit', which we now recognize as oxygen but his work was largely ignored for almost a century. Both Priestley and Scheele independently isolated oxygen but Priestley was confused about its nature, believing that it was 'unphlogisticated air', and Scheele's report was delayed because of publication problems. It was left to the brilliant French chemist Lavoisier (Fig. 1.4) to clearly describe the three respiratory gases. In 1777 he stated:

Eminently respirable air [he later called it oxygine] that enters the lung, leaves it in the form of chalky aeriform acids [carbon

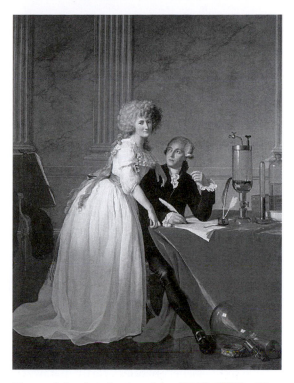

Figure 1.4 Antoine Lavoisier (1747–1794) with his wife Marie-Anne (1759–1836), who was his laboratory assistant. From the painting by David, 1780.

dioxide] . . . in almost equal volume. . . . Respiration acts only on the portion of pure air that is eminently respirable . . . the excess, that is its mephitic portion [nitrogen], is a purely passive medium which enters and leaves the lung . . . without change or alteration. The respirable portion of air has the property to combine with blood and its combination results in its red color.

Carbon dioxide had been discovered earlier by Joseph Black (1728–99) while he was a medical student although he used the term 'fixed air'.

1.9 FIRST BALLOON ASCENTS AND THE RECOGNITION OF SEVERE ACUTE HYPOXIA

The Montgolfier brothers, Joseph (1740–1810) and Jacques (1745–99), invented the man-carrying balloon, first using heated air, and later hydrogen. The first free ascent of a manned balloon took place in Paris in 1783. It was not long before these adventurous balloonists became aware of the deleterious effects of high altitude on the body. For example, Alexandre Charles (1746–1823) (of Charles' law) ascended in a hydrogen-filled balloon in December 1783 and reported 'In the midst of the inexpressible rapture of this contemplative ecstasy, I was recalled to myself by a very extraordinary pain in the interior of my right ear. . . .' He correctly attributed this to the effects of air pressure.

However, more ominous effects were soon noted. Jean Blanchard (1753–1809) claimed to have ascended to an altitude of over 10 000 m in 1785 (although the altitude was contested) and reported that 'Nature grew languid, I felt a numbness, prelude of a dangerous sleep. . . .' However, much more dramatic were the events in 1862 when James Glaisher (1809–1903) and Henry Coxwell (1819–1900) rose to an altitude which was estimated to exceed 10 000 m. Glaisher became partly paralyzed and then unconscious, and Coxwell lost the use of his hands, and could only open the valve of the balloon by seizing the cord with his teeth. Glaisher also reported losing his sight before his partial paralysis.

The most famous and tragic balloon ascent was by three French aeronauts, Gaston Tissandier (1843–99), Joseph Crocé-Spinelli (1843–75) and Theodore Sivel (1834–75), in their balloon Zénith in 1875. Paul Bert (see below) had recommended that they take oxygen but they had too little and there were difficulties in inhaling it. Tissandier's report (1875) is dramatic.

> Towards 7500 meters, the numbness one experiences is extraordinary. . . . One does not suffer at all; on the contrary. One experiences inner joy, as if it were an effect of the inundating flood of light. One becomes indifferent. . . . Soon I wanted to seize the oxygen tube, but could not raise my arm. . . . Suddenly I closed my eyes and fell inert, entirely losing consciousness.

When the balloon ultimately reached the ground, Sivel and Crocé-Spinelli were dead, having perished as a result of the severe hypoxia. The disaster caused a sensation in France.

1.10 MOUNTAIN SICKNESS IN MOUNTAINEERS

During the nineteenth century, mountaineering became popular particularly in the European Alps. The result was many descriptions of acute mountain sickness, some of which seem to us today to be greatly exaggerated. One of the first was from the great German naturalist Alexander von Humboldt (1769–1859) when he reached very high altitudes on two volcanoes in South America in 1799. On Chimborazo, at an altitude of about 5540 m, he stated that the whole party felt 'a discomfort, a weakness, a desire to vomit, which certainly arises as much from the lack of oxygen in these regions as from the rarity of the air.' Another early account was by Horace-Bénédict de Saussure (1740–99) on Mont Blanc (4807 m) in 1787. When he was near the summit he stated:

> I therefore hoped to reach the crest in less than three quarters of an hour; but the rarity of the air gave me more trouble than I could have believed. At last I was obliged to stop for breath every fifteen or sixteen steps. . . . This need of rest was absolutely unconquerable; if I tried to overcome it, my legs refused to move. . .

Numerous other reports of the deleterious effects of high altitude while climbing mountains are given in the first chapter of Paul Bert's book *La Pression Barométrique* (1878).

1.11 PAUL BERT AND THE PUBLICATION OF *LA PRESSION BAROMÉTRIQUE*

The French environmental physiologist Paul Bert (1833–86) is often cited as the father of modern high altitude physiology and medicine. The publication of his great book *La Pression Barométrique* in 1878 was certainly an important landmark. One of his principal findings was that the deleterious effects of exposure to low pressure could be attributed to the low P_{O_2}. He did this by exposing experimental animals to a low pressure of air on the one hand (hypobaric hypoxia), and to gas mixtures at normal pressure but with a low oxygen concentration (normobaric hypoxia) on the other. In this way he showed that the critical variable was the P_{O_2}. *La Pression Barométrique* is essential reading for anybody with a serious interest in the history of high altitude medicine and physiology. A good English translation is available (Bert, 1878). For one thing, there is a long introductory section on the history as Bert saw it, and this makes fascinating reading today. Bert wrote with a charming style and urbane wit. The book not only deals with the medical and physiological effects of low pressure but high pressure as well.

Many of Bert's studies were carried out at the Sorbonne in Paris which was equipped with both low pressure and high pressure chambers (Fig. 1.5). At one stage he tested the three French balloonists Tissandier, Crocé-Spinelli and Sivel who were referred to above and he actually warned them that they had insufficient oxygen but the warning letter arrived too late.

La Pression Barométrique includes many interesting passages. For example, it contains the first graphs of the oxygen and carbon dioxide dissociation curves in blood. Bert also speculated that polycythemia might occur at high altitude and this was shown a short time later by compatriots including Viault (1890). At one point Bert speculated on the possible reduction of metabolism in frequent visitors to high altitude and people who live permanently there. This short section will be cited partly because it gives a good feel for the style of Bert and his pungent wit.

We see that very probably, in the habitual conditions of our life, we commit excesses of oxygenation as well as of nourishment, two kinds of excess, which are correlative. And just as peasants, who eat much less than we do, but utilizing all that they absorb, produce in heat and work a useful result equal, if not superior, to that of city dwellers; just as a Basque mountaineer furnished with a piece of bread and a few onions makes expeditions which require of the member

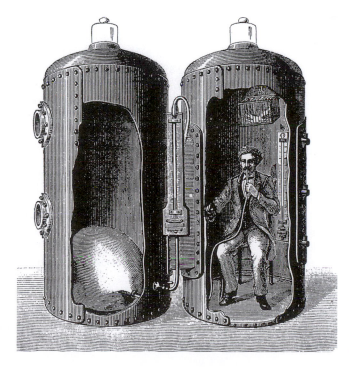

Figure 1.5 Low pressure chambers used by Paul Bert at the Sorbonne. From Bert (1878).

of the Alpine Club who accompanies him the absorption of a pound of meat, so it may be that the dwellers in high places finally lessen the consumption of oxygen in their organism, while keeping at their disposal the same quantity of vital force, either for the equilibrium of temperature, or the production of work. Thus we could explain the acclimatization of individuals, of generations, of races.

(Bert 1878, p. 1004 in the English translation)

1.12 HIGH ALTITUDE LABORATORIES

1.12.1 Observatoire Vallot

Towards the end of the nineteenth century the pace of discoveries in high altitude medicine and physiology accelerated rapidly partly as the result of the publication of *La Pression Barométrique*. This was a period when two high altitude laboratories were established. The first was the Observatoire Vallot on Mont Blanc which was installed in 1890. Joseph Vallot (1854–1925) conceived the idea of placing a small building at an altitude of about 4350 m, which is about 460 m below the summit of Mont Blanc. With typical French panache he was not satisfied with a simple hut, but in addition there were a comprehensive laboratory, a well-appointed kitchen, and attractive interior decorations including a French tapestry of courtly ladies in the eighteenth century style. The laboratory was used for research in several of the physical sciences, including astronomy and glaciology, but physiological studies were also carried out including some of the first observations of periodic breathing at high altitude (Egli-Sinclair 1893). The Observatoire Vallot is still in use today although it has been considerably modified. Access is challenging because usually a night has to be spent at the Grands Mulets (3050 m) followed by a climb over the snow and ice the next day. Alternatively, a helicopter ascent is possible.

In 1891, a young physician, Dr Jacottet, died in the Observatoire Vallot from what was almost certainly high altitude pulmonary edema. A description of the illness including the post-mortem findings is in Mosso's book *Life of Man on the High Alps* (Mosso 1898) referred to in the next section.

1.12.2 Capanna Margherita

Shortly after the construction of the Observatoire Vallot, an even higher structure was placed on one of the peaks of Monte Rosa in Italy at an altitude of 4559 m. The original hut was completed in 1893 and 10 years later it was enlarged by the influential Italian scientist Angelo Mosso (1846–1910) to include a laboratory for physiological and medical studies. The structure owes its name to Queen Margherita of Savoy who was a lover of alpinism and a generous patron of science. In fact, she visited the Capanna in 1893 and spent the night there.

Mosso was a physiologist with very broad interests, particularly in the area of exercise and environmental physiology. Some of the early studies in the Capanna Margherita were reported in his book *Fisiologia dell'uomo sulle Alpi: studii fatti sul Monte Rosa* (Mosso 1897), and this was translated into English as *Life of Man on the High Alps* (Mosso 1898). Among the projects carried out at the Capanna were some on periodic breathing, and also total ventilation at high altitude. In fact, Mosso believed that the deleterious effects of high altitude were related to the low carbon dioxide levels in the blood rather than the reduced P_{O_2} as previously proposed by Paul Bert. Mosso coined the term 'acapnia' to describe this condition which he thought was important in the development of acute mountain sickness. An interesting event at the Capanna was the illness of an Italian soldier, Pietro Ramella, who developed what was thought to be a respiratory infection and from which he recovered. In retrospect, this may have been high altitude pulmonary edema as was the case with Jacottet at the Observatoire Vallot. The Capanna Margherita has been enlarged over the years and

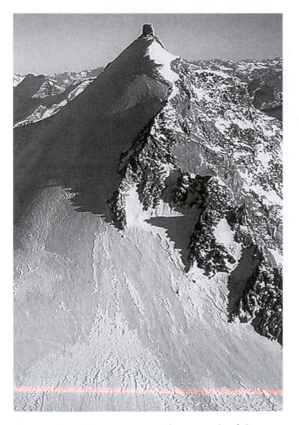

Figure 1.6 Contemporary photograph of the Capanna Margherita on one of the peaks of Monte Rosa. It is the site of an active research program on high altitude medicine and physiology.

is the site of a very active research program at the present time (Fig. 1.6).

1.13 EARLY SCIENTIFIC EXPEDITIONS TO HIGH ALTITUDE

In the early 1900s the tradition began of organizing expeditions to high altitude locations to carry out medical and physiological research. One of the first was organized by Nathan Zuntz (1847–1920), Professor of Animal Physiology in Berlin, who was the first author of an influential book on high altitude physiology published in 1906 (Zuntz *et al.* 1906). The expedition was to Tenerife in the Canary Islands and experiments were carried out at the Alta Vista hut at an altitude of 3350 m. Among the members of the

expedition were Joseph Barcroft (1872–1947) and C.G. Douglas (1882–1963) and they made an interesting observation on the alveolar gases and acclimatization. Barcroft was the only member of the party who showed no significant fall in alveolar P_{CO_2} at the Alta Vista hut; that is, he was the only person who did not exhibit an increase in ventilation, and he was also the only person who was incapacitated by acute mountain sickness. By contrast, the alveolar P_{CO_2} of Douglas fell from 41 to 32, and that of Zuntz fell from 35 to 27 mmHg and both of these members had no mountain sickness. This was corroborative evidence that mountain sickness was caused by the low P_{O_2} as suggested by Paul Bert, rather than the low P_{CO_2} as proposed by Angelo Mosso.

A very important expedition took place in 1911 when an Anglo-American group led by J.S. Haldane (1860–1936) went to Pikes Peak just outside Colorado Springs where there was a hotel on the summit at an altitude of 4300 m (Fig. 1.7). One of the advantages of Pikes Peak was a cog railway all the way to the summit. The expedition was carefully planned so that there were measurements at a lower altitude prior to the ascent. Then, a rapid ascent was made and the party stayed on the summit where extensive data were collected. Finally, measurements were made again when the participants returned to low altitude. Many important observations were made. The hyperventilation that accompanies ascent to high altitude was documented with the alveolar P_{CO_2} falling to about two-thirds of its sea level value over 2 weeks on the summit. Periodic breathing was confirmed. The polycythemia was studied with the percentage of hemoglobin in the blood increasing over several weeks on the summit to values between 115 and 154% of normal as measured by color changes in the blood. All the measurements were reported in a long paper (Douglas *et al.* 1913).

The members of the expedition also believed that they had obtained evidence for oxygen secretion at high altitude. In fact, the report stated that the arterial P_{O_2} at rest was as much as 35 mmHg above the alveolar value on the summit, whereas at or near sea level the two values were the same. The investigators proposed

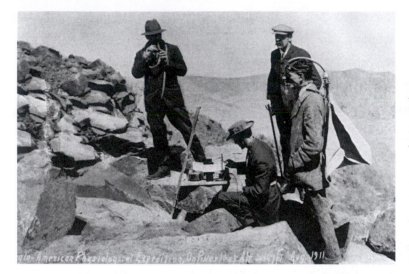

Figure 1.7 Members of the Anglo-American Pikes Peak Expedition of 1911. Left to right: Henderson taking samples of alveolar gas, Schneider sitting and recording his respiration, Haldane standing, and Douglas wearing a 'Douglas bag' to collect expired gas during exercise. From Henderson (1939).

that oxygen secretion was the most important factor in acclimatization. To this day it is not clear where this large error was made in the measurements.

Oxygen secretion was an important controversy around this time and Haldane actually believed in it until his death in 1936. In fact, the second edition of his book on respiration (Haldane and Priestley 1935) has a whole chapter devoted to the evidence for oxygen secretion. Haldane had originally developed the notion after visiting Christian Bohr (1855–1911) in Copenhagen who was a great champion of oxygen secretion. However, the error was exposed in the view of most physiologists by August Krogh (1874–1949) and his wife Marie (1874–1943) in a series of papers published in 1910.

Mabel FitzGerald (1872–1973) was invited to join the Pikes Peak expedition but did not spend any time in the laboratory for reasons that are not entirely clear. Instead, she visited various mining camps in Colorado at altitudes between 1500 and 4300 m where she measured the alveolar P_{CO_2} in acclimatized miners and produced data on acclimatization to moderate altitudes that are still extensively cited (FitzGerald 1913, Fitzgerald 1914). Although she studied at Oxford University for a number of years it was not the custom then to give degrees to women. However, the university relented in 1972 when she was 100 years old and awarded her an honorary MA degree.

Another classical expedition to high altitude was the International High Altitude Expedition to Cerro de Pasco, Peru which took place in 1921–22 under the leadership of Joseph Barcroft (1872–1947). An attractive feature of this location at an altitude of about 4330 m was that it could be reached by railway from Lima, and the expedition fitted out a railway baggage van as an efficient laboratory (Fig. 1.8). Again, there was a very extensive scientific program and the report occupied 129 pages (Barcroft *et al.* 1923). The topic of oxygen secretion was investigated but no support for it was found. In fact, the P_{O_2} in arterial blood measured by a bubble equilibration method was about 3 mmHg lower than that in alveolar gas. There was an increase in red blood cell concentration by about 20–30% over the sea level value. The arterial oxygen saturation fell during exercise at high altitude and this fall was correctly attributed to the failure of the P_{O_2} to equilibrate between alveolar gas and pulmonary capillary blood because of diffusion limitation. Extensive measurements of neuropsychological function showed that this was impaired at high altitude. In fact, Barcroft made the famous statement 'All dwellers at high altitude are persons of impaired physical and mental powers.'

One of the novel features of this expedition was its studies of permanent residents of high altitude. Cerro de Pasco was a substantial mining town with a large permanent population. It

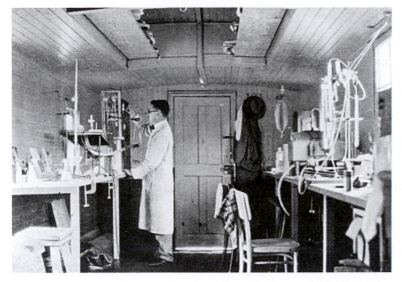

Figure 1.8   Laboratory of the International High Altitude Expedition to Cerro de Pasco, Peru, 1921–22. This was set up in a railroad car. From Barcroft *et al.* (1923).

was shown that the red cell concentrations in the permanent residents had values of 40–50% above what would be expected at sea level, that is substantially higher than the newcomers to high altitude. It was also found that the permanent residents of Cerro tended to have lower arterial oxygen saturations of 80–85%, one of the first intimations that highlanders have lower ventilations than newcomers to high altitude.

In 1935 the International High Altitude Expedition to Chile took place under the scientific leadership of D.B. Dill (1891–1986). A number of measurements were made at a mining camp, altitude 5334 m, and these resulted in a classical paper entitled 'Blood as a physicochemical system. XII. Man at high altitudes' (Dill *et al.* 1937). Extensive measurements of exercise were carried out showing, for example, that in one of the members the maximal oxygen consumption fell from 3.72 to 1.80 L min^{-1} at the altitude of the high camp (compared with sea level) while the maximal heart rate fell from 190 to 132 beats min^{-1}. A particularly interesting finding made by Edwards (1936) was that in well-acclimatized subjects the maximal levels of blood lactate were remarkably low, certainly much lower than in acute hypoxia or in subjects without acclimatization. This so-called 'lactate paradox' has been observed on many occasions since and is still not fully understood.

1.14 PERMANENT RESIDENTS OF HIGH ALTITUDE

A large number of people live permanently at high altitude. For example, about 140 million people live at altitudes above 2500 m (WHO 1996) and it has been estimated that each year some 40 million travel to similar altitudes for work or recreation. The high altitude populations are mainly in underdeveloped regions of the world, including the South American Andes, the Tibetan plateau and, to a lesser extent, Ethiopia. Partly as a result of this, these large populations have not received the attention they deserve.

Just as many people regard Paul Bert as the father of modern high altitude physiology, Carlos Monge Medrano (1884–1970) merits the title of father of the study of permanent high altitude residents. He started the influential Peruvian school in Lima and this was subsequently continued by Alberto Hurtado Abadilla (1901–83) and Monge's son, Carlos Monge Cassinelli (1921–2006). The Peruvian school remains very active today with high altitude scientists such as Fabiola León-Velarde, and there are also groups in Argentina, Bolivia, Chile, China and Tibet who are now doing extensive work on high altitude residents.

Mention was made earlier of Barcroft's unguarded statement that 'All dwellers at high altitude are persons of impaired physical and mental powers' (Barcroft 1925). Monge took great exception to this and in his influential book *Acclimatization in the Andes* (Monge M. 1948) he referred to 'the incredible statement of Professor Barcroft, the Cambridge physiologist, who after staying 3 months at Cerro de Pasco. . . .' Monge made the point that because of the 'climatic aggression' of high altitudes as he referred to it, Andean man should not be assessed using the same criteria as people who live near sea level. In fact, at one stage, Monge attributed Barcroft's statement to the fact that the latter had mountain sickness at the time!

Monge made extensive studies of the ability of permanent residents of the Andes to withstand the hypoxia and cold of the environment. Nevertheless, he is best known for his work on chronic mountain sickness, also known as Monge's disease, which he set out in his book *La Enfermedad de los Andes* (Monge M. 1928). In this he describes the condition associated with severe polycythemia, cyanosis and a variety of neuropsychological complaints including headache, dizziness, somnolence and fatigue. Initially the condition was thought to be polycythemia vera but was later shown to be distinct.

Alberto Hurtado (1901–83) was a physiologist who trained under Monge and who made extensive studies of the high altitude residents of Morococha at an altitude of 4550 m. Typically, the arterial Po_2 was only 45 mmHg with a corresponding arterial oxygen saturation of 81%. However, interestingly, because of the polycythemia which raised the hemoglobin concentration to nearly 20 g dL^{-1}, the arterial oxygen concentration was actually above the normal sea level value. The son of Carlos Monge Medrano, Carlos Monge Cassinelli (1921–2006) was a biologist with broad interests in high altitude including comparative physiology. However, he was very interested in the relationships between high altitude, polycythemia and chronic mountain sickness and many of his studies were reported in a classical book (Winslow and Monge C. 1987).

1.15 HIGH ALTITUDE STUDIES FROM THE LAST 60 YEARS

There have been such a wealth of high altitude studies during this period that it is impossible to

do them justice, and furthermore many of them will be alluded to in subsequent chapters of this book and so only a brief summary is given here. Many of the studies have concentrated on the effects of extreme altitude.

In 1944, Charles Houston (1913–2009) and Richard Riley (1911–2001) carried out a remarkable study known as Operation Everest I at the US Naval School of Aviation Medicine in Pensacola, Florida. Four volunteers lived continuously in a low pressure chamber for 35 days and were gradually decompressed to the equivalent of the altitude of Mount Everest. The project was justified to the Navy on the grounds that it was relevant to improving the tolerance of aviators to high altitudes. Alveolar gas and arterial blood studies were carried out and the most striking finding was that it was possible for resting, partly acclimatized subjects to survive for 20 minutes or so at a simulated altitude that actually exceeded the summit of Mount Everest. This came about because they were using the Standard Atmosphere which predicts a substantially lower pressure on the summit than actually exists.

A major high altitude physiologist at this time was L.C.G.E. Pugh (1909–94) who was a participant of the expedition to make the first successful ascent of Everest in 1953. During 1952, Pugh and others conducted physiological studies on the nearby mountain Cho Oyu to clarify some of the logistics of tolerating extreme altitude, including ventilation rates, maximal oxygen consumptions, effects of oxygen breathing, hydration, food and clothing. Pugh's contributions were a major factor in the ultimate success of the expedition when Edmund Hillary (1919–2008) and Tenzing Norgay (1914–86) became the first people to reach the highest point in the world.

In 1960–61 Pugh was the scientific leader of the Himalayan Scientific and Mountaineering Expedition, now universally known as the Silver Hut Expedition. The reason for the name is that the scientists wintered for several months at an altitude of 5800 m in a wooden structure painted silver (Fig. 1.9). The extensive scientific program was largely devoted to studies of exercise, pulmonary gas exchange, the control of ventilation, polycythemia, the electrocardiogram

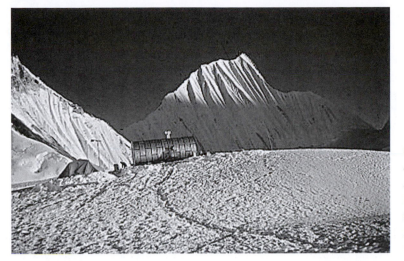

Figure 1.9 Main laboratory of the Himalayan Scientific and Mountaineering Expedition, 1960–61. The Silver Hut was at an altitude of 5800 m about 16 km south of Mount Everest.

and neuropsychological function (Pugh 1962a). Many of the studies are referred to in later chapters of this book.

In 1981 the American Medical Research Expedition to Everest set out to obtain the first data from the Everest summit itself and made measurements that so far have not been repeated. Among the remarkable findings were alveolar P_{O_2} and P_{CO_2} values of 35 and 7–8 mmHg and an arterial pH (based on the measured alveolar P_{CO_2} and blood base excess) of over 7.7. The barometric pressure on the summit was 253 mmHg., and the maximal oxygen consumption measured using the summit-inspired P_{O_2} was just over 1 L min^{-1}.

Four years later Houston and John Sutton (1941–96) carried out Operation Everest II at a US Army facility in Natick, Massachusetts which was basically similar to Operation Everest I in design but much more sophisticated in the measurements that could be made. Again the volunteers were gradually decompressed to the barometric pressure on the Everest summit and a large series of measurements that could not be made in the field were completed. These included cardiac catheterization which showed substantial increases in pulmonary artery pressures with ascent, particularly on exercise.

An interesting aspect was that after a few days the pulmonary hypertension could not be reversed by giving oxygen, suggesting that some remodeling of the pulmonary circulation had taken place. Other important information was obtained on pulmonary gas exchange, changes in skeletal muscle by biopsy, and neuropsychological changes. Another simulated ascent of Mount Everest using a low pressure chamber was carried out in 1997 (called Operation Everest III (COMEX '97)) and, again, important new information was obtained in a number of areas.

In 2007 the Caudwell Xtreme Everest Expedition was led by Michael Grocott. It had the distinction of collecting arterial blood samples from four climbers at an altitude of 8400 m. These showed an arterial P_{O_2} as low as 19.1 mmHg. In addition, extensive studies were carried out on 220 subjects who trekked into the Everest base camp (Grocott *et al.*, 2010).

In 2010, several groups reported the discovery of genetic changes in Tibetans compared with Han Chinese. One gene that was shown to be upregulated was *EPAS1* which codes for the hypoxia inducible factor HIF2alpha. The significance of this advance is the subject of intense research at the present time (Beall *et al.*, 2011).

2

The atmosphere

SUMMARY

Most of the medical problems that occur at high altitude are caused by the low partial pressure of oxygen in the atmosphere which in turn is due to the decrease in barometric pressure as altitude increases. The relationship between barometric pressure and altitude is therefore important, especially in regions of the world such as the Andes and Himalayas where large numbers of people reside at high altitude. Recent work has clarified the pressure–altitude relationship with much better accuracy than previously. Considerable confusion occurred in the past by assuming that the relationship follows the standard atmosphere. In fact, the pressures are usually substantially higher at a given altitude because the relationship between barometric pressure and altitude is latitude-dependent, and most of the high mountains of the world are relatively near the equator. At extreme altitudes, the variation of barometric pressure with season is believed to be sufficient to affect human performance. This is particularly true of the summit of Mount Everest where climbers are near the limit of tolerance to hypoxia. Other atmospheric factors, such as temperature, humidity and solar radiation, are also important.

2.1 INTRODUCTION

It has been known since the time of Paul Bert and the publication of *La Pression Barométrique* (Bert 1878) that most of the deleterious effects of high altitude on humans are caused by hypoxia. This, in turn, is a direct result of the reduction in atmospheric pressure. Yet in spite of the fact that Bert's book appeared over 130 years ago, there is still confusion in the minds of some physicians and physiologists about the relationship between barometric pressure and altitude, particularly at extreme heights. For example, some environmental physiologists are still surprised to learn that the barometric pressure at the summit of Mount Everest is considerably higher than that predicted by the standard pressure–altitude tables used by the aviation industry, and that humans can reach the summit without supplementary oxygen only because the tables are inapplicable.

Although most of the undesirable effects of high altitude are due to hypoxia, under some circumstances additional deterioration results from cold, dehydration, solar radiation, and perhaps ionizing radiation. However, most of these hazards of the environment can be avoided by proper clothing or shelter. Only hypoxia is unavoidable unless, of course, supplementary oxygen is available. The low barometric pressure in itself has no physiological sequelae unless the decompression is rapid, for example in the case of the explosive decompression that occurs when a window fails in a pressurized aircraft. Rapid decompression causes so-called barotrauma as a result of the very rapid enlargement of airspaces within the body including the lungs and middle ear cavity. Such accidents can also occur in ascent from deep diving, but are not considered here.

That low pressure per se is innocuous was not always realized. Indeed, early theories of mountain sickness included a number of exotic explanations based on the reduced pressure itself (Bert 1878, pp. 342–7 in the 1943 translation). One was weakening of the coxofemoral articulation; it was thought that barometric pressure was an important factor in pressing the head of the femur into its socket and that, at high altitudes, the necessary increase in action of the neighboring muscles resulted in fatigue. Another hypothesis was that superficial blood vessels would dilate and rupture if the barometric pressure which normally supported them was reduced. Indeed, modern-day medical students occasionally raise issues of this kind when they are first introduced to high altitude physiology. A further theory was that distension of intestinal gas would interfere with the action of the diaphragm and also impede venous return to the heart. All these theories overlook the fact that, when humans ascend to high altitude, all the pressures in the body fall together. In other words, although the pressure outside the superficial blood vessels falls, the pressure inside the vessels falls to the same extent and therefore the pressure differences across the vessels are unchanged.

2.2 BAROMETRIC PRESSURE AND ALTITUDE

2.2.1 Historical

A general historical introduction can be found in Chapter 1, but some additional background material related to the atmosphere is included here. A fuller discussion is in West (1998). The notion that air has weight and therefore exerts a pressure at the surface of the earth eluded the ancient Greeks and had to wait until the Renaissance. Galileo (1638) was well aware of the force associated with a vacuum and therefore the effort required to 'break' it, but he thought of this in the context of a force required to break a copper wire by stretching it, that is, the cohesive forces within the substance of the wire. It was left to Galileo's pupil Torricelli to realize that the force of a vacuum is due to the weight of the atmosphere. In addition, he wondered whether the air pressure became less on the tops of high mountains where the air 'begins to be distinctly rare . . .' as he put it. Torricelli made the first mercury barometer, though barometers filled with other liquids had apparently been constructed previously, for example by Gaspar Berti in 1639. These had limitations because of the effect of the vapor pressure of the liquid.

A landmark experiment took place in 1648 when the French philosopher and mathematician Blaise Pascal (1623–62) suggested that his brother-in-law, F. Périer, take a barometer to the top of the Puy-de-Dôme (1463 m) in central France to see whether the pressure fell (Pascal 1648). The results were communicated to Pascal in a delightful letter by Périer in which he described how the level of the mercury barometer fell some three pouces (about 75 mm) during the ascent of '500 fathoms' of altitude (probably about 900 m). The experiment had elaborate controls. For example, the Reverend Father Chastin, 'a man as pious as he is capable', stood guard over one barometer in the town of Clermont while Périer and a number of observers (including clerics, counselors and a doctor of medicine) took another to the top of the mountain. On returning, it was found that the first barometer had not changed, and Périer even checked it again by filling it with the same mercury that he had taken up the mountain. Another observation was made the next day on the top of a high church tower in Clermont, and this also showed a fall in pressure, though of much smaller extent.

A few years later, Robert Boyle carried out experiments with the newly invented air pump and wrote his influential book *New Experiments Physico-Mechanicall Touching the Spring of the Air, and its Effects*. In the second edition of this book, published in 1662, he formulated his famous law, which states that gas volume and pressure are inversely related (at constant temperature) (Boyle 1662). Recent commentaries on both the original book and Boyle's law are available (West 1999b; West 2005).

An influential analysis of the relationships between altitude and barometric pressure was made by Zuntz *et al.* (1906). They pointed out the important effect of temperature on the pressure–altitude relationship noting that, on a fine warm day, the upcurrents carry air to high altitudes and thus increase the sea level barometric pressure. Indeed, this is the basis for weather prediction based on barometric pressure.

Zuntz *et al.* (1906, pp. 37–9) gave the following logarithmic relationship for determining barometric pressure at any altitude:

$$\log b = \log B - \frac{h}{72\ (256.4 + t)}$$

where h is the altitude difference in meters, t is the mean temperature (°C) of the air column of height h, B is the barometric pressure (mmHg) at the lower altitude, and b is the barometric pressure at the higher altitude. Note that this expression implies that the higher the mean temperature, the less rapidly does barometric pressure decrease with altitude. In addition, if temperature were constant, $\log b$ would be proportional to negative altitude, that is, the pressure would decrease exponentially as altitude increased. Zuntz *et al.* cite Hann's *Lehrbuch der Meteorologie* where the pressure–altitude relationship is given in a slightly different form (Hann 1901).

The expression by Zuntz *et al.* was used by FitzGerald (1913) in her study of alveolar P_{CO_2} and hemoglobin concentration in residents of various altitudes in the Colorado mountains during the Anglo-American Pikes Peak expedition of 1911. She showed that barometric pressures calculated from the Zuntz formula agreed closely with pressures observed in the mountains when a sea level pressure of 760 mmHg and a mean temperature of the air column of 115°C were assumed. Kellas (2001) used the same expression to predict barometric pressures in the Himalayan ranges, obtaining a value of 251 mmHg for the summit of Mount Everest, assuming a mean temperature of 0°C. This was almost the same as the pressure of 248 mmHg given by Bert (Bert 1878, Appendix 1) in contrast to the erroneously low values used 70 years after Bert because of the inappropriate application of the standard atmosphere (section 2.2.3). However, a major difficulty with the use of the Zuntz formula is the sensitivity of the calculated pressure to temperature and the fact that the mean temperature of the air column is not accurately known. For example, the barometric pressure on the summit of Mount Everest was calculated by Kellas to be 267 mmHg for a mean temperature of 115°C, but only 251 mmHg for a mean temperature of 0°C.

2.2.2 Physical principles

Barometric pressure decreases with altitude because the higher we go, the less atmosphere there is above us pressing down by virtue of its weight. Various units for barometric pressure are available. In this book mmHg are used. One mmHg is equal to 0.133 kPa. The barometric pressure at sea level for the standard atmosphere is 760 mmHg or 101.325 kPa. Other units are 1013.25 millibars (mbar) or 14.696 pounds per square inch (psi).

If the atmospheric air was incompressible, as is very nearly the case for a liquid, barometric pressure would decrease linearly with altitude, just as it does in a liquid. However, because the weight of the upper atmosphere compresses the lower gas, barometric pressure decreases more rapidly with height near the earth's surface. If temperature were constant, the decrease in pressure would be exponential with respect to altitude, but because the temperature decreases as we go higher (at least, in the troposphere), the pressure falls more rapidly than the exponential law predicts.

The relationships between pressure, volume and temperature in a gas are governed by simple laws. These derive from the kinetic theory of gases which states that the molecules of a gas are in continuous random motion, and are only deflected from their course by collision with other molecules, or with the walls of a container.

When they strike the walls and rebound, the resulting bombardment results in a pressure. The magnitude of the pressure depends on the number of molecules present, their mass and their speed:

- Boyle's law states that, at constant temperature, the pressure (P) of a given mass of gas is inversely proportional to its volume (V), or PV = constant (at constant temperature). This can be explained by the fact that as the molecules are brought closer together (smaller volume), the rate of bombardment on a unit surface increases (greater pressure).
- Charles' law states that at constant pressure, the volume of a gas is proportional to its absolute temperature (T), or V/T = constant (at constant pressure). The explanation is that a rise in temperature increases the speed and therefore the momentum of the molecules, thus increasing their force of bombardment on the container. Another form of Charles' law states that at constant volume, the pressure is proportional to absolute temperature. (Note that absolute temperature is obtained by adding 273 to the Celsius temperature. Thus 37°C = 310 K.)
- The ideal gas law combines the above laws thus: $PV = nRT$, where n is the number of gram molecules of the gas and R is the 'gas constant'. When the units employed are mmHg, liters and Kelvin, then $R = 62.4$. Real gases deviate from ideal gas behavior to some extent at high pressures because of intermolecular forces, which are neglected in the derivation of the ideal gas law.
- Dalton's law states that each gas in a mixture exerts a pressure according to its own concentration, independently of the other gases present. That is, each component behaves as though it were present alone. The pressure of each gas is referred to as its partial pressure. The total pressure is the sum of the partial pressures of all gases present. In symbols: $P_x = PF_x$, where P_x is the partial pressure of gas x, P is the total pressure and F_x is the fractional concentration of gas x. For example, if half the gas is oxygen, $FO_2 = 0.5$. The fractional concentration always refers to dry gas.
- The kinetic theory of gases explains their diffusion in the gas phase. Because of their random motion, gas molecules tend to distribute themselves uniformly throughout any available space until the partial pressure is the same everywhere. Light gases diffuse faster than heavy gases because the mean velocity of the molecules is higher. The kinetic theory of gases states that the kinetic energy ($0.5\ mv^2$) of all gases is the same at a given temperature and pressure. From this it follows that the rate of diffusion of a gas is inversely proportional to the square root of its density (Graham's law).

On the basis of different rates of diffusion, one might expect that very light gases such as helium would separate and be lost from the upper atmosphere. This does happen to some extent at extreme altitudes. However, at the altitudes of interest to us, say up to 10 km, convective mixing maintains a constant composition of the atmosphere.

Vertically, the atmosphere can be divided on the basis of temperature variations into the troposphere, the stratosphere, and regions above that. The troposphere is the region where all the weather phenomena take place and is the only region of interest to high altitude medicine. Here, the temperature decreases approximately linearly with altitude until a low of about −60°C is reached. The troposphere extends to an altitude of about 19 km at the equator but only to about 9 km at the poles. The average upper limit is about 10 km.

Above the troposphere is the stratosphere where the temperature remains nearly constant at about −60°C for some 10–12 km of altitude. The interface between the troposphere and stratosphere is known as the tropopause.

Beyond the stratosphere, temperatures again vary with altitude. One of the important components of this region is the ionosphere where the degree of ionization of the molecules makes short-wave radio propagation possible.

2.2.3 Standard atmosphere

With the development of the aviation industry in the 1920s it became necessary to develop a barometric pressure–altitude relationship that could be universally accepted for calibrating altimeters, low pressure chambers and other devices. Although it had been recognized for many years that the relationship between pressure and altitude was temperature dependent and, as a result, latitude dependent, there were clear advantages in having a model atmosphere that applied approximately to mean conditions over the surface of the earth. This is often referred to as the ICAO Standard Atmosphere (ICAO 1964) or the US Standard Atmosphere (NOAA 1976). These two are identical up to altitudes of interest to us.

The assumptions of the standard atmosphere are a sea level pressure of 760 mmHg, sea level temperature of +15°C and a linear decrease in temperature with altitude (lapse rate) of 6.5°C km^{-1} up to an altitude of 11 km (Table 2.1). Haldane and Priestley (1935, p. 323) gave the following expression for the pressure–altitude relationship of the standard atmosphere in the second edition of their textbook *Respiration*:

$$\frac{P_0}{P} = \left(\frac{288}{288 - 1.98H} \right)^{5.256}$$

where P_0 and P are the pressures in mmHg at sea level and high altitude, respectively, and H is the height in thousands of feet. A more rigorous description is given in the *Manual of the ICAO Standard Atmosphere* (ICAO 1964).

It should be emphasized that this standard atmosphere was never meant to be used to predict the actual barometric pressure at a particular location. Rather, it was developed as a model of more or less average conditions within the troposphere with full recognition that there would be local variations caused by latitude and other factors. Nevertheless, the standard atmosphere has assumed some importance in respiratory physiology because it is universally used as the standard for altimeter calibrations, and it has frequently been inappropriately used to predict the pressure at various specific points of the earth's surface, particularly on high mountains.

Haldane and Priestley (1935) clearly understood that the standard atmosphere predicted barometric pressures considerably lower than those given by the expression of Zuntz *et al.* (1906), which had been shown by FitzGerald to predict accurately pressures in the Colorado mountains when a mean air column temperature of +15°C was assumed.

Nevertheless, some physiologists have used the standard atmosphere for predicting the pressure at great altitudes, for example

Table 2.1 Barometric pressures (in mmHg) from the standard atmosphere (ICAO 1964) and a model atmosphere (West 1996a): the latter is a better fit for most sites where high altitude physiology and medicine are studied

Altitude		Standard pressure		Model atmosphere	
Kilometers	Feet	Barometric pressure	Inspired P_{O_2}[a]	Barometric pressure	Inspired P_{O_2}
0	0	760	149	760	149
1	3281	674	131	679	132
2	6562	596	115	604	117
3	9843	526	100	537	103
4	13 123	462	87	475	90
5	16 404	405	75	420	78
6	19 685	354	64	369	67
7	22 966	308	54	324	58
8	26 247	267	46	284	50
9	29 528	231	38	247	42
10	32 810	199	31	215	35

[a]The P_{O_2} of moist inspired gas is 0.2094 (P_B – 47).

on Mount Everest (Houston and Riley 1947; Riley and Houston 1951; Rahn and Fenn 1955; Houston *et al.* 1987). The barometric pressure calculated in this way for the Everest summit (altitude 8848 m) is 236 mmHg, which is far too low. In retrospect, one of the reasons for the indiscriminate use of the standard atmosphere was undoubtedly its very frequent employment in low pressure chambers during the very fertile period of research on respiratory physiology during World War II.

Climbers using altimeters from sports shops, including those on some wristwatches, should be aware that these use the standard atmosphere to convert barometric pressure to altitude. The difference between the readings given by these altimeters and the true altitude up to about 3000 m is unimportant for navigation in the mountains. From 4000 to 5000 m a climber should add 3% to the altimeter reading to get a truer altitude. From 5000 to 6000 m the change is 4%, from 6000 to 8000 m the change is about 5%, and above 8000 m it is 6–7%. Of course, if the altimeter also measures and reads pressure, the best solution is to relate this to altitude using the model atmosphere equation.

2.2.4 Variation of barometric pressure with latitude

The limited applicability of the standard atmosphere is further clarified when we look at the relationship between barometric pressure and altitude for different latitudes (Fig. 2.1). This shows that the barometric pressure at the earth's surface and at an altitude of 24 km is essentially independent of latitude. However, in the altitude range of about 6–16 km, there is a pronounced bulge in the barometric pressure near the equator both in winter and summer. Since the latitude of Mount Everest is 28°N, the pressure at its summit (8848 m) is considerably higher than would be the case for a hypothetical mountain of the same altitude near one of the poles.

The cause of the bulge in barometric pressure near the equator is a very large mass of very cold air in the stratosphere above the equator (Brunt

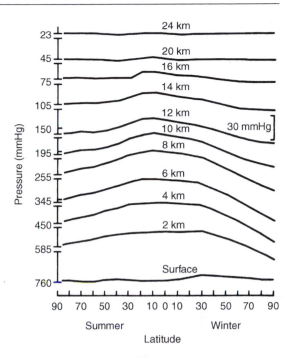

Figure 2.1   Increase of barometric pressure near the equator at various altitudes in both summer and winter. Vertical axis shows the pressure increasing upwards according to the scale on the right. The numbers on the left show the barometric pressures at the poles for various altitudes; the altitude of Mount Everest is 8848 m. (From Brunt 1952.)

1952, p. 379). In fact, paradoxically, the coldest air in the atmosphere is above the equator. This is brought about by a combination of complex radiation and convective phenomena which result in a large up-welling of air near the equator. Another corollary of the same phenomenon is that the height of the tropopause is much greater near the equator than near the poles. These latitude-dependent variations of pressure are of great physiological significance for anyone attempting to climb Mount Everest without supplementary oxygen, because they result in a barometric pressure on the Everest summit which is considerably higher than that predicted from the model atmosphere. By the same token, a climber at a high latitude such as Mount McKinley (Denali) is at a considerable disadvantage because of the low barometric pressure, especially in the winter months.

2.2.5 Variation of barometric pressure with season

Not only does barometric pressure alter with latitude, but there are marked variations according to the month of the year. For example, Fig. 2.2 shows the mean monthly pressures for an altitude of 8848 m as obtained from radiosonde balloons released from New Delhi, India, over a period of 15 years. Delhi has about the same latitude as Everest. Note that the mean pressures were lowest in the winter months of January and February (243.0 and 243.7 mmHg, respectively) and highest in the summer months of July and August (254.5 mmHg for both months). The monthly standard deviation showed a range of 0.65 mmHg (July) to 1.66 mmHg (December). The daily standard deviation was as low as 1.54 in the summer and as high as 2.92 in the winter. The standard deviation shown in Fig. 2.2 is the mean of the monthly standard deviation for the 12 months of the year.

The single measurement of barometric pressure (253.0 mmHg) made by Pizzo on the summit of Mount Everest on 24 October 1981 (West *et al.* 1983a) is also shown in Fig. 2.2. This was 4.3 mmHg higher than that predicted from the data shown in Fig. 2.1, which is twice the daily standard deviation of barometric pressure for the month of October. It should be added that Pizzo had an exceptionally fine day for his summit climb, the temperature on the summit being measured as −9°C, much higher than expected for that altitude (section 2.3.1).

Figure 2.3 combines the effects of latitude and month of the year on the barometric pressure at an altitude of 8848 m. The data are for the northern hemisphere, and the pressures for the months of January (midwinter), July (midsummer) and October (preferred month for climbing in the post-monsoon period) are compared. The profile for the month of May, which is the usual month for reaching the summit in the pre-monsoon season, is almost the same as that for October.

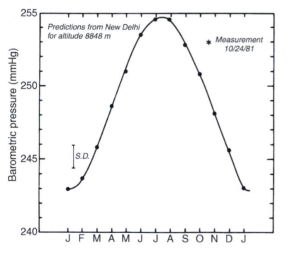

Figure 2.2 Mean monthly pressures for 8848 m altitude as obtained from weather balloons released from New Delhi, India. Note the increase during the summer months. The mean monthly standard deviation (SD) is also shown. The barometric pressure measured on the Everest summit on 24 October 1981 (*) was unusually high for that month. (From West *et al.* 1983a.)

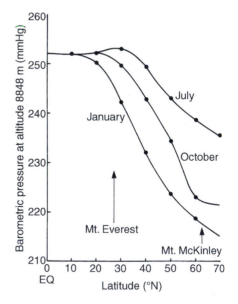

Figure 2.3 Barometric pressure at the altitude of Mount Everest plotted against latitude in the northern hemisphere for midsummer, midwinter, and the preferred month for climbing in the post-monsoon period (October). Note the considerably lower pressures in the winter. The arrows show the latitudes of Mount Everest and Mount McKinley. (From West *et al.* 1983a.)

The data are the means from all longitudes (Oort and Rasmusson 1971). The data clearly show the marked effects of both latitude and season on barometric pressure. It is interesting that in midsummer the pressure reaches a maximum near the latitude of Mount Everest (28°359N). Figure 2.3 shows that if Mount Everest was at the latitude of Mount McKinley (63°N), the pressure on the summit would be very much lower.

Radiosonde balloons are released from meteorological stations all over the world twice a day, and the resulting data on the relationship between barometric pressure and altitude are available from constant pressure charts. Details on how to obtain these are given in West (1993a). Using these data it can be shown that the barometric pressure on the Everest summit was 251 mmHg when Messner and Habeler made their first ascent without supplementary oxygen in 1978. In August 1980, Messner made the first solo ascent without supplementary oxygen and he was fortunate that the barometric pressure was unusually high at 256 mmHg. When Sherpa Ang Rita made the first winter ascent on 22 December 1987, the barometric pressure was only 247 mmHg.

2.2.6 Barometric pressure–altitude relationship for locations of importance in high altitude medicine and physiology

We have seen that the standard atmosphere generally underestimates the pressures on the high mountains which are of interest to people concerned with high altitude medicine and physiology. Recently, it has been possible to define the barometric pressure–altitude relationship in the Himalayan and Andean ranges with some accuracy, and it transpires that the relationship holds for many other locations where high altitude medicine and physiology are studied.

As already stated, the first direct measurement of barometric pressure on the Everest summit was obtained by Pizzo in 1981 during the course of the American Medical Research Expedition to Everest (West *et al.* 1983a). The value was 253 mmHg, as shown in Fig. 2.2. During the same expedition, careful measurements of barometric pressure were

made at two other locations on Mount Everest where the altitudes were accurately known. These were the base camp (altitude 5400 m) and Camp 5, just above the South Col (altitude 8050 m). These points lay very close to a straight line on a log pressure–altitude plot and therefore allowed the barometric pressure–altitude relationship at very high altitudes on Mount Everest to be accurately described for the first time (Fig. 2 in West *et al.* 1983a). This relationship is of great physiological interest because, as discussed in Chapter 13, the pressure near the summit is so low that the P_{O_2} is very near the limit for human survival.

More recently, additional measurements have been made at very high altitudes on Mount Everest (West 1999a). Another direct measurement was made on the summit in May 1997 and this agreed within 1 mmHg of Pizzo's measurement of 253 mmHg. In addition, a large number of measurements were reported from a barometer that telemetered information from the South Col (altitude 7986 m). When these points were added

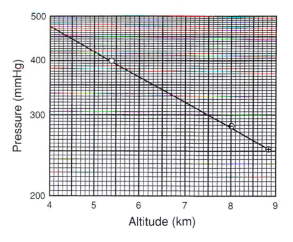

Figure 2.4   Barometric pressure–altitude relationship for Mount Everest. The circles show data from the 1981 American Medical Research Expedition to Everest. The cross at the summit altitude (8848 m) is from the 1997 NOVA expedition. The cross at an altitude of 7986 m is from measurements made by the Massachusetts Institute of Technology in 1998. The standard deviations are too small to show on the graph. The line corresponds to the model atmosphere equation: $P_B = \exp(6.63268 - 0.1112\,h - 0.00149\,h^2)$ where h is in kilometers. (From West 1999a.)

to those obtained during the 1981 expedition (Fig. 2.4), they greatly increase our confidence in the barometric pressure–altitude relationship.

Two other pieces of data have more recently come to light. Charles Corfield made a single measurement of the barometric pressure on the Everest summit at 10 a.m. on 5 May 1999. He used a Kollsman aneroid barometer and the value was 253 mmHg (personal communication). The air temperature was −18°C, and this had been shown not to affect the calibration of the barometer. The other data point comes from measurements made on the South Col by the Italian Ev-K2-CNR program. They reported 52 measurements of barometric pressure on 29 and 30 September and 1 October 1992 (personal communication). The mean value was 383.0 mbar (287 mmHg). This is the same pressure as that found by the MIT group in August 1997 (West 1999a). These two additional pieces of data fit very well with the other measurements listed above.

2.2.7 Model atmosphere equation

It is now possible to provide a barometric pressure–altitude relationship that accurately predicts the pressure at most locations of interest to high altitude medicine and physiology (West 1996a). The data are shown in Fig. 2.5. The prediction is particularly good if the locations lie within 30° of the equator, and especially if the pressure is measured in the summer months. Since many studies of high altitude medicine and physiology are carried out in locations and times that fulfill these criteria, the relationship is very useful in practice. The equation of the line is

$$P_B = \exp(6.63268 - 0.1112\,h - 0.00149\,h^2)$$

where P_B is the barometric pressure (in mmHg) and h is the altitude in kilometers. This has been called the model atmosphere equation, and is useful for theoretical calculations in high altitude physiology such as predicting the effects of oxygen enrichment at different altitudes. Procedures for

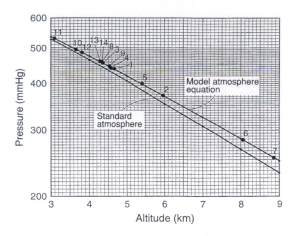

Figure 2.5   Barometric pressure–altitude relationship corresponding to the model atmosphere equation. Note that it predicts the altitudes of many locations of interest in high altitude medicine and physiology very well. The lower line shows the standard atmosphere which predicts pressures that are too low. The locations and measured pressures are as follows: (1) Collahuasi mine, Chile, 438 mmHg; (2) Aucanquilcha mine, Chile, 372 mmHg; (3) Vallot observatory, France, 452 mmHg; (4) Capanna Margherita, Italy, 440 mmHg; (5) Mount Everest Base Camp, Nepal, 400 mmHg; (6) Mount Everest South Col, 284 mmHg; (7) Mount Everest summit, 253 mmHg; (8) Cerro de Pasco, Peru, 458 mmHg; (9) Morococha, Peru, 446 mmHg; (10) Lhasa, Tibet, 493 mmHg; (11) Crooked Creek, California, 530 mmHg; (12) Barcroft laboratory, California, 483 mmHg; (13) Pikes Peak, Colorado, 462 mmHg; (14) White Mountain summit, California, 455 mmHg. (From West 1996a.)

both the standard and model atmospheres are available on the web at <http://physiology ucsd. edu/ /convert.html>.

2.2.8 Barometric pressure and inspired Po_2

As we have seen, the composition of the atmosphere is constant up to altitudes well above those of medical interest so it is safe to assume that the concentration of oxygen in dry air is approximately 20.94%. However, the effects of water vapor on the inspired P_{O_2} become increasingly important at higher altitudes.

When air is inhaled into the upper bronchial tree, it is warmed and moistened and becomes saturated with vapor at the prevailing temperature. The water vapor pressure at 37°C is 47 mmHg and this, of course, is independent of altitude. Thus the P_{O_2} of moist inspired gas is given by the expression

$$PI_{,O_2} = 0.2094 \, (P_B - 47)$$

where P_B is barometric pressure. This equation shows how much more important water vapor pressure becomes at very high altitudes. For example, at sea level, the water vapor pressure at 37°C is only 6% of the total barometric pressure. However, on the summit of Mount Everest, where the barometric pressure is about 250 mmHg, the water vapor pressure is nearly 19% of the total pressure, and the inspired P_{O_2} is correspondingly further reduced (see Table 2.1).

It has been pointed out from time to time that a relatively small reduction in body temperature at extreme altitude would confer a substantial increase in inspired P_{O_2}. For example, if the body temperature fell from 37 to 35°C where the water vapor is 42 mmHg, the P_{O_2} of moist inspired gas would be increased from 42.5 to 43.5 mmHg. This increase of 1 mmHg would be beneficial because the arterial P_{O_2} would increase by approximately the same extent, and since the oxygen dissociation curve is very steep at this point, there would be an appreciable gain in arterial oxygen concentration. However, there is no evidence that body temperature falls at extreme altitude. Nor is it reasonable to assume that the temperature in the alveoli where gas exchange takes place would be significantly less than the body core temperature.

2.2.9 Physiological significance of barometric pressure at high altitude

Since the barometric pressure directly determines the inspired P_{O_2}, it is clear that the variations of barometric pressure with latitude and season, as described in sections 2.2.4 and 2.2.5, will affect the degree of hypoxemia in the body. For example, a climber on Mount McKinley in Alaska, which is situated at a latitude of 63°N, will be exposed to a considerably lower barometric pressure on the summit than would be the case for a mountain of the same height located in the tropics (see Fig. 2.3).

The reduction in inspired P_{O_2} resulting from the lower barometric pressure will not only reduce exercise performance but may also increase the risk of altitude illness. In fact, there is some evidence that this may be the case at the comparatively modest altitudes of Summit County, Colorado (2650–2950 m) as reported by Reeves et al. (1994). They found that barometric pressure and environmental temperature averaged 8 mmHg and 23°C lower in winter compared with summer months. While the number of visits to the Summit Medical Center (2773 m) was nearly the same in the two periods, the proportion of patients with high altitude pulmonary edema was higher in winter, though interestingly there was no difference in the incidence of acute mountain sickness. Cold seemed to be more important than barometric pressure.

The variations of barometric pressure with latitude and season become particularly significant from a physiological point of view at extreme altitudes such as near the summit of Mount Everest. For example, it has been argued that if the pressure on the Everest summit conformed to the standard atmosphere, it would be impossible to climb the mountain without supplementary oxygen (West 1983). In addition, the variation of barometric pressure with month of the year shown in Fig. 2.2 indicates that it would be considerably more difficult to reach the summit without supplementary oxygen in the winter as a result of the reduced inspired P_{O_2}, quite apart from the obvious difficulties of lower temperatures and high winds. Although there have now been many ascents of Everest without supplementary oxygen in the pre- and post-monsoon seasons, only one person has made a winter ascent without supplementary oxygen. This was Sherpa Ang Rita on 22 December 1987 when the barometric pressure was 247 mmHg based on radiosonde balloon data for that date. Therefore, the pressure was much higher than it typically becomes in midwinter, for example in late January (see Fig. 2.2). A total of 13 climbers have now reached the Everest summit during the winter but apparently supplementary oxygen was used in all cases (Salisbury and Hawley, 2007). This topic is considered in more detail in Chapter 13.

2.3 FACTORS OTHER THAN BAROMETRIC PRESSURE AT HIGH ALTITUDE

2.3.1 Temperature

Temperature falls with increasing altitude at the rate of about 1°C for every 150 m. This lapse rate is essentially independent of latitude. The consequence is that on a very high mountain, such as Mount Everest, the average temperature near the summit is predicted to be about −40°C. Most climbers choose the warmer months of the year. In May, a temperature of −27°C was measured at an altitude of 8500 m on Everest (Pugh 1957), although Pizzo obtained a temperature of −9°C on the summit in October (West *et al.* 1983a). In the winter the temperatures are much lower. However, even then they do not approach the extremely low temperatures seen in northern Canada or Siberia during midwinter.

More important than temperature per se is the wind chill factor. Moore and Semple (2011) have calculated two indices related to cold injury on Mount Everest using a meteorological dataset. They found that throughout the year the typical wind chill equivalent temperature on the summit is always less than −30°C, and the typical facial frostbite time is always less than 20 minutes. During the spring climbing season, typical values are −50°C and 5 minutes. The authors stated that the barometric pressure on the summit is a good predictor of these indices with a low pressure being associated with a low temperature and short frostbite time. Cold injury is common in the mountains and is discussed in Chapter 24.

2.3.2 Humidity

Absolute humidity is the mass of water vapor per unit volume of gas at the prevailing temperature. This value is extremely low at high altitude because the water vapor pressure is so depressed at the reduced temperature. Thus even if the air is fully saturated with water vapor, the actual amount will be very small. For example, the water vapor pressure at +20°C is 17 mmHg but only 1 mmHg at −20°C.

Relative humidity is a measure of the amount of water vapor in the air as a percentage of the amount that could be contained at the prevailing temperature. This value may be low, normal or high at altitude. The disparity between absolute and relative humidities is explained by the fact that even saturated air is unable to contain much water vapor because of the very low temperature. If this air is warmed without allowing additional water vapor to form, its relative humidity falls.

The very low absolute humidity at high altitude frequently causes dehydration. First, the insensible water loss caused by ventilation is great because of the dryness of the inspired air. In addition, the levels of ventilation may be extremely high, especially on exercise (Chapter 12), and this increases water loss. For example, near the summit of Mount Everest, the total ventilation is increased some five-fold compared with sea level for the same level of activity. Pugh (1964b) calculated that during exercise at 5500 m altitude, the rate of fluid loss from the lungs alone was about 2.9 g water per 100 L of ventilation (body temperature and pressure, saturated with water vapor, or BTPS). This is equivalent to about 200 mL of water per hour for moderate exercise.

However, it is likely that Pugh's calculation gives erroneously high values because the temperature of expired gas is below body temperature, and the gas is probably not fully saturated with water even at this lower temperature (Loewy and Gerhartz 1914; Burch 1945; Webb 1951; Ferrus *et al.* 1980). Using an equation given by Ferrus *et al.* (1984), Milledge (1992) calculated that the water loss is only about 30–40% of that calculated assuming that the expired gas is fully saturated at body temperature in a climber at extreme altitude. Actual measurements during climbing at extreme altitude would be valuable.

There is evidence that the dehydration resulting from these rapid fluid losses does not produce as strong a sensation of thirst as at sea level. As a result, it is necessary for climbers to drink large quantities of fluids at high altitude to remain hydrated even though they have little desire to do so. For people climbing 7 hours a day at altitudes over 6000 m, 3–4 L of fluid are required in order to maintain a urine output of 1.5 L day^{-1} (Pugh 1964b). Even so, it appears that people living at very high altitude are in a state of chronic volume depletion (Blume *et al.* 1984). In a group of subjects living at an altitude of 6300 m during the American Medical Research Expedition to Everest, serum osmolality was significantly increased compared with sea level despite the fact that ample fluids were available and the lifestyle in terms of exercise and diet was not exceptional (Blume *et al.* 1984).

2.3.3 Atmospheric ozone

Ozone (O_3) is a potentially toxic gas and an important constituent of smog. Ozone can cause inflammation of mucous membranes and bronchi, cough, throat irritation, bronchoconstriction and dyspnea. It is interesting therefore that increased concentrations have been recorded in the European Alps (Stohl *et al.* 2000) and at very high altitudes on Mount Everest (Zhou *et al.* 2006; Bonasoni *et al.* 2008; Semple and Moore 2008). Surface measurements in the Mount Everest region have exceeded 140 ppb during an 8-hour exposure (Semple and Moore 2009). Two mechanisms for the increased concentrations have been identified on Mount Everest. One is ozone penetrating from the stratosphere in the pre-monsoon period, and the other is ozone from the troposphere during monsoon periods. The latter may be related to the so-called Asian Brown Clouds resulting from pollution in South East Asia (Ramanathan *et al.* 2007).

2.3.4 Solar radiation

The intensity of solar radiation increases markedly at high altitude for two reasons. First, the much thinner atmosphere absorbs fewer of the sun's rays, especially those of short wavelength in the near ultraviolet region of the spectrum. Second, reflection of the sun from snow greatly increases radiation exposure.

The reduced density of the air causes an increase in incident solar radiation of up to 100% at an altitude of 4000 m compared with sea level (Elterman 1964). The fact that mountain air is so dry is another important factor because water vapor in the atmosphere absorbs substantial amounts of solar radiation.

The efficiency with which the ground reflects solar radiation is known as its albedo. This varies from less than 20% at sea level to up to 90% in the presence of snow at great altitudes (Buettner 1969). Mountaineers are familiar with the extreme intensity of solar radiation, especially on a glacier in a valley between two mountains. Here, the sunlight is reflected from both sides as well as from the snow or ice on the glacier and the heat can be very oppressive despite the great altitude. A consequence of this is the extreme variation in temperature which has been noted in camps under these conditions.

2.3.5 Ionizing radiation

The intensity of cosmic radiation increases at high altitude because there is less of the earth's atmosphere to absorb the rays as they enter from space. This is the reason why cosmic radiation laboratories are often located on high mountains. It has been shown that, at an altitude of 3000 m, the increased cosmic radiation results in an increased radiation dose to a human being of approximately 0.0007Gy year^{-1} (70 mrad year^{-1}). This should be considered in relation to the normal background radiation dose from all sources of 0.0005–0.004 Gy year^{-1} (50–400 mrad year^{-1}). The increased ionizing radiation of high altitude has been cited as one of the factors causing acute mountain sickness (Bert 1878), but there is no scientific basis for this assertion.

3

Geography and the human response to altitude

SUMMARY

The highland areas of the world support considerable populations. The climate is harsh and methods of cultivation have to be adapted to the terrain. Terracing has been brought to a fine art in the mountain regions, although the South American altiplano and the Tibetan plateau allow normal methods of cultivation. Animal husbandry and mining are important, and tourism is becoming increasingly popular and can contribute significantly to the economy of mountainous regions.

Mountains often form boundaries between cultures. Highland peoples have developed a physique that enables them to survive under severe conditions of cold and hypoxia. Commerce in high valleys without roads depends on porters and without their remarkable capacity to carry loads the economy would remain static. Acclimatization to hypoxia is complex and far-reaching and depends on the severity and rate at which oxygen lack is imposed (Chapter 5). Local cold tolerance but not general cold acclimatization occurs, and protection is mainly by cultural methods, clothing and shelter.

3.1 INTRODUCTION

Although the expression 'high altitude' has no precise definition, the majority of individuals have certain clinical, physiological, anatomical and biochemical changes which occur at levels above 3000 m. Individual variation is, however, considerable and some people are affected at levels as low as 2000 m. For sea level visitors, an altitude of 4600–4900 m represents the highest acceptable level for permanent habitation; for high altitude residents 5800–6000 m is the highest so far recorded (West 1986a). Indeed, the highest permanent human habitation is probably the town of La Rinconada, a town of 29 678 inhabitants (GeoNames 2010) in southern Peru, at an altitude of 5100 m (West 2002). Although even altitude residents are affected by the altitude, the limit of permanent habitation is probably dictated by economic, rather than physiological, factors. Above 5000 m, even in the tropics, crops cannot be grown and animals cannot be pastured all year round. Nomadic and semi-nomadic peoples regularly take their flocks to pastures higher than 5000 m but these are not permanent dwellings.

The main areas of the world above 3000 m are:

- The Tibetan plateau
- The Himalayan range and its valleys
- The Tien Shan and Pamir
- The mountain ranges of east Turkey, Iran, Afghanistan and Pakistan
- The Rocky Mountains and Sierra Nevada of the USA and Canada
- The Sierra Madre of Mexico
- The Andes of South America
- The European Alps
- The Pyrenees between Spain and France
- The Atlas Mountains of North Africa
- The Ethiopian highlands
- The mountains of East and South Africa
- The plateau and mountains of Antarctica
- Parts of New Guinea and other small regions such as Hawaii, Tenerife and New Zealand.

The three main regions that support large populations are the Tibetan plateau and Himalayan valleys, the Andes of South America and the Ethiopian highlands.

3.1.1 European Alps

The early development of all branches of mountain science resulted from the increasing ability to travel in these inhospitable regions, due to developments in mountaineering and skiing.

The word 'alp' is based originally on a Celtic word meaning 'high mountain': the modern use of this word meaning 'high pasture' dates from the Middle Ages.

The history of the European Alps is the story of how this region, constrained by its geographical position and topography, became a vital and indispensable link in the communications of the whole of Europe.

The discovery of 'Similaun Man', some 5000 years old, at a height of 3210 m shows that considerable altitudes were reached by local people when crossing from one valley to another. The deposition of gold bracelets to propitiate the mountain gods was common from prehistory to the Middle Ages and many offerings have been found in the neighborhood of the Great St Bernard Pass.

The native population was neither static nor homogenous, but it was the Romans who established the main framework of communication in this region. However, their roads had little impact on the essential pasturalism of the Alpine economy and the mountains themselves were feared by the Romans as the abode of dragons and evil forces. The people, with their susceptibility to goitre, were not much admired either.

It was not until the nineteenth century that gradual easing of communications opened up the whole region to the outside world and ignorance turned to knowledge and understanding (Snodgrass 1993).

3.1.2 Himalayas and Tibetan plateau

The Himalayas form a topographically extremely complex region, extending 1500 miles from Nanga Parbat (8125 m) in the west to Namcha Barwa (7756 m) in the east. At their western extremity they are part of a confused mass of peaks, passes and glaciers where the western Kun Lun, Karakoram, Pir Panjal and Pamirs form an area the size of France. The Himalayas contain the world's highest mountain, Mount Everest (8848 m), and many other peaks over 7500 m. The main range forms the watershed between Central Asia and India, and there are middle ranges at intermediate altitudes. The outer Himalayas (up to 1500 m) form foothills rising from the plains of India.

The Tibetan plateau is an area occupied by Tibetans, who have a well-defined culture. It extends in the south to the Himalayas and high Himalayan valleys. To the west the plateau is demarcated by the northward curve of the Himalayas which continues into Kashmir, Baltistan and then to Gilgit and the Karakoram. To the north the peaks (up to 7700 m) of the Kun Lun range, 1500 miles long, mark off the plateau of Tibet from Xinjiang (Chinese Turkestan). To the east it extends to the Koko Nor or Qinghai Lake and, further south, the valleys of Qinghai and Sikiang and the gorge country of south-east Tibet.

The area covers about 1.5 million square miles and is the largest and highest plateau in the world, much of it at an altitude of 4600–4900 m. It presents an enormous range of climate and topography. The major climatic contrast is between the southern side of the Himalayas and the high valleys exposed to the summer Indian monsoon with very high rainfall, particularly in the east, and the aridity and low rainfall of the Tibetan plateau. The change is so abrupt that in some passes in the eastern Himalayas, vegetation may change from tropical to subarctic within a few yards.

Tibetans have been subject to influences from China, India, Central Asia and the Middle East for many centuries (Stein 1972). Permanent buildings are found up to 3500 m with nomadic populations at higher levels. Neolithic human remains have been found near Lhasa (Ward 1990, Ward 1991). Aldenderfer (2011) discusses the question, how long have people been living on this plateau? He says, 'Although the data are sparse, both archaeology and genetics suggest that the plateau was occupied in the Late Pleistocene, perhaps as early as 30,000 yr ago'. However, there were almost certainly later migrations, but there is evidence of permanent settlements dating from about 6500, 5900 and 3750 years ago.

With increasing numbers of Han Chinese immigrants there are more than three million people living at over 3000 m. It is estimated that the amount of this land available for agriculture is only 5% of the total. The opening of the Golmud to Lhasa rail link in July 2006 means that it is possible now to travel from all parts of China to Lhasa by rail. This has been a prodigious enterprise. The link is 1100 km, three-quarters of it at altitudes over 4000 m (West 2004). The numbers of Han Chinese at altitude in Tibet, as visitors or immigrants, are bound to increase as a result. This immigrant population is at higher risk of altitude illness than Tibetans (Chapters 19–21).

3.1.3 Andes of South America

The highland zone extends from Colombia in the north to central Chile in the south, and is flanked by an arid desert on its west, with a deeply eroded escarpment to the east, which adjoins the Amazon basin.

The central Andean region has three broadly defined areas running parallel with the Pacific Ocean: the cordillera occidentale, the altiplano, a broad undulating plain at 4000 m in the middle, and the cordillera orientale in the east.

The earliest archeological evidence for human occupation dates back 20 000 years (MacNeish 1971) and has been found at Ayacucho, Peru at 2900 m; other early finds are recorded in central Chile, Venezuela and Argentina. However, this date and the evidence for it has been questioned by Lynch (1990) who suggests a maximum date as 12 000 years ago. The skeleton of a man who lived 9500 years ago has been found at Lauricocha (4200 m) in Peru (Hurtado 1971). It is widely accepted that all South American indigenous peoples migrated into the American continent from the Mongolian area via the Bering land bridge.

The pre-Inca civilizations were situated mainly along the Pacific coast and the population subsisted mainly on seafood. Little is known of the highland population during this period.

Both agriculture and stock raising dominate the subsistence economy, with the upper limit of agriculture at 4000 m and the upper limit of vegetation at 4600 m. Mining is carried out at even greater altitudes and tourism is increasingly popular.

3.1.4 Ethiopian highlands

No well-circumscribed highland zone exists. The country is intersected by a number of rift valley systems, establishing a connection between the African rift valley in the south and the Red Sea. The valley systems divide the country into three reasonably well-defined regions: the western highlands, the eastern highlands and the rift valley itself with the lowland area.

The northern part of the western highlands, the Amhara highlands, attains the greatest altitude (2400–3700 m). Much of Ethiopian history centers on this area, which has been settled for many centuries. It is inhabited by the largest of Ethiopia's many population groups, the Amharas and Tigraeans, who are the descendants of people who came from southern Arabia prior to 1000 BCE (Sellassie 1972).

Gondar (3000 m), in the Amhara highlands, with a population of 200 000, became the second largest city in Africa, and it remained the capital of Ethiopia until the middle of the first century, when Addis Ababa was founded.

Much of the population of Ethiopia lives above 2000 m, and in the highland area two types of cultivation, by plough and by hoe, predominate. Teff, a type of grass which produces a small seed, is grown up to 3000 m and is the mainstay of the agricultural economy.

3.2 POPULATION

Most of the high altitude areas of the world are in the economically least developed regions and for this reason population numbers in relation to altitude are difficult to obtain. Although the total population living in mountainous regions is estimated at 400 million, the majority live at low altitude in the valleys. De Jong (1968) 'guessed' that between 13 and 14 million people lived at altitudes above 3000 m. The World Health Organization published data indicating that 89.3 million people lived at altitudes above 2500 m, 25.9 million above 3500 m and 5.4 million of these at altitudes above 4500 m (WHO Publication, Table 1, data from 2004).

In South America large populations have lived at high altitude since prehistory and the Andean population at the time of the Spanish conquest was estimated as between 4.5 and 7.5 million. In 1980 it was considered that between 10 and 17 million were living at over 2500 m and in Peru 30–40% of the population of 4 million lived at or above this height, with 1.5% living at over 4000 m.

In Asia and Africa the estimates are less accurate. On the Tibetan plateau, which consists of the autonomous region of Tibet (Xizang) and Qinghai province, the population is estimated as between 4 and 5 million. Lhasa (3658 m), in 1986, had about 130 000 inhabitants, mainly Tibetan, but recent immigration of Han Chinese has increased this number. Relatively small groups, nomads (at up to 5450 m) and miners (at up to 6000 m), live at higher levels. Fairly large numbers live at altitudes exceeding 3000 m in the upper valleys of eastern Tibet, and in Nepal about 60 000 live above this level, with a number of villages in Dolpo being at 5000 m (Snellgrove 1961). In Ethiopia about 50% of the total population of 26 million live above 2000 m. Small populations in Mexico, the USA and the former USSR live above 3000 m, for instance in Kyrgyzstan.

In tropical latitudes permanent settlements are usually placed where both pasture and timber can be used and the upper limit of habitation may fall between the two. Further from the equator the upper limit falls below the timber line and variation in temperature becomes seasonal; the upper pasturelands are thus used for a semi-nomadic economy. Permanently inhabited villages are found at lower levels, with isolated groups of buildings or shelters on the pastures occupied for the grazing season and evacuated during the winter. Considerable migration may occur and part of the population may always be on the move. One mine, now closed, was worked at 5950 m in South America; although the miners lived at rather lower altitudes, the caretakers lived there permanently (West 1986a).

Highland populations, being strategically placed between prosperous lowland centers, play a vital role in trade. Because they are physiologically well adapted they are capable of crossing high mountain passes with heavy loads and use their animals to carry produce. Major mountain passes have for centuries been arteries for trade, the movement of people and ideas, and the dissemination of disease.

3.3 TERRAIN

Although mountain country varies widely, there are two distinct types: the high, flat, plateaux (Tibet and the altiplano of South America) and deep valleys (Himalayas and Andes) (Fig. 3.1).

Plateaux can support large populations and large towns but they may be isolated by virtue of distance from lowland cities, which are usually the center of government, commerce and industry.

In mountain valleys, because flat ground is at a premium, populations tend to be smaller, with groups perched on slopes and ridges far from one another. The placing of houses in sunny

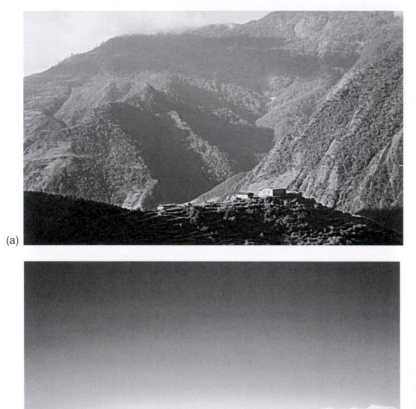

(a)

(b)

Figure 3.1 Contrasting terrain and climate at altitude. (a) Typical mountainous country on southern slopes of the Himalayas. (b) The north Tibetan plateau with the Kun Lun range in the background

positions is more difficult and isolation within the community is common. Communications are easily severed by land slips, avalanches and other natural disasters. The funneling effect of valleys on wind may increase its velocity with an ensuing stunting effect on vegetation and trees. This also restricts the placing of houses, as does the availability of water and the possibility of natural disasters.

3.4 CLIMATE

The climate near the ground at high altitude has several basic features. At any given latitude, seasonal variation of monthly temperature is less at high altitude than at sea level and, as the equator is reached, seasonal variation virtually disappears. Diurnal variations are considerable, and can show a range of 30°C. This is because of high levels of long-wave radiation that occur in cloudless skies during the day and escape to clear skies at night. In overcast conditions the diurnal variation decreases.

With increasing altitude the temperature falls. There is no uniform value for decline, or lapse rate, although the figure 1°C for every 150 m is usually given.

Solar radiation is an important factor in maintaining thermal balance in humans at extreme altitude. High winds are also a feature of mountains.

3.4.1 Rainfall

In Asia, the monsoon flows from east to west across India, cooling as it is forced to ascend by the Himalayas. Water vapor condenses and falls as rain, and as it passes to the west the monsoon becomes depleted of water; the eastern Himalayas are thus very wet, the western dry. In Darjeeling the annual rainfall is 2000–3000 mm a year; in the central Himalayas at Simla it is 1500 mm, but in the west at Ladakh it is only 75 mm. The Karakoram is arid whereas the eastern Himalayan region is tropical.

There is also considerable north–south variation with subarctic species on the Tibetan plateau and tropical species often only a few hundred yards away to the south. This is particularly marked on some passes in the eastern Himalayas. On the plateau, although 'monsoon' clouds are seen on the Tangulla range, about 700 km north of Lhasa, precipitation is small. In the deserts of the Tarim basin and Tsaidam to the north of the Tibetan plateau, annual rainfall may be less than 100 mm.

In the Andes the Pacific coastal strip is desert. The western slopes of the Andes are dry, cacti and eucalyptus trees flourish and only a few high mountains are snow covered. The eastern slopes which descend to the Amazon basin become progressively more humid and tree covered.

3.4.2 Temperature

The fall in temperature globally with altitude has been discussed in Chapter 2. However, the temperature of mountain regions is very variable and records of the observatory on the summit of Ben Nevis (1300 m) between 1884 and 1901 show that the mean temperature over these 17 years was −0.1°C; the lowest temperature was −17°C and the highest +19°C.

In North America, Alaska and the Yukon a number of peaks of 6000 m lie within the Arctic Circle. Temperatures of −30°C at 5500–6000 m have been recorded, with gale force winds, in the winter (Mills 1973b).

In the European Alps, the average temperature was −13°C during a winter expedition up to 4000 m, carried out over several days, in the Bernese Oberland, Switzerland (Leuthold *et al.* 1975); gale force winds were not uncommon. Temperatures on the summit of Everest (8848 m) in winter are probably of the order of −60°C; in summer the average temperature would be about −30°C. Hillary recorded a temperature of −27°C at 8500 m on Everest at 3 a.m. on 29 May 1953, the day the first ascent was made (Ward 1993b). On the other hand, on 24 October 1981 Pizzo measured a temperature of −8.8°C on Everest summit.

In Lhasa (3658 m) there are about 100 days a year when the temperature is around 10°C; in summer it may rise as high as 27°C but in the winter it falls to −15°C.

In Antarctica, the lowest recorded temperature is −88.2°C and the highest 15.2°C. The dangers of cold injury, therefore, are likely to complicate accidents or illness in mountain regions.

3.4.3 Solar radiation

Although temperature falls with altitude there is increased exposure to solar radiation (Chapter 2). The amount of radiation absorbed by the body depends on clothing and posture. The clear mountain air permits an increased degree of direct radiation which is enhanced by indirect radiation reflected from the snow. The altitude of the sun is also important (Chrenko and Pugh 1961). The solar heat absorbed depends on the type of clothing; dark clothing absorbs more radiation than light-colored clothing.

3.4.4 Ultraviolet radiation

There is an increase in the level of ultraviolet radiation at high altitude. Snow reflects up to 90% of ultraviolet radiation, compared with 9–17% reflected from ground covered by grass (Buettner 1969), so in snow-covered terrain the combination of direct (incident) and reflected ultraviolet radiation is considerable.

3.5 ECONOMICS

Most mountain communities depend on animal husbandry and agriculture; mining is important in some regions but, more recently, tourism has assumed a greater significance.

Animal husbandry predominates in regions above the limit of agriculture. On the Tibetan plateau, there are immense herds of yak, sheep and goats herded by nomads. Similar nomadic culture was traditional in mountainous regions of central Asian countries, such as Kyrgyzstan, although now most herdsmen are semi-nomadic, living in town or village houses in the winter and in their traditional felt-covered tents (yurts) in the summer. In the bitter climate nomadic pastoralism is the only viable and economic way of life and this may have started between 9000 and 10 000 years ago. The survival of the animals depends exclusively on natural fodder, which creates problems as the sedges and grasses have only a short growing season between May and September. Because there are no areas on the plateau where grass will grow in the winter they cannot escape the climate and, as extensive migration would weaken the stock, only short distances, up to 40 miles, are traversed. Each family has a 'home base', which is sometimes a house, and migrates to set areas whose boundaries, though not fenced, are all well known. On the Tibetan plateau, tents made of yak and sheep's wool are used as dwellings. Further north, camels are common (Goldstein and Beall 1989). In the upper Himalayan valleys the pattern is similar, with flocks spending the summer on pastures up to 5000 m, but below the snow line; in the winter they return to more permanent and protected locations at 4000 m.

The llama (*Lama glama*) and yak (*Bos grunniens*) are extremely important to the economy of the populations of the South American altiplano, and of Tibet and the Himalayan valleys. Both these species show genetic adaptation to high altitude (Chapter 18).

The limiting factor in agriculture is the number of months that the soil becomes frost-free. The type of crop may influence the size of population. Potatoes introduced into the high Himalayan valleys of Nepal between 1850 and 1860 increased the population of Sola Khumbu in the Everest region from 169 households in 1836 to 596 in 1957 (Fuhrer-Haimendorf 1964, p. 10). Immigrants came from Tibet over the Nangpa La, a glacier pass of 5800 m, and, because food was more abundant, were able to adopt the religious life and built many new monasteries. Increasing the productivity of the land, as well as the area under cultivation in Tibet, may change the pattern of life near the centers of population under the present Chinese-organized regime.

Level land may have to be manufactured in the form of terraces. This technique to produce land for agriculture from even steeply sloping hillsides is found in almost all mountainous areas but especially in the Himalayas and Andes. The terraces range in size from a few square feet to a relatively large area, but which is usually too small for pasture (Fig. 3.2). Irrigation may involve ingenious construction of water conduits from surrounding streams. The task of building and maintaining terraces is considerable, especially

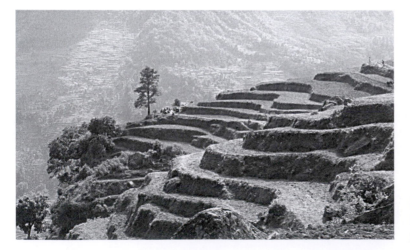

Figure 3.2 Typical terraces in Nepal after harvesting, late autumn

as manure has to be carried up and placed manually. Despite this, terracing is a marked feature of populated mountain valleys and, as it involves ownership and maintenance by groups rather than individuals, the social implications are important. High grazing pasture (alps) is also communal pasture land and this too has social overtones.

Mining, which is often carried out above the pasture level or in rocky terrain, may involve the building of special towns and roads. In Tibet, gold mining has been carried out for centuries, often at 5000 m. However, shallow trenches were used and no deep mines were worked. Recently, a gold mine has been established at 4500 m in northern Chile, and a new copper mine, Toromocho in Peru, has ore as high as 4900 m. In mines at high altitude in Chile there are no resident high altitude populations. The miners live at low altitude with their families and commute to the mine for a period of a week or 10 days followed by the same period off duty at low altitude. Thus they never fully acclimatize nor are they unacclimatized. This intermittent exposure to altitude has been of interest to physiologists (Richalet *et al.* 2002 and is further discussed in Chapter 28).

Tourism, particularly skiing, may involve developing an area which has no natural amenities except good snowfields and glaciers. In 2001 about 25 000 tourists visited the Everest region out of about 100 000 trekkers and almost 300 000 tourists to Nepal.

3.6 LOAD CARRYING

Loads are carried by all who visit mountainous regions. In the valleys of the Himalayas professional porters carry much of the merchandise and the economy depends on them, together with yak and mule transport (Fig. 3.3a).

Observations by Pugh in 1952 and 1953 on the march into Everest (Pugh 1955b) suggest that loads of 40–50 kg, with an addition of 10 kg personal baggage, are carried routinely by porters for 10–12 hours over 10–12 miles each day. Often ascents and descents of 1000–1200 m are made, with loads of tea or paper weighing over 60 kg occasionally being carried.

As the body weight of porters is usually 45–60 kg, and the average height just over 150 cm, each porter carries his own weight in merchandise.

Where possible, loads are carried in a conical, light but strong, wicker basket, 22 by 30 cm at the base and 50 by 70 cm at the top, with a height of 60 cm (Fig. 3.3b). Larger sizes are available for carrying bulky loads such as leaf mould. Loads are supported by a strap passing over the forehead and under the lower end of the basket. When in position the upper end of the basket is level with the top of the porter's head. The center of gravity therefore is as close as possible to a vertical line passing through the center of the pelvis, thus reducing the torque on the spine. The advantage of the head band is that it allows direct transmission of the load to the vertebral column, with muscles being used for balancing rather than support, as when shoulder straps are used. This method of carrying has to be learnt as a child, and the neck muscles in all such Himalayan porters are extremely well developed. In East Africa, heavy loads are carried in this way or just balanced on the head. It has been suggested that this method of load carrying, if practiced from childhood, is more economic, in terms of oxygen consumption, than the Western method in a rucksack (Maloiy *et al.* 1986). Minetti *et al.* (2006) found Nepalese porters to have greatly increased performance in load carrying compared with Caucasian mountaineers. This was especially true of uphill walking (+60% in speed and +39% in mechanical power) but they showed greater efficiency also in downhill walking when carrying a load. The authors thought the porters' superior performance could be partly explained by better balance control; they had less oscillations of the trunk than the mountaineers, due presumably to skill acquired over a lifetime of load carrying. Thus they did not waste energy in the unproductive muscle contraction needed by the mountaineers to keep their balance.

Marching technique depends on the weight of the load. With loads of 50 kg, stops are made every 2–3 minutes, with rests lasting 0.5–1.0 minutes after a distance of 70–250 m has been covered, depending on the gradient. With lighter loads, rests for 2–3 minutes every 10 minutes are normal. Longer pauses are made every hour.

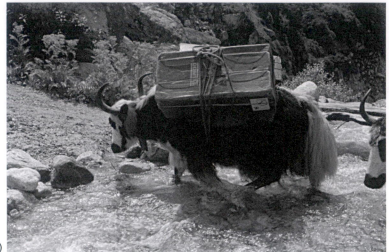

(a)

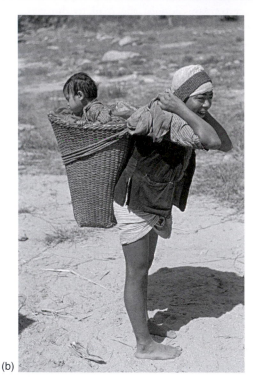

(b)

Figure 3.3   Load carrying in the Himalayas. (a) A yak carrying expedition equipment. (b) A young Nepalese porter with typical basket and head strap carrying his young sister and a load

During rests, the loads are supported on a T-stick about 1 m long, and the porter does not sit down. When longer rests are taken, loads are placed on the top of stone walls conveniently placed beside the track, usually in the shade of a large tree.

At about 3700 m, porter loads are reduced to 25 kg (gross weight 35 kg) which are carried to 5700 m. Exhaustion, when it occurs, is due to overwork; that is, not enough rest days. Few porters have any interest in climbing mountains and so tend to give up when the effects of hypoxia appear.

With high altitude Sherpas, load carrying ability is considerable. Without supplementary oxygen on Everest in 1933 eight porters carried loads weighing 10–15 kg to an altitude of 8300 m, as they did on the Swiss Everest Expedition in 1952.

Low altitude porters carry their own food, eating tsampa (pre-cooked barley) or ata (wheat flour), which is made into a paste or dough, three times a day. Four seers (4 kg) of tsampa is the standard ration for each man for 3.5 days, equivalent to 3500 kcal (14.6 MJ) man^{-1} day^{-1}.

Mountaineers also carry considerable loads to high altitude but use shoulder straps, climb more slowly and stop less frequently.

3.7 PORTERS' HEALTH AND WELFARE

In the early days of Himalayan climbing and trekking, Sherpas were employed as porters above an altitude of about 3000–3500 m. Sherpas had clothing appropriate to the cold and were physiologically adapted to high altitudes. With increasing wealth, Sherpas moved up the social scale becoming guides and staff members of expeditions and treks, so low altitude porters were employed at higher altitudes for which they had neither clothing nor adaptation (Fig. 3.3b). To make matters worse, they were employed as casual labour, and expedition and trek leaders, in many cases, felt little or no responsibility for their welfare. Porters have to provide their own food, clothing and shelter. Traditionally, most commercial portering was done at lower altitudes, going from one village to another where shelter could be found, but treks and expeditions often need to take routes far from any village. In recent years a number of charities have been set up to provide clothing and shelter at least on some of the more popular trek routes and to encourage trekking companies to take responsibility for their porters.

A common scenario is illustrated by the following case:

A young porter from lowland Nepal, carrying about 40 kilos of material, fell ill at Lobuche (5018m). This was his first trip to the Everest region. He was used to carrying much heavier loads in his home region so he could not understand why he had such a hard time carrying this load here. He actually had symptoms of acute mountain sickness (AMS) at Pheriche (4280m) but did not want to lose his job so, without complaining, continued to ascend to Lobuche where his headache became very severe with nausea and vomiting. He also started walking like a drunk. He was so tired that he was the last one to arrive at Lobuche. His trekking Sirdar realized he was very ill and promptly had him sent down to Pheriche from Lobuche. He came to the aid post at Pheriche completely disoriented with an arterial saturation in the low 70s%. He was treated with high flow oxygen from the oxygen concentrator, steroids and nifedipine after a diagnosis of both high altitude cerebral and pulmonary edema (HACE and HAPE). His companions that brought him "dumped" him in the care of the aid post and went back up, despite requests from the staff that someone should remain behind with the patient to help look after him.

Luckily his condition improved rapidly and in 2 days time he was ready to head down to his lowland home. On later questioning the trip leader in charge of the group said that he thought that Nepalese adjusted to altitude very well and that it was mostly the Westerners who fell ill. Supplied by Dr B. Basnyat (personal communication).

Lowland porters are just as prone to altitude illness as are tourists from the West and to other illnesses, such as gastrointestinal and respiratory diseases. Again, those employing porters have a responsibility for these aspects of their welfare. Basnyat and Litch (1997) collected data on porter illnesses from a 22-day trek in the Mansalu area of Nepal, at altitudes up to 5100 m. The illness rate was similar in the porter group as in Western trekkers (52 and 55%) but lower in the trek staff, Sherpas (13%). However, there were, of course, greater numbers of porters than trekkers (102 compared with 22). Most of the illnesses were not altitude diseases, but among the latter, again the rate in porters was similar to the trekkers, and evacuation was required for 5% of the party, all from the porter group.

3.8 HOUSES AND SHELTER

Cultural mechanisms that provide a comfortable microclimate and reduce heat loss have been developed in all high altitude communities. The ideal house should be draught-free with a low ratio of surface area to volume and well constructed of material which diminishes the daily extremes of temperature. The roof should be well insulated.

In the Andes, the adobe (dried mud) building has the first meter or so of the walls made of stone, the roof is of tile, grass or tin and walls are plastered with mud to provide an airtight structure; the roof is tightly fitted and the floor may be wood or dirt. Because of the method of construction the diurnal change is reduced (Baker 1966). In the Himalayas the thermal protection of stone structures built for semi-nomadic occupation appears to be less. Traditional Sherpa houses often have only one floor, with stone walls and wooden roofs held on with stones. The ground floor is without windows and provides quarters for animals; the first floor is for human habitation. Windows usually have no glass, but have wooden shutters, and an open fire is placed in the center of one side, but this provides only a transient increase in temperature. Nowadays, in places like Namche Bazaar, where the benefits of greatly increased tourism have increased wealth, better housing with glass in the windows is to be found. However, in areas less popular with trekkers, such as the Rolwaling Valley, traditional Sherpa houses are still common.

In north Bhutan houses are similarly constructed but animals are kept in a yard. Cracks between stones in both Bhutanese and Sherpa houses are filled with earth. Tibetan houses may be of more than one floor and are often in terraces. Glass is rare and the houses are heated by an open fire or stove. Nomads have tents with a loose wide weave which enables warm air to be entrapped but allows egress of smoke from open fires and is waterproof. However, some semi-nomadic families have a stove with a chimney.

In Central Asia the nomads traditionally live in yurts. These tent-like structures have a wooden frame, the tunduk, covered with felt. The floor and walls are covered with rugs. Yurts are circular with an opening in the center of the conical roof allowing smoke to escape. This opening can be covered or 'cowled' against the prevailing wind. The yurt can be quickly dismantled and transported on pack animals, yaks, camels or horses.

3.9 CLOTHING

Because of the generally low temperature and loss of heat, particularly due to radiation and convection, clothing with good insulation is necessary to provide a warm microclimate. Trapped, still air is the best insulation and wool is the best naturally available insulating material; it resists compacting and loses only 40% of its insulating value when wet. Garments that are loosely woven entrap more air than those that are tightly woven.

A multiple layered system for garments is preferable to one thick layer because insulation can be varied at will, thus minimizing perspiration. The outer layer should be as impermeable to wind as possible. A sheepskin coat is the best naturally available garment that has many of these characteristics, and is usually worn with cotton or wool undergarments.

In general, Andean clothing conforms to the above model and natural clothing is adequate for the conditions encountered. Measurements of insulation of normal clothing without hats, shawls and ponchos showed values for men slightly less than those for women. The greatest increase in surface temperature occurred in the hands and feet. At night, Andean highlanders, who use a bedding of skins, can maintain their metabolic rate by light shivering that does not disturb sleep.

In the high Himalayan valleys and Tibet, clothing assemblies are similar. The main garment is a thick sheepskin 'chupa' with long, wide sleeves which, when extended, keep the hands warm; gloves are never used. Normally the garment is gathered around the waist by a belt and hitched up to the knees so that there is a pocket for loose objects in front of the chest. When the belt is loosened the garment extends to the ground and thus can be used as a sleeping robe; often in warm conditions one or both shoulders are left bare. Under this is a woolen shirt and often long woolen, cotton or sheepskin trousers. Soft leather boots with decorative wool leggings extending to the knees are packed with grass, straw or leaves, but a Tibetan often may walk in bare feet in the snow or through streams. Some wear a felt hat or balaclava and, to prevent snow blindness, yak hair is put in front of the eyes if goggles are not available (Desideri 1712–27; Moorcroft and Trebeck 1841, Vol. 1 p. 399). Other methods used by Tibetans include blackening the eyelids and wearing masks with tiny eye holes, the rims of which are blackened (MacDonald 1929, p. 182). Cotton clothing is favored at high temperatures and low altitudes, but nomads wear wool or sheepskin. Many now wear wool sweaters and

leather boots. Tibetan nomads sleep resting on their elbows and knees with all their clothes piled on their backs (Holditch 1907; Duff 1999). This 'fetal position' diminishes surface area and therefore heat loss; contact with the ground is also minimal.

Some Tibetan lamas have developed the ability to 'warm without fire'. The central core temperature is kept raised under cold conditions, both by increasing the metabolic rate, probably by continuous light shivering, and also by the practice of g-tum-mo yoga (an advanced form of Tibetan yoga), which appears to involve peripheral vasodilatation (Pugh 1963; Benson *et al.* 1982).

4

Genetics and high altitude

SUMMARY

The topic of genetics in relation to high altitude is a fast-moving area and justifies its own chapter in this new edition. In the past many people commented on the superior exercise ability of highlanders such as Tibetans and Andeans but, of course, only recently has it become possible to determine the genetic basis if this exists. One of the first areas of research was the effects of polymorphism of the *ACE* gene. These variants are believed to influence athletic ability although their importance at high altitude is still uncertain. A major advance was the discovery of hypoxia-inducible factors which are now known to play major roles in the expression of genes related to hypoxia. At high altitude they alter erythropoiesis, the ventilatory response to hypoxia and hypoxic pulmonary vasoconstriction among other functions. An exciting advance has been the discovery of genetic changes in Tibetans, being reported in no less than seven independent publications in 2010. Research in this area is moving rapidly but it is clear that a major gene is *EPAS1* which codes for HIF-2α and therefore has a large variety of physiological effects. Studies of genetic changes in other high altitude populations, such as those in the South American Andes and Ethiopia, are ongoing. Another important area is the role of genetic factors in high altitude diseases. Different susceptibilities of individuals, families and populations suggest that genetic factors play a role and a large number of candidate genes are under investigation. Finally, the remarkable phenotype differences between Tibetans and Andeans are reviewed. The fact that these two groups of highlanders who have both adapted so successfully to high altitude have very different physical make-ups is tantalizing and is provoking much research.

4.1 INTRODUCTION

Genetic change in relation to high altitude comprises one of the newest and fastest growing topics in high altitude medicine and physiology and has attracted a great deal of research. As a result it has now progressed sufficiently to justify its own chapter. A convenient starting point is the recognition that polymorphism of the *ACE* gene affects physical performance. In fact, the first publication in 1998 claimed that the insertion allele of the gene was associated with elite endurance performance among high altitude mountaineers (Montgomery *et al.* 1998) although, as we shall see, this conclusion has been questioned. The discovery of hypoxia-inducible factors (HIF), which we now recognize play a major role in the body's response to hypoxia, occurred in 1992 (Semenza and Wang 1992). Finally, the dramatic demonstration of genetic changes in Tibetans compared with Han Chinese was not reported until 2010 by several groups working independently. At the time of writing, progress in this last area is so fast that the term frenetic comes to mind. Other related topics include possible genetic factors in high altitude diseases, and the fascinating phenotypical differences between residents of Tibet and the Andes.

The rate of advance is such that a textbook like this cannot possibly keep up with the latest work. Nevertheless, it is valuable to summarize the development of the topic, particularly for the general reader. Much of this new work is very technical, and some readers may not have the scientific background to understand the details. The chapter is heavily referenced for those who want to consult the original papers and some of the reviews.

4.2 HISTORY

The study of genetic changes in humans is very recent compared with most of the material in this book. A watershed discovery was the structure of DNA in 1953 by Watson and Crick (1953) but the human genome was not sequenced until 2001 (Lander *et al.* 2001; Venter *et al.* 2001). However, there are many references in the older literature to human adaptation to high altitude, and references to the fact that highlanders seemed to have a different biological make-up compared with lowlanders.

Bert (1878) in his typically urbane fashion wrote that:

Just as a Basque mountaineer furnished with a piece of bread and a few onions makes expeditions which require of the member of the Alpine club who accompanies him the absorption of a pound of meat, so it may be that dwellers in high places finally lessen the consumption of oxygen in their organism,

while keeping at their disposal the same quantity of vital force.

Kellas was one of the first people to recognize the superior performance of Sherpas at high altitude (these people are Tibetans who crossed into Nepal many years ago). He used them as partners on some of his high climbs after his first expedition in 1907 when he took two Swiss guides but both were badly affected by mountain sickness (Kellas 1912). Barcroft in his account of the International High Altitude Expedition to Cerro de Pasco in 1921–22 remarked both on the extraordinary physical ability of the indigenous people, but also on their remarkable phenotype such as their very large chests (Barcroft *et al.* 1923).

Monge in his classical book *Acclimatization in the Andes* devoted a great deal of space to the special characteristics of the Peruvian Quechua highlanders (Monge 1948). He was adamant that these people should not be judged by the standards of lowlanders, and he was incensed by Barcroft's comments that 'all dwellers at high altitudes are persons of impaired physical and mental powers'. Monge's response was that 'Andean man being different from sea-level man, his biological personality must be measured with a scale distinct from that applied to the men of the lower valleys and plains'. So there were many references to the fact that highlanders were different from lowlanders in the early literature but, of course, there was no way of studying the genetic basis if indeed one existed.

As indicated above, the origin of high altitude genetics can perhaps be traced to the recognition of possible effects of polymorphism of the *ACE* gene on athletic performance in 1998, the discovery of HIF in 1992, and the very recent dramatic demonstration of genetic differences between Tibetans and Han Chinese in 2010. The prospects of further research are exciting indeed.

4.3 POLYMORPHISM OF THE *ACE* GENE

Polymorphism refers to the natural variation in a gene caused by a change in the DNA sequence. It often occurs with a fairly high frequency in the general population but generally has no adverse effects on the individual. *ACE* is angiotensin-converting enzyme. It degrades vasodilator kinins and converts angiotensin I to the powerful vasoconstrictor angiotensin II. The renin–angiotensin system (RAS) is not just an endocrine regulator but also has a variety of functions within local tissue and cells. Polymorphic variants have been identified for many components of RAS, and here we deal with insertion and deletion (I and D) polymorphism of the *ACE* gene. The insertion or deletion allele refers to the presence or absence of a 250 base pair DNA fragment within the gene. In white North Americans, the distribution of II, ID and DD genotypes is approximately 29, 40 and 31%, and other ethnic groups show different distributions (Mathew *et al.* 2001). This is consistent with variations in the genetic background of different racial groups generally.

The I allele has been demonstrated to be associated with endurance-orientated events, notably in triathlons. On the other hand, the D allele is associated with strength and power-orientated performance, and has been found in significant excess among elite swimmers. However, exceptions to these associations occur.

In the initial description of *ACE* gene polymorphism in relation to physical performance, it was claimed that the insertion allele of the gene was associated with elite endurance performance among high altitude mountaineers. For example, 33 mountaineers with a history of ascending beyond 7000 m without supplementary oxygen were studied and it was found that among the 15 climbers who had ascended beyond 8000 m without oxygen none were homozygous for the D allele. Six of them had the II allele and nine had the ID allele (Montgomery *et al.* 1998).

Additional studies appeared to confirm an association between the I allele and performance at extreme altitude. For example, 141 mountaineers who had participated in expeditions to peaks above 8000 m completed a questionnaire and provided a buccal swab for *ACE* I/D genotyping, and it was reported that the I allele was associated with the maximum altitudes achieved (Thompson *et al.* 2007). Another study reported an association between the presence of the I allele and success in reaching the summit of Mont Blanc (4807 m) (Tsianos *et al.* 2005). There was also a report

that the I allele was more prevalent in Sherpas, suggesting that this might be one of the genetic factors giving them an advantage at high altitude (Droma *et al.* 2008).

A possible reason for the association between the I allele and exceptional performance at high altitude could be that these climbers are less prone to high altitude illnesses. However, in a study of 83 mountaineers who stayed overnight in the Capanna Margherita (altitude 4559 m) and developed symptoms of acute mountain sickness, there was no difference in the *ACE* polymorphism. Furthermore, the same investigators reported 76 mountaineers who had participated in previous studies in which 38 had developed high altitude pulmonary edema, and again there was no link between the symptoms and the frequency of the *ACE* gene polymorphism (Dehnert *et al.* 2002a). Other possible links between *ACE* gene polymorphism and physiological changes at high altitude have been explored without success. For example, 63 athletes exposed to an altitude of 2200 m failed to demonstrate a relationship between the *ACE* genotype and erythropoietic response to altitude (González *et al.* 2006).

A recent extensive review concludes that the I allele may relate to improved endurance performance and enhanced oxygen utilization in general, while the D allele is apparently associated with gains in strength with training and the associated acquisition of increased muscle bulk in response to muscle strength training (Puthucheary *et al.* 2011). In this review the link with high altitude tolerance is downplayed. The paper includes a large table summarizing the results of some 54 studies on the effects of *ACE* polymorphism on physical performance and the interested reader will find a wealth of information there.

4.4 HYPOXIA-INDUCIBLE FACTORS

4.4.1 Description of hypoxia-inducible factors

Hypoxia-inducible factors are transcription factors that respond to changes in available oxygen in the cellular environment. A transcription factor is a protein that binds to specific DNA sequences in a gene. This allows it to control the flow, that is transcription, of genetic information from DNA to messenger RNA (mRNA). It does this by helping or hindering RNA polymerase binding to DNA. Increasing the rate of gene transcription is referred to as upregulation, while decreasing the rate of gene transcription is called downregulation. There are some additional proteins such as co-activators that also play a role in transcription of DNA but if these do not contain DNA-binding domains they are not classified as transcription factors.

Most oxygen-breathing species express the transcriptional factor HIF-1. In other words this has been highly conserved. It is a heterodimer, that is it is made up of two macromolecules, in this case an alpha and beta subunit known as HIF-1α and HIF-1β subunits. HIF was originally discovered as a protein that bound to the hypoxia response element (HRE) of the *EPO* gene under hypoxic conditions (Semenza and Wang 1992). The *EPO* gene encodes erythropoietin, the hormone controlling red cell production. HIF-1 plays a critical role in a large number of responses of the cell to hypoxia. For example, in cellular hypoxia the transcription of several hundred mRNAs is increased and the expression of an equal number of mRNAs is decreased.

4.4.2 HIF responses to hypoxia

The response of HIF-1 to normoxia and hypoxia is complicated (Fig. 4.1). As stated above, HIF-1 is a heterodimer consisting of HIF-1α and HIF-1β subunits. HIF-1β is constitutively expressed, that is it is transcribed continually. By contrast, the HIF-1α subunit is found at very low levels under normoxic conditions as shown in the left half of Fig. 4.1. Under normoxic conditions HIF-1α is hydroxylated by prolyl hydroxylase domain (PHD) proteins. The hydroxylated HIF-1α then interacts with the von Hippel–Lindau (VHL) protein using molecular oxygen. This then leads to the addition of ubiquitin (Ub), which is a small regulatory protein found in almost all tissues and which plays an important role in the degradation of unneeded proteins. The result is proteasomal degradation, that is the proteins are broken up by

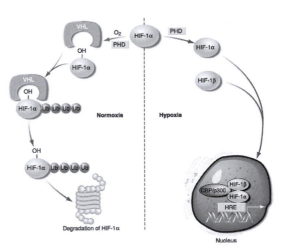

Figure 4.1 Regulation of HIF-1 by hypoxia. In normoxia (left panel), hydroxylation of HIF-1α by prolyl hydroxylase domain proteins (PHD) using molecular oxygen leads to interaction with von Hippel–Lindau (VHL) and addition of ubiquitin (Ub) resulting in proteasomal degradation. In hypoxia (right panel), HIF-1α is not targeted for degradation and it moves to the nucleus where it binds with HIF-1β and combines with co-activators at the hypoxia response element (HRE) to effect gene transcription. (Reprinted with permission of the American Thoracic Society. Copyright 2012 American Thoracic Society. Shimoda, L.A. and Semenza, G.L. (2011) HIF and the lung: role of hypoxia-inducible factors in pulmonary development and disease. *American Journal of Respiratory and Critical Care Medicine* **183**, 152–6.)

severing the peptide bonds. The residues can be used for synthesizing new proteins.

Now turning to the right-hand part of Fig. 4.1, under hypoxic conditions PHD activity is decreased and this results in stabilization of HIF-1α. It then translocates to the nucleus where it binds with HIF-1β and recruits co-activator proteins to the HIF binding site with the HRE. The HRE is a specialized short sequence of DNA of 50 or less base pairs. The result is activation of transcription of various target genes.

Several years after the discovery of HIF-1α, a closely related protein was identified and named HIF-2α. The processing of HIF-2α is similar to that of HIF-1α as shown in Fig. 4.1. However,

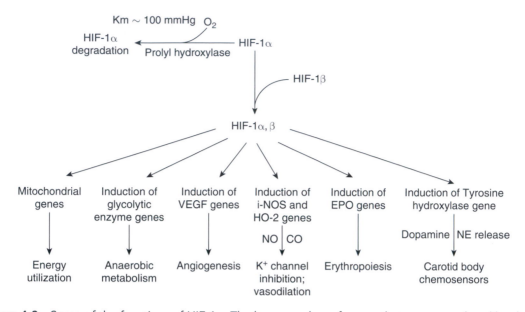

Figure 4.2   Some of the functions of HIF-1α. The large number of genes that are upregulated by the mechanism shown in Fig. 4.1 results in extensive physiological effects. (From Wilson *et al.* 2005, with permission.)

although HIF-1α is found in all nucleated cells, HIF-2α has a much more restricted pattern of expression.

As indicated above, a large number of target genes are upregulated by HIF. Some of the consequences are shown in Fig. 4.2. As can be seen, the physiological consequences of HIF production include the regulation of vascular endothelial growth factor (*VEGF*) genes resulting in angiogenesis, *EPO* genes controlling erythropoiesis, and the genes for tyrosine hydroxylase which alter the sensitivity of the carotid body to hypoxia. HIF is therefore a master switch in the general response of the body to hypoxia.

4.4.3 Congenital Chuvash polycythemia

This unusual condition is of interest because of the light it throws on the HIF pathway shown in Fig. 4.1. The Chuvash Republic is a small area in the east of Russia, and some of its residents have a congenital form of polycythemia associated with genetic abnormalities. High hemoglobin concentrations of 22.6 ± 1.4 g/dL^{-1} have been reported while platelet and white blood cell counts are normal (Sergeyeva *et al.* 1997). The affected people are homozygous for a missense mutation, that is a change in a single nucleotide that results in a codon that codes for the wrong amino acid. The consequence is partial impaired binding of the VHL protein to hydroxylated HIF-1α subunits. This results in HIF activity that is inappropriately elevated for a given level of P_{O_2}. In addition to the very high red cell concentrations, these people have changes in the control of ventilation and pulmonary vascular tone. Hypoxia-induced changes in respiration and pulmonary vascular pressures occur at higher P_{O_2} levels than in normal people indicating a generalized defect in oxygen sensing (Smith *et al.* 2006). There are also altered metabolic responses to exercise (Formenti *et al.* 2010).

4.4.4 Regulation of cellular metabolism by HIF

It has been found that HIF-1 is expressed in very primitive animals such as the worm *Caenorhabditis elegans* that lacks specialized respiratory or circulatory systems. This suggests that HIF was initially developed to allow individual cells to survive in low oxygen environments. Consistent with this, HIF-1 assists cell survival under hypoxic conditions by switching metabolism from oxidative to glycolytic. This is done by upregulating the genes that increase the flux of glucose to pyruvate, such as pyruvate dehydrogenase kinase, genes that inactivate pyruvate dehydrogenase that converts pyruvate to acetyl-CoA, and genes that increase lactate dehydrogenase that converts pyruvate to lactate (Kim *et al.* 2006). Glycolysis is a relatively inefficient path for the production of adenosine triphosphate (ATP) compared with oxidative metabolism. The latter produces 18 times as much ATP per mole of glucose compared with glycolysis.

This discovery of the role of HIF-1 in cellular metabolism has some interesting implications. Surprisingly, HIF-1α null fibroblasts (that is with both copies of the gene missing) produce higher ATP levels at 1% O_2 than wild-type cells at 20% O_2. This demonstrates that under these severely hypoxic conditions, oxygen is not limiting ATP production. However, under these conditions, the HIF-1α null cells die as a result of the build up of reactive oxygen species (ROS). It has therefore been suggested that the advantage of switching to glycolysis is to prevent excess mitochondrial generation of ROS (Semenza 2012). If this occurred it would interfere with mitochondrial electron transport under hypoxic conditions. This work raises the question of whether cells switch to glycolysis because insufficient oxygen is available, or because oxidative metabolism under hypoxic conditions leads to a lethal concentration of ROS.

4.4.5 HIF and hypoxic pulmonary hypertension

Chronic alveolar hypoxia (for example as occurs at high altitude) causes hypoxic pulmonary vasoconstriction that progresses to vascular wall remodeling. This includes thickening of the vessel wall as a result of the proliferation of smooth muscle and fibroblasts, and also extension of smooth muscle cells into previously nonmuscular precapillary arterioles.

Recently, a role for HIF-1α and HIF-2α in the development of hypoxic pulmonary hypertension

has been investigated. It is known that increases in intracellular calcium ion concentration and intracellular pH contribute to the growth and contraction of pulmonary artery smooth muscle cells under hypoxic conditions. There is evidence that the increase in intracellular pH is related to an increased activity and expression of the sodium/hydrogen ion exchanger isoform 1 (NHE1) (Rios *et al.* 2005). In addition, the increase in intracellular calcium ion concentration is due to the increased expression of canonical transient receptor potential (TRPC) proteins and enhanced calcium ion entry through non-selective cation channels (Wang *et al.* 2006). Both the increase in intracellular pH and calcium ion concentration are mediated by HIF-1 (Shimoda *et al.* 2001).

It is now known that digoxin, a drug that has been used to treat heart failure for a very long time, inhibits HIF-1. To test the possible therapeutic value of this drug in hypoxic pulmonary hypertension, mice were injected with digoxin or saline and exposed to room air or ambient hypoxia for 3 weeks. It was shown that the digoxin-treated animals had attenuation of the development of right ventricular hypertrophy, pulmonary vascular remodeling, and increases in intracellular calcium and pH in the pulmonary artery smooth muscle cells. There was also a fall in right ventricular pressures (Abud *et al.* 2012). These exciting results suggest a possible role for digoxin in the treatment of high altitude pulmonary hypertension. Presumably, William Withering (1741–99) who first discovered the active ingredient of foxglove in the treatment of heart failure would be just as surprised as we are.

4.4.6 HIF and intermittent hypoxia

Intermittent hypoxia commonly occurs at high altitude. For example, many people at high altitude have periodic breathing during sleep that sometimes includes periods of many seconds of apnea. In fact, periodic breathing is almost universal in lowlanders above about 5000 m. Another pattern of intermittent hypoxia is seen in mine workers who commute to high altitude. For example, the workers of the Collahuasi mine in north Chile live in Iquique at sea level but are bused up to the mine where they work at an altitude as high as 4500 m although they sleep at the lower altitude of 3800 m. A common pattern is to spend a week at the mine followed by a week at sea level with the pattern being repeated for many months or years.

It is therefore interesting that the patterns of HIF production are affected by intermittent hypoxia. Studies have been carried out on animals exposed to patterns of intermittent hypoxia that are similar to those that occur in many people who suffer from obstructive sleep apnea. It is known that these people who cycle between hypoxia and re-oxygenation dozens of times during the night have increased sympathetic activation and increased levels of catecholamines that lead to systemic hypertension. Rats exposed to intermittent hypoxia for 35 days (lowest O_2 concentration 3–5%) developed systemic hypertension and left ventricular hypertrophy (Fletcher *et al.* 1992).

As already discussed, HIF-1α is expressed at low levels under normoxic conditions, and it is also induced by chronic intermittent hypoxia. However, it is remarkable that the results of intermittent hypoxia on HIF-1α and HIF-2α are diametrically opposed. In experiments on rats it was found that intermittent hypoxia upregulated HIF-1α but downregulated HIF-2α (Nanduri *et al.* 2009). This is particularly surprising given the similar structures of HIF-1α and HIF-2α. These different effects of intermittent hypoxia on the two transcription factors were found both in tissue from rats exposed to intermittent hypoxia and in cells in culture. The results are all the more surprising because continuous hypoxia upregulates both HIF-1α and HIF-2α in the cell cultures. Thus intermittent hypoxia has a differential effect upon these two structurally related HIF transcriptional activators. These studies also showed that the downregulation of HIF-2α in rats exposed to intermittent hypoxia could be inhibited by calpain proteases (calpain is a protein belonging to a family of calcium-dependent proteases). This may have implications for the prevention of the pathology caused by intermittent hypoxia (Nanduri *et al.* 2009).

4.4.7 HIF and lung injury

Acute lung injury such as that caused by the acute respiratory distress syndrome results in severe hypoxemia accompanied by pathological changes in the pulmonary capillaries and lung edema. The possible role of HIF in these changes has been briefly studied although a clear pattern has not emerged as yet. In a hypoxic ischemia/reperfusion model using isolated ferret lungs, levels of HIF-1α mRNA and protein were increased during hypoxic ischemia. These were associated with an increase in VEGF which was thought to be a mediator of the increased pulmonary vascular permeability in this model (Becker *et al.* 2000). By contrast, another study using both endothelial cell cultures and also mice lacking one HIF-1α allele found downregulation of HIF-1α and adenosine kinase in this model of lung injury (Morote-Garcia *et al.* 2008).

4.4.8 HIF and cancer

Most solid cancerous tumors outrun their blood supply with the result that the center of the lesion is hypoxic. It is therefore not surprising that HIF-1α is upregulated in these tumors. In addition, there may be loss of function of the VHL protein which results in increased expression of both HIF-1α and HIF-2α. There is consequently considerable interest in the use of chemotherapeutic agents against cancer that function as HIF-1 inhibitors. This is a very active area of research.

4.4.9 HIF and ischemia

Patients with coronary artery disease often develop collateral vessels in response to narrowing of a coronary artery, and patients with collaterals are likely to have smaller infarcts if the main vessel is occluded (Resar *et al.* 2005). It has been shown that patients with coronary artery disease who have collateral vessels have an increased frequency of a single nucleotide polymorphism (SNP) affecting HIF-1α. This change in HIF-1α was associated with stable exertional angina rather than a serious myocardial infarction (Hlatky *et al.* 2007).

4.5 GENETIC CHANGES IN TIBETANS

4.5.1 Early evidence of phenotype differences in Tibetans

Anecdotal evidence of the exceptional exercise ability of Sherpas (who were originally Tibetans) at high altitude were alluded to in section 4.2. For example, Kellas recognized this before 1920, and Sherpas played important roles in the early expeditions to Mount Everest. Tensing Norgay Sherpa along with Edmund Hillary were the first people to reach the summit. Later during the Silver Hut expedition of 1960–61, one Sherpa was studied at an altitude of 5800 m and it was found that he had a considerably higher maximal oxygen consumption than the maximal value for any of the Westerners. Furthermore, the Sherpa's maximum heart rate was 186 beats min^{-1} whereas the mean value for the Westerners was only 143.

Another clear difference is the lower hemoglobin concentrations of Tibetans or Sherpas compared with Westerners and Han Chinese. Some of the earliest measurements were made by Pugh (1954) when he found lower hemoglobin concentrations in Sherpas on the expeditions to Cho Oyu in 1952 and Everest in 1953. The comparisons were with the European climbers. More recently, Wu et al. (2005) found substantially lower hemoglobin concentrations in Tibetans compared with Han Chinese at the same altitude. These lower hemoglobin concentrations are consistent with the lower prevalence of chronic mountain sickness in Tibetans compared with Han Chinese, Europeans and Andeans (Moore 2001).

Another striking difference is the much lower degree of hypoxic pulmonary vasoconstriction in Tibetans compared with North Americans and Andeans (Groves et al. 1993). This is consistent with the higher plasma nitric oxide (NO) concentrations in Tibetans compared with Americans because NO is a pulmonary vasodilator (Erzurum et al. 2007). Another difference between Tibetans and others including Andeans, Europeans and Han Chinese is the higher birth weight of infants for the same altitude (Moore 2001). This is consistent with the higher

uterine blood flow that has been measured in pregnant Tibetan women. Finally, Tibetan infants born at high altitude have higher arterial oxygen saturations than corresponding Han Chinese (Niemeyer et al. 1995).

All of these observations suggested that there may be genetic changes in Tibetans compared with Han Chinese and other people (Moore 2001) but, of course, no progress could be made on this front until the dawn of genomics in 2010. But then there was an explosion of new findings.

4.5.2 Description of genetic changes

In 2010–11, there were no fewer than seven publications on genetic changes in Tibetans (Aggarwal et al. 2010; Beall et al. 2010; Bigham et al. 2010; Simonson et al. 2010; Yi et al. 2010; Peng Y et al. 2011; Xu et al. 2011). Many of these are very technical and would be challenging for the average reader. A somewhat simplified, less technical account is presented here and all the references are given so that the original publications can be consulted. Only three of this extensive series of papers will be discussed in any detail.

First, we should appreciate that the challenge is daunting. It involves determining the potential roles of about 25 000 genes scattered among the three billion DNA bases that make up the human genome. The approach taken by Beall et al. (2010) was to scan the entire human genome looking for regions that were differently represented in Tibetans compared with Han Chinese. They looked at over 500 000 SNPs and found that eight of these had variants that were significantly increased in Tibetans. The size of the project can be appreciated from the fact that there were about 30 authors' names on the paper from a number of universities including Case Western Reserve, Oxford and several Chinese institutions. It was found that all eight of the overrepresented variants were on chromosome 2 close to the EPAS1 gene. This abbreviation stands for endothelial PAS domain protein 1, and it is known that the gene encodes for HIF-2α as was described in section 4.4.4. In addition to this primary study, variants of EPAS1 were correlated with lower hemoglobin concentrations in two additional groups of Tibetans.

The authors argued that the change in *EPAS1* could be critical in high altitude adaptation in Tibetans because the resulting reduced erythropoietic response helped to avoid the development of chronic mountain sickness. There are also other deleterious effects of a high hematocrit, such as flow abnormalities in the microcirculation including rouleaux formation that can interfere with oxygen delivery. In addition, the increase in viscosity increases vascular resistance including that in the lung. As indicated in Fig. 4.1, HIFs are involved in the regulation of numerous genes and pathways so the reduced erythropoietin response, although apparently clearly advantageous, may be only the tip of the iceberg for high altitude adaptation.

Simonson *et al.* (2010) took a different approach. The work was carried out at the University of Utah in Salt Lake City, and included extensive collaboration with Qinghai University located in Xining in Western China. Xining is on one of the primary access routes to the Tibetan plateau and it has had a vigorous program in high altitude biology for several years. The project included comparisons of Tibetans with lowland Asian populations, including those in China and Japan. The approach was to focus on a subset of candidate genes that were thought to have a high probability of being involved in adaptation to high altitude. These genes were chosen from Gene Ontology and Panther databases which are involved in oxygen delivery pathways including NO metabolism. The investigators looked for chromosomal regions exhibiting a strong signal of positive selection that contained any of the 247 genes. Ten genes were identified and six of these were related to the HIF system, including *EPAS1* as identified by Beall *et al.* (2010). In addition, they found two other genes, *EGLN1* and *PPARA,* which were associated with hemoglobin concentration, this again being consistent with the phenotype described above. In particular, the protein encoded by *EGLN1* is known to be involved in HIF-1α-mediated gene expression.

The third study that will be briefly reviewed was by Yi *et al.* (2010). This had no less than

60 authors from the University of California, Berkeley, University of California, Davis and China. The approach was somewhat different again. The investigators limited the analysis of the whole human genome to 50 exomes of Tibetans. The term exome refers to that part of the gene formed by all the exons, that is the coding portions of the genes that are expressed. Using this strategy the investigators were able to include the coding sequences of 92% of all the genes. Again, the *EPAS1* gene among others was identified as a strong candidate for natural selection. In fact, the frequency of one variant of the *EPAS1* gene differed between Tibetans and Han Chinese by 78% (87 versus 9%). This variant was associated with hemoglobin concentration and erythrocyte count, again consistent with the phenotype information discussed earlier.

An interesting conjecture raised by Yi *et al.* (2010) was that the Tibetan and Han Chinese populations diverged less than 3000 years ago. If this were true it would probably be the most rapid example of Darwinian evolution that has ever been observed in humans. The only other contender for this honor is the selection for lactose tolerance seen, for example in northern Europeans, that benefited populations who kept cattle. However, this assertion of the rapidity of the change has been strongly challenged, for example by Aldenderfer (2011), who has studied the anthropological evidence for the date of settlements in Tibet. Nevertheless, the study by Yi *et al.* concluded that there are very strong selective pressures that resulted in the genetic differences.

In addition to the three studies briefly described above, several others have been reported and these will be just mentioned here. Interested readers should refer to the original publications. Bigham *et al.* (2010) obtained additional support for the role of *EPAS1* in Tibetan adaptation by carrying out high density scans of genomes from natives of three regions of Tibet. Peng *et al.* (2011) carried out SNP typing of 50 people from seven Tibetan communities using the Affymetrix chip 6.0 array that was also used by Bigham *et al.* (2010). Xu *et al.* (2011) compared genome-wide allele frequencies of Tibetans and Han Chinese and identified *EPAS1* and *EGLN1* as important. These investigators also re-analyzed the data from

Yi *et al.* (2010), Beall *et al.* (2010) and Simonson *et al.* (2010). The fact that this large number of essentially independent studies provided such an extensive amount of agreement greatly increases our confidence in the results.

An interesting feature of these studies is that none so far has detected any variance in *HIF-1A*, the gene that encodes for HIF-1α. As we have seen, HIF-1α is thought to be a central mediator of responses to hypoxia and its omission is something of a puzzle. One possible explanation is that HIF-1α controls critical responses that have limited latitude for variation whereas perhaps HIF-2α serves the role of a more adaptable regulator.

As stated earlier, the pace of research in this area is so rapid that the brief account given here will soon be superseded. Nevertheless, a discussion of the early findings is useful to gain a perspective.

4.6 GENETIC CHANGES IN ANDEAN POPULATIONS

More people live at very high altitudes in the South American Andes than anywhere else in the world and so it is natural to ask whether they also have genetic responses to altitude. However, fewer studies have been reported on the Andean highlanders so far. One reason for this is that since the Spanish conquest in the sixteenth century, there has been substantial admixture of European genes with those of the original high altitude inhabitants. This is in contrast to Tibet where much less admixture has occurred.

Bigham *et al.* (2010) investigated the genomes of two Andean populations, the Quechua and Aymara. They reported more chromosomal regions showing evidence of positive selection in Andeans than in Tibetans (37 versus 14) with none of the regions shared. They concluded that the genetic basis for altitude adaptation was dissimilar in the two populations. However, they did detect evidence for selection of the *EGLN1* gene in Andeans. We can expect much more attention to be given to Andeans in the near future. Highlanders in Ethiopia are another important group that are beginning to be studied (Scheinfeldt *et al.* 2012).

4.7 GENETICS AND HIGH ALTITUDE DISEASES

Whether genetic factors can help to predict susceptibility to high altitude diseases is an interesting and important subject but research is at an early stage. Much of what we know to date has been reviewed by a group at the University of British Columbia (Rupert and Koehle 2006; MacInnis *et al.* 2010; MacInnis *et al.* 2011). The primary diseases of interest are acute mountain sickness (AMS), high altitude pulmonary edema (HAPE), high altitude cerebral edema (HACE), high altitude pulmonary hypertension (HAPH) (previously known as subacute mountain sickness), and chronic mountain sickness (CMS).

Evidence for a genetic basis for altitude illness can be inferred from patterns of susceptibility. These include individual patterns, familial patterns and population patterns. Individual patterns of susceptibility have been recognized for many years although often on an anecdotal rather than scientific basis. For example, Bärtsch *et al.* (2001) noted that previous history of high altitude disease is one of the best predictors of subsequent illness. In fact, the use of HAPE susceptible and HAPE nonsusceptible individuals has been an important tool in high altitude medical research. Dehnert *et al.* (2002a) studied a group of 76 mountaineers who ascended to the Capanna Margherita at 4559 m altitude. Approximately half of the group had a previous history of HAPE and 66% of these developed the condition on ascent. By contrast, there were no cases of HAPE among those without a previous history. In a study of people who summited on Mt Whitney (4420 m), Wagner *et al.* (2006) found that a history of AMS was a risk factor for developing the condition. These studies are consistent with individual susceptibility playing a role although they do not distinguish between genetic factors on the one hand or some environmental or development factor on the other. In some cases physiological measurements can point to risk factors. For example, it has been known for many years that people with a high pulmonary artery pressor response to hypoxia are more likely to develop HAPE (Hultgren *et al.* 1971; Dehnert *et al.* 2005). Therefore genes that may result in pulmonary hypertension are of interest.

Familial patterns of susceptibility have been described on several occasions. For example in an early study, Hultgren *et al.* (1961) described two Peruvian families where the siblings developed HAPE following an ascent to 3760 m. Norboo *et al.* (2004) described another family with a high incidence with three of the four people developing HAPE. A number of other examples of familial susceptibility are listed in Table 1 of MacInnis *et al.* (2010). This includes a striking description of a family in which an 11-year-old boy, his father, paternal grandfather, aunt, uncle and cousin all had a history of HAPE on ascending to altitude.

Population patterns of susceptibility also suggest a genetic basis. There is now extensive experience suggesting that Han Chinese have a much higher incidence of AMS than Tibetans on ascent to high altitude and this would be consistent with the discussion of genetic changes in Tibetans in section 4.5. Wu *et al.* (2005) documented the higher frequency of AMS in Han Chinese than Tibetans. This was also highlighted in a study of workers on the Qinghai–Tibet Railroad which reaches an altitude of 5000 m (Wu *et al.* 2009). There is considerable evidence that CMS is less common in Tibetans than in similarly exposed Andeans, as discussed in the section 4.8.

Turning to the possible role of individual genes in susceptibility to high altitude diseases, the possible influence of polymorphism of the *ACE* gene was briefly discussed in section 4.3. For example, Aldasher *et al.* (2012) reported that highlanders in a Kyrgyz population had a preponderance of the ID genotype. However, a compilation of the large number of studies of candidate genes in relation to high altitude disease is too long to be given here. The interested reader should consult Table 2 of MacInnis *et al.* (2010) which includes no less than four pages of very technical data.

4.8 PHENOTYPE DIFFERENCES BETWEEN TIBETANS AND ANDEANS

This final section does not deal directly with genetic differences but a related fascinating topic.

This is the fact that the two most successful groups of humans who have adapted to high altitude, the Tibetans and Andeans, have very different phenotypes. Presumably some of these differences have a genetic base, but this has not been determined as yet. The fact that these two groups of highlanders have such different physical characteristics is truly remarkable.

4.8.1 Ventilation

Beall (2000) reported a lower resting ventilation in Aymara compared with Tibetans as shown in Fig. 4.3. Here the resting ventilation in L min^{-1} is plotted against the age of the subjects over a large range from less than 20 to 90 years of age. Males are shown by the filled circles and females by the open circles. Note that the resting ventilations of the Aymara are uniformly low. In addition, those of females tend to be less than those of

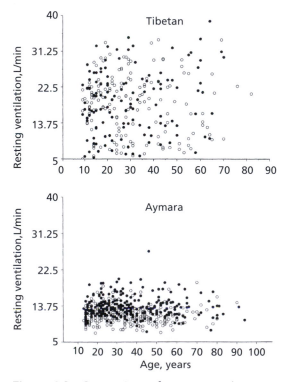

Figure 4.3   Comparison of resting ventilation in Tibetans and Aymara plotted against age. Males, filled circles; females, open circles. (From Beall 2000, with permission.)

males. This is somewhat surprising because many measurements of resting ventilation at high altitude indicate that females have higher values. For example, FitzGerald (1914) in her early studies of alveolar P_{CO_2} in the Colorado mountains found that women had a lower P_{CO_2} than men at the same altitude indicating that they had higher ventilations.

A striking feature of Fig. 4.3 is the large range of resting ventilations in Tibetans, and the corresponding fact that many Tibetans have higher resting ventilations than Aymara. Additional analysis of these data where Tibetans and Andeans are compared at the same altitude confirms that there is a difference between the two populations for resting ventilation (Beall 2000).

The reason for these differences in ventilation is clarified when we look at the ventilatory responses to hypoxia for the two populations, as shown in Fig. 4.4. Actually, this looks similar to Fig. 4.3 in that the Aymara have a fairly uniformly low hypoxic ventilatory response over the large age range, whereas there is much more variability for Tibetans. However, many Tibetans have much higher hypoxic ventilatory responses than Aymara for a given age. The difference in resting ventilation between Tibetans and Aymara appears to be adequately explained by the differences in hypoxic ventilatory response. Furthermore, the relatively high response of the Tibetans may well be due to the genetic factors described earlier. Tibetans have upregulation of the *EPAS1* gene that codes for HIF-2α, and there is evidence that this transcription factor results in induction of tyrosine hydroxylase gene which increases the chemosensitivity of the carotid body.

4.8.2 Blood changes

Figure 4.5 shows arterial oxygen saturations measured by pulse oximetry plotted against altitude for Tibetans (filled circles) and Andeans (open circles). The triangles show results for Americans and Europeans. On the basis of the higher ventilations and hypoxic ventilatory response of the Tibetans we would expect a higher arterial oxygen saturation, and this seems to be true above 4000 m but two open circles between 3000 and 4000 m are not in agreement. The data show samples of 10 or more highlanders with a mean age from 10 to 50 years of age.

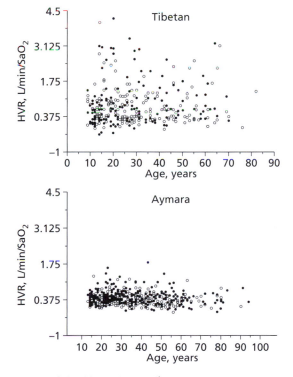

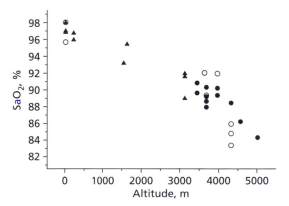

Figure 4.4 Hypoxic ventilatory response in Tibetans and Aymara plotted against age. Males, filled circles; females, open circles. (From Beall 2000, with permission.)

Figure 4.5 Arterial oxygen saturation plotted against altitude for Tibetans (filled circles), Andeans (open circles) and Europeans (filled triangles). (From Beall 2000, with permission.)

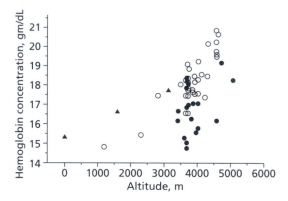

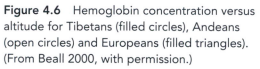

Figure 4.6 Hemoglobin concentration versus altitude for Tibetans (filled circles), Andeans (open circles) and Europeans (filled triangles). (From Beall 2000, with permission.)

Figure 4.6 shows hemoglobin concentrations plotted against altitude with Tibetans being the filled circles and Andeans being the open circles. There is a reasonably clear demonstration that Andeans have higher hemoglobin concentrations and this is consistent with the earlier discussion of the relatively low hemoglobins in Tibetans, presumably related to the regulation of erythropoietin by HIF-2α that is coded by the *EPAS1* gene.

The data on the four traits, resting ventilation, hypoxic ventilatory response, oxygen saturation and hemoglobin concentration shown in Figs 4.3, 4.4, 4.5 and 4.6 show considerable scatter. Beall (2000) carried out additional statistical analysis of the data and found that the first two traits were more than 0.5 standard deviation higher than the Aymara means. In addition, the Tibetan means were more than 1 standard deviation lower than the Aymara means for the last two traits. Also, Beall calculated the 'effect size' for the four traits, that is the difference in the mean values of 20 to 29-year-old males divided by their pooled standard deviation. The result showed that the effect sizes of resting ventilation and hypoxic ventilation response are large and positive, that is the Tibetan means are larger than Aymara means, and the effect sizes of arterial oxygen saturation and hemoglobin concentrations are large and negative, that is Tibetan means are smaller than Aymara means.

4.8.3 Hypoxic pulmonary vasoconstriction

Figure 8.11 shows the relationship between mean pulmonary artery pressure and arterial P_{O_2} in Tibetans, Andeans and North Americans (Groves *et al.* 1993). The increase in pressure as the P_{O_2} falls is caused by hypoxic pulmonary vasoconstriction, and the causative variable is the alveolar P_{O_2} although the arterial value was measured. Note the striking difference between Andeans and Tibetans. The Andean response is not very different from that in North Americans but the Tibetans have a strikingly reduced or 'blunted' pulmonary vasoconstriction response. A low response is beneficial at high altitude because the high pulmonary artery pressure, particularly on exercise, causes right ventricular hypertrophy. In addition, it can be the main factor in the development of high altitude pulmonary edema.

Information about the mechanism of the differences in hypoxic pulmonary vasoconstriction comes from measurements of nitric oxide concentrations in plasma. Erzurum *et al.* (2007) found substantially lower plasma NO concentrations in Tibetans compared with North Americans. Nitric oxide is a powerful vasodilator in the pulmonary circulation. HIF is known to result in the induction of *iNOS* and *HO-2* genes that inhibit calcium channels in vascular smooth muscle cells, and this results in inhibition of hypoxic pulmonary vasoconstriction.

It is interesting that the reduced hypoxic pulmonary vasoconstriction is not limited to Tibetans but is also seen in some animals in that region. For example, Ishizaki *et al.* (2005) reported lower pulmonary artery pressures in yaks (*Bos grunniens*) at sea level, 2260 and 4500 m altitudes.

Altitude acclimatization and deterioration

5

SUMMARY

Altitude acclimatization is the physiological process which takes place in the body on exposure to hypoxia at altitude (or in a chamber). It comprises a number of responses by different systems in the body, which mitigate, to a degree, the effects of the fall in oxygen partial pressure. In this way the tissues of the body are defended against this fall to a remarkable degree. Advantageous though this process is, it does not restore performance to that at sea level. Probably the most important change is the increase in breathing (minute ventilation) due to stimulation of the peripheral chemoreceptor (carotid bodies) by hypoxia and changes in the chemical control of breathing. Another is the well-known increase in hemoglobin concentration in the blood. The time courses of these responses vary but most of the changes take place over a period of days up to a few weeks. These changes restore oxygen delivery to the tissues though at a lower partial pressure. Individuals vary in the speed and extent to which they can acclimatize. Apart from past history of acclimatization, there are no good predictors of future performance. A recent interest is in the effect of intermittent hypoxia. Intermittent hypoxia in sufficient dose, can produce some of the changes of acclimatization.

Adaptation is a term used to describe the changes which take place over generations by natural selection enabling animals and humans to function better at altitude.

Deterioration is a condition that is evident after some time spent at extreme altitude. It develops over weeks above about 5500 m, and over days above 8000 m. It is characterized by loss of appetite, weight loss, lethargy, fatigue, slowness of thought and poor judgment.

5.1 THE PHYSIOLOGICAL RESPONSE TO HYPOXIA

5.1.1 Introduction

The response of the body to hypoxia depends crucially on the rate as well as the degree of hypoxia. For instance, the effect on a pilot of sudden loss of oxygen supply in an unpressurized aircraft at the height of the summit of Mount Everest is quite different from the effect of similar altitude on a climber who has spent some weeks at altitude. The pilot would probably lose consciousness in a few minutes (Fig. 5.1) whereas

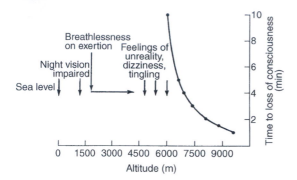

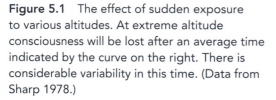

Figure 5.1   The effect of sudden exposure to various altitudes. At extreme altitude consciousness will be lost after an average time indicated by the curve on the right. There is considerable variability in this time. (Data from Sharp 1978.)

the climber, though very breathless, will not only remain conscious but also be able to work out his route and climb slowly upward.

The symptoms of acute hypoxia are few and subtle (Fig. 5.1). The effect of acute, often severe, hypoxia has been studied intensively since Paul Bert first pointed out the danger of ascent to high altitude to early balloonists (Chapter 1). Figure 5.1 shows the effect of sudden exposure to various increasing altitudes. At modest altitude breathlessness may be felt on exertion and some rise in heart rate noticed but the main effect is on the central nervous system. At levels as low as 1500 m night vision is impaired (Pretorius 1970). At 4000–5000 m some tingling of the fingers and mouth may be noticed but, although the subject would now definitely be hypoxic, there is very little subjective sensation to indicate this fact. Above about 5000 m some subjects may become unconscious and above 7000 m most will do so (Sharp 1978). There is considerable individual variation in response to acute hypoxia. Figure 5.1 shows the average time to loss of consciousness after sudden exposure to given altitudes. It will be seen that, on acute exposure to the altitude equivalent to the summit of Everest, the unacclimatized subject remains conscious for only about 2 minutes.

By contrast, the effect of hypoxia on an acclimatized person is much less. The main symptom is shortness of breath on exertion. The preferred rate of climbing among mountaineers is at about 50% $Vo_{2,max}$. This typically requires a ventilation of about 50 L min^{-1} at sea level, whereas at 6300 m the ventilation for this work rate will be about 160 L min^{-1}, close to the maximum voluntary ventilation at sea level. The difference between the pilot and the climber is due to a series of adaptive changes in the body known as acclimatization.

Oxygen, being such a vital substrate for mammalian life, it is not surprising that hypoxia causes many deleterious effects on many systems in the body. Some of these changes are addressed in later chapters; the term acclimatization is reserved for those changes resulting from hypoxia that are considered beneficial.

5.1.2 Definition of altitude acclimatization

To mountaineers, acclimatization is the process by which they become more comfortable at altitude and find they can perform better than when they first arrived at a particular altitude. Subjectively, there is both relief of symptoms of acute mountain sickness (AMS) and a return of some of their climbing performance lost on arrival at altitude. For physiologists, altitude acclimatization is, strictly, the sum of all the beneficial changes in response to altitude hypoxia, but it is often defined by the increase in ventilation and the consequent reduction in Pco_2 (and increase in Po_2). However, this is not a satisfactory measure since other processes are involved.

5.1.3 Rate of acclimatization

The changes involved in acclimatization occur in various systems and with varying time courses. These are illustrated in Fig. 5.2, which shows the futility of the frequently asked question, 'How long does it take to become acclimatized?'

However, the most important changes are in the cardiorespiratory system and the blood with

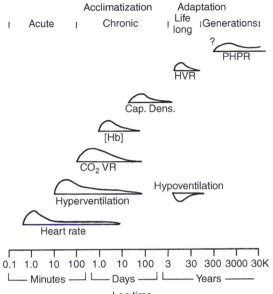

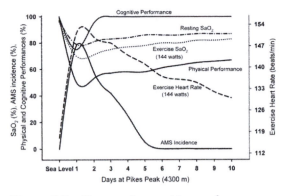

Figure 5.3 Changes in cognitive performance, resting Sa,o_2, exercise Sa,o_2, physical performance, exercise heart rate and incidence of acute mountain sickness (AMS) in lowlanders ascending directly to 4300 m. (From Muza et al 2010 with permission.)

Figure 5.2 Time course of a number of acclimatization and adaptive changes plotted on a log time scale, the curve of each response denoting the rate of change, which is fast at first then tails off. Included are: heart rate, hyperventilation and hypoventilation, the carbon dioxide ventilatory response (HCVR), hemoglobin concentration ([Hb]), changes in capillary density (Cap. Dens.), hypoxic ventilatory response (HVR) and pulmonary hypoxic pressor response (PHPR)

time courses of days or a few weeks. Figure 5.3 shows the changes in a number of physiological systems over the first 10 days of altitude 4300 m (Muza *et al.* 2010).

Early changes in acclimatization were studied in six lowlanders by Lundby *et al.* (2004). Subjects were studied at sea level (normoxic and acute hypoxia) and after 2 and 8 weeks acclimatization at 4100 m in Bolivia. Local high altitude residents were also studied at altitude. Some results from this study are shown in Fig. 5.4 for rest (Fig. 5.4a) and maximum exercise (Fig. 5.4b). It can be seen that the hematocrit rises during the first 2 weeks to close to the high altitude residents' value and is no higher at 8 weeks (see below). The Pa,o_2

continues to rise for 8 weeks and is still below that of the high altitude residents. Changes in Pa,co_2 appear to be complete at 2 weeks while the alveolar to arterial Po_2 difference $((A–a)PO_2)$ rises with acute hypoxia, is greater at 2 weeks and falls slightly at 8 weeks. The high altitude residents have very low values for this parameter. The situation at maximum work rate is similar except that the Pa,co_2 continues to fall due to increased exercise ventilation. The improvement in Pa,o_2 is impressive and no doubt contributes to the improved performance so frequently noted by mountaineers during the course of an expedition.

In some cases the changes of acclimatization involve a biphasic response; for instance, the heart rate response to hypoxia shows a rise within a few minutes, followed by a fall over weeks at altitude (Chapter 9). The change measured can include two responses with different time courses. For instance, minute ventilation involves the rapid hypoxic ventilatory response within a few minutes, followed by slow changes in both central and peripheral chemoreceptor response over 1–20 days (Chapter 6). Similarly, the well-known increase in hemoglobin concentration is due to a rapid decrease in plasma volume, followed by a slow increase in red cell mass (Chapter 9).

(a)

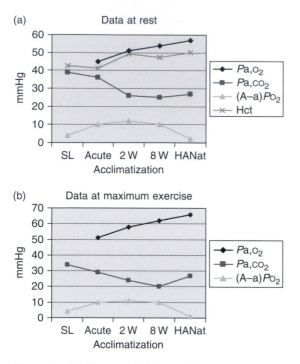

(b)

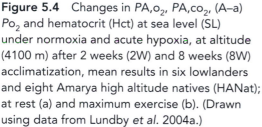

Figure 5.4   Changes in PA,O_2, PA,CO_2, (A–a) PO_2 and hematocrit (Hct) at sea level (SL) under normoxia and acute hypoxia, at altitude (4100 m) after 2 weeks (2W) and 8 weeks (8W) acclimatization, mean results in six lowlanders and eight Amarya high altitude natives (HANat); at rest (a) and maximum exercise (b). (Drawn using data from Lundby *et al.* 2004a.)

5.1.4 Hypoxia: is there a difference between hypobaric and normobaric hypoxia?

Since the studies of Paul Bert (Bert 1878), it has been accepted that the effects of hypoxia are due to the reduced partial pressure of oxygen (PO_2) and are the same however this reduction is achieved. Hypoxia can be produced either by lowering the barometric pressure, hypobaric hypoxia, as happens in a decompression chamber or when we ascend to high altitude, or by reducing the percentage of oxygen ($O_2\%$) in the inhaled gas mixture, normobaric hypoxia.

Apart from the effects of hypoxia, hypobaria has some physiological effects, especially if imposed suddenly upon the subject. These relate to possible bubble formation in the blood and tissues as in decompression sickness experienced by divers coming to the surface too fast and also in aircrew subject to explosive decompression at great altitudes. However, in the case of travelers taking some hours or mountaineers taking days to reach altitude this is not a problem though it cannot be ruled out in chamber studies where rates of ascent may be fast enough to cause micro-bubble formation.

There is also the physical effect of reduced air density in hypobaric hypoxia. This will reduce the work of breathing (per liter) and may affect rates of diffusion of gas in the respiratory airways. This latter effect has to be taken into account when studying exhaled nitric oxide (NO) (Hemmingsson and Linnarsson 2009). Thus hypobaric hypoxia may result in enhanced axial back diffusion of NO because of the reduced gas density and an associated increased alveolar NO uptake into the blood as compared with normobaric hypoxia. This mechanism may partly account for the suggestion that real altitude training (living high, training low (LHTL)) gives better results in sea level performance than simulated (normobaric) hypoxia (Bonetti and Hopkins 2009).

A number of studies have addressed this question and have reported some differences in the effect of these two types of hypoxia. Borel *et al.* (1998) studied anesthetized cats. They found no differences between hypo- and normobaric hypoxia with respect to Pa,O_2 or Pa,CO_2 but that ventilation was reduced due to reduced breath frequency. They wondered whether the dead space was reduced.

Roach *et al.* (1996) studied nine subjects exposed to 9 hours of either normobaric or hypobaric hypoxia equivalent to 4564 m, or to normoxic hypobaria (increased $O_2\%$ at lowered pressure). They found that AMS scores were significantly higher in hypobaric hypoxia than in normobaric hypoxia.

Loeppky *et al.* (1997) carried out a similar study but this time looking at ventilation. They found that after 3, 6 and 9 hours normobaric hypoxia resulted in 26% higher ventilation than hypobaric hypoxia but $P_{ET}CO_2$ was higher than in hypobaria. In a later study (Loeppky *et al.* 2005), the authors extended these results, confirming the effect on AMS scores and finding differences in fluid balance and in some endocrine responses. The reduction in plasma volume was less in hypobaria, especially in subjects with AMS. Aldosterone levels were elevated and anti-diuretic hormone reduced compared with hypobaria. They found no differences in Sa,o_2.

Savourey *et al.* (2003) looked for differences in cardiorespiratory variables between the two forms of hypoxia (altitude equivalent 4500 m) given for 40 minutes. They found that hypobaric hypoxia resulted in lower ventilation, lower Pa,o_2, Sa,o_2, Pa,co_2, and higher pH, suggesting that there is a problem in gas exchange under hypobaric hypoxia not present in normobaric hypoxia. Conkin and Wessel (2008) have reviewed the literature and conclude that there is, 'an independent effect on hypoxia and AMS' of hypobaria itself. They propose equations, incorporating barometric pressure and F_Io_2 to construct 'iso hypoxic' lines, i.e. lines of equal 'hypoxic stress' with respect to equal Pa,o_2 and probability of AMS.

However, the data currently available are sparse and inconsistent. But it does seem that normobaria produces less AMS and lower V_E than hypobaria of the same P_Io_2. The mechanism is not clear but presumably involves the reduction in gas density with hypobaria, leading to reduced work of breathing and changes in gas diffusion rates. This in turn leads to lower Pa,o_2, Sa,o_2 and Pa,co_2. For further discussion of this topic see Millet *et al.* (2012).

5.2 ACCLIMATIZATION AND ADAPTATION

5.2.1 Acclimatization

The term altitude acclimatization refers to the process whereby lowland humans and animals respond to the reduced partial pressure of oxygen (Po_2) in the inspired air. It refers only to the changes in response to hypoxia seen as beneficial as opposed to changes which result in illness such as AMS. Acclimatization is then a series of physiological responses. Other changes, resulting in illness, are pathological.

The processes of acclimatization all tend to reduce the fall in Po_2 as oxygen is transported

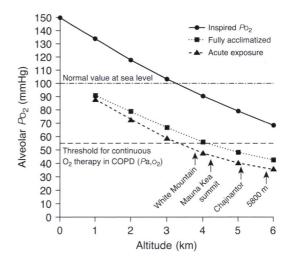

Figure 5.5 PA,o_2 of unacclimatized (acute exposure) and acclimatized subjects at altitudes from 1000 to 6000 m. Also plotted, as dashed lines, are the normal sea level PA,o_2 of 100 Torr, and the value at which patients with chronic obstructive pulmonary disease (COPD) are entitled to continuous oxygen therapy, 55 Torr. Note that even acclimatized subjects are below this latter value when above altitudes of about 4000 m. (From West 2004b, with permission.)

through the body from the outside air to the tissues. However, even in the best acclimatized individual the tissue Po_2 is not restored to the sea level value and performance remains impaired. This is illustrated in Fig. 5.5, which shows the inspired Po_2 and arterial Po_2 (Pa,o_2) of a subject exposed to acute hypoxia and after acclimatization. Also shown are the normal Pa,o_2 at sea level and the Pa,o_2 at which continuous O_2 therapy is advised for patients with chronic obstructive lung disease. It can be seen that even acclimatized subjects are below this level at altitudes above 4000 m.

5.2.2 Adaptation

People born and bred at altitude have certain characteristics which distinguish them from even well-acclimatized lowlanders. There is debate about whether these are due to environmental, operating during early growth, or genetic causes. The term adaptation is used for characteristics thought to be due to natural selection, working on the gene pool. Adaptation, in this sense, has certainly taken place in animals such as the yak and llama. In the case of the yak, one example is the loss of the hypoxic pulmonary pressor response which seems to be due to a single dominant gene (Harris 1986). There is evidence of a similar adaptation in Tibetans resident at high altitude for generations (see Chapter 4).

5.3 THE OXYGEN TRANSPORT SYSTEM

5.3.1 Introduction

Figure 5.6 shows the oxygen transport system at sea level and at high altitude. This diagram can be used as a 'table of contents' of changes due to acclimatization, which will be followed in succeeding chapters. Po_2 falls at each stage as oxygen is transported from outside air, ambient Po_2 to inspired, to alveolar, to arterial, to mixed venous which approximates to the mean tissue Po_2. This forms a staircase or cascade of Po_2. The process of acclimatization can be thought of as reducing each step in this cascade.

5.3.2 Ambient to inspired Po_2 (PI,O$_2$)

The ambient Po_2 of dry air at sea level is about 160 mmHg (20.9% of 760 mmHg the barometric pressure). At an altitude of 5800 m, in the example shown in Fig. 5.6, the barometric pressure is just half that at sea level (Chapter 2) so the ambient Po_2 is also half the sea level value, 80 mmHg. The drop seen in the figure from ambient to inspired Po_2 of about 10 mmHg is due to the addition of water vapor to the inspired air as it is wetted and warmed to body temperature in the nose, mouth, larynx and trachea. The water vapor pressure at body temperature is 47 mmHg, and this displaces almost 10 mmHg Po_2. This physical cause of Po_2 reduction is beyond the control of the body and so applies equally at altitude, although its effect is proportionately more important there.

5.3.3 Inspired to alveolar Po_2 (PA,O$_2$)

At sea level there is a drop of about 50 mmHg at this point in the oxygen transport system. This drop can be thought of as being due to the addition of carbon dioxide and the uptake of oxygen and so depends, in part, on the metabolic rate. However, it also depends on alveolar ventilation and for a given O_2 uptake and CO_2 output the size of this reduction is entirely due to ventilation. A doubling of ventilation results in a halving of this drop. If ventilation were infinite there would be no reduction and alveolar gas would be fresh air. After acclimatization at 5800 m resting alveolar ventilation is approximately doubled and this step in the system, as shown in Fig. 5.6, is halved.

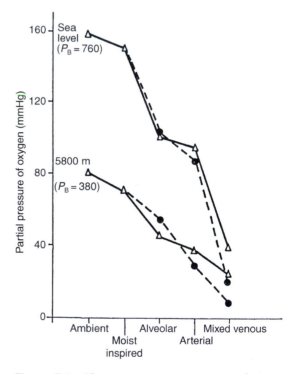

Figure 5.6 The oxygen transport system from outside air through the body at sea level and at an altitude of 5800 m. P_B, barometric pressure; Δ, rest; ●, maximum exercise. Ref Pugh 1964a (Pugh, L.G.C.E. (1964a) Man at high altitude, *Scientific Basis of Medicine, Annual Review*, pp. 32–54, 1964.)

This increase in ventilation is one of the most important aspects of acclimatization and the mechanisms underlying it. The changes in control of breathing, are dealt with in Chapter 6.

Figure 5.6 shows also the effect of exercise on the oxygen transport system (the dashed lines). At sea level the PA,o_2 is little changed by exercise but at altitude the increase of ventilation is far greater in response to exercise than at sea level, so that with exercise the PA,o_2 is increased and PA,co_2 decreased (Chapter 12).

5.3.4 Alveolar to arterial Po_2 (Pa,o_2)

Oxygen passes across the alveolar-capillary membrane by diffusion resulting in a small pressure drop but in the normal lung this accounts for less than 1 mmHg. The total alveolar–arterial $(A–a)Po_2$ gradient at sea level is 6–10 mmHg. The major part of this gradient is due to ventilation/perfusion ratio (V/Q) inequalities. Even in the healthy lung the matching of ventilation to blood flow is not perfect. In lung disease such as emphysema or pulmonary embolism this mismatching results in much greater $(A–a)Po_2$ gradients and results in significant hypoxemia. For a full discussion of this important topic see West 1986b.

At altitude, at rest there is little change in the $(A–a)Po_2$ gradient from its value at sea level. The V/Q ratio inequality is modestly reduced, because of the increase in pulmonary artery pressure due to hypoxia (Chapter 8), reducing the gravitational effect on the distribution of blood flow in the lung. This was thought not to cause an increase in the diffusing capacity of the lung during acclimatization (West 1962). However, a recent study of trekkers to Everest Base Camp has found an increase in lung diffusing capacity and membrane diffusing capacity (Agostoni et al. 2011).

On exercise at high altitude, however, the $(A–a)Po_2$ gradient increases significantly and becomes important in limiting exercise performance. This is shown as the dashed line in Fig. 5.6. This diffusion limitation, shown by West et al. (1962) is explored more fully in Chapters 7, 12 and 13.

5.3.5 Arterial to mixed venous Po_2 (Pv,o_2)

The last drop in Po_2 shown in Fig. 5.4 from arterial to mixed venous is due to the uptake of oxygen in the systemic capillaries. Its magnitude is influenced by the metabolic rate, the cardiac output and the oxygen carrying capacity of the blood, i.e. the hemoglobin concentration ([Hb]). Probably the best known aspect of acclimatization is the increase in [Hb].

A modest increase in [Hb] is probably beneficial in that it increases the oxygen carrying capacity of the blood and at altitudes up to about 4000 m this is sufficient to balance the reduction in oxygen saturation due to reduced Pa,o_2 and restore the oxygen content of arterial blood to sea level values (though now at a lower Po_2). However, the increase in viscosity of the blood is the price paid and this increases vascular resistance and contributes to raised pulmonary arterial pressure. This certainly happens in patients with chronic mountain sickness where hematocrits of over 80% are seen. If the rise in vascular resistance is too great, the cardiac output falls and so oxygen delivery is reduced. It has been shown that reducing the hematocrit in these patients never reduces exercise performance and may increase it (Winslow and Monge 1987a). There is also the increased risk of vascular disorders. A report on the effect of hemodilution in lowlanders at 5260 m showed that lowering the [Hb] by 24% had no effect on $Vo_{2,max}$ (Calbet et al. 2002). With moderate, physiological, increases in [Hb] there seems to be a close reciprocal relationship between [Hb] and blood flow so that oxygen delivery to particular organs, e.g. working muscles or brain, remains constant over a range of [Hb] and Vo_2. The question of optimum hemoglobin value is further considered in Chapter 9.

The in vitro oxygen dissociation curve is shifted slightly to the right at moderate altitudes due to an increase in 2,3-diphosphoglycerate. However, the position of the in vivo curve is uncertain because of uncertainties about the in vivo pH (Winslow and Monge 1987b). There is probably some degree of respiratory alkalosis which offsets the effect of the 2,3-diphosphoglycerate. At extreme altitude, above about 7000 m, there is quite severe respiratory alkalosis and therefore a definite leftward shift in the dissociation curve. This is beneficial to the climber at least as far as oxygen delivery to working muscles is concerned. This is because more oxygen is loaded into the blood in the lungs while the unloading of oxygen in the muscles is only slightly reduced. This in turn is because the difference in position of the curves for normal and higher pH, at very low Po_2, is so small. (See Chapter 10, for a fuller discussion of the position of the oxygen dissociation curve and the graphical representation, Fig. 10.1.)

Cardiac output increases with acute hypoxia but decreases as [Hb] increases with continued stay at altitude over the first 1–2 weeks. These changes, as well as other effects on the vascular system, are discussed in Chapter 8. At the tissue level there is an increase in the density of capillaries due to a reduction in diameter of muscle fibers (Chapter 11).

Taking the body as a whole, the mixed venous Po_2 can be thought of as reflecting the mean tissue Po_2. It will be seen, in Fig. 5.6, that the effect of these processes of acclimatization is to maintain this critical Po_2 as near as possible to the sea level value. Beyond this there is the possibility of adaptation at the tissue level involving the microcirculation and then intracellular mechanisms. These form the subject of Chapter 11.

5.4 PRACTICAL CONSIDERATIONS AND ADVICE

A very real problem in the study of acclimatization is that there is no single measure of the process. Respiratory acclimatization is very important and can be followed by measuring minute ventilation or the alveolar or end-tidal Pco_2. The ventilation rises with acclimatization and the Pco_2 falls exponentially over the first few days at altitude. However, climbers find that their performance continues to improve over a longer period; presumably changes in other systems underlie this further acclimatization. This problem of how to measure the degree of acclimatization coupled with the very great individual variation in the rate and final degree of acclimatization means that we still do not have answers to apparently simple questions such as, 'Does exercise speed acclimatization?' There is also the problem that the time of early and rapid acclimatization is also the risk period for AMS. It is hard and perhaps futile, to try and separate the effect of any given strategy on preventing AMS and on speeding acclimatization since the two are inextricably commingled. Thus the advice given here is as much about preventing AMS as with acclimatization itself. Also, in the absence of hard data, anecdotal evidence has to be relied on.

5.4.1 Rate of ascent

A rate of ascent which is slow enough to avoid AMS should be chosen. This will inevitably be dictated, in part, by the terrain, availability of camp sites, etc. A rule of thumb often given is that above 3000 m each night's camp should be about 300 m above the previous one and that every 2–3 days a rest day be added when the party remains based at the same site for two nights. This is an unnecessarily slow ascent rate for many individuals but will prove too fast for a substantial minority (see Chapter 19 for more discussion and references). Where a greater height gain has to be made, then a rest day should be taken. During the 'rest' day trips to higher altitude and back are considered beneficial by experienced climbers, probably because the greater altitude and exercise stimulates acclimatization. However, it should be noted that there is some evidence that exercise is a risk factor for AMS (Roach *et al.* 1999).

5.4.2 Individual variability and acclimatization

As mentioned, there is great individual variation in the rate and degree of acclimatization. Some may acclimatize rapidly to moderate altitude but then find that they simply cannot tolerate an altitude above say 7000 m. Others may take time to acclimatize but then go well to extreme altitude. Usually, as with susceptibility to AMS, past experience is a good guide to future performance but apart from this there are no reliable predictors for good acclimatization.

5.4.3 Age, gender and experience

There are not a lot of data to answer the oft-asked question about the effects of age or gender on acclimatization. If anything, older people are less susceptible to AMS than the young providing they are healthy and they seem to acclimatize just as well. There does not seem to be any important difference between and men and women in this respect. Children have about the same incidence of AMS as adults and one recent paper suggests that previous history is less reliable in them than in adults for predicting future susceptibility to AMS (Rexhaj *et al.* 2011). There is a strong impression that experienced mountaineers acclimatize better than novices. (See Chapters 26 and 27 for further discussion of acclimatization in women, children and the elderly.)

5.4.4 Pre-acclimatization by continuous hypoxia

There is increasing interest in methods by which people can achieve some degree of acclimatization before going to the mountains. There is no doubt that living in a chamber for a number of days at simulated altitude will achieve acclimatization (Richalet *et al.* 1992). There is an impression that the degree of acclimatization is not as great as that achieved in the mountains, perhaps because of the lack of exercise. West (1998) argues the case for this being true for the long-term studies of Operation Everest I and II. In any case, incarceration in a chamber for days or weeks is not practicable or acceptable for most climbers. Those in a position to get up to moderate altitudes, about 2000 m for a night or two and hike to higher altitudes in the day, such as in the European Alps or the Rockies shortly before a trek or expedition to the great ranges, will probably benefit in terms of acclimatization (Muza *et al.* 2010).

5.4.5 Pre-acclimatization by intermittent hypoxia

Intermittent hypoxia (IH) has been used to see if this stimulus could result in some degree of acclimatization. IH can be achieved by spending a few hours a day in a chamber, sometimes with exercise, i.e. training under hypoxia, or, alternatively, sleeping in a hypoxic environment, e.g. at altitude but coming down to train at low altitude, that is, 'living high, training low', a pattern popularized by Levine and Stray-Gunderson (1997). Their proposals were an attempt to improve performance of athletes for sea level races but the effect of such a pattern of hypoxic exposure can also result in some of the changes of acclimatization (see below). Instead of actually commuting up and down athletes and researchers can achieve a similar effect by breathing a low oxygen percentage in a normobaric chamber, or by using a machine to provide low oxygen percentage in the inspired gas via a mask. These machines can be programed to give any pattern of bursts of hypoxia or normoxia. End points of these studies are usually changes in cardiorespiratory or blood measurements or athletic performance. Whether these indirect measures of acclimatization translate into improvement in performance at altitude is not clear. Savourey *et al.* (1998) studied the effect of 8 hours daily for 5 days at 4500 m equivalent altitude on various hormones and biochemical measures but found very little effect with this dose of pre-acclimatization. Garcia *et al.* (2000) had their subjects breath 13% oxygen (equivalent to 3800 m) for 2 hours daily for 12 days. They found the hypoxic ventilatory response (HVR) increased significantly reaching a peak at 5 days but there was no change in ventilation, Pco_2 or Sa,o_2.

Townsend *et al.* (2002) studied trained endurance athletes for 20 days, under LHTL, i.e. sleeping in a normobaric chamber in low O_2% equivalent to 2650 m. A control group underwent the same training but with no nocturnal hypoxia. Results showed that HVR was increased by LHTL. Resting ventilation, tested in normoxia, was not significantly changed by the exposure, but $P_{ET}co_2$ was decreased in both hypoxic groups, though only by about 2.5 Torr.

A recent study by Pialoux *et al.* (2009) also found a significant increase in acute HVR in subjects exposed to 6 hours of hypoxia a day for 4 days. They also found an increase in reactive oxygen species without a compensatory increase in antioxidant activity.

The effect of IH on the erythropoietic system has been studied by a number of workers. Garcia *et al.* (2000) found a reticulocytosis but no change in [Hb] or hematocrit. Schmidt (2002) reviewed this topic and concluded that the effect of IH depended upon the intensity and duration of the hypoxia, both with respect to the length of each burst and the total duration of exposure. Short hypoxic episodes like sleep apnea seem to result in only small increases in [Hb] concentration due mainly to reduction in plasma volume. There seems to be a critical threshold of about 90 minutes cumulative hypoxia. Athletes, using longer periods of hypoxia, such as sleeping in hypoxia, show increases in plasma erythropoietin concentration, transferin receptor and reticulocyte count (Koistinen *et al.* 2000) but an increase in red cell mass has not been found. A more recent study (Gore *et al.* 2006) using quite severe IH of 4000–5500 m equivalent altitude for 3 hours a day 5 days a week for 4 weeks again found an increase in erythropoietin concentration but no increase in red cell mass.

Burtscher *et al.* (2008) have reviewed 21 studies of IH and its effect on pre-acclimatization. They concluded that, '1–4 h of daily exposures for 1–5 weeks to simulated altitudes of about 4,000 m seem to initiate ventilatory and autonomic nervous system adaptations to high altitude with the potential to reduce AMS development'. They considered that for protocols of short duration there was no difference between rest and exercise in hypoxia though for longer protocols exercise might enhance exercise performance at altitude. They also included their own observational study in which 67 out of 141 trekkers were given pre-trek IH of 1–2 hours for 5 days before going on trek. Mild AMS was reported in 10% of the pre-acclimatization group while 30% of the control group had mild to severe AMS. Of course this was not a blind trial. They included a case report of a HAPE (high altitude pulmonary edema) susceptible woman given pre-trek IH, which seemed to prevent HAPE.

It seems that intermittent hypoxia does effect some of the changes seen in acclimatization, e.g. HVR and hence ventilation and P_{CO_2} depending upon the 'dose' of hypoxia. Also, erythropoietin levels are increased but not apparently red cell mass. AMS may also be reduced by pre-trek IH.

The topic of altitude training, either real or simulated, for sea level competitive athletics is further considered in Chapter 29.

5.4.6 Carry-over acclimatization

If pre-acclimatization is attempted, how quickly should a climber get out to the mountains? In other words, how long does acclimatization last? There are little hard data to guide us, though one study by Lyons *et al.* (1995) showed that a group of subjects who had been at 4300 m for 3 weeks retained some beneficial effect after 8 days at low altitude compared with a group who had had no altitude exposure. A later study by the same group (Beidleman *et al.* 1997) with a similar protocol put some quantification on this carry-over effect. After 8 days at sea level they calculated that on average 92% of the effect on S_{a,O_2} was retained, 74% of plasma volume and 58% of the lactic acid concentration at 75% $V_{O_2,max}$ exercise. For intermittent hypoxia in the study of Townsend *et al.* (2002) quoted above, the HVR increased by 50% over pre-hypoxia values and declined 30% by 2 days after cessation of IH. However, Katayama *et al.* (2001) found most of the effect of IH on HVR, the ventilatory equivalent, and S_{a,O_2} to be still present 1 week after stopping IH. The review paper by Muza *et al.* (2010) mentioned above, also discusses this topic.

These studies support anecdotal experience. The effect of acclimatization probably falls off exponentially with time over perhaps 2 or 3 weeks, although some feel there is some residual benefit even after months at sea level. It is likely that the time course of the 'off' transients are different for different systems involved in the acclimatization process.

5.5 ALTITUDE DETERIORATION

5.5.1 Introduction

The term high altitude deterioration was first used by members of early Everest expeditions to denote deterioration in mental and physical condition as a result of prolonged stay at altitude. De Filippi (1912) noted the condition during an expedition to the Karakoram. He writes:

> The atmosphere of the expedition did work some evil effect revealing itself only gradually after several weeks of life above 17500 feet in a slow decrease of appetite and consequent lack of nourishment without, however, any disturbance of digestive function.

In this way he distinguished the condition from acute mountain sickness, though the mechanisms, at least of anorexia, may be common to both conditions.

It is well known among climbers that staying at extreme altitudes for long is deleterious. Altitudes above 8000 m have been called 'The Death Zone' and summit bids on peaks over this height are wisely planned so as to spend as short a time as possible in this zone. Deterioration can frequently be attributed to factors such as dehydration, starvation, physical exhaustion and cold. However, in the absence of such factors it seems that hypoxia per se can cause deterioration if sufficiently severe (Pugh, 1962). Many of the symptoms and signs are seen in prolonged chamber experiments such as Operation Everest II (Houston *et al.* 1987; Rose *et al.* 1988). The altitude at which this becomes manifest is about 5000–6000 m, with considerable individual variation. Highlanders can probably tolerate prolonged periods at a higher altitude better than can most lowlanders (West 1986a). For lowlanders, there is probably a maximum altitude for prolonged residence at about this altitude. The experience of spending the winter at 5800 m (the Silver Hut, 1960) suggested this was above the critical altitude. Above this altitude deterioration limits the time that can be spent. The higher the altitude, the more rapid is the deterioration.

5.5.2 Symptoms and signs

High altitude deterioration (in the absence of dehydration, starvation, etc.) is characterized by weight loss, poor appetite, slow recovery from fatigue, lethargy, irritability and an increasing lack of will-power to start new tasks (Ward 1954). There is slowing of mental processes, dulling of affect and impaired cognitive function. There may be low systemic blood pressure.

ANOREXIA AND WEIGHT LOSS

Loss of appetite soon after arrival at altitude is part of the symptomatology of acute mountain sickness but after acclimatization, appetite is regained at altitudes below about 5500 m. Above this altitude there is usually further loss of appetite which tends to increase the longer is the time spent at these extreme altitudes. At 5800 m in the Silver Hut all subjects lost weight at the rate of 0.45–1.36 kg per week (Pugh 1962a). The anorexia tends to be worse in the mornings and for certain types of food, with considerable individual variation. This anorexia results in reduced calorie intake, a negative calorie balance and weight loss. There may also be a degree of malabsorption. Weight loss is the most well-attested, objective sign of deterioration. The mechanisms underlying this weight loss are considered further in Chapter 15.

FATIGUE, SLOW RECOVERY FROM EXERTION

Other symptoms of deterioration, fatigue and slow recovery from exertion, are more subjective and difficult to measure. In the 1970s we made an attempt to find a biochemical basis for the reported symptoms of slow recovery from exhausting exercise at altitude. We followed the resynthesis of muscle glycogen after depletion by exercise at sea level under normoxia (air breathing) and hypoxia (breathing 12% O_2). We found that, although the rate of resynthesis was not significantly slowed by hypoxia in the muscle overall, there was an enhancement of the difference between the type I and type II fibers. This suggested that hypoxia depresses glycogen synthesis in type I though not type II fibers (Milledge *et al.* 1977). This might contribute to the slowness of recovery from severe exercise at high altitude. However, fatigue and lassitude are felt even in the absence of exercise, so there is probably a central effect as well.

SLOWING OF MENTAL PROCESS, DULLING OF AFFECT AND IMPAIRED COGNITIVE FUNCTION

There have been numerous studies of cognitive function at altitude though not many at extreme altitude. They have mostly shown some impairment of some tests involving memory (reviewed by Raichle and Hornbein 2001 and in Chapter 17), and also speech deterioration with increasing altitude (Leiberman *et al.* 1995). An effect of severe hypoxia, often not appreciated by the subject, is to cause a slowing of mental and physical function. For instance, well-learned acts, such as strapping on crampons, take much longer at extreme altitude. Similarly, mental tasks, such as calculating the remaining supply time of an oxygen cylinder, though still possible, take longer than at low altitude. A recurring theme in accounts of life at extreme altitude is the lethargy, which gets worse with time. There is a great disinclination to get started on a task. The climber, normally a very active man, just wishes to lie dozing in his tent. The emotions too seem to be dulled and the capacity to initiate a new plan in the face of the unexpected is reduced. Ward reported after the 1953 Everest Expedition, that at camp 7 on the Lhotsi face, the sight of the exhausted Tom Bourdilon provoked nothing more than the comment, 'Poor old Tom, he's had it!' Ward himself had no doubt that at lower altitude, attempts would have been made to help the exhausted climber (Pugh and Ward 1956). Insight and judgment are impaired and no doubt contribute to fatalities at extreme altitude.

SLEEP

Sleep is disrupted at altitude by more frequent arousals than at sea level and the architecture of sleep is changed with less time spent in REM (rapid eye movement) sleep (Weil and White 2001). Periodic breathing may contribute to this and becomes more frequent the higher the altitude. The climber is conscious that he has not slept well and feels unrefreshed in the morning. This sleep deprivation may contribute to the psychological element of deterioration. A more detailed description of sleep at altitude is given in Chapter 14.

LOW SYSTEMIC BLOOD PRESSURE

The blood pressure (BP) response to altitude is either no change or a slight rise initially, falling back to sea level values with acclimatization. However there have been a few reports that at, or returning from, extreme altitude, the BP was low. Pugh and Ward (1956) reported from the 1953 Everest Expedition on a number of climbers returning to their camp from higher on the mountain. One had a BP of 86/66, a second 80/60 and a third 115/90. In Operation Everest II, Reeves noted in his diary about one subject at the simulated altitude of the summit, 'Roger Gough's study today underscored an observation that we have noted repeatedly at these very hypoxic levels. Namely, that when the subjects were not exercising, their arterial blood pressure falls (there was an arterial line in place). In Roger's case, systolic pressure would fall to 80 or less' (quoted by Houston *et al.* 1991). The mechanism is unknown. Pugh (personal communication) suggested it might be due to adrenal insufficiency but there is no evidence for this. These observations are only anecdotes and we clearly need more research. If extreme altitude does cause hypotension this could also contribute to the fatigue characteristic of altitude deterioration.

6

Control of breathing at high altitude

SUMMARY

Of all the changes that take place in the physiology of a person acclimatizing to altitude, those resulting in an increase in ventilation are probably the most important. There are changes in both the hypoxic ventilatory response (HVR) and the hypercapnic ventilatory responses (HCVR). The changes in HVR are more difficult to measure but it is now accepted that HVR increases with time at altitude over a period of days to a few weeks. The changes in HCVR were characterized over 50 years ago and include a shift to the left and a steepening of the carbon dioxide response line. That is, a person when acclimatized responds to a lower P_{CO_2} and is more sensitive to carbon dioxide than when unacclimatized. The time course of the changes in HCVR is exponential, with almost half taking place in the first 24 hours and most of the change being complete in about 2 weeks at a given altitude. These changes in the chemical control of breathing underlie the well-known increase in ventilation and result in a lower P_{CO_2} and higher P_{O_2} characteristic

of acclimatization. The mechanism underlying the increased carbon dioxide sensitivity may be due to the documented reduction in bicarbonate concentration in cerebrospinal fluid (CSF), blood and, presumably, brain extracellular fluid (ECF). The mechanisms of the increase in HVR are debatable but probably include changes in both the peripheral chemoreceptors and central processing of the signal in the brain.

Hypoxic ventilatory response does not predict susceptibility to acute mountain sickness (AMS), though subjects susceptible to high altitude pulmonary edema (HAPE) do have low HVRs. High altitude residents have similar HCVR but generally have blunted HVR compared to acclimatized lowlanders. Some studies have found a correlation between HVR and performance at extreme altitude but some elite climbers have HVR in the normal range. Among high altitude residents, Sherpas and Andean peoples tend to have low HVR while Tibetans have higher HVR than Andean altitude residents but lower than Han Chinese. All three altitude populations perform very well at altitude compared to lowlanders.

6.1 INTRODUCTION

The increase in ventilation that takes place in the first few days at altitude is one of the most important aspects of the acclimatization process. It results in higher alveolar and arterial P_{O_2} and lower P_{CO_2} than would have been obtained if the ventilation were unchanged. The cause of this increased ventilation is a change in the chemical control of breathing. Interest in the mechanisms underlying these changes goes back to the early years of the twentieth century. Haldane, who had shown that the level of carbon dioxide in the body was stable at sea level, soon realized that altitude resulted in depression of P_{CO_2} due to increased ventilation. While Haldane and his companions were on the Pikes Peak Expedition of 1911, he suggested that his colleague Mabel FitzGerald measure the alveolar P_{CO_2} in residents at mining camps at various altitudes in Colorado. She found that the P_{CO_2} fell linearly with altitude (FitzGerald 1913). At that time the mechanism for detecting hypoxia was unknown. Heymans and Heymans (1927, father and son) discovered that the carotid body detected hypoxia (see section 6.3). Since then physiologists have continued to investigate these mechanisms and their work is reviewed in this chapter.

There are two sensing systems for the chemical control of breathing: the peripheral chemoreceptors (the carotid and aortic bodies) and central chemoreceptors situated in the medulla. There are three chemical drives to ventilation: hypoxia, pH and carbon dioxide. The peripheral chemoreceptors principally sense hypoxia, though they also respond to carbon dioxide and pH, whereas the central chemoreceptors respond principally to changes in P_{CO_2} sensed by the induced change in pH.

6.2 HYPOXIC VENTILATORY RESPONSE

6.2.1 Introduction

The hypoxic ventilatory response (HVR) is the increase in ventilation brought about by acute hypoxia. This is not a simple linear response and

is complicated by the effect of ventilation on P_{CO_2}. As ventilation rises in response to hypoxia, P_{CO_2} falls and pH rises. Thus the carbon dioxide drive to breathing is reduced and the hypoxic response is masked unless measures are taken to prevent this fall in P_{CO_2}.

If the inspired P_{O_2} is reduced acutely, i.e. over a period of a few minutes, either by breathing a low oxygen mixture or by decompression in a hypobaric chamber, the minute ventilation is increased. However, this increase in ventilation varies greatly from individual to individual and does not usually begin until the inspired P_{O_2} is reduced to approximately 100 mmHg (equivalent to about 3000 m altitude) (Rahn and Otis 1949). This corresponds to an alveolar P_{O_2} of about 50 mmHg. Thereafter, as inspired P_{O_2} is further reduced ventilation increases more rapidly.

The relationship of ventilation to P_{O_2} is hyperbolic, as shown in Fig. 6.1. However, if arterial saturation is measured by an oximeter the relationship between it and ventilation is found to be approximately linear (Fig. 6.1). The P_{a,O_2} at

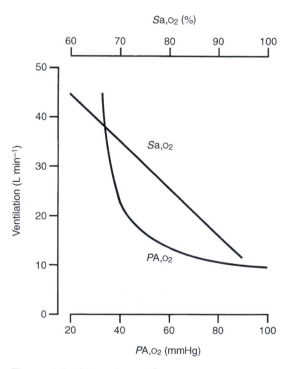

Figure 6.1 Hypoxic ventilatory response to decreasing P_{A,O_2} and to decreasing arterial oxygen saturation (S_{a,O_2}).

which ventilation starts to increase corresponds to the P_{O_2} at which the oxygen dissociation curve begins to steepen, thus HVR protects arterial oxygen content increasing ventilation as saturation begins to fall.

The actual effect of acute hypoxia on ventilation will depend upon whether P_{CO_2} is allowed to fall or not. Unless the experimental arrangement allows control of $PA,_{CO_2}$, a rise in ventilation will result in a fall of P_{CO_2}. This is the normal situation as a person ascends to altitude and HVR measured in this way is termed poikilocapnic. As P_{CO_2} is reduced some drive to breathing will be lost so that the full hypoxic response is not seen. In order to see the full HVR, P_{CO_2} is usually held constant and the response measured is termed the isocapnic HVR.

6.2.2 Time course of ventilatory response to hypoxia: minutes to days

There are three phases to this response, as shown in Fig. 6.2, where P_{CO_2} is used as a (reciprocal) measure of ventilation:

- In the first few seconds to about 10 minutes there is an increase in ventilation (and fall in P_{CO_2}) if the hypoxia is sufficiently severe.

- From about 20 to 30 minutes there is a reduction of ventilation back towards the control value (a rise in P_{CO_2}). This is called the hypoxic ventilatory decline (HVD) or 'roll off'. For a fuller discussion of this phenomenon see Smith *et al.* (2001). Bascom *et al.* (1990) showed that HVR declined during this period reaching a nadir at about 5 minutes. Vovk *et al.* (2004) have shown that HVR recovers after this 5-minute decline, over the next 36 minutes to pre-hypoxia control values. However, Garcia *et al.* 2000 found this decrease in ventilation in the absence of a change in HVR. They found that the slope of the ventilation/$Sa,_{O_2}$ line was unchanged but its intercept decreased. Clearly, the mechanism of HVD is unclear.

- There is further increase in ventilation (reduction in P_{CO_2}) from about 30 minutes to some days and continuing at a decreasing rate up to about 2 weeks at a given altitude. This is termed respiratory acclimatization and is due to an increase in HVR and hypercapnic ventilatory response (HCVR) as discussed in further sections of this chapter.

6.3 PERIPHERAL CHEMORECEPTORS

Before considering HVR further, the transduction of the hypoxic response will be briefly considered. A transducer effects the conversion of one mode of signal to another, in this case from $Pa,_{O_2}$ to a neural signal by the carotid body.

6.3.1 Historical

The stimulating effect of oxygen lack on respiration had been known for many years before it became apparent at the turn of the twentieth century that, under normal sea level conditions, carbon dioxide was the main chemical stimulus to ventilation.

In the late 1920s, the father and son team of Heymans and Heymans in Belgium, using complex cross-circulation experiments in dogs, localized the main sensing organ for hypoxia to the carotid body (Heymans and Heymans

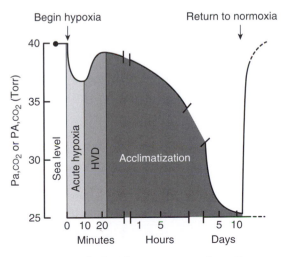

Figure 6.2   Idealized time course of ventilatory acclimatization, using P_{CO_2} as an index of ventilation. (From Smith *et al.* 2001 with permission.)

1927). Not long afterwards Comroe (1938) showed that the aortic bodies have a similar function. These bodies are known collectively as the peripheral chemoreceptors. However, in most animals, including humans, the main organ for transduction of the hypoxic signal are the carotid bodies and if these are removed or denervated, acute hypoxia actually results in depression of ventilation.

6.3.2 Anatomy and physiology of the carotid body

The human carotid body weighs about 10 mg and is situated just above the bifurcation of the common carotid artery. It has an extremely rich blood flow for its mass and oxygen consumption, and thus it extracts only a very small percentage of the oxygen in the blood presented to it. This explains how it is able to respond to arterial P_{O_2} (or saturation) and not to oxygen content. Thus it responds to hypoxemia but not anemia or reduced flow. This is appropriate since an increase in ventilation would not help the organism overcome the tissue hypoxia caused by anemia or low cardiac output, but does help in a hypoxic environment.

MECHANISM OF RESPONSE TO ACUTE HYPOXIA

An enormous amount of research work has been carried out on the carotid body. It is now generally accepted that the glomus cell (type I), the characteristic cells of the carotid body, is the site of chemoreception and that modulation of neurotransmitter release from the glomus cells by physiological and chemical stimuli affects the discharge rate of the carotid body afferent fibers. Undoubtedly the signal is modified, enhanced or suppressed by parts of the system not involved with the primary sensing process. The information on the arterial P_{O_2} travels via the carotid sinus nerve and cranial nerve IX to the respiratory centers in the brain, which then affect their output and thus breathing rate and minute ventilation.

There have been a number of good reviews of the mechanisms by which hypoxemia is sensed by the carotid body and transmitted as increased neural discharge (Lahiri and Cherniack 2001; Wilson *et al.* 2005; Prabhakar and Jacono 2005; and most recently by Teppema and Dahan, 2010). Hypoxia may slow down mitochondrial electron transport owing to the presence of a reduced affinity cytochrome in the oxygen transport chain. This could stimulate neurotransmitter release from glomus cells by progressive breakdown of the mitochondrial electrochemical gradient and release of mitochondrial calcium into the cytoplasm. The elevated intracellular calcium would then cause release of the neurotransmitter. Metabolic blockers which interfere with electron transport and oxidative phosphorylation would have a similar effect (Mulligan *et al.* 1981; Biscoe and Duchen 1990). However, the reduction in P_{O_2} at which the carotid body increases its firing rate is far higher than the P_{O_2} at which mitochondrial electron transport begins to fail (Teppema and Dahan 2010).

As shown in Fig 6.3, a primary oxygen sensor within the glomus cell detects hypoxia and communicates with potassium channels, closing

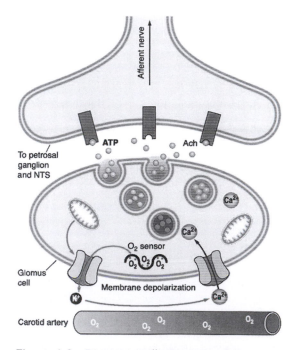

Figure 6.3 Diagram to illustrate possible mechanism of the transduction of the hypoxic signal to a neural impulse. (From Teppema and Dahan 2010, with permission.)

them. This results in membrane depolarization and the opening of calcium channels. Mitochondria, sensing hypoxia via a haem protein, may also communicate with these potassium channels. The depolarization and Ca^{2+} influx results in release of neurotransmitters (acetylcholine and adenosine triphosphate (ATP)), which excite nerve endings of the carotid sinus nerve.

There is also evidence that non-mitochondrial enzymes such as NADPH oxidases, nitric oxide (NO) synthase and heme oxygenases may be involved in the hypoxia sensing process. These proteins could contribute to transduction via generation of reactive oxygen species, NO and/or carbon monoxide (Prabhakar and Overholt 2000).

Dopamine is the most abundant transmitter found in the carotid body. Hypoxia increases the rate of release of dopamine from glomus cells. Norepinephrine (noradrenalin) and 5-hydroxytryptamine, are next in abundance. There are also small quantities of acetylcholine and enkephalin-like peptides in some glomus cells. Substance P, endothelin-1, adenosine and purinergic receptors are also present and may be involved in modulating the hypoxic response (Wilson *et al.* 2005).

It should be noted that, although the most important function of the peripheral chemoreceptors (carotid and aortic bodies) is to respond to hypoxia, they do also respond to an increase in Pa,CO_2 and decrease in arterial pH. The greatest response to PCO_2 is via the central chemoreceptors in the brain stem (see section 6.13.1); a study by Fatemian *et al.* 2003 suggested that subjects who had had both carotid bodies removed, had about 36% lower HCVR than normal subjects.

CHRONIC HYPOXIA

Anatomically, chronic hypoxia results in hypertrophy of the carotid body in animals and man probably due to up regulation of growth factors e.g. vascular endothelial growth factor (VEGF) (Prabhakar and Jacono 2005). Physiologically there is an increase in sensitivity over a period of about 30 minutes to some weeks. The mechanism of this involves a number of

systems including those mentioned above and no doubt others. It is likely that during this period gene induction is involved (see section 6.5.1).

6.4 HVR AT SEA LEVEL

6.4.1 Methods for measuring HVR

A number of different methods have been used to measure HVR, each having its advantages and disadvantages. Probably the most popular method for studies involving large numbers of subjects is the rebreathing method using an oximeter to measure oxygen saturation continuously as hypoxia is increased (by rebreathing) while the PCO_2 is held constant (Rebuck and Campbell 1974).

Previously, steady-state methods have been used, e.g. Cunningham *et al.* (1957), Severinghaus *et al.* (1966a) in which the subject breathed a hypoxic mixture until ventilation was steady, typically 10–20 minutes. All these methods measure the isocapnic HVR. Single breath methods have also been used, e.g. Dejours *et al.* (1959) in which a single breath of altered PO_2 was given and the change in tidal volume in the following few breaths observed. Single breath methods were thought to reflect the activity of peripheral and not central chemoreceptors and would not be influenced by HVD. There would also be no time for a significant change in PCO_2. The steady-state methods would reflect the activity of both central and peripheral chemoreceptors and the effect of HVD depending upon how long the 'steady state' was held. They are also influenced by changes in cerebral blood flow (CBF) which alter the arterial–venous blood-gas difference so that the central chemoreceptors may see a change in PCO_2 even if end-tidal PCO_2 is held constant. The simple and popular progressive hypoxia test is likely to be influenced by both sets of chemoreceptors, HDV and CBF.

It should also be born in mind that posture influences the HVR (but not HCVR). Usually the subject is seated. The supine position results in a 52% reduction in HVR and microgravity a reduction of 46%, presumably by the same mechanism, that of an increase in the blood pressure in the carotid baroreceptors (Prisk *et al.* 2000) since it is known that there is interaction of baroreceptor and chemoreceptor reflexes (Somers *et al.* 1991).

No method is free of criticism on one count or another and there is no concensus as to the preferred method. A useful review has been published by Duffin (2007) and on the history of the subject by Severinghaus (2008).

6.4.2 Variability of HVR: effect of age, specific groups and drugs

The range of HVR found in healthy sea level residents is wide. The coefficient of variation varies between 23 and 72% in different studies (Cunningham *et al.* 1964; Weil *et al.* 1970; Rebuck and Campbell 1974).

Various groups of subjects at sea level have been shown to have lower HVRs than controls, for instance endurance athletes (Byrne-Quinn *et al.* 1971) and swimmers (Bjurstrom and Schoene 1986). With increasing age HVR becomes lower (Kronenberg and Drage 1973; Chapman and Cherniak 1986; Poulin *et al.* 1993). Alcohol (Sahn *et al.* 1974), respiratory depressant drugs and anesthetics inhibit HVR (Davis *et al.* 1982).

The thiol disulfide redox state (REDST) has an effect on HVR (and erythropoietin production) as shown by treatment with *N*-acetyl-cysteine. Hildebrandt *et al.* (2002) showed that HVR was more than doubled after 6 days' treatment with the drug compared with placebo. This treatment greatly increased the REDST and the increase in HVR showed a significant correlation with the increase in REDST state. They suggest that the reduction in HVR with age may be due to the effect of age on REDST.

6.5 HVR AT HIGH ALTITUDE AND INTERMITTENT HYPOXIA

6.5.1 HVR and acclimatization

During the first few days at altitude, respiratory acclimatization takes place. This is shown by an increase in ventilation and a decrease in PA,CO_2. PA,O_2 falls immediately on exposure to acute

altitude and then rises (as PA,CO_2 falls) over the next few days. The rise in ventilation on acute exposure to hypoxia is mediated by the HVR (by definition) but further increase in ventilation is due to changes in HCVR (see section 6.12) and HVR with more time at altitude (see below).

The peripheral chemoreceptors are essential for normal respiratory acclimatization, and animals which have had their carotid bodies denervated fail to acclimatize normally (Forster *et al.* 1981; Lahiri *et al.* 1981; Smith *et al.* 1986). After denervation these animals have raised Pa,CO_2, which rises further with acute hypoxia. With chronic hypoxia, at least in some cases, there is a small fall in Pa,CO_2 which has been taken by some workers as evidence of acclimatization (Sorensen and Mines 1970). This and other evidence suggests that chronic hypoxia produces some effect on ventilation via mechanisms other than the carotid body, possibly via cerebral metabolism. All agree, however, that denervated animals appeared ill at altitude and a proportion die.

It might be expected that exposure to hypoxia of some days or months would result in attenuation or sensitization of the HVR. Michel and Milledge (1963) found an increase in the hypoxic parameter *A* in three out of four subjects after 1–3 months at 5800 m. Parameter *A* is the 'shape' parameter of the hyperbola relating PA,O_2 to ventilation (Fig. 6.1). The larger the value the greater is the response. There was no change in the other hypoxic parameter, *C* (the PO_2 at which theoretically ventilation becomes infinite, the PO_2 asymptote of the hyperbola). Cruz *et al.* (1980) also found an increase in parameter *A* after 74 hours of altitude exposure; this was not seen in subjects whose PA,CO_2 was not allowed to fall.

Yamaguchi *et al.* (1991) and Sato *et al.* (Sato *et al.* 1992; Sato *et al.* 1994) found a significant increase in HVR in lowland subjects after acclimatization at 3730–4860 m compared with pre-exposure values. Masuda *et al.* (1992) measured HVR serially in seven lowland subjects after arrival at Lhasa (3658 m) as they acclimatized over 27 days. They found a small decrease in HVR over the first 3–5 days then a considerable increase from day 5 to 27. It seems that there are significant differences in response in different subjects especially in the first few days at altitude, and that this may be associated with their susceptibility or resistance to acute mountain sickness (AMS) (see section 6.6 and Bartsch *et al.* 2002). These differences may account for some of the variability in results from different studies.

Robbins's group in Oxford has carried out a series of chamber studies in which the inspired gases can be controlled so as to keep the subject's end-tidal P_{CO_2} constant. Thus they are able to study the changes in HVR with hypoxia over first 8 hours and later 48 hours with or without the confounding effect of respiratory alkalosis mentioned above. They found that HVR did increase even under isocapnia (Howard and Robbins 1995). They also showed that acclimatization had taken place even with isocapnia in that ventilation was raised under acute hyperoxia (Tansley *et al.* 1998). Using a 48-hour chamber exposure, under either isocapnic or poikilocapnic hypoxia, the increase in hypoxic sensitivity started within 12 hours and reached a peak at about 36 hours. That there was no difference between isocapnic and poikilocapnic results suggests that the respiratory alkalosis (due to reduced P_{CO_2}), normal in early acclimatization, is not an important part of the mechanism for the increase of HVR.

This increase in HVR over the period of a few days to a few weeks could explain the further increase in ventilation over this period of altitude exposure. The mechanism for this increase in HVR is not clear. A study in awake goats using selective inhibitors indicates that 5-HT is not essential for this aspect of ventilatory acclimatization (Herman *et al.* 2001). The possibility that HVD might change during acclimatization was considered by Sato *et al.* over a 3-day and a 2-week exposure (Sato *et al.*1992; Sato *et al.* 1994) and they found no change. Hupperets *et al.* (2004) extended this period to 8 weeks at a similar altitude (3900 m) and also found that HVD did not change.

Kline *et al.* (2002) studied the importance of the hypoxia-inducible factor-1α (HIF-1α) in the changes in HVR with acclimatization. In this study, transgenic mice, with one chromosome for HIF-1α knocked out, heterozygous (homozygous knock-out mice die *in utero*), were compared with wild-type mice. Whereas there was no difference in response to acute hypoxia, the effect of chronic hypoxia (3 days at 0.4 atm) was different. The wild-type mice showed the expected increase in HVR, the knock-out mice showed reduced

HVR. They showed this result both in terms of ventilation, especially respiratory rate, and in sinus nerve activity, indicating it was an effect in the carotid body as opposed to a purely central effect. HIF-1α induces transcription of many genes that are influenced by hypoxia, including those mentioned above. It may also be the mechanism by which hypoxia effects the potassium channel activity in glomus cells leading to depolarization and increases in calcium concentration and neurotransmitter release (Prabhakar 2000). HIF-1α clearly has a global role as the master regulator of oxygen homeostasis (see Chapter 9, section 9.4.1 for further discussion of HIF-1). Gassmann *et al.* (2009) showed, in mice, that enhanced erythropoietin (EPO) in the brainstem increased the HVR. This effect was abolished by an EPO antagonist (soluble EPO receptor). The effect was more pronounced in female than male mice. Another study from the same group (Soliz *et al.* 2009) using transgenic mice, overexpressing the *EPO* gene, found the same effect. They then went on to conduct a small 'proof of concept' study in humans. Subjects were given EPO before being exposed to 10% oxygen. HVR was increased in both male and female subjects but the effect was greater in women than men.

Malik *et al.* (2005) found a clue as to a gene that might be responsible for the increase in HVR with acclimatization, the immediate–early gene, *fos B*. This is a member of a family of transcription factor genes active in the brain which are inducible by a variety of stimuli including drugs, hormones and interestingly, repetitive behavior, as well as hypoxia. They found that mice lacking this gene had the same HVR as wild-type mice, but while the latter increased their ventilation and HVR with chronic hypoxia (3 days at 0.4 atm), the mutant mice failed to increase their ventilation or their HVR.

The question of the role of HVR in effecting the change in carbon dioxide response and brain extracellular bicarbonate concentration is considered in section 6.13.

6.5.2 HVR and intermittent hypoxia

With the increase in the use of intermittent hypoxia (IH) in athletic training and also interest in clinical conditions such as obstructive sleep apnea, there have been a number of studies in which the effect of various forms of IH have been used and the effect on HVR observed.

Serebrovskaya and colleagues (1999) gave their subjects three, 5-to-6-minute rebreathing sessions per day, separated by two 5-minute breaks, for 14 days. During the procedure the end-tidal P_{O_2} progressively decreased from 105–100 mmHg to 50–40 mmHg during the first week and to 40–35 mmHg during the second week as subjective tolerance to hypoxia increased. End-tidal P_{CO_2} (PET_{CO_2}) was kept constant. They found that the HVR increased by 43% after the training compared with pre-training control values.

Garcia *et al.* (2000) using 2 hours a day of hypoxia (3800 m equivalent) for 12 days found HVR increased to 193% above control by day 5 but then declined to 70% above control by day 12. Katayama *et al.* (2001) showed that as little as 1 hour of hypoxia (4500 m equivalent) per day for 7 days significantly increased HVR while Townsend *et al.* (2002) in their study of trained athletes 'living high–training low' also found an increase in HVR that was dose dependent. That is, the groups having most hypoxia had greatest increase in HVR and this continued to increase with the number of nights spent in hypoxia. They were also able to show a decrease in PET_{CO_2} of about 3 torr in normoxia, though no measured change in ventilation. Katayama *et al.* (2007) confirmed that IH increased HVR but interestingly, this did not result in an increase in exercise ventilation. Peng *et al.* (2006) using HIF-1α knock-out mice, have shown that the increase in HVR induced by IH is HIF-1 dependent.

It seems that IH definitely results in an increase in HVR though whether the change is more, less or about the same as an equivalent dose of hypoxia given continuously, is not clear. The effects of IH on other aspects of the physiology of hypoxia are addressed in other chapters.

6.5.3 HVR and altitude residents

Chiodi (1957) reported that altitude residents in the Andes had higher $PA,_{CO_2}$ than acclimatized lowlanders. Severinghaus *et al.* (1966a) showed that Andean Indians born and living at altitude

had a blunted HVR and similar findings were reported in Sherpas, natives to high altitude in the Himalayas (Lahiri and Milledge 1967; Milledge and Lahiri 1967).

Steady-state inhalation experiments typical of a lowlander and a Sherpa are shown in Fig. 6.4. The 'opened-out fan' of CO_2 response lines of the lowlander indicates a brisk HVR whereas the 'closed fan' of the Sherpa shows that changing

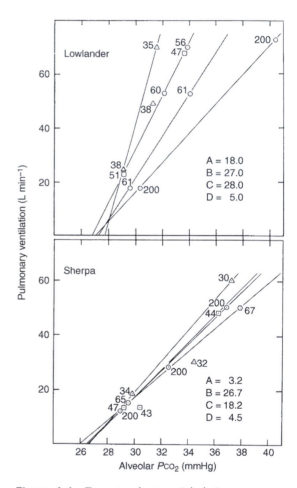

Figure 6.4 Two steady-state inhalation experiments typical of a lowlander (upper panel) and a Sherpa highlander (lower panel). The numbers refer to the P_{O_2} of each point. There is no significant difference in hypercapnic ventilatory response (HCVR) but the 'closed fan' of the Sherpa indicates very little hypoxic ventilatory response (HVR). Letters A–D refer to the parameters relating HVR (A and C) and HCVR (B and D). (From Milledge and Lahiri 1967.)

PA,O$_2$ between 200 and 30 mmHg has very little effect on ventilation. These early reports have been confirmed and Lahiri (1977) has reviewed the data from these studies. There is considerable variability among these people, the HVR varying from almost zero response to values within the lowlander range. One study (Hackett *et al.* 1980) claimed that Sherpas did not show this blunted HVR. However, even this study showed that HVR was lower in Sherpas with the longest altitude exposure. More recently, Zhuang *et al.* (1993) found HVR in Tibetan subjects at 3658 m to be less than in acclimatized Han Chinese at the same altitude.

One large study compared Tibetan with Andean high altitude residents directly. Beall *et al.* (1997a) studied 320 Tibetans and 552 Andean subjects. They found resting ventilation to be higher in Tibetans by a factor of about 1.5, and their HVR to be roughly double that of the Andean subjects. Comparison of these two populations is discussed further in Chapter 18.

Weil *et al.* (1971) showed blunting of HVR in North Americans born and living at Leadville, Colorado (3100 m), HVR being only 10% of that found in the sea level controls. In residents, the blunting of HVR was dependent on the time of residence at altitude. Roughly 50% reduction in HVR was found at about 10 years. In conclusion, compared with lowlanders, Tibetans, Sherpas and Caucasians born and brought up at altitude have reduced HVR while Andean high altitude residents have even lower HVR.

6.5.4 Lowlanders resident at high altitude

Early studies of lowland subjects resident for a few years at high altitude suggested that HVR remained unchanged indefinitely (Sorensen and Severinghaus 1968; Lahiri *et al.* 1969). However, in a study of lowlanders resident at altitude for decades (Weil *et al.* 1971) it was shown that blunting did take place slowly.

6.5.5 Highlanders resident at sea level

The HVR was found not to change in high altitude natives who came down to live at low altitude for 10 months (Lahiri *et al.* 1969), but Vargas *et al.* (1998), also in South America, in two studies found no difference in HVR between high and low altitude natives measured at low altitude. In one study the high altitude natives had been at altitude (>3000 m) for an average of 14 years and had resided at sea level for at least 20 years. In the other study they had lived above 3500 m for at least 20 years and at sea level for no more than 5 years. This study was followed up more recently by a group from Lima and Oxford. Gamboa *et al.* (2003) considered the possibility that HVR might differ according to whether the test used a sufficiently short hypoxic exposure to avoid HVD (see section 6.2.2) or not. They found that high altitude natives, from altitudes above 3500 m, resident at low altitude for more than 5 years, when compared with low altitude natives had blunted HVR using a 10-minute hypoxic exposure; but using a more acute hypoxic exposure (50 seconds for each step change of oxygen) most of the difference disappeared. These findings may explain some of the differences in results of previous studies of this topic. Why high altitude natives appear to have greater HVD than sea level natives is not clear.

6.5.6 The development of blunted HVR

Lahiri *et al.* (1976) found evidence in Andean Indians that HVR was normal in children and became blunted only as they grew into adulthood at altitude. They suggested the rate of blunting was more rapid the higher the place of residence. Weil *et al.* (1971) showed that in North American subjects in Leadville, Colorado, blunted HVR also developed but only after decades of high altitude residence.

In cats, this blunting is seen after 3–5 weeks if the hypoxia is sufficiently severe. Tatsumi *et al.* (1991) showed blunting of HVR after this time at a simulated altitude of 5500 m. They also found that HVR, measured by recording from the carotid sinus nerve, was blunted. They considered that both central and peripheral parts of the system contributed to the reduction in overall HVR.

These findings prove that the blunting of the HVR takes many years to develop in humans and is due to environmental rather than genetic factors.

6.6 HVR AND ACUTE MOUNTAIN SICKNESS

Acute mountain sickness is a condition affecting otherwise fit people on ascending rapidly to altitude. For details of symptomatology, etiology and treatment see Chapter 19. It would seem axiomatic that a brisk HVR by increasing ventilation reduces the degree of hypoxia and must be protective against AMS. There is some evidence that this may be the case, but it is by no means overwhelming.

Hu *et al.* (1982) showed that six good acclimatizers (no history of AMS) had brisk HVR while four poor acclimatizers (subjects who had AMS on going to altitude) had blunted responses. Richalet *et al.* (1988) found that in 128 climbers going to altitude on various expeditions, a measure of HVR carried out before departure indicated that a low response was a risk factor for AMS. However, high altitude residents and peoples native to high altitude have blunted HVR (see section 6.5.2) and yet tend to be less subject to AMS than lowlanders. In climbers resident at low altitude, of varying altitude experience, Milledge *et al.* (1988, 1991) found no correlation between HVR, measured before expeditions to Everest, Mount Kenya and Bolivia, and the symptom score for AMS in the first few days after arrival at altitude.

Masuda *et al.* (1992) found an initial decrease in HVR 1–5 days after arrival at Lhasa (3700 m) followed by an increase and suggested that this might explain why these first few days are the time of risk for AMS. Bartsch *et al.* (2002) examined the correlation of HVR (both iso- and poikilocapnic) measured at sea level, with subsequent development of AMS at 4559 m. They found none. However, they also measured HVR on the first few days after arrival at 4559 m and showed that there was a significant correlation between the change in HVR from the sea level value, to that measured on the first day at altitude, and the AMS symptom score on the next day.

That is, subjects who increased their HVR, tended to be resistant to AMS, while those who, on the second day had AMS, had shown a decrease in HVR on the first day at altitude (see Fig. 6.5). In most of the studies quoted, HVR was measured with only a few minutes of hypoxia thus measured HVR of the initial phase of the response (section 6.2.2) whereas any correlation with AMS could be expected only with the third phase of the response. Burtscher *et al.* (2004) argued this point and studied 63 AMS-susceptible, and 87 non-susceptible subjects. They found that the Sa_{O_2} of the AMS-susceptible group averaged 4.9% lower than non-susceptible after 20–30 minutes of hypoxia (poikilocapnic). Modeling gave an 86% correct identification of AMS susceptibility. Probably some measure of HVR is a factor in susceptibility to AMS.

These studies all considered a correlation, or lack of it, between HVR and simple or benign AMS. The relationship of HVR and HAPE seems clearer. Hackett *et al.* (1988b) studied seven male patients with HAPE and found HVR was low, especially in those with the most severe hypoxemia. Bandopadhyay and Selvamurthy (2003) also reported that HVR was lower in a group of soldiers who had suffered from HAPE.

Hohenhaus *et al.* (1995) measured HVR in 30 subjects proved to be HAPE-susceptible compared with a control group. They concluded that a low

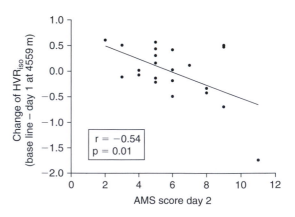

Figure 6.5 Changes in isocapnic hypoxic ventilatory response (HVR) between baseline and day 1 at altitude (4559 m) versus Lake Louise acute mountain sickness (AMS) scores on day 2. (From Bartsch *et al.* 2002 with permission.)

HVR is associated with an increased risk of HAPE but not with simple AMS. HAPE-susceptible subjects have a greater hypoxic pulmonary vascular response (HPVR) than HAPE-resistant subjects (see Chapter 21). A low HVR means that their PA,O_2 is likely to be lower than others at a given altitude, especially on exercise (see section 6.7), thus raising their pulmonary artery pressure even higher.

6.7 HVR AND ALTITUDE: PERFORMANCE

Apart from AMS, some people 'go well' at extreme altitude whereas others, just as athletically fit, seem much more adversely affected. In general, there is a correlation between freedom from AMS and good altitude performance but there are many exceptions. Individuals homozygous for the I allele of the angiotensin converting enzyme (*ACE*) gene are greatly over-represented in climbers who have reached 7000 m without supplementary oxygen (Montgomery *et al.* 1998) whereas this association is not found as a factor for resistance/susceptibility to AMS (Koehle *et al.* 2006; Kalson *et al.* 2009). There has been much more work in this field which is further discussed in Chapter 4 (section 4.3) and a recent comprehensive review (Puthucheary *et al.* 2011).

Again, it would seem advantageous for a mountaineer to have a brisk HVR in order to maintain a better oxygen supply to the working muscles. However, the evidence for this is conflicting.

Climbers with a brisk HVR were found to suffer greater impairment of mental performance at altitude (Hornbein *et al.* 1989), presumably as a result of reduced brain blood flow due to lower Pa,CO_2 (see Chapter 17 for details of this work).

Schoene (1982) showed that 14 high altitude climbers had significantly higher HVR than 10 controls. During the 1981 American Medical Research Expedition to Everest, Schoene *et al.* (1984) extended this work, showing again that the HVR measured before and on the expedition correlated well with performance high on the mountain (Fig. 6.6). They also showed that, at altitude (6300 m), the fall in oxygen saturation on exercise is greater in subjects with a low HVR and least in those with a brisk response. This effect is

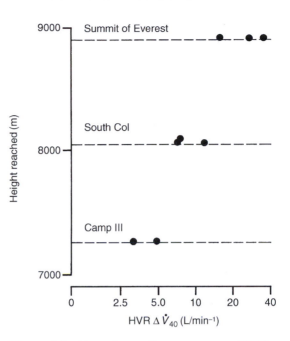

Figure 6.6 Hypoxic ventilatory response (HVR) and height reached on Mount Everest by eight mountaineers on the American Medical Research Expedition to Everest 1981. (Redrawn from data of Schoene *et al.* 1984.)

most obvious at extreme altitude when the Pa,O_2 is well onto the steep part of the O_2 dissociation curve. In part of this study subjects breathed a low oxygen mixture which brought out this effect even more clearly. Thus, subjects with a blunted HVR are not only more hypoxic at rest but have even greater hypoxia on exercise than brisk responders. This is because there is a correlation between HVR and exercise ventilatory response (Martin *et al.* 1978). On the other hand, Bernardi *et al.* (2006) found that compared with climbers who needed O_2 to reach the summit of Everest or K2, climbers who succeeded without O_2 had a lower HVR (measured after 15 days' acclimatization). They attributed this to their greater ventilatory reserve, that is the difference between their ventilation at a given Sa,O_2 percent and their maximum voluntary ventilation.

Matsuyama *et al.* (1986) found that five climbers who reached an altitude of 8000 m on Kangchenjunga (8486 m) had a higher HVR than five climbers who did not.

However, the blunted HVR in peoples native to high altitude who perform at least as well as lowlanders argues against the necessity for a brisk HVR. They have probably adapted in other ways, such as having larger lungs with higher diffusing capacities and may have developed differences in metabolism (Chapter 18). There is also evidence of not so brisk HVR in top-level climbers. On the British Mount Kongur Expedition, four elite climbers were found to have lower HVR than four scientists on the same expedition (Milledge *et al.* 1983c). Schoene *et al.* (1987) studied one of the two climbers to first reach the summit of Mount Everest without supplementary oxygen and found him to have a low HVR. Oelz *et al.* (1986) also showed that six elite climbers who had all reached at least 8400 m without supplementary oxygen had HVRs no different from controls. In a prospective study of 128 climbers going on expeditions to the great ranges, Richalet *et al.* (1988) found that a measure of HVR did not correlate with the height reached, whereas maximal oxygen consumption ($V_{O_{2,max}}$) measured at sea level did.

Serebrovskaya and Ivashkevich (1992) found that subjects with the highest HVR had higher physical capacity at moderate altitude but tolerated extreme hypoxia less well, in that the P_{O_2} at which they had a disturbance of consciousness was higher than subjects with less brisk HVR. This may be explained by the fact that because of their hyperventilation their P_{CO_2} would be lower and therefore their cerebral blood flow would be lower leading to more severe brain hypoxia. Possibly, in lowlanders for physical performance, a brisk HVR is advantageous at moderate and high altitude but not at extreme altitude.

6.8 HVR AND SLEEP

A feature of sleep at high altitude is periodic breathing. This not only disturbs sleep, the subject often waking with a distressing sensation of suffocation, but also results in quite profound hypoxia for short but repeated periods following the apneic phase of the periodic breathing (see Chapter 14). It may be that these short but repeated periods of profound hypoxia are more detrimental than a steady moderate hypoxia, although the peak and average S_{a,O_2} tend to be higher during periodic breathing (Salvaggio *et*

al. 1998). Lahiri *et al.* (1984) have shown that to produce periodic breathing a brisk HVR is needed, so in this respect a brisk HVR may be a disadvantage (see Chapter 14).

6.9 HVR AT ALTITUDE: CONCLUSIONS

Animals that have had their carotid bodies denervated appear sick on being taken to altitude and have a high mortality, so an HVR sufficient to at least counter the central depressant effect of hypoxia is clearly beneficial. Whether a very brisk HVR is more advantageous than a more modest response is questionable. Relative hypoventilation at altitude is possibly a risk factor for AMS (see Chapter 19) but the HVR measured at sea level is only one factor in determining the ventilation after a day or two at altitude. The speed of respiratory acclimatization (rate of change in both HVR and HCVR) may be more important than the sea level HVR (Fig 6.5).

In subjects with a brisk HVR it seems likely that periodic breathing will begin at lower altitudes and be present for more of the night than in subjects with a more blunted HVR. Mental performance at altitude and even after return to sea level may be more impaired in subjects with a brisk HVR (see Chapter 17).

Lowlanders with little or no altitude experience may possibly acclimatize faster and be freer of AMS if they are endowed with a brisk HVR. Highlanders, with decades of altitude living, probably develop adaptations at the tissue level, which allow them to dispense with this 'emergency' response to hypoxia and avoid the need for such hyperventilation. They therefore avoid the extra energy cost.

Highly experienced climbers may also have made some progress towards this adaptation and so may not require a brisk HVR to avoid mountain sickness and perform well at altitude.

6.10 ALVEOLAR GASES AND ACCLIMATIZATION

It has been pointed out that if P_{I,O_2} is progressively reduced over a few minutes there is very little effect on ventilation until PI,O_2 has fallen to about 100 mmHg (equivalent to about 3000 m). However, in residents at altitudes lower than this, ventilation is increased. This effect of chronic hypoxia in increasing ventilation (over and above that due to acute hypoxia) is an important aspect of respiratory acclimatization.

Minute ventilation at rest is not easy to measure accurately because the placing of a mouthpiece or a mask on a subject itself tends to increase ventilation. Therefore it is usual to use PA,CO_2 as an index of ventilation, since during steady state there is a close (inverse) relationship between PA,CO_2 and ventilation.

The classical description of the effect of altitude on alveolar gases is by Rahn and Otis (1949) on the oxygen/carbon dioxide diagram (Fig. 6.7). Alveolar gases in subjects acutely exposed to varying PI,O_2 in a decompression chamber are compared with results from residents at various altitudes culled from the literature.

It will be seen that in chronic hypoxia PCO_2 falls in a linear fashion from sea level up to altitudes of about 5400 m, above which PCO_2 falls more rapidly so that the line dips down, that is with increasing altitude, PCO_2 falls but PO_2 falls very little. These are altitudes above the highest permanent habitation and points are from climbers who have been there for some days or weeks. At this altitude complete acclimatization is probably not possible; the physiology is further discussed in Chapter 13.

Figure 6.7 also shows that at about 3600 m the difference in alveolar gases between the two lines, i.e. acclimatized and unacclimatized subjects, is greatest. The PA,CO_2 is 10–12 mmHg lower in acclimatized subjects, indicating an increase in ventilation of over 40% compared with unacclimatized subjects.

6.11 ACUTE NORMOXIA IN ACCLIMATIZED SUBJECTS

If acclimatized subjects are returned to normal (sea level) PO_2 either by rapid return to sea level or by breathing a gas mixture appropriately enriched with oxygen, their ventilation is reduced and the PA,CO_2 rises but does not return to sea level values. The remaining elevation of ventilation and depression of PA,CO_2 has been termed 'ventilatory deacclimatization from hypoxia' (VDH). The increase in PI,O_2 turns off most of the hypoxic drive and the residual hyperventilation indicates the changes in CO_2 response induced by acclimatization. This VDH is most accurately measured when ventilation is recorded during exercise.

Figure 6.8 shows results from two typical experiments (Milledge 1968). It will be seen that by breathing sea level PI,O_2 the increase in ventilation

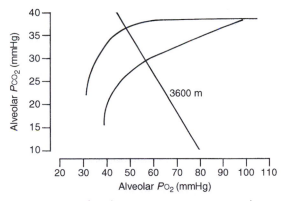

Figure 6.7 Alveolar gas concentrations and altitude. The upper line represents the PO_2 and PCO_2 found in subjects actually exposed to increasing hypoxia in a chamber. The lower line is from residents at various altitudes and from acclimatized mountaineers. (After Rahn and Otis 1949.)

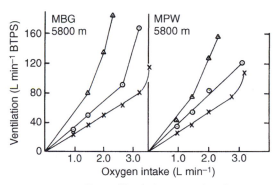

Figure 6.8 Effect of breathing sea level PI,O_2 on exercise minute ventilation in two acclimatized subjects (○) compared with their ventilation during air breathing at altitude (△) and at sea level (×). (Milledge 1968.)

at altitude compared with sea level is reduced by only 40–50% at any given submaximal work rate. This suggests that about half the increase in ventilation is due to the hypoxic stimulus (HVR being increased by acclimatization) and half due to the changes in control of breathing, principally in the response to CO_2, due to acclimatization.

If subjects are returned abruptly to sea level, as after a long chamber experiment, this continued hyperventilation persists for some days. The time course of this VDH is similar to that of acclimatization and has been assumed to be due to similar mechanisms being turned on and off. However, the view that there may be different mechanisms involved is gaining ground (Smith et al. 2001) and a chamber study in humans found that VDH was similar in subjects whose P_{CO_2} was allowed to drop (poikilocapnic) compared with those maintained isocapnic during a 48-hour exposure to hypoxia to subjects (Tansley et al. 1998).

6.12 CARBON DIOXIDE VENTILATORY RESPONSE AND ACCLIMATIZATION

An important aspect of respiratory acclimatization is the change in carbon dioxide ventilatory response measured either by the steady state (Lloyd et al. 1958) or by a rebreathing method (Reed 1967).

The effect of time at altitude on the HCVR is shown in Fig. 6.9, which is from the work of Kellogg (1963). The steady-state method was used in three subjects to measure the HCVR before

ascent to White Mountain. The measurement was repeated a few hours after arrival by road at 4350 m and thereafter at intervals as indicated on the figure. It will be seen that the HCVR line shifts progressively leftwards and steepens.

This increase in HCVR was confirmed at higher altitude by Michel and Milledge (1963) and recently again by Fan et al. (2010). Voluntary hyperventilation of only 6 hours' duration breathing air has a significant effect in shifting the carbon dioxide response curve to the left.

6.13 MECHANISM FOR RESETTING HCVR

6.13.1 Central chemoreceptors

Although the peripheral chemoreceptors are sensitive to changes in P_{CO_2} and hydrogen ion concentration, the main sensor for changes in P_{CO_2} is the central medullary chemoreceptor. This is a paired region of the central nervous system (CNS) situated just beneath the surface of the fourth ventricle in the medulla. Work by Mitchell (1963) showed that this area is sensitive to changes in hydrogen ion concentration in the brain ECF. Such changes are brought about primarily by changes in arterial P_{CO_2}. More recent work indicates that, in addition, there are other sites in the brainstem also chemosensitive and respond to changes in [H] (Nattie 2002).

The blood–brain barrier is readily permeable to dissolved carbon dioxide, less permeable to

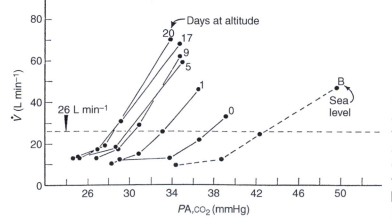

Figure 6.9 Effect of acclimatization on hypercapnic ventilatory response (HCVR) at an altitude of 4340 m. $\dot{V}$, ventilation. (Reproduced with permission from Kellogg 1963.) Values for $[HCO_3^-]$, $[H^+]$ and P_{CO_2} are for levels in the cerebrospinal fluid.

hydrogen ions and even less to bicarbonate. Thus, a rise in $Pa,_{CO_2}$ is rapidly reflected in CSF P_{CO_2} and causes a rapid increase in CSF hydrogen ion concentration. Increases in hydrogen ion concentration sensed by the chemoreceptors result in increased stimulation of the respiratory center and an increase in ventilation.

6.13.2 The importance of CSF bicarbonate

The chemoreceptors sense the hydrogen ion concentration in the brain ECF (or possibly some other extracellular or intracellular compartment) but since this cannot be sampled, the following discussion centers on the CSF acid–base changes which can be measured. See section 6.15.1 for further discussion of the differences between these two compartments.

The Henderson–Hasselbalch equation, which defines the relationship between P_{CO_2}, bicarbonate and pH (hydrogen ion concentration), is shown in Fig. 6.10. This indicates that for hydrogen ion concentration to be held constant, a change of bicarbonate concentration must be followed by a change of P_{CO_2} in the same direction. Assuming the sensitivity of the central chemoreceptors to hydrogen ion concentration remains constant, a reduction in bicarbonate concentration will result in an increase in hydrogen ion concentration

which will stimulate the central chemoreceptor and cause a rise in ventilation. This, in turn, will lower the P_{CO_2} and restore the hydrogen ion concentration to normal, but now with a lower P_{CO_2}. Thus a reduction in CSF bicarbonate concentration has the effect of resetting the chemoreceptor to start responding at a lower P_{CO_2} (a shift to the left of the HCVR line). A rise in CSF bicarbonate concentration has the opposite effect and is seen in patients with chronic obstructive pulmonary disease (COPD) and hypercapnia. If the chemoreceptor responds to log hydrogen ion concentration (i.e. pH), then changes in P_{CO_2} at low values, e.g. 20–21 mmHg, will have twice the effect as that at normal values, i.e. 40–41 mmHg. This would then explain the steepening of the HCVR seen in acclimatized subjects.

These effects are shown in Fig. 6.10. This is a theoretical representation of the effect on HCVR of a reduction in CSF bicarbonate concentration. A typical HCVR line at sea level is shown on the right. The CSF bicarbonate concentration is 24 mmol L^{-1}. If the CSF bicarbonate concentration is reduced to 17 mmol L^{-1} the chemoreceptor now 'sees' an increased hydrogen ion concentration and ventilation is stimulated until hydrogen ion concentration is reduced to the previous value. The resulting P_{CO_2} values are plotted and joined by a line giving the new HCVR on the left. This looks very similar to the actual effect of acclimatization on HCVR.

It is suggested that the mechanism of the change in HCVR is a reduction in CSF bicarbonate concentration. Evidence for this is provided by the experiments of Pappenheimer *et al.* (1964) in which they perfused the cerebral ventricles of awake goats with artificial CSF, varying the pH and bicarbonate concentration. They showed that by simply reducing the bicarbonate concentration in the CSF, the HCVR was shifted to the left.

6.13.3 Reduction in CSF bicarbonate concentration at altitude

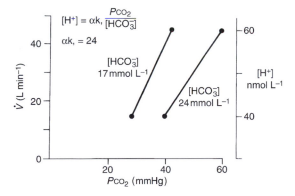

Figure 6.10   Calculated effect of reducing cerebrospinal fluid (CSF) [HCO_3^-] on the hypercapnic ventilatory response HCVR using the Henderson–Hasselbalch equation and assuming (CSF) pH is held constant by ventilatory induced changes in P_{CO_2}. $\dot{V}$, ventilation.

In lowlanders going to an altitude of 3800 m the CSF bicarbonate concentration is reduced from a mean sea level value of 24.7 mmol L^{-1} to 20.4 mmol L^{-1} on the second day at altitude and

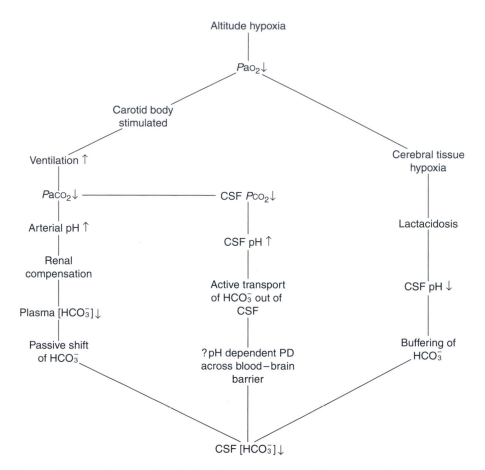

Figure 6.11 Possible mechanisms by which altitude hypoxia could cause a reduction in CSF [HCO_3^-]. PD, potential difference.

20.1 mmol L^{-1} on day 8 (Severinghaus *et al.* 1963). Similar results (mean 20.1 mmol L^{-1}) were found at 4880 m (Lahiri and Milledge 1967). Residents at high altitude had similar values, 19.1–21.3 mmol L^{-1} (Severinghaus and Carcelan 1964; Lahiri and Milledge 1967; Sorensen and Milledge 1971). Thus, the reduction in CSF bicarbonate concentration of 4.5 mmol L^{-1} measured at altitude might explain the shift of the HCVR line to the left, though respiratory acclimatization probably also involves contributions from other mechanisms, such as changes in HVR (see section 6.5.1). The mechanism for the reduction in bicarbonate and the importance of CNS pH was discussed at length in previous editions of this textbook. However, the consensus of opinion now seems to emphasize the changes in HVR rather than in CO_2 response as the more important element in the hyperventilation of altitude acclimatization. To quote Smith *et al.* (2001):

> Regulation of CNS [H+] as a mechanism of ventilatory acclimatization to hypoxia is an elegant hypothesis with considerable logical appeal. However, it has been difficult to establish any major role for CNS [H+] in the control of ventilatory acclimatization… when the entire time course of the process is considered.

6.14 DYNAMIC CARBON DIOXIDE RESPONSE

Carbon dioxide is eliminated only during expiration; during inspiration it is retained. Therefore, the level of carbon dioxide in the blood leaving the lungs must oscillate in time with breathing. During exercise these oscillations will be increased. Yamamoto and Edwards (1960) suggested that these oscillations might be a signal to which the peripheral chemoreceptors could respond over and above the mean level of carbon dioxide in the arterial blood and might help explain the hyperpnea of exercise. The response to this putative signal of change in carbon dioxide with time is called the dynamic carbon dioxide ventilatory response. Datta and Nickol (1995) showed that this response could be demonstrated in exercising humans (it had been shown previously in anesthetized cats) by measuring the ventilation during the injection of a small bolus of carbon dioxide either early or late in inspiration. Ventilation was found to be greater with early pulses. Collier et al. (2008) confirmed the effect of early boluses of CO_2 and showed that this response is most clearly seen after acclimatization especially after ascent to very high altitude (>7000 m). In one study it was seen in acute hypoxia, but not in another study. It was weak or absent on first arrival at altitude. This provides evidence that the ventilatory response of the peripheral chemoreceptor for dynamic changes in CO_2 is increased with acclimatization, as it is for hypoxia (section 6.5.1).

6.15 LONGER-TERM ACCLIMATIZATION

6.15.1 Highlanders

People native to high altitude have slightly lower ventilation and higher Pa,CO_2 than acclimatized newcomers (Chiodi 1957). This is probably due to their blunted HVR (see section 6.5.3). The HCVR of Andean natives (Severinghaus et al. 1966a), Sherpas (Milledge and Lahiri 1967) and Tibetans (Shi et al. 1979) has the same slope as that of lowlanders at the same altitude. The position of the carbon dioxide ventilatory response line may be to the right (Severinghaus et al. 1966a) or not significantly different from lowlanders (Milledge and Lahiri 1967). That is, there is little difference between highlanders and lowlanders in their carbon dioxide ventilatory response.

6.15.2 Lowlanders

Although most of the respiratory acclimatization takes place within the first few hours and days at altitude, there may be further changes over the following weeks. In humans, there is a further increase in ventilation and Pa,O_2 with a further decrease in Pa,CO_2 (Forster et al. 1974), though in other animals, e.g. pony and goat, the Pa,CO_2 reaches the lowest point at 8–12 hours and then rises. The rat responds like humans with continued fall in Pa,CO_2 up to 14 days (Dempsey and Forster 1982). There is no significant change in acid–base balance over this period to account for this further ventilatory adaptation. This further increase in ventilation is probably due to an increase in HVR, due to changes in both sensitivity of the carotid body over this period (see section 6.5.1) and in changes in control of ventilation from higher centers, such as has been demonstrated in cats by Tenney and Ou (1977). This might be due to activation of genes such as fos B (Malik 2005) (section 6.5.1).

7

Pulmonary gas exchange

SUMMARY

Important changes in pulmonary gas exchange occur at high altitude. The most obvious feature is the hyperventilation resulting from hypoxic stimulation of the peripheral chemoreceptors. The hyperventilation reduces the alveolar P_{CO_2} and helps to maintain the alveolar P_{O_2} in spite of the inevitable fall associated with the reduced P_{O_2} of inspired gas. As an example of the extent of the hyperventilation that can occur, climbers on the summit of Mount Everest increase their alveolar ventilation some five-fold and drive the alveolar P_{CO_2} down to less than 10 mmHg. The degree of hyperventilation is very different depending on whether subjects are exposed to acute hypoxia, or whether they have the advantages of acclimatization. With acute hypoxia there may be no increase in ventilation up to altitudes of about 3500 m. However, in acclimatized subjects, essentially any increase in altitude above sea level results in a rise in alveolar ventilation and a fall in alveolar P_{CO_2}. Diffusion of oxygen across the blood-gas barrier is challenged at high altitude. Diffusion limitation of oxygen transfer across the blood-gas barrier occurs during exercise at even moderate altitudes and at rest at extreme altitude. This is one of the few situations when diffusion limitation for oxygen is seen in the normal lung. Diffusion across the blood-gas barrier is enhanced if the oxygen affinity of hemoglobin is increased, and it is of interest that this occurs at extreme altitude because of the severe respiratory alkalosis. Lowlanders who go to high altitude have a small increase in diffusing capacity caused partly by the polycythemia. Highlanders may have higher diffusing capacities than lowlanders possibly because of the accelerated growth of the lung in a hypoxic environment. The reduction in arterial P_{O_2} caused by ventilation–perfusion inequality is less at high altitude than at sea level because of the steeper slope of the oxygen dissociation curve. Very high altitudes, particularly associated with exercise, cause ventilation–perfusion inequality possibly because of the development of subclinical pulmonary edema. There is some evidence that gas exchange in the placenta is enhanced in residents of high altitude.

7.1 HISTORICAL

Some aspects of the effects of high altitude on pulmonary gas exchange, particularly the hyperventilation and the cyanosis, have been recognized ever since the early days of the balloonists. For example, in 1804, the eminent French scientist Louis Joseph Gay-Lussac ascended to an altitude of what was thought to be 7020 m in a balloon and reported that his breathing was difficult, and his pulse and respiration were high. There were also reports of discoloration of the hands and face presumably the result of cyanosis. In fact, during the ill-fated flight of the *Zénith* referred to in Chapter 1, Tissandier reported that Sivel's face was black. On the other hand, the early balloonists did not complain as much about difficulties with breathing including breathlessness as did high altitude climbers, and this is consistent with the fact that acute hypoxia does not result in as large a ventilatory response as prolonged hypoxia, as we shall see below.

Early mountain climbers were well aware of the shortness of breath at high altitudes. During an early ascent of Mont Blanc by the Swiss physicist Horace-Bénédict de Saussure in 1787, he complained that 'the rarity of the air gave me more trouble than I could have believed. At last I was obliged to stop for breath every 15 or 16 steps . . . .' In fact, on the summit he complained that he was 'constantly forced to interrupt my work and devote myself entirely to breathing.' The eminent climber Edward Whymper, during the first ascent of Chimborazo (6420 m) in 1880, gave a colorful description of shortness of breath stating that:

we were unable to satisfy our desire for air, except by breathing with open mouths. . . . Besides having our normal rate of breathing largely accelerated, we found it impossible to sustain life every now and then giving spasmodic gulps, just like fishes when taken out of water.

Some of the most striking accounts of breathlessness at high altitude came from the early expeditions to Mount Everest. For example, in 1924, at an altitude of about 8380 m, E.F. Norton stated that:

our pace was wretched. My ambition was to do twenty consecutive paces uphill without a pause to rest and pant elbow on bent knee; yet I never remember achieving it – thirteen was nearer the mark.

His companion T. Howard Somervell was even more breathless stating 'From taking three or four breaths to a step we were reduced to having to take ten or more.' Finally, Reinhold Messner, who with Peter Habeler made the first ascent of Everest without supplementary oxygen in 1978, stated when he was on the summit 'I have nothing more to do than breathe. . . . I am nothing more than a single, narrow, gasping lung.'

It is remarkable that in spite of so many anecdotal accounts of hyperventilation at high altitude, some of the most eminent physiologists claimed that it did not occur. For example, Paul Bert stated that hyperventilation does not occur at high altitude and wrote:

what is really certain is that . . . a dweller in lofty altitudes, does not even try to struggle against the decrease of oxygen in his arterial blood by speeding up his respiration successively, as was first supposed. The observations of Dr. Jourdanet are conclusive.

(Bert 1878)

Possibly this error can be traced to the fact that Bert worked exclusively with low pressure chambers that only allowed short-term observations of the effects of acute hypoxia. However, even Angelo Mosso, who had the advantage of studying long-term residents at the Capanna Margherita, reported that although respiratory frequency was increased at high altitude, total ventilation was decreased. He reached this erroneous conclusion because he converted the volumes to standard conditions (0°C and 1000 mmHg in his case) rather than to body temperature and pressure, saturated with water vapor (BTPS).

Turning now to the role of diffusion in pulmonary gas exchange, the controversy over oxygen secretion constitutes one of the most colorful episodes in the history of high altitude medicine. The debate was briefly alluded to in Chapter 1. An early proponent of the secretion hypothesis was the Danish physiologist Christian Bohr. In a paper published in 1891 he compared the P_{O_2} and P_{CO_2} of alveolar gas with that of gas in a tonometer equilibrated with arterial blood taken at the same time (Bohr 1891). In some instances the alveolar P_{O_2} was found to be as much as 30 mmHg below, and the P_{CO_2} as much as 20 mmHg above, the arterial blood values. Bohr's conclusion was: 'In general, my experiments have shown definitely that the lung tissue plays an active part in gas exchange; therefore the function of the lung can be regarded as analogous to that of the glands.' Bohr referred to the secretion ability of the lung as its 'specific function', and claimed that the active secretion of oxygen and carbon dioxide by the lung could use large amounts of oxygen, up to 60% of the total requirements of the body.

August Krogh was one of Bohr's students and assisted him in his experiments on gas secretion from 1899 to 1908. However, Krogh gradually became persuaded that passive diffusion rather than active secretion could account for the experimental data and in 1910 published a landmark paper on this topic. Since Bohr was his major professor and very jealous of the secretion theory, the introductory section of Krogh's paper required an unusually delicate touch. Part of it reads:

> I shall be obliged in the following pages to combat the views of my teacher Prof. Bohr on certain essential points. . . . I wish here not only to acknowledge the debt of gratitude which I, personally, owe to him, but also to emphasize the fact . . . that the real progress, made during the last twenty years in the knowledge of the processes in the lungs, is mainly due to his labours. . . .

The British physiologist J.S. Haldane visited Bohr in Copenhagen and also became convinced of the secretion theory, at least as far as oxygen was concerned. For example, in 1897, Haldane and Lorraine Smith (1897) wrote: 'The absorption of oxygen by the lungs thus cannot be explained by diffusion alone.' Haldane argued that oxygen secretion would be particularly beneficial at high altitudes, and in order to test the hypothesis the Anglo-American expedition to Pikes Peak was organized in 1911. Arterial P_{O_2} was calculated by an indirect method following the inhalation of carbon monoxide, and the results appeared to strongly support the secretion hypothesis. However, the theory was also attacked by Marie Krogh (wife of August) when she developed a method for measuring the diffusing capacity of the lung using

small concentrations of carbon monoxide. Her results indicated that the normal lung was capable of transferring very large amounts of oxygen by passive diffusion even when the inspired P_{O_2} was greatly reduced.

Another physiologist who did not accept the secretion story was Joseph Barcroft. He conducted a heroic experiment on himself by living in a sealed glass chamber filled with hypoxic gas for 6 days (Barcroft et al. 1920). His left radial artery was exposed 'for an inch-and-a-half' and blood was taken for measurements of oxygen saturation. There was a 'somewhat dramatic moment' when the first blood sample was drawn because it 'looked dark'. Measurements on the blood then showed that diffusion was the only mechanism necessary for oxygen transfer across the blood-gas barrier during hypoxia.

Barcroft and his colleagues subsequently tested the secretion hypothesis further on the International High Altitude Expedition to Cerro de Pasco (4330 m) in the Peruvian Andes in 1921–22. The diffusing capacity of the lung for carbon monoxide was measured on five members of the expedition both at sea level and at Cerro de Pasco, and only a small increase was found. Barcroft therefore argued that the tendency for the arterial oxygen saturation to fall during exercise at high altitude could be explained by the failure of equilibration of P_{O_2} between alveolar gas and pulmonary capillary blood (Barcroft et al. 1923). This was one of the first direct demonstrations of diffusion limitation of oxygen at high altitude, a finding that has been confirmed many times since.

It is remarkable that J.S. Haldane remained a staunch supporter of oxygen secretion all his life. In the second edition of his book *Respiration*, written with J.G. Priestley and published in 1935, a year before Haldane's death, a whole chapter was devoted to evidence for oxygen secretion (Haldane and Priestley 1935). Haldane gradually shifted his position as evidence mounted against the secretion hypothesis. He initially thought that oxygen secretion occurred under all conditions, but later argued that it only became significant at high altitude, and later still that it only occurred after a period of acclimatization. His obsession with this theory seems strange to us now, but

Haldane was something of a vitalist, believing that not all the phenomena of living creatures could be fully explained by classical chemistry and physics (Sturdy 1988).

7.2 EFFECTS OF HYPERVENTILATION ON GAS EXCHANGE

The most important feature of pulmonary gas exchange at high altitude is the increase in alveolar ventilation and its consequences. The importance of hyperventilation is emphasized if we look at its role at extreme altitude, for example on the summit of Mount Everest. First, we need to refer to two simple equations governing pulmonary gas exchange. The first is the alveolar ventilation equation:

$$\dot{V}_A = \frac{\dot{V}_{CO_2}}{PA,co_2} \times K$$

where $\dot{V}_A$ is alveolar ventilation, $\dot{V}_{CO_2}$ is the CO_2 production, and PA,co_2 is the alveolar partial pressure of carbon dioxide. This equation states that if the rate of CO_2 production is constant, the alveolar ventilation and alveolar Pco_2 are inversely related. For example, if the alveolar ventilation is doubled, the Pco_2 is halved.

The second equation is the alveolar gas equation:

$$PA,o_2 = PI,o_2 - \frac{PA,co_2}{R} + F$$

where PA,o_2 and PA,co_2 are the alveolar partial pressures of oxygen and carbon dioxide, respectively; PI,o_2 is the inspired partial pressure of oxygen; R is the respiratory exchange ratio; and F is a correction factor that is generally small during air breathing.

At sea level the normal alveolar ventilation equation results in an alveolar Pco_2 of about 40 mmHg. If we insert this value into the alveolar gas equation, assuming an inspired Po_2 of 150 and a normal respiratory exchange ratio at rest of 0.8, the alveolar Po_2 is given by

$$150 - \frac{40}{0.8} = 100 \text{ mmHg}$$

Now suppose we apply this equation to a climber on the summit of Mount Everest where the barometric pressure is, say, 250 mmHg (see Fig. 2.2). The Po_2 of moist inspired gas is given by

$$PI,o_2 = 0.2904(P_B - 47)$$

where 0.2094 is the fractional concentration of oxygen, P_B is the barometric pressure, and 47 mmHg is the water vapor partial pressure. This gives an inspired Po_2 of about 43 mmHg. If we now assume that both the alveolar ventilation and the CO_2 production of the climber at rest are unchanged compared with sea level, his alveolar Pco_2 is 40 mmHg. The alveolar gas equation then gives an alveolar Po_2 of

$$43 - \frac{40}{0.8} = -7 \text{ mmHg}$$

which, of course, is absurd. However, if the climber now increases his alveolar ventilation five-fold thus reducing his alveolar Pco_2 to 8 mmHg, the alveolar gas equation gives

$$PA,o_2 = 43 - \frac{8}{0.8} = 33 \text{ mmHg}$$

While this value is very low, it is just sufficient to maintain life. This simple calculation shows the crucial importance of hyperventilation at high altitude. The mechanism of the hyperventilation is hypoxic stimulation of the peripheral chemoreceptors as discussed in Chapter 6.

7.3 ACUTE HYPOXIA COMPARED WITH ACCLIMATIZATION

There is a striking difference between the degree of hyperventilation that occurs when subjects are exposed acutely to hypoxia on the one hand, and when they are acclimatized to high altitude on the other. One of the classical studies was performed

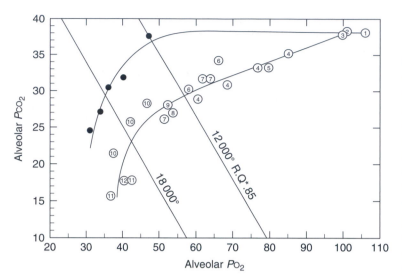

Figure 7.1   Oxygen–carbon dioxide diagram showing the alveolar gas composition in subjects acutely exposed to high altitude (upper line) and after acclimatization (lower line). The two diagonal lines are for a respiratory exchange ratio (RQ) of 0.85 for altitudes of 12 000 ft (3660 m) and 18 000 ft (5490 m). The numbers in the circles show the sources of the data (see original article). (From Rahn and Otis 1949.)

by Rahn and Otis (1949) and their original results are shown in Fig. 7.1. The data on subjects exposed acutely to high altitude (upper line) were obtained using low pressure chambers. The data for the acclimatized line come from a number of sources including lowlanders who spent various periods at a given altitude, and in some cases permanent residents at high altitudes.

It can be seen that with acute exposure to high altitude there is typically no change in alveolar P_{CO_2}, which implies no change in alveolar ventilation, up to an altitude of about 12 000 ft or about 3600 m. By contrast, acclimatized subjects show a fall in alveolar P_{CO_2} indicating an increase in alveolar ventilation for any increase in altitude. Note that altitude itself is not shown explicitly on the graph but the intersection of the diagonal RQ lines with the lower horizontal axis indicates the inspired P_{O_2} which falls as altitude increases.

In Fig. 7.2 the P_{O_2} data are redrawn so that they are now plotted against altitude.

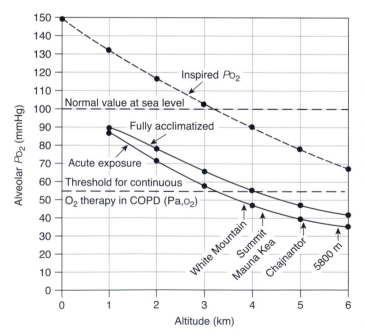

Figure 7.2   Alveolar P_{O_2} at high altitudes following acute exposure (lower line) and full acclimatization (upper line). The values come from the measurements shown in **Fig. 7.1** and there is considerable individual variation. The altitudes of several observatories where astronomers work are also shown. Note that fully acclimatized astronomers on the summit of Mauna Kea (4200 m) have an alveolar P_{O_2}, and therefore an arterial P_{O_2}, lower than the accepted threshold for continuous oxygen therapy in patients with chronic obstructive pulmonary disease (COPD) at sea level.

This plot shows more clearly the relentless fall in alveolar P_{O_2} with increasing altitude for both acute exposure and full acclimatization. However, acclimatization results in an increase in ventilation which lowers the alveolar P_{CO_2} and thus increases the alveolar P_{O_2} at any given altitude according to the alveolar gas equation shown earlier. The altitudes can be read off the horizontal axis and some important high altitude sites are identified. The summit of Mauna Kea in Hawaii at an altitude of 4200 m is the site of several large telescopes and many astronomers are exposed to this altitude. Additional telescopes are located on the Chajnantor plateau in north Chile at an altitude of 5050 m, including the extremely large radio telescope (Atacama Large Millimeter Array). Other high altitude sites near Chajnantor up to an altitude of 5800 m are being considered for astronomy.

Figure 7.2 emphasizes that, in spite of the hyperventilation that occurs at high altitude, severe alveolar hypoxia and therefore arterial hypoxemia may occur. As an example, astronomers on Mauna Kea, even if they are fully acclimatized, have an alveolar P_{O_2} on average less than 55 mmHg. Their arterial P_{O_2} will therefore be a little lower. Forster (1986) reported that the mean arterial P_{O_2} on the first day at 4200 m was 42 mmHg rising to 44 mmHg on day 5. The severity of the hypoxemia is further indicated by the fact that an arterial P_{O_2} of 55 or less is the accepted criterion for continuous oxygen administration at sea level if that degree of arterial hypoxemia is caused by chronic obstructive pulmonary disease. This emphasizes the severe hypoxemia that occurs even in fully acclimatized subjects at these altitudes. In fact, astronomers at Mauna Kea never become fully acclimatized because of the limited time they spend there.

Figures 7.1 and 7.2 emphasize the advantages of acclimatization in raising the alveolar P_{O_2} at high altitude. However, it is interesting that permanent residents of high altitude often have lower alveolar P_{O_2} values and higher alveolar P_{CO_2} values than fully acclimatized lowlanders. This is discussed in Chapter 6, section 6.15.1.

7.4 PHYSIOLOGY OF DIFFUSION IN THE LUNG

7.4.1 Fick's law of diffusion

Fick's law of diffusion states that the rate of transfer of a gas through a sheet of tissue is proportional to the area of the tissue and to the difference in gas partial pressure between the two sides, and inversely proportional to the tissue thickness. The area of the blood-gas barrier in the human lung is some 50–100 m^2, and the thickness is less than 0.3 µm in many places, so the dimensions of the barrier are well suited to diffusion.

In addition, the rate of gas transfer is proportional to a diffusion constant which depends on the properties of the tissue and the particular gas. The constant is proportional to the solubility of the gas and inversely proportional to the square root of its molecular weight. This means that carbon dioxide diffuses about 20 times more rapidly than oxygen through tissue sheets since its solubility is about 24 times greater at 37°C and the molecular weights of carbon dioxide and oxygen are in the ratio of 1.375 to 1.

Fick's law can be written as

$$\dot{V}_{gas} = \frac{A}{T} D (P_1 - P_2)$$

where $\dot{V}$ is volume of gas per unit time, A is area, T is thickness, D is the diffusion constant, and P_1 and P_2 denote the two partial pressures.

For a complex structure such as the blood-gas barrier of the human lung, it is not possible to measure the area and thickness during life. Instead, we combine A, T and D and rewrite the equation as

$$\dot{V}_{gas} = D_L (P_1 - P_2)$$

where D_L is the diffusing capacity of the lung.

The gas of choice for measuring the diffusing capacity of the lung is carbon monoxide (at very low concentrations) because the affinity of this gas for hemoglobin is so great that the partial pressure in the capillary blood is extremely small (except in smokers) and thus the uptake of the gas is solely limited by the diffusion properties of the blood-gas barrier. (The complication caused by finite reaction rates is considered below.) Thus if we rewrite the above equation as

$$D_L = \frac{\dot{V}_{CO}}{P_1 - P_2}$$

where P_1 and P_2 are the partial pressures of alveolar gas and capillary blood, respectively, we can set P_2 to zero. This leads to the equation for measuring the diffusing capacity of the lung for carbon monoxide:

$$D_L = \frac{\dot{V}_{CO}}{PA,co}$$

In words, the diffusing capacity of the lung for carbon monoxide is the volume of carbon monoxide transferred in mL min⁻¹ mmHg⁻¹ of alveolar partial pressure.

7.4.2 Reaction rates with hemoglobin

Early workers assumed that all of the resistance to the transfer of oxygen from the alveolar gas into the capillary blood could be attributed to the diffusion process within the blood-gas barrier. However, when the rates of reaction of oxygen with hemoglobin were measured using a rapid reaction apparatus, it became clear that the rate of combination with hemoglobin might also be a limiting factor. If oxygen is added to deoxygenated blood, the formation of oxyhemoglobin is quite fast, being well on the way to completion in 0.2 s. However, oxygenation occurs so rapidly in the pulmonary capillary that even this rapid reaction significantly delays the loading of oxygen by the red cells and can be regarded as a resistance. Thus the uptake of oxygen can be regarded as occurring in two stages:

1. Diffusion of oxygen through the blood-gas barrier (including the plasma and red cell interior)
2. Reaction of the oxygen with hemoglobin (Fig. 7.3)

In fact, it is possible to sum the two resulting resistances to produce an overall resistance (Roughton and Forster 1957).

We saw above that the diffusing capacity of the lung is defined as

$$D_L = \frac{\dot{V}_{gas}}{P_1 - P_2}$$

that is, the flow of gas divided by the pressure difference. It follows that the inverse of D_L is pressure difference divided by flow and is therefore analogous to electrical resistance. Consequently, the resistance of the blood-gas barrier in Fig. 7.3 is shown as $1/D_M$ where M denotes membrane. The rate of reaction of oxygen with hemoglobin can be described by θ, which gives the rate in mL min⁻¹ of oxygen which combine with 1 mL blood mmHg⁻¹ P_{O_2}. This is analogous to the 'diffusing capacity' of 1 mL of blood and, when multiplied by the volume of capillary blood (V_c), gives the effective 'diffusing capacity' of the rate of reaction of oxygen with hemoglobin. Again its inverse, $1/(\theta V_c)$, describes the resistance of this reaction.

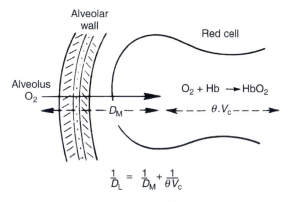

Figure 7.3 The measured diffusing capacity of the lung (D_L) is made up of two components, one due to the diffusion process itself (D_M), and one attributable to the time taken for oxygen to react with hemoglobin (θV_c).

It is possible to add the resistances offered by the membrane and the blood to obtain the total resistance. Thus the complete equation is

$$\frac{1}{D_{\mathrm{L}}} = \frac{1}{D_{\mathrm{M}}} + \frac{1}{\theta V_{\mathrm{C}}}$$

In practice, the resistances offered by the membrane and blood components are approximately equal in the normal lung.

7.4.3 Rate of oxygen uptake along the pulmonary capillary

By using Fick's law of diffusion, and data on reaction rates of oxygen with hemoglobin, it is possible to calculate the time course of P_{O_2} along the pulmonary capillary as the oxygen is loaded by the blood. The application of Fick's law to this situation is not trivial because of the chemical bond which forms between oxygen and hemoglobin. This means that the relationship between P_{O_2} and oxygen concentration in the blood is nonlinear, as shown by the oxygen dissociation curve. This problem was first solved by Bohr (1909) and the numerical integration procedure which he developed is known as the Bohr integration. A further complication occurs because, as oxygen is being taken up, carbon dioxide is given off, and this alters the position of the oxygen dissociation curve. A full treatment of this latter process should take into account not only the rate of diffusion of carbon dioxide through the blood-gas barrier, but also the rates of reaction of carbon dioxide in blood. Since not all the rate constants are known under all the required conditions, some assumptions and simplifications are necessary.

Figure 7.4 shows a typical time course calculated for the lung of a resting subject at sea level (Wagner and West 1972; West and Wagner 1980). The diffusing capacity of the blood-gas barrier itself (D_{M}) was assumed to be 40 mL min^{-1} mmHg^{-1}, and the time spent by the blood in the pulmonary capillary was taken as 0.75 s (Roughton 1945). Other assumptions include a resting cardiac output of 6 L min^{-1} and oxygen uptake of 300 mL min^{-1}.

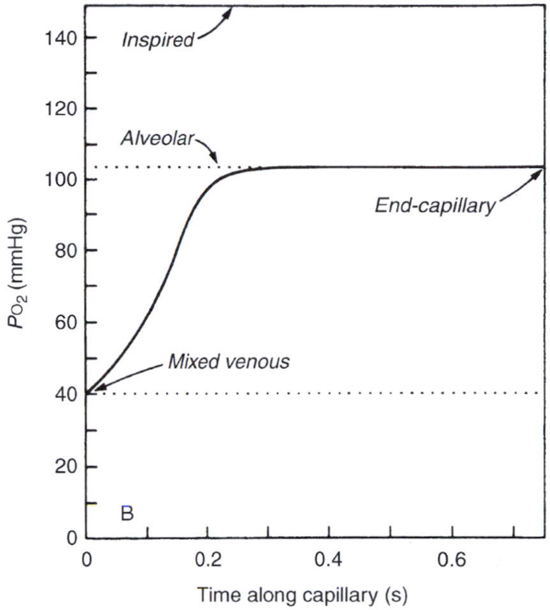

Figure 7.4   Calculated time course for P_{O_2} in the resting human pulmonary capillary at sea level. Note that there is ample time for equilibration of the P_{O_2} between alveolar gas and end-capillary blood. $\dot{V}_{O_2}$ 300 mL min^{-1}; D_{M,O_2} 40 mL min^{-1} mmHg^{-1}. (From West and Wagner 1980.)

Note that the blood comes into the lung with a P_{O_2} of 40 mmHg and the P_{O_2} rapidly rises to almost the alveolar P_{O_2} level by the time the blood has spent only about one-third of its available time in the capillary. The rate of rise of P_{O_2} in the latter two-thirds of the capillary is extremely slow, and there is a negligible P_{O_2} difference between alveolar gas and end-capillary blood.

This time course can be contrasted with that calculated for a resting climber breathing air on the summit of Mount Everest (Fig. 7.5). Again, the membrane diffusing capacity of the blood-gas barrier was assumed to be 40 mL min^{-1} mmHg^{-1} based on measurements made on acclimatized lowlanders at an altitude of 5800 m (West 1962a). The oxygen uptake was taken to be 350 mL min^{-1}, and other blood and alveolar gas variables were taken from measurements made on the American Medical Research Expedition to Everest (West *et al.* 1983b). The time spent by the blood in the pulmonary capillary was assumed to be unchanged at 0.75 s because this is determined

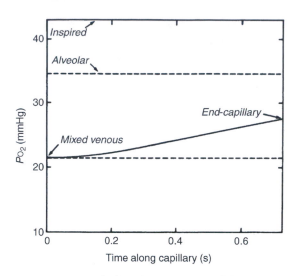

Figure 7.5 Calculated time course of the Po_2 along the pulmonary capillary for a climber at rest on the summit of Mount Everest. Note that there is considerable diffusion limitation of oxygen uptake with a large alveolar end-capillary Po_2 difference. P_B 253 mmHg; $\dot{V}_{O_2}$ 350 mL min^{-1} (From West *et al.* 1983b.)

by the ratio of capillary blood volume to cardiac output (Roughton 1945). The capillary blood volume was shown to be unchanged at 5800 m (West 1962a), and the cardiac output is also the same as at sea level according to the measurements of Pugh (1964c) (Chapter 8, section 8.3).

It can be seen that the oxygen profile is very different at this extreme altitude. The blood comes into the lung with a Po_2 of only about 21 mmHg, and the Po_2 rises very slowly along the pulmonary capillary, reaching a value of only about 28 mmHg at the end. Thus there is a large Po_2 difference of some 7 mmHg between alveolar gas and capillary blood. This indicates marked diffusion limitation of oxygen transfer. It can be shown that this diffusion limitation becomes more striking as the oxygen consumption is increased by exercise. Diffusion limitation at extreme altitude is discussed further in section 7.6.

The very different time courses for Po_2 shown in Figs 7.4 and 7.5 represent the extremes between sea level and the highest point on Earth for resting humans. At intermediate altitudes, the difference between alveolar and end-capillary Po_2 will be considerably reduced at rest and may be negligibly

small. However, exercise at high altitude will always tend to cause diffusion limitation of oxygen transfer as originally demonstrated by Barcroft *et al.* (1923).

Whether carbon dioxide elimination is ever limited by diffusion is still unknown. This is partly because some of the reaction rates of carbon dioxide in blood remain uncertain.

7.4.4 Diffusion and perfusion limitation of oxygen transfer

It is clear from Fig. 7.4 that a resting subject at sea level has no diffusion limitation of oxygen transfer because there is no Po_2 difference between alveolar gas and end-capillary blood. Under these conditions, the amount of oxygen which is taken up by the blood is determined by the pulmonary blood flow. This means that oxygen uptake is perfusion limited.

By contrast, Fig. 7.5 shows a situation where oxygen uptake is, in part, diffusion limited. This is indicated by the large Po_2 difference between alveolar gas and end-capillary blood. However, under these conditions, oxygen uptake is also partly perfusion limited because increasing pulmonary blood flow will increase oxygen uptake, other things being equal.

At first sight, the substantial diffusion limitation of oxygen transfer shown in Fig. 7.4 might be attributed to the low alveolar Po_2, and therefore the smaller driving gradient for oxygen diffusion. However, this is not correct. The conditions under which diffusion and perfusion limitation occur have been clarified by Piiper and Scheid (1980). They used a simplified model with several assumptions including linearity of the oxygen dissociation curve in the working range. This situation is approached during conditions of severe hypoxia when the lung is operating very low on the oxygen dissociation curve.

Using this simplified model, Piiper and Scheid showed that the total transfer rate $\dot{M}$ of a gas is given by the expression

$$\dot{M} = (P_A - P_V)\,\dot{Q}\beta\left[1 - \exp\left(\frac{-D}{\dot{Q}\beta}\right)\right]$$

where P_A and P_V are the partial pressures of oxygen in the alveolar gas and venous blood, respectively,

$\dot{Q}$ is cardiac output, D is the diffusing capacity, and β is the slope of the oxygen dissociation curve (assumed to be linear). The total conductance, G, for gas exchange between alveolar gas and capillary blood may be defined as the transfer rate divided by the total effective partial pressure difference $(P_A - P_V)$, or

$$G = \dot{Q}\beta \left[1 - \exp\left(\frac{-D}{\dot{Q}\beta}\right) \right]$$

This expression clarifies the factors responsible for diffusion and perfusion limitation. The equation shows that if D is very much larger than $\dot{Q}\beta$, the expression inside the large brackets tends to 1, and gas transfer is limited by perfusion only. In this case, the (perfusive) conductance is given by $G = \dot{Q}\beta$. The relative difference between the conductance without diffusion limitation and the actual conductance is an index of diffusion limitation, L_{diff} as shown in Fig. 7.6.

By contrast, diffusion limitation occurs if $\dot{Q}\beta$ is so large that it greatly exceeds D, or to put it in another way, D becomes relatively very small. In this case the (diffusive) conductance is given by $G = D$. The relative difference between the conductance without perfusion limitation and the actual conductance is an index of perfusion limitation. Zero on the vertical axis of Fig. 7.6 indicates complete perfusion limitation.

Figure 7.6 shows that oxygen uptake is entirely perfusion limited in hyperoxia (extreme right of diagram) and that this is also true for the uptake of inert gases (those that do not combine with hemoglobin) such as nitrogen and sulfur hexafluoride. However, oxygen transfer during hypoxia becomes diffusion limited to some extent (middle of diagram) and this is particularly the case during exercise when oxygen consumption is greatly increased. For carbon monoxide, gas transfer is essentially diffusion limited under all conditions (left of diagram).

The above analysis emphasizes that an important factor leading to diffusion limitation is an increase in β; that is, the slope of the blood-gas dissociation curve. This is the reason why the uptake of carbon monoxide is entirely diffusion limited; the slope of its dissociation curve is extremely large. An increased slope of the oxygen dissociation curve tending to diffusion limitation occurs for three reasons at high altitude:

1. The lung is working on a low part of the oxygen dissociation curve which is very steep.
2. The polycythemia of high altitude increases the change in blood oxygen concentration per unit change in P_{O_2}.

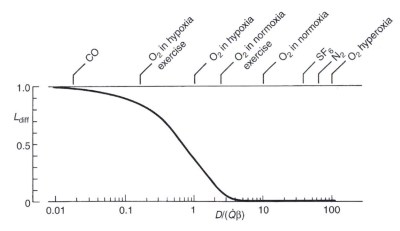

Figure 7.6   Conditions under which diffusion limitation of gas transfer in the lung occurs. L_{diff} is a measure of diffusion limitation; when its value is 1.0, gas transfer is entirely diffusion limited. It can be seen that L_{diff} is greatest for carbon monoxide, and least for oxygen under hyperoxic conditions. D, diffusing capacity; $\dot{Q}$, pulmonary blood flow; β, solubility of the gas in blood, or slope of its dissociation curve. See text for details. (Modified from Piiper and Scheid 1980.)

3. The left shift of the curve caused by the respiratory alkalosis increases its slope. In fact, at extreme altitude, oxygen begins to resemble carbon monoxide to some extent.

For readers who prefer an intuitive explanation to the more formal analysis given above, the essential conclusion can be stated as follows. Diffusion limitation is likely when the 'effective solubility' of the gas in pulmonary capillary blood (that is, the slope of the dissociation curve) greatly exceeds the solubility of the gas in the tissues of the blood-gas barrier. This condition is met for carbon monoxide which has an enormous affinity for hemoglobin, and is approached for oxygen at high altitude because of the steepness of its dissociation curve at low Po_2 values, and the increased blood hemoglobin concentration.

An analogy is the rate at which sheep can enter a field through a gate. If the gate is narrow but the field is large, the number of sheep that can enter in a given time is limited by the size of the gate. This is the situation at high altitude because the steepness of the oxygen dissociation curve allows a lot of oxygen to be loaded for a small rise in arterial Po_2. However, if both the gate and the field are small (or both are big) the number of sheep is limited by the size of the field. This is the case at sea level.

7.4.5 Oxygen affinity of hemoglobin and diffusion limitation

It can be shown that increasing the affinity of hemoglobin for oxygen expedites the loading of oxygen in the pulmonary capillary under conditions of diffusion limitation at high altitude. The oxygen affinity of hemoglobin is conveniently expressed by the P_{50}, that is the Po_2 for 50% saturation of the hemoglobin. The normal value for adult human hemoglobin is about 27 mmHg.

Numerical analysis shows that increasing the affinity (leftward shift of the oxygen dissociation curve) results in more rapid equilibration between the Po_2 of alveolar gas and pulmonary capillary blood. A simplified way of looking at this is that the left-shifted curve keeps the blood Po_2 low

in the initial stages of oxygen loading and thus maintains a large Po_2 difference between alveolar gas and capillary blood during much of the oxygenation time. This increased Po_2 difference therefore maintains the driving pressure and accelerates loading.

However, a left-shifted oxygen dissociation curve interferes with the unloading of oxygen in peripheral capillaries because, for a given Po_2 in venous blood (required to maintain the diffusion head of pressure to the tissues), the blood unloads less oxygen. It is therefore not intuitively obvious whether the advantages of a left-shifted curve in assisting the loading of oxygen in the pulmonary capillaries outweigh the disadvantages of unloading the oxygen in the peripheral capillaries.

Several pieces of evidence suggest that a high oxygen affinity of hemoglobin is beneficial under hypoxic conditions. For example, the llama and vicuna, animals native to the Peruvian highlands, have left-shifted oxygen dissociation curves (Fig. 7.7), as do some burrowing animals whose environment becomes oxygen depleted (Hall *et al.* 1936). The human fetus, which is believed to have

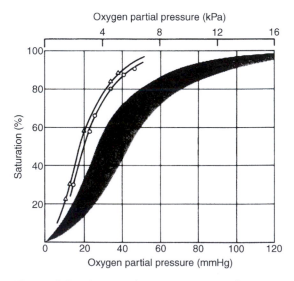

Figure 7.7 Oxygen dissociation curves for blood of llama (circle) and vicuna (triangle) compared with other mammals. The left-shifted curve for these high altitude native animals indicates an increased affinity of the hemoglobin for oxygen which assists in oxygen loading along the pulmonary capillaries. (From Hall *et al.* 1936.)

arterial P_{O_2} in the descending aorta of less than 25 mmHg, has a greatly increased oxygen affinity by virtue of its fetal hemoglobin which has a P_{50} at pH 7.4 of about 17 mmHg. Experimental studies have shown that rats with artificially left-shifted oxygen dissociation curves tolerate severe acute hypoxia better than rats with normal dissociation curves (Eaton *et al.* 1974). Again, Hebbel *et al.* (1978) described a family in which two of the four children had an abnormal hemoglobin (Andrew-Minneapolis) with a P_{50} of 17 mmHg. These two siblings had a higher $V_{O_2,max}$ at an altitude of 3100 m than the two with normal hemoglobin.

Numerical modeling gives some basis for these findings by showing that the increased oxygen affinity of the hemoglobin improves oxygenation in the pulmonary capillaries under conditions of diffusion limitation more than it interferes with the release of oxygen by peripheral capillaries (Bencowitz *et al.* 1982). Table 7.1 lists some of the strategies used by animals (including humans) to increase the oxygen affinity of their hemoglobin under hypoxic conditions.

Climbers at very high altitude tend to have an increased arterial blood pH, which causes a leftward shift of the oxygen dissociation curve. This is caused by a respiratory alkalosis which is only partially compensated and was the case for

Table 7.1 Strategies for increasing oxygen affinity in chronic hypoxia

Strategy	Subject
Different sequence in globin chain	Human fetus, bar-headed goose, toadfish
Decrease in red cell 2,3-DPG	Fetus of dog, horse, pig
Decrease in ATP	Trout, eel
Different hemo-globin, small Bohr effect	Tadpole
Mutant hemoglobin (Andrew-Minneapolis)	Family in Minnesota
Respiratory alkalosis	Climber at extreme altitude

2,3-DPG, 2,3-diphosphoglycerate; ATP, adenosine triphosphate.

members of the 1981 American Medical Research Expedition to Everest who spent several weeks at an altitude of 6300 m. The mean arterial pH of three subjects was 7.47 (Winslow *et al.* 1984), which is well above the normal range.

At extreme altitudes, there is an extraordinary degree of respiratory alkalosis. For example, when Pizzo took alveolar gas samples on the summit of Mount Everest, there is good evidence that his arterial pH exceeded 7.7. This value is based on a measured alveolar P_{CO_2} of 7.5 mmHg, and a base excess measured in venous blood taken on the following morning of -5.9 mmol L^{-1}. This extreme respiratory alkalosis would cause a marked leftward shift of the oxygen dissociation curve with a calculated *in vivo* P_{50} of about 19 mmHg. Thus a climber on the summit of Mount Everest develops conditions rather similar to those in the human fetus where the arterial P_{O_2} is less than 30 mmHg and the P_{50} is less than 20 mmHg.

7.5 PULMONARY DIFFUSING CAPACITY AT HIGH ALTITUDE

7.5.1 Acclimatized lowlanders

Barcroft and his colleagues measured the diffusing capacity for carbon monoxide in five members of the expedition to Cerro de Pasco in the Peruvian Andes in 1921–22. They used the single breath method which had recently been described by Krogh (1915) and the measurements were made at rest. There was no consistent change from the sea level values though the investigators believed that there was a slight tendency for the diffusing capacity to rise. They pointed out, however, that this change would not be an important element in acclimatization (Barcroft *et al.* 1923). Subsequent investigators have confirmed the absence of change or found only a very small (less than 10%) increase in diffusing capacity for carbon monoxide in resting subjects after periods of up to several months at altitudes of up to 4560 m (Kreuzer and van Lookeren Campagne 1965; DeGraff *et al.* 1970; Guleria *et al.* 1971; Dempsey *et al.* 1978).

Measurements on exercising subjects at altitudes up to 5800 m showed that after 7–10 weeks of acclimatization, there was an increase in pulmonary diffusing capacity of 15–20% (Fig. 7.8). However, this small change could be wholly accounted for by the increased rate of reaction of carbon monoxide with hemoglobin due to hypoxia and by the increased blood hemoglobin concentration (West 1962a).

The mechanism of this increase can be explained by reference to Fig. 7.3. The 'resistance' attributable to the rate of combination of oxygen with hemoglobin is given by $1/(\theta V_c)$ where θ is the rate of reaction of carbon monoxide with hemoglobin, and V_c is the volume of blood in the pulmonary capillaries. It has been found experimentally that the value of θ varies depending on the ambient P_{O_2}. At low P_{O_2} values, θ is increased and therefore the resistance to oxygen transfer is decreased. An additional factor is the increased blood hemoglobin concentration which, for a given value of V_c, increases the amount of hemoglobin present. Thus these factors completely accounted for the small observed increase in diffusing capacity for carbon monoxide at high altitude and indicated that there was no change in the diffusion properties of the lung itself after 7–10 weeks of acclimatization at an altitude of 5800 m.

The diffusing capacity for carbon monoxide at high altitude has been shown to be reduced in subjects with acute mountain sickness (AMS) (Ge et al. 1997). The measurements were made 2 days after arrival at 4700 m. The subjects with AMS also showed a lower vital capacity and arterial P_{O_2}, and an increased alveolar–arterial P_{O_2} gradient (based on arterialized capillary blood) than subjects without AMS. The mechanism was thought to be subclinical pulmonary edema. In another study, subjects with a history of high altitude pulmonary edema (HAPE) were found to have a lower diffusing capacity for carbon monoxide during hypoxia and exercise than a HAPE-resistant group (Steinacker et al. 1998). The HAPE-susceptible group also had smaller increases in stroke volume, cardiac output and ventilation during exercise. Enhanced pulmonary vasoconstriction was suggested as the mechanism of the lower diffusing capacity.

Interestingly, the diffusing capacity measured during submaximal exercise was reduced following a Himalayan expedition to 4900 m and above compared with measurements made prior to the expedition (Steinacker et al. 1996). The fall in diffusing capacity was about 14% and this was accompanied by a reduction in cardiac index of about 16% and $\dot{V}_{O_2,max}$ of about 5%. A possible explanation was the wasting of skeletal muscle which resulted in a reduced cardiac output and therefore diffusing capacity on exercise.

In a recent study, Agostini et al. (2011) measured the diffusing capacity for carbon monoxide $D_{L_{CO}}$ and its components D_M and V_c on 33 lowlanders before and after a 9-day trek to the Everest Base Camp, altitude 5400 m, and 2 weeks of residence there. There were increases in $D_{L_{CO}}$, D_M and alveolar volume, but no change in V_c. A surprising finding was an average increase in D_M, normalized for alveolar volume, from 10.9 to 16.0 mL min^{-1} $mmHg^{-1}$. The authors suggested that this might be due to increased sympathetic tone. The results seem to be at variance with most previous studies.

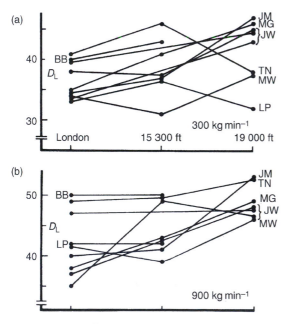

Figure 7.8 Diffusing capacities (D_L) in mL min^{-1} $mmHg^{-1}$ measured at sea level (London), 15 300 ft (4700 m) and 19 000 ft (5800 m) in acclimatized lowlanders exercising at: (a) 300 kg min^{-1} and (b) 900 kg min^{-1}. Note the moderate increase in diffusing capacity of carbon monoxide with altitude. (From West 1962.)

7.5.2 Highlanders

Several studies have shown that people who live permanently at high altitude (high altitude natives or highlanders) have pulmonary diffusing capacities that are about 20–50% higher than the predicted values for lowlanders, or compared with lowlander controls (Fig. 7.9). One of the first investigations was by Velásquez (1956) who studied 12 native residents of Morococha (altitude 4550 m) and showed that the diffusing capacity for oxygen was consistently higher than in similar subjects at sea level. Remmers and Mithoefer (1969) found that Andean Indians at an altitude of 3700 m had a diffusing capacity for carbon monoxide which was some 50% higher than predicted. High diffusing capacities have also been reported in Caucasians living at an altitude of 3100 m (DeGraff *et al.* 1970; Dempsey *et al.* 1978). The increased diffusing capacities were demonstrated both during rest and exercise.

A potential problem in such studies is the appropriateness of the predicted values for diffusing capacity. For example, in the study by Remmers and Mithoefer (1969), predicted values were obtained from Caucasian North Americans and were applied to the South American high altitude Indian population. This may introduce errors because of ethnic differences in body build. However, in other studies, such as that by Dempsey *et al.* (1971), diffusing capacities were compared between lowlanders and highlanders in similar ethnic groups (Fig. 7.9).

The increased diffusing capacities can presumably be explained by the larger lungs which result in an increased alveolar surface area and capillary blood volume. Barcroft *et al.* (1923) commented on the remarkably large chest development of the Peruvian natives in Cerro de Pasco and these early investigators made chest radiographs to confirm this. The radiographs showed that the ratio of chest width to height was greater in the high altitude natives than in the Anglo-Saxon lowlanders (expedition members). Children who are raised at altitudes of 3000 m have been shown to have increased lung volumes and diffusing capacities (de Meer *et al.* 1995). It has also been shown experimentally that

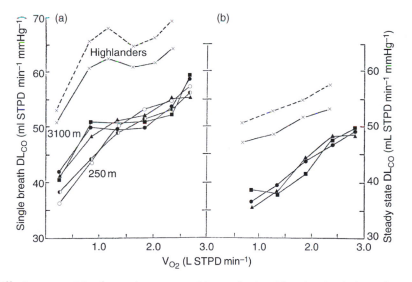

Figure 7.9 Diffusing capacities for carbon monoxide as obtained by the single breath method (a) and steady-state method (b) in three groups of subjects: lowlanders at 250 m (open circle and half-filled circle), lowlanders sojourning at 3100 m (closed circle, triangle and square indicate different periods at this altitude), and native highlanders at 3100 m. The broken line indicates the measured data for highlanders; the continuous line shows the results after correction for $1/\theta$. All the measurements are on Caucasians, the 3100 m data being from Leadville, Colorado. Note the higher diffusing capacities of the highlanders both at rest and on exercise. (From Dempsey *et al.* 1971.)

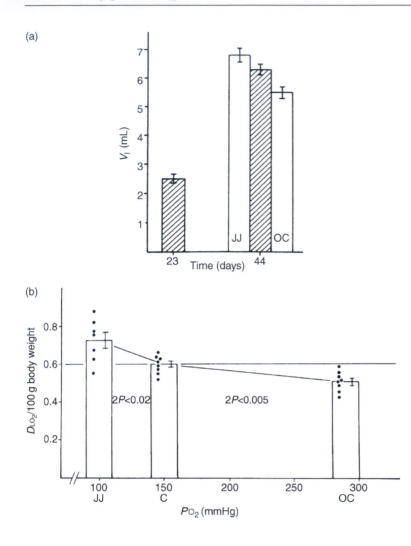

Figure 7.10 (a) Increase in lung volume V_l from day 23 to day 44 of life in three groups of rats exposed to an altitude of 3450 m (JJ), sea level (cross-hatched), and 40% oxygen at sea level (OC). Note that lung volume increased most in the hypoxic and least in the hyperoxic animals. (b) Pulmonary diffusing capacity estimated morphometrically in the same three groups of animals at the 44th day. Note that the diffusing capacities reflected the changes in lung volume. C shows a control group. (From Burri and Weibel 1971.)

animals exposed to low oxygen partial pressures during their active growth phase develop larger lungs and bigger diffusing capacities than animals reared in a normoxic environment (Fig. 7.10) (Bartlett and Remmers 1971; Burri and Weibel 1971). Beagles raised at an altitude of 3100 m had higher diffusing capacities and lung tissue volume than a control group at sea level (Johnson et al. 1985). In a subsequent study on foxhounds, it was shown that exposure of pups to 3800 m for only 5 months resulted in higher diffusing capacities in the adults (McDonough et al. 2006). These studies provide an adequate explanation for the observed high diffusing capacities, and would also account for the persistence of an increased diffusing capacity for carbon monoxide in highlanders after a prolonged period spent

at sea level as observed by Guleria et al. (1971). However, Lechner et al. (1982) presented evidence that the lungs only grow faster in a hypoxic environment and the end result is the same lung volume as in normoxic animals. This discrepancy is unresolved.

The impact of pregnancy on the diffusing capacity for carbon monoxide was measured in pregnant and nonpregnant Peruvian women by McAuliffe et al. (2003). One group lived at sea level and the other at 4300 m. The diffusing capacities were corrected for the hemoglobin concentration. At sea level, the diffusing capacities of pregnant and nonpregnant women were similar though smaller than those of the women at high altitude consistent with the results discussed earlier.

7.6 DIFFUSION LIMITATION OF OXYGEN TRANSFER AT HIGH ALTITUDE

One reason for the importance of pulmonary diffusion at high altitude is that it may be a limiting factor in oxygen uptake and therefore exercise ability. A considerable amount of evidence now supports this.

One of the first groups to suggest diffusion limitation of oxygen uptake at altitude was Barcroft and his colleagues (Barcroft *et al.* 1923). They concluded from their measurements of pulmonary diffusing capacity for carbon monoxide at an altitude of 4300 m, that P_{O_2} equilibration between alveolar gas and the blood at the end of the capillary was not achieved, especially on exercise. Subsequently, Houston and Riley (1947) measured alveolar–arterial P_{O_2} differences in four subjects who spent 32 days in a low pressure chamber in which the pressure was gradually reduced from 760 to 320 mmHg (Operation Everest I). Measurements were made during rest and during relatively low levels of exercise (oxygen uptakes less than 1200 mL min^{-1} at simulated high altitude). During exercise, the alveolar–arterial P_{O_2} difference was increased to about 10 mmHg, which they correctly ascribed to diffusion limitation.

During the Silver Hut Expedition of 1960–61, measurements of arterial oxygen saturation by ear oximetry were made on five subjects who lived for 4 months at an altitude of 5800 m ($P_B = 380$ mmHg) in a prefabricated hut. The average arterial oxygen saturation at rest was 67% and this fell at work levels of 300 and 900 kg m min^{-1} to 63 and 56%, respectively (West *et al.* 1962). The progressive fall in arterial oxygen saturation as the work level was raised occurred in the face of an increasing alveolar P_{O_2} and was strong evidence for diffusion limitation of oxygen transfer. Alveolar–arterial differences were calculated and nine measurements at the maximal exercise level gave a mean P_{O_2} difference of 26 mmHg with a standard deviation of 4 mmHg. Calculations based on the Bohr integration procedure showed that the results were consistent with a maximum pulmonary diffusing capacity for oxygen of about 60 mL min^{-1} mmHg^{-1}.

Further evidence for diffusion limitation of oxygen transfer during exercise at very high altitudes was obtained on the 1981 American Medical Research Expedition to Everest. Fifteen subjects spent up to 4 weeks at an altitude of 6300 m ($P_B = 350$ mmHg) and arterial oxygen saturation was measured by oximeter at rest and during increasing levels of work (Fig. 7.11). Again, there was a progressive fall in arterial oxygen saturation as the work level was increased from rest to 1200 kg min^{-1}, equivalent to an oxygen consumption of about 2.3 L min^{-1}. The calculated alveolar–arterial P_{O_2} difference at this highest work level was 21 mmHg (West *et al.* 1983c).

Figure 7.11 also shows that additional measurements were made with subjects breathing 16% and 14% oxygen at this very high altitude. The latter gave an inspired P_{O_2} of 42 mmHg, equivalent to that encountered by a climber breathing air on the summit of Mount Everest. Note the very abrupt fall in arterial oxygen saturation as work rate was increased at the inspired P_{O_2} of the highest altitude on Earth. Two subjects performed maximum exercise while

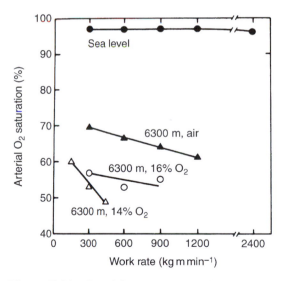

Figure 7.11 Arterial oxygen saturation as measured by ear oximetry plotted against work rate at sea level and 6300 m altitude. The two lower lines were obtained with subjects breathing 16% and 14% oxygen at 6300 m. Note the fall in oxygen saturation with work rate at high altitude. (From West *et al.* 1983c.)

breathing 14% oxygen and in one of them the oximeter reading fell to less than 10% oxygen saturation at one point during the experiment! Although the calibration of the oximeter at such values is unreliable, the actual saturation must have been extremely low.

7.7 VENTILATION/PERFUSION INEQUALITY

Ventilation/perfusion inequality is a major cause of impaired gas exchange at sea level in lung diseases such as chronic obstructive pulmonary disease, interstitial lung disease and acute respiratory failure. At high altitude, ventilation/perfusion inequality also becomes important in the presence of lung disease caused, for example, by high altitude pulmonary edema or pulmonary thromboembolism.

In the absence of obvious lung disease, ventilation/perfusion inequality generally plays a minor role at high altitude. In fact, there is some evidence that the topographical inequality of ventilation/perfusion ratios is actually improved by ascent. The reason is that the increase in pulmonary artery pressure caused by hypoxic pulmonary vasoconstriction causes a more uniform distribution of blood flow in the lung (Dawson 1972) and, other things being equal, this will improve the relationships between ventilation and blood flow. However, the degree of ventilation/perfusion inequality in the normal lung caused by the topographical differences of ventilation and blood flow is so small that this must be a minor effect.

There is evidence that ventilation/perfusion inequality can develop at extreme altitude especially on exercise. These measurements were made by Wagner and his colleagues in a simulated ascent of Mount Everest (Operation Everest II). The measurements of ventilation/perfusion inequality were made using the multiple inert gas elimination technique (Wagner *et al.* 1974). Inert gas exchange is not diffusion-limited, even during maximal exercise.

Figure 7.12 shows the increase in ventilation/perfusion inequality caused both by increasing altitude and increasing work level in the 40-day

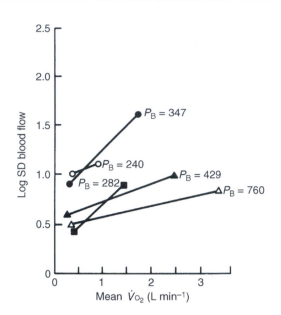

Figure 7.12 Relationship between the degree of ventilation/perfusion inequality in the lung and oxygen uptake in subjects during a simulated ascent of Mount Everest in a low pressure chamber (Operation Everest II). The ordinate shows the log SD of blood flow which is a measure of ventilation/perfusion inequality. Note that both a reduction of barometric pressure (P_B, measured in mmHg) and increase in work rate tended to increase the degree of ventilation/perfusion inequality. (From Wagner *et al.* 1987.)

low pressure chamber experiment (Wagner *et al.* 1987). The vertical scale shows the mean log standard deviation of the blood flow distribution which is one measure of the degree of ventilation/perfusion inequality. It can be seen that this index was about 0.5 during rest at sea level but increased slightly when the oxygen consumption was raised to over 3 L min^{-1} during exercise at sea level. At very high altitude, where the barometric pressure was 347 mmHg, the standard deviation at rest rose to approximately 0.9 and it increased further to over 1.5 with exercise. The explanation of these intriguing data is uncertain but may be subclinical pulmonary edema. There was also evidence that rapid ascent was more likely to result in ventilation/perfusion inequality than slow ascent, suggesting that inadequate acclimatization may have been an important factor. It is now known that both subclinical and alveolar edema can occur in some human athletes, even at sea level. For a review see Hopkins (2010).

Using these independent measurements of the amount of ventilation/perfusion inequality present, it was possible to separate the contribution of diffusion limitation and ventilation/perfusion inequality to the observed increase of the alveolar–arterial P_{O_2} difference at high altitude. The results are shown in Fig. 7.13. The arterial P_{O_2} was directly measured on arterial blood samples. It can be seen that the measured alveolar–arterial P_{O_2} difference increased to a mean of about 13 mmHg during maximal exercise at a barometric pressure of 347 mmHg where the oxygen consumption was a little over 2 L min^{-1}. At higher simulated altitudes, the maximum alveolar–arterial P_{O_2} differences were smaller. This can be explained by the smaller maximum oxygen uptakes, and the fact that the subjects were operating on the lower, steeper region of the oxygen dissociation curve.

Also shown in Fig. 7.13 are the predicted alveolar–arterial P_{O_2} differences for the degree of ventilation/perfusion inequality measured at the same time by means of the multiple inert gas elimination technique. These predicted P_{O_2} differences decreased as the altitude increased despite the broadening of the distributions of ventilation/perfusion ratios as shown in Fig. 7.11. Again, the reason is that the P_{O_2} values are lower on the oxygen dissociation curve where its slope is steeper. The data allow the total alveolar–arterial P_{O_2} difference to be divided into two components, one caused by ventilation/perfusion inequality, and the rest presumably attributable to diffusion limitation. The results show that, at sea level, essentially all of the alveolar–arterial P_{O_2} difference was attributable to ventilation/perfusion inequality up to an oxygen consumption of nearly 3 L min^{-1}. Above that high exercise level, some diffusion limitation apparently occurred. By contrast, at a barometric pressure of 429 mmHg, the measured alveolar–arterial P_{O_2} difference exceeded that predicted from the amount of ventilation/perfusion inequality when the oxygen uptake was above about 1 L min^{-1}. This was also true at a barometric pressure of 347 mmHg. At the higher simulated altitudes, with barometric pressures of 282 and 240 mmHg, almost all of the observed alveolar–arterial P_{O_2} difference during exercise could be ascribed to diffusion limitation.

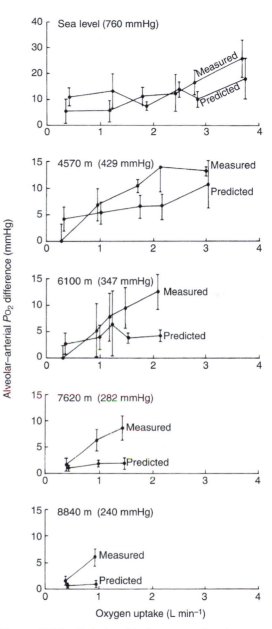

Figure 7.13   Relationship between alveolar–arterial P_{O_2} difference and the oxygen uptake in Operation Everest II (compare Fig. 7.12). The predicted difference refers to that calculated from the measured amount of ventilation/perfusion inequality. Note that, at the highest altitudes, the measured differences considerably exceeded the predicted values, indicating diffusion limitation of oxygen uptake. For the measurements at 240 mmHg, the subjects breathed an oxygen mixture to give an inspired P_{O_2} of 43 mmHg. (From Wagner *et al.* 1987.)

These elegant studies beautifully elucidate the role of diffusion in the hypoxemia of high altitude during exercise.

7.8 DIFFUSION IN THE PLACENTA AT HIGH ALTITUDE

The fetus derives its oxygen via the placenta rather than the lung. Gas exchange in the placenta is much less efficient than in the lung and, for example, the P_{O_2} in the descending aorta of the human fetus at sea level is believed to be less than 25 mmHg. The fetus must be even more hypoxic at high altitude and it is known that birth weight is reduced at high altitude, and that smaller birth weights at high altitude are associated with increased infant morbidity and mortality (Lichty et al. 1957; Moore et al. 1998a).

An interesting question is whether the diffusion properties of the placenta are improved at high altitude, just as the diffusing capacity of the lung in high altitude natives is apparently raised. There is some evidence for this. Reshetnikova et al. (1994) examined 10 normal term placentas from women in Kyrghyzstan up to altitudes of 2800 m and found that there was an increase in capillary volume, and that the harmonic mean thickness of the maternal–fetal barrier fell from 6.9 μm in controls to 4.8 μm at high altitude. They calculated that the morphometric diffusing capacity of the villous membrane for oxygen was significantly increased, by about 80%. Zhang et al. (2002) reported that in human placentas at high altitude, the small blood vessels were dilated and were less frequently associated with perivascular cells than in an ethnically matched lowland population. Other evidence of structural differences at high altitude was obtained by Tissot van Patot et al. (2003) who showed that fetal capillary density increased at 3100 m compared with 1600 m. However, Mayhew (1991) found somewhat different results in placentas from populations living at 3600 m compared with 400 m altitude in Bolivia. Although there was some improvement in diffusion properties on the maternal side of the placenta, these did not extend to the fetal side. In another study, no differences were found in capillary surface area or length, and it was concluded that high altitude pregnancy is not accompanied by increased angiogenesis (Mayhew 2003).

8

Cardiovascular system

SUMMARY

Important changes in the cardiovascular system occur at high altitude. Cardiac output increases following acute exposure to high altitude, but in acclimatized lowlanders and high altitude natives, most measurements show the cardiac output for a given work rate is the same as at sea level. Nevertheless, because of the polycythemia, hemoglobin flow is increased.

Heart rate at rest and for a given work rate is higher than at sea level, with the result that stroke volume is reduced at high altitude. However, this is not caused by reduced myocardial contractility; on the contrary, this is preserved up to very high altitudes in normal subjects. Abnormal heart rhythms, such as premature ventricular or atrial contractions, are unusual despite the severe hypoxemia. However, sinus arrhythmia accompanying periodic breathing is very common at high altitude.

Changes in systemic blood pressure are variable. Generally, there is a small increase in pressure during the first few days at altitude and several studies report an increase when lowlanders move to high altitude. However, in some instances patients with hypertension at sea level have developed a reduction in pressure on ascent to altitude.

Pulmonary hypertension is striking at high altitude, in both newcomers and high altitude natives, particularly on exercise. Tibetans have smaller degrees of pulmonary hypertension than other highlanders. This is also the case in some animals native to high altitude. The hypertension is relieved by oxygen breathing when the exposure to high altitude is acute, but after a few days the response to oxygen is less presumably because of vascular remodeling. Right ventricular hypertrophy and corresponding electrocardiographic changes are seen. Newborn infants sometimes develop right heart failure at high altitude and this also occurs in young soldiers stationed at extreme altitudes.

8.1 INTRODUCTION

The cardiovascular system is an essential link in the transport of oxygen from the air to the mitochondria, and it therefore has an important role in acclimatization and adaptation to the oxygen-depleted environment of high altitude. However, some aspects of the cardiovascular system at high altitude have not been as extensively studied as their importance may suggest. One reason for this is the difficulties of measurement, especially the invasive investigations necessary to reliably measure cardiac output and pulmonary artery pressure. However, echocardiographic assessment of tricuspid regurgitation is increasingly used to estimate systolic pulmonary artery pressure.

In this chapter we look at available data on many aspects of the cardiovascular system, although, as will be seen, there are still many areas of ignorance.

8.2 HISTORICAL

Early travelers to high altitudes frequently complained of symptoms related to the cardiovascular system. Many of these accounts were collected by Paul Bert and set out in the first chapter of his classical book *La Pression Barométrique* (Bert 1878, p. 29 in the 1943 translation). For example, he quotes the great explorer Alexander von Humboldt at an altitude of 2773 'fathoms' (about 5070 m) on Chimborazo in the South American Andes complaining that 'blood issued from our lips and eyes'. Many other travelers gave accounts of bleeding from the mouth, eyes and nostrils, and they often attributed this to the low barometric pressure which, they argued, did not balance the pressures within the blood vessels. This is fallacious reasoning because all vascular pressures fall along with the ambient atmospheric pressure (Chapter 2, section 2.1). These early reports of bleeding are intriguing because this is not a typical feature of mountain sickness as we see it today.

Another common complaint of these early mountain travelers was cardiac palpitations, especially on exercise. Typical is the passage quoted by Bert (Bert 1878, p. 37 in 1943 translation) from the explorer D'Orbigny who stated when he was on the crest of the Cordilleras that 'at the least movement, I felt violent palpitations'. The most observant travelers measured their pulse rate and noted that mild exercise such as horse riding caused it to increase dramatically although it was normal at rest. Cloves of garlic were frequently eaten to relieve these symptoms, which often seem exaggerated to the modern reader.

An interesting historical vignette was the occurrence of peripheral edema in cattle while grazing at high altitude in Utah and Colorado early in the twentieth century (Hecht *et al.* 1962). The condition is known as brisket disease because the edema is most prominent in that part of the animal between the forelegs and neck (brisket). The condition is caused by right heart failure as a result of severe pulmonary hypertension caused by hypoxic pulmonary vasoconstriction. Right heart failure also occurs in some newborn infants at high altitude, especially in Han children born in Tibet (Sui *et al.* 1988). A somewhat similar condition has been described in Indian soldiers stationed at very high altitudes near the border with Pakistan (Anand *et al.* 1990). These conditions are further discussed in Chapter 22.

Early climbers on Mount Everest who became fatigued were sometimes diagnosed as having 'dilatation' of the heart. This was thought to be one of the signs of failure to acclimatize. As late as 1934, Leonard Hill stated that 'degeneration of the heart and other organs due to low oxygen pressure in the tissues, is a chief danger which the Everest climbers have to face' (Hill 1934).

8.3 CARDIAC FUNCTION

8.3.1 Cardiac output

It is generally accepted that acute hypoxia causes an increase in cardiac output both at rest and for a given level of exercise compared with normoxia. These responses are seen at sea level following inhalation of low oxygen mixtures, and on acute exposure to high altitude (Asmussen and Consolazio 1941; Keys *et al.* 1943; Honig and Tenney 1957; Kontos *et al.* 1967; Vogel and Harris 1967). There is also evidence that, in well-acclimatized lowlanders at high altitude, the relationship between cardiac output and work rate returns to the sea level value (Pugh 1964d; Reeves *et al.* 1987). On the other hand, there is some uncertainty about the changes following short periods of acclimatization.

Perhaps the first systematic studies of cardiac output at high altitude were made by Douglas, Haldane and their colleagues (Douglas *et al.* 1913) on the Anglo-American Pikes Peak Expedition where they made measurements on themselves by means of ballistocardiography. No consistent changes in stroke volume of the heart were noted. They therefore concluded that cardiac output at rest was proportional to heart rate, which they showed increased over the first 11 days at 4300 m and subsequently decreased towards normal. Barcroft and his colleagues (Barcroft *et al.* 1923) used an indirect Fick technique to measure cardiac output in their study of themselves at Cerro de Pasco in the Peruvian Andes at an altitude of 4330 m. They reported essentially no difference in acclimatized subjects compared with sea level.

Grollman (1930) made an impressive series of measurements on Pikes Peak in 1929 using the acetylene rebreathing method. He reported that resting cardiac output increased soon after reaching high altitude, with a maximum value approximately 5 days later. However, by day 12 it had returned to its sea level value. Similar changes were found by Christensen and Forbes (1937) during the International High Altitude Expedition to Chile.

More recent investigators have reported similar findings. Figure 8.1 shows the increase in resting cardiac output during the first 40 hours of acute exposure to simulated high altitude (Vogel and Harris 1967). Klausen (1966) found an increase in cardiac output following ascent to an altitude of 3800 m but after 3–4 weeks it had returned to its sea level value. Similar findings were reported by Vogel and his colleagues (Vogel *et al.* 1967) on Pikes Peak at an altitude of 4300 m. However, Alexander *et al.* (1967) reported a decrease in cardiac output during exercise after 10 days at 3100 m compared with sea level. The decrease was caused by a fall in stroke volume. Reductions in cardiac output (compared with sea level) after several days at high altitude were also reported by Wolfel *et al.* (1994) and Sime *et al.* (1974).

In well-acclimatized lowlanders at high altitude, and in high altitude natives, cardiac output in relation to work level is the same as at sea level. Pugh (1964d) showed this relationship during the Silver Hut Expedition at an altitude of 5800 m where the measurements were made by the acetylene rebreathing technique (Fig. 8.2). Further measurements were made by Cerretelli (1976a) at the Everest Base Camp where the subjects had acclimatized for 2–3 months. Reeves *et al.* (1987) reported the same finding on subjects during Operation Everest II where a remarkable series of measurements was made, using cardiac catheter studies in a hypobaric chamber, down to an inspired PO_2 of 43 mmHg, equivalent to that of the Everest summit (Fig. 8.3). Similar results were found in Operation Everest III (COMEX '97) (Boussuges *et al.* 2002). Since the maximal work level is greatly reduced at high altitude it

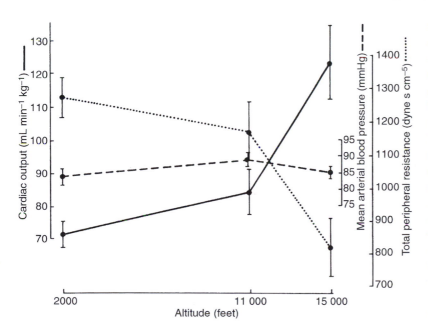

Figure 8.1 Cardiac output (solid line), mean systemic arterial pressure (dashed line), and calculated peripheral resistance (dotted line) during acute exposure to a simulated altitude of 2000 ft (610 m), 11 000 ft (3353 m) and 15 000 ft (4572 m). Measurements were made on 16 subjects after 10, 20, 30 and 40 hours at each altitude. The results from the different altitude exposures were pooled. Mean ± SE indicated by vertical bars (1 dyne = 10^{-5} N). (From Vogel and Harris 1967.)

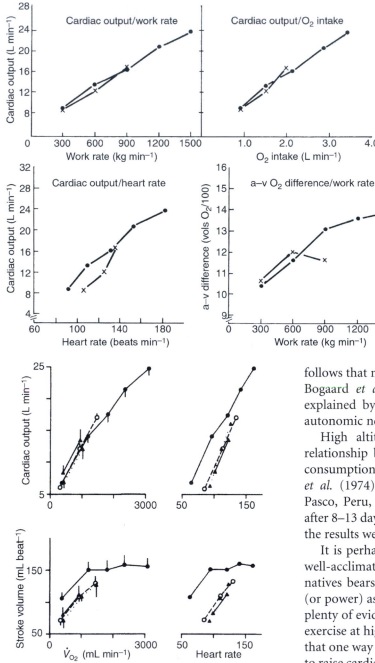

Figure 8.2 Cardiac output in relation to work rate and related variables as obtained from four well-acclimatized subjects during the Silver Hut Expedition. Note that the cardiac output/work rate relationship is the same at an altitude of 5800 m (×, barometric pressure 380 mmHg) as at sea level (●). (From Pugh 1964a.)

Figure 8.3 Cardiac output (by thermodilution) and stroke volume plotted against oxygen uptake ($\dot{V}_{O_2}$) and heart rate at barometric pressures of 760 (●, $n = 8$), 347 (○, $n = 6$), 282 (▲, $n = 4$) and 240 (▲, $n = 2$) mmHg during Operation Everest II. For the measurements at 240 mmHg, the subjects breathed an oxygen mixture to give an inspired P_{O_2} of 43 mmHg. (From Reeves et al. 1987.)

follows that maximal cardiac output is also lower. Bogaard et al. (2002) showed that this is not explained by alterations in the function of the autonomic nervous system.

High altitude natives also show the same relationship between cardiac output and oxygen consumption during exercise as at sea level. Vogel et al. (1974) studied eight natives of Cerro de Pasco, Peru, at an altitude of 4350 m and again after 8–13 days at Lima (sea level) and showed that the results were almost superimposable (Fig. 8.4).

It is perhaps surprising that cardiac output in well-acclimatized lowlanders and high altitude natives bears the same relationship to work rate (or power) as it does at sea level. After all, there is plenty of evidence of severe tissue hypoxia during exercise at high altitude, and at first sight it seems that one way of increasing the tissue P_{O_2} would be to raise cardiac output and thus peripheral oxygen delivery. However, in a theoretical study, Wagner (1996) argued that although increasing cardiac output improves calculated maximal oxygen consumption at sea level, the improvement becomes progressively less as altitude increases. In fact, calculations done for a subject on the summit of Mount Everest show that maximal oxygen consumption ($\dot{V}_{O_2,max}$) was essentially unchanged

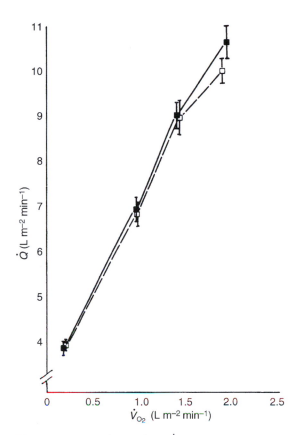

Figure 8.4 Cardiac index ($\dot{Q}$) against oxygen uptake ($\dot{V}O_2$) (both related to body surface area) in high altitude natives at 4350 m (□) and again after 8–13 days at sea level (■). (From Vogel *et al.* 1974.)

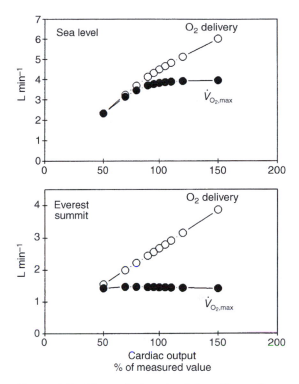

Figure 8.5 Theoretical study of the effects of changing cardiac output on maximal oxygen consumption ($\dot{V}O_{2,max}$) at sea level and at extreme altitude. Note that although $\dot{V}O_{2,max}$ improves at sea level, there is essentially no change at extreme altitude. This is explained by diffusion limitation in the lung and tissues. (From Wagner 1996.)

as cardiac output was increased from 50 to 150% of its expected value (Wagner 1996) (Fig. 8.5).

A similar picture emerged when hemoglobin concentration was varied between 50 and 150% of its expected value. Note that in the case of both cardiac output and hemoglobin concentration, calculated oxygen delivery to the tissues was greatly increased. The reason for the lack of improvement in $\dot{V}O_{2,max}$ with increases in cardiac output and hemoglobin concentration (and therefore oxygen delivery) is that diffusion impairment of oxygen, both in the lungs and in the muscles, reduces its availability. At medium altitudes, the calculated improvement in $\dot{V}O_{2,max}$ that accompanies an increase in cardiac output or hemoglobin concentration is intermediate between the values at sea level and extreme altitude. Reeves (2004) has also discussed the limited value of increasing cardiac output and

hemoglobin concentration at high altitude. Calbert *et al.* (2002) reported that the increase in hemoglobin concentration accompanying acclimatization to 5260 m did not increase $\dot{V}O_{2,max}$ or peak cardiac output.

Although cardiac output in relation to work level is unchanged in acclimatized subjects at high altitude, and in high altitude natives, hemoglobin flow is appreciably increased because of the polycythemia. As long ago as 1930, Grollman suggested that the return of cardiac output to its sea level value was related in some way to the increase in hemoglobin concentration of the blood (Grollman 1930).

8.3.2 Heart rate

Acute hypoxia causes an increase in heart rate both at rest and for a given level of exercise, just as is the case for cardiac output. The higher the altitude, the greater the increase in heart rate. At simulated altitudes of 4000–4600 m where acute exposure depresses the arterial Po_2 to 40–45 mmHg, resting heart rates increase by 40–50% above the sea level values (Kontos *et al.* 1967; Vogel and Harris 1967). Benoit *et al.* (2003) showed that when normal subjects are exposed to acute hypoxia, the lowest peak heart rates are seen in those people who have the lowest arterial oxygen saturations.

In acclimatized subjects at high altitude, resting heart rates return to approximately the sea level value up to an altitude of about 4500 m, although there is some individual variation (Rotta *et al.* 1956; Peñaloza *et al.* 1963). On exercise, heart rate for a given work rate or oxygen consumption exceeds the sea level value. Figure 8.6 shows comparisons of heart rate at sea level

and at an altitude of 5800 m in four subjects from the Himalayan Scientific and Mountaineering Expedition who had spent several months at that altitude (Pugh 1964d). It can be seen that the sea level values were generally lower than the high altitude measurements. However, in three of the four subjects the data points crossed at the highest work level that was tolerated at the high altitude. In other words, at the highest work level the heart rate was actually less than at sea level for the same power output. However, in every instance, this crossover was associated with a reduction in measured oxygen consumption, suggesting that at the high work rate, an increasing amount of work was being accomplished anaerobically.

Maximal heart rate, that is the heart rate at maximal exercise, is reduced in acclimatized subjects at high altitude. This is clearly seen from Fig. 8.6. In Operation Everest II, maximal

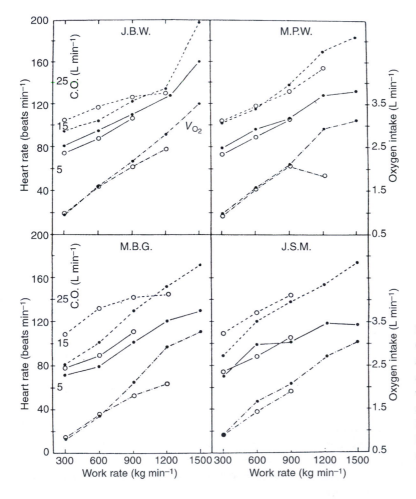

Figure 8.6 Heart rate (HR, – – –), cardiac output (CO, -), and oxygen uptake (Vo_2, -.-.) against work rate in four well-acclimatized subjects at an altitude of 5800 m. Measurements taken at sea level (●) and 5800 m (○, P_B 380 mmHg). (From Pugh 1964d.)

heart rates decreased from 160 ± 7 at sea level to 137 ± 4 at a simulated altitude of 6100 m, 123 ± 6 at 7620 m and 118 ± 3 at 8848 m (Reeves *et al.* 1987). For a given work level, heart rates were greater at high altitude compared with sea level, though, interestingly, there seemed to be little difference between the measurements made at barometric pressures of 347, 282 and 240 mmHg, as shown in Fig. 8.7. This is possibly a reflection of the limited degree of acclimatization of the subjects at the highest altitudes (West 1988a). The difference between field and chamber studies was emphasized by Lundby and van Hall (2001), who showed that although peak heart rate was reduced at an altitude of 8750 m on Mount Everest, the heart rates were considerably higher than found in chamber experiments. In Operation Everest III (Comex '97) maximal heart rates were also reduced compared with sea level values (Richalet *et al.* 1999). Lundby *et al.* (2001) confirmed that the peak heart rate fell as the altitude is increased.

Richalet (1990) has argued that the reduction of maximal heart rate in acclimatized subjects at high altitude represents a physiological

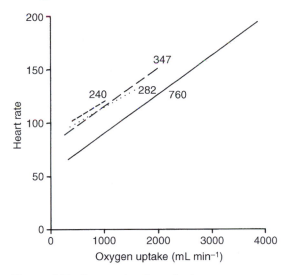

Figure 8.7 Regression lines for heart rate on oxygen uptake at barometric pressures of 760, 347, 282 and 240 mmHg during Operation Everest II. For the measurements at 240 mmHg, the subjects breathed an oxygen mixture to give an inspired P_{O_2} of 43 mmHg. (From Reeves *et al.* 1987.)

adaptation which reduces cardiac work under conditions of limited oxygen availability. There is good evidence that hypoxia induces downregulation of β-adrenergic receptors in animal hearts (Voelkel *et al.* 1981; Kacimi *et al.* 1992) and the role of the autonomic nervous system in controlling heart rate and cardiac output is well established. Short periods of exposure to hypoxia increase the plasma concentration of epinephrine and norepinephrine (Richalet 1990) and the increase in heart rate caused by hypoxia is abolished by beta-blockers (Kontos and Lower 1963). Mazzeo *et al.* (2003) emphasized the various roles of β-adrenergic stimulation in response to exercise at 4300 m. Lundby *et al.* (2001b) reported that dopamine D_2 receptors are not involved in the hypoxia-induced decrease in maximal heart rate.

However, the reduction of maximal heart rate in acclimatized subjects at high altitude can be interpreted differently. Since heart rate is actually increased both at rest and at a given work level compared with sea level (except perhaps at the highest work level; Fig. 8.6), it seems reasonable to regard the reduced maximal heart rate simply as a reflection of the reduced maximal work level. For example, it hardly makes sense that a climber on the summit of Mount Everest where the $\dot{V}_{O_2,max}$ is only about 1 L min^{-1} should have a maximal heart rate as high as the same person at sea level when the $\dot{V}_{O_2,max}$ is 4–5 L min^{-1}.

Oxygen breathing in acclimatized subjects at high altitude reduces the heart rate for a given work level (Pugh *et al.* 1964d). This is shown in Fig. 12.4 where it can be seen that the heart rate for a given work level was actually lower than the corresponding measurements at sea level. A possible explanation for the reduction below the sea level value is the fact that the arterial P_{O_2} at this altitude of 5800 m with 100% oxygen breathing is higher than at sea level, and also that these subjects had much higher hemoglobin levels than at sea level because of the high altitude polycythemia. It is known that heart rate for a given work rate at sea level is inversely related to hemoglobin concentration (Richardson and Guyton 1959).

8.3.3 Stroke Volume

Since stroke volume is determined by cardiac output divided by heart rate, its changes at high altitude can be deduced from those variables described in the last two sections.

Acute hypoxia causes approximately the same increase in cardiac output as in heart rate. The result is no consistent change in stroke volume. This is true for both rest and exercise (Vogel and Harris 1967).

After a few weeks' exposure to high altitude, the cardiac output response to work rate is the same as at sea level (Figs 8.2 and 8.3) but heart rate remains high (Figs 8.6 and 8.7). This means that stroke volume is reduced. The fall in stroke volume has been attributed to depression of myocardial function as a result of myocardial hypoxia (Alexander *et al.* 1967) but, as the next section shows, myocardial contractility is apparently well maintained up to extremely high altitudes in young healthy subjects. The reduction of stroke volume was also confirmed in Operation Everest II where it was shown that oxygen breathing did not increase stroke volume for a given pulmonary wedge or filling pressure. This suggested that the decline in stroke volume was not caused by severe hypoxic depression of contractility (Reeves *et al.* 1987). A possible contributing factor is a fall in plasma volume. A reduction in stroke volume during ascent was also well documented in Operation Everest III (Comex '97) (Boussuges *et al.* 2000). However, Calbert *et al.* (2004) found that plasma volume expansion did not increase maximal cardiac output or oxygen consumption in lowlanders acclimatized to an altitude of 5260 m.

Studies of high altitude natives at an altitude of 4350 m gave results similar to those found in acclimatized lowlanders. Cardiac output against oxygen consumption at high altitude was almost identical to the sea level measurements (Fig. 8.4), whereas heart rate was higher at high altitude and stroke volume was up to 13% less (Vogel *et al.* 1974).

8.3.4 Myocardial contractility

As indicated above, stroke volume is reduced at high altitude both in acclimatized lowlanders and in high altitude natives compared with sea level. The reduced stroke volume could be caused by either reduced cardiac filling or impaired myocardial contractility. A fall in filling pressures could result from either an increased heart rate or a reduction of circulating blood volume, or both.

During Operation Everest II, it was possible to measure both right atrial mean pressure (filling pressure for the right ventricle) and pulmonary wedge pressure (as an index of the filling pressure of the left ventricle). Both these measurements tended to fall as simulated altitude increased (Reeves *et al.* 1987). It was interesting that the right atrial pressures tended to be low despite pulmonary hypertension (section 8.5). In general, the relationship between stroke volume and right atrial pressure was maintained. This finding suggests maintenance of contractile function. In addition, as indicated above, oxygen breathing did not increase stroke volume for a given filling pressure, suggesting that the reduced stroke volume was not caused by hypoxic depression of contractility.

Additional evidence to support the finding of normal myocardial contractility came from a two-dimensional echocardiography study during Operation Everest II (Suarez *et al.* 1987). It was found that the ventricular ejection fraction, the ratio of peak systolic pressure to end-systolic volume, and mean normalized systolic volume at rest were all sustained at a barometric pressure of 282 mmHg, corresponding to an altitude of about 8000 m. Indeed, the surprising observation was made that during exercise at the level of 60 W, the ejection fraction was actually slightly higher (79% ± 2% compared with 69% ± 8%) at a barometric pressure of 282 mmHg compared with sea level. The conclusion was that, despite the decreased cardiac volumes, the severe hypoxemia and the pulmonary hypertension, cardiac contractile function appeared to be well maintained. Preservation of left ventricular contractility in spite of the severe hypoxia at simulated high altitude was also well documented in Operation Everest III (COMEX '97) using echocardiographic and Doppler techniques (Boussuges *et al.* 2000). Further confirmation of this finding was shown by Bernheim *et al.* (2007) even when the pulmonary artery pressure was grossly elevated by altitude in high altitude pulmonary edema (HAPE)-susceptible subjects. Their study involved a comparison of such subjects with controls at rest and on exercise, at sea level and altitude (4559 m). Using Doppler ultrasound, they showed that measures of left ventricular function were unchanged from sea level value, at altitude, even on exercise and even in HAPE-susceptible subjects whose RV pressure gradient at rest was 43 (± 9) mmHg.

However, a recent study from the Caudwell Xtreme Everest Expedition found that in 14 climbers studied with echocardiography before and immediately after return from Everest, there was evidence of diastolic dysfunction in that there was a reduction in peak left ventricular filling rates and mitral flow (Holloway et al. 2011). They also found a reduction in left ventricular muscle mass of 11% compared with a loss of body weight of 3%; though loss of total muscle mass was likely to have been greater (Chapter 15, section 15.4). In this study ^{31}P magnetic resonance was also used to measure cardiac phosphocreatine (PCr)/ATP (adenosine triphosphate) ratios. There was a reduction in this measure of cardiac energetics of 18%. Reduced cardiac PCr/ATP ratio was found by Hocharchka et al. (1996) in Sherpa subjects and by Weiss et al. (1990) in patients with coronary artery disease when exercising, suggesting that it is probably a universal response to hypoxia of cardiac muscle.

8.3.5 Abnormal rhythms

Abnormal rhythms (apart from sinus arrhythmia during periodic breathing) are uncommon at high altitude and perhaps this is surprising in view of the very severe arterial hypoxemia. A resting climber on the summit of Mount Everest has an arterial P_{O_2} of around 30 mmHg (West et al. 1983b; Sutton et al. 1988; Richalet 2010) or lower; Grocott et al. (2009) found a range from 29.5 to 19.1 (mean 24.5) mmHg in five climbers, 352 m below the summit. During exercise, the arterial P_{O_2} falls even further, principally because of diffusion limitation across the blood-gas barrier in the lung (West et al. 1983b; Sutton et al. 1988) (see Chapter 6). Thus the myocardium is exposed

to extremely low oxygen levels and it is known that the hypoxic myocardium is prone to rhythm abnormalities (Josephson and Wellens 1984).

In an electrocardiographic study of 19 subjects during the 1981 American Medical Research Expedition to Everest, only one subject had premature ventricular contractions and these were recorded at an altitude of 5300 m. Another climber showed premature atrial contractions at 6300 m (Karliner et al. 1985). One subject on the 1960–61 Silver Hut Expedition showed premature ventricular contractions after exercise at an altitude of 5800 m (Fig. 8.8). However, no other member of the expedition showed any dysrhythmia (Milledge 1963). Occasional premature ventricular contractions and premature atrial contractions have been observed by others (Cummings and Lysgaard 1981). One report suggests that cardiac arrhythmias may become more frequent with aging (Alexander 1999). Thus it appears that extreme hypoxia of the otherwise normal myocardium causes little abnormal rhythm, even at the most extreme altitudes. This conclusion is consistent with the maintenance of normal myocardial contractility even during the extreme hypoxia of very great altitudes (Reeves et al. 1987), as discussed in section 8.3.4.

There is a report that permanent inhabitants of mountainous regions (altitude 2800–4000 m) have a higher prevalence of cardiac arrhythmias than low altitude dwellers at rest. However, the rhythm disturbances were less on exercise (Mirrakhimov and Meimanaliev 1981). There are also studies in animals claiming that intermittent hypoxia protects the myocardium against ischemic arrhythmias (Meerson et al. 1987; Asemu et al. 1999).

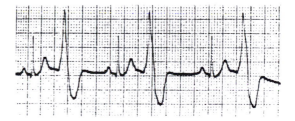

Figure 8.8 Electrocardiogram showing premature ventricular contractions occurring after exercise at 5800 m. (From Milledge 1963.)

Sinus arrhythmia accompanying the periodic breathing of sleep is very common at high altitude (Chapter 14). Indeed, the periodic slowing of the heart can be reliably used to identify the presence of periodic breathing at sea level (Guilleminault *et al.* 1984) and was used in this way with a Holter monitor to detect periodic breathing in climbers at an altitude of 8050 m during the American Medical Research Expedition to Everest (West *et al.* 1986). It is likely that the most extreme arterial hypoxemia for a given altitude occurs during the periodic breathing of sleep following the periods of apnea. It is not surprising that occasional premature ventricular and premature atrial contractions are then sometimes seen. For example, during the four sleep studies at 8050 m, one individual had occasional premature ventricular contractions, another had atrial bigeminy and a third had occasional premature atrial beats (Karliner *et al.* 1985).

A recent study by Woods *et al.* (2008) used implantable loop recorders in nine subjects on a trek in Nepal to over 6300 m. They found that above 5000 m all subjects showed sinus tachycardia and marked sinus arrhythmia on exercise. One subject had an episode of atrial flutter, one of non-conducted p waves and one marked ST depression. Of the seven episodes of arrhythmia reported, six occurred during climbing above 4300 m and the seventh was during strenuous exercise at 2800 m when the $S_a,_{O_2}$ was 84%. Prior to the expedition these subjects did some very strenuous hill walking in the UK and showed no arrhythmias at this low altitude. This is the first time that this type of recorder has been used in this sort of setting. It allows the capture of any arrhythmia over a period of many days, so the incidence of arrhythmia is low. However, the average age of these subjects was 30 years. One can only suppose that in more elderly subjects going to altitude the incidence will be higher and could possibly account for the occasional unexplained sudden death at high altitude.

8.3.6 Coronary circulation

The myocardium normally extracts a large proportion of the oxygen from the coronary arterial blood, with the result that the venous P_{O_2} has one of the lowest values of all organs in the body. Acute hypoxia has been shown to increase coronary blood flow in proportion to the fall in arterial oxygen concentration (Hellems *et al.* 1963). It is perhaps surprising therefore that coronary blood flow has been shown to be reduced in permanent residents of high altitude compared with people at sea level. Moret (1971) measured coronary flow in two groups of people at La Paz (3700 m) and Cerro de Pasco (4375 m) and compared them with a group at sea level. The flow per 100 g of left ventricle was some 30% less in the high altitude natives. A reduction of coronary blood flow of about the same magnitude in lowlanders 10 days after ascent to high altitude (3000 m) was found by Grover *et al.* (1970).

Despite this, there appears to be little evidence of myocardial ischemia in people living at high altitude (Arias-Stella and Topilsky 1971). These authors showed that casts of the coronary vessels had a greater density of peripheral ramifications than those of sea level controls. This might be part of the explanation for the apparent low incidence of angina and other features of myocardial ischemia.

8.4 SYSTEMIC BLOOD PRESSURE

Acute hypoxia (up to 40 hours at rest) causes essentially no change in the mean systemic arterial blood pressure in humans, at least up to altitudes of 4600 m (Kontos *et al.* 1967; Vogel and Harris 1967). This is in contrast to the dog, in which acute hypoxia results in a rise of mean arterial pressure (Kontos *et al.* 1967). However, when lowlanders move to high altitude there is frequently an increase in blood pressure for the first few weeks. In one study of 32 subjects who moved to an altitude between 3500 and 4000 m, 31 of them had an increase in resting blood pressure, and this persisted for some 3 weeks at altitude but returned to normal after descent (Kamat and Banerji 1972). In another study of four sea level residents who moved to an altitude of 4350 m, the mean arterial blood pressure rose from about 100 to about 128 mmHg after arrival and this persisted for 10 days (Vogel *et al.* 1974).

In a further report there was a rise in systemic blood pressure in 11 subjects who ascended to 4300 m and it was shown that propanolol given to some of the subjects reduced the rise in pressure suggesting that increased sympathetic activity was a causative factor (Wolfel *et al.* 1994).

In a group of 24 trekkers ascending to Everest Base Camp, the mean blood pressure rose from 130/80 at sea level to 140/90 at 5300 m (Levett *et al.* 2011).

In contrast to these increases in systemic blood pressure shortly after moving to high altitude, people who reside there for several years apparently have a decrease in both systolic and diastolic pressure (Marticorena *et al.* 1969; Hultgren 1970). These studies included 100 lowlanders who moved to altitudes of about 3800 to 4300 m for between 2 and 15 years. There is also a report that a stay of 1 year at an altitude of 4500 m resulted in a decrease of systemic systolic and diastolic pressures (Rotta *et al.* 1956).

There is some evidence that patients with systemic hypertension who move to high altitude are improved. Penaloza (1971) found that some patients with systemic hypertension who moved to an altitude of 3750 m had a reduction in their level of systemic blood pressure. This finding is consistent with a study of the prevalence of systemic hypertension at altitudes of 4100 to 4360 m in Peru, compared with two communities at sea level. This showed a prevalence of hypertension in men at least 12 times greater at sea level than at high altitude (Ruiz and Penaloza 1977). The difference was even more marked in women.

In high altitude natives living at 4350 m, Vogel *et al.* (1974) found that the mean brachial arterial blood pressure was consistently higher during exercise than in the same subjects at sea level. By contrast, the increase in mean systemic arterial pressure which occurs during the course of heavy exercise is apparently the same in acclimatized lowlanders as it is in sea level residents.

Syncope occasionally occurs at high altitude in otherwise healthy individuals (Nicholas *et al.* 1992; Perrill 1993; Freitas *et al.* 1996; Westendorp *et al.* 1997). This has been seen mainly in young adults, often within 24 hours of arrival at altitude, and commonly after a meal including alcohol. Imbalance of the sympathetic–parasympathetic systems is the probable cause.

8.5 PULMONARY CIRCULATION

8.5.1 Pulmonary hypertension

One of the most striking cardiovascular changes at high altitude is the occurrence of pulmonary hypertension caused by an increase in pulmonary vascular resistance. This is seen in subjects exposed to acute hypoxia, in acclimatized lowlanders at high altitude, and in most high altitude natives. The pulmonary hypertension of acute hypoxia is reversed by oxygen breathing, but this is not the case in acclimatized lowlanders or high altitude natives.

In normal subjects at sea level who are given low oxygen mixtures to breathe, mean pulmonary artery pressure almost always increases. In early studies, Motley *et al.* (1947) reported an increase of 13–23 mmHg as a result of breathing 10% oxygen in nitrogen for 10 minutes. This study followed the initial demonstration by von Euler and Liljestrand (1946) that the pulmonary arterial pressure in the cat increased when the animals breathed 10% oxygen. The increase in pulmonary vascular resistance is caused by vasoconstriction, mainly or solely as a result of contraction of smooth muscle in small pulmonary arteries.

Extensive studies of the effects of acute hypoxia on the pulmonary circulation have been made in humans and in a variety of animals. Figure 8.9 shows a typical study by Barer *et al.* (1970) in anesthetized cats in which the left lower lobe of the lung was made hypoxic and its blood flow was plotted against the alveolar P_{O_2}. Note the typical nonlinear stimulus–response curve. When the alveolar P_{O_2} was altered in the region above 100 mmHg, little change in blood flow and therefore vascular resistance was seen. However, when the alveolar P_{O_2} was reduced to approximately 70 mmHg, a marked increase in vascular resistance occurred, and at very low P_{O_2} values approaching those of mixed venous blood, the local blood flow was almost abolished.

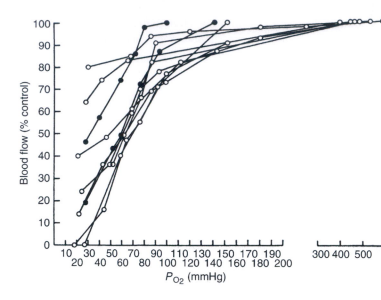

Figure 8.9 Blood flow from left lower lobe of open-chest anesthetized cats plotted against the P_{O_2} of the pulmonary venous blood from the lobe. The lobe was ventilated with different inspired gas mixtures while the rest of the lung was breathing air (○) or 100% oxygen (●). (From Barer *et al.* 1970.)

There are differences among species in the stimulus–response curves. Tucker and Rhodes (2001) carried out an extensive review of a series of species and noted that sheep and dogs typically have small responses whereas cattle and pigs have large increases in pulmonary artery pressure. The response is related to the degree of muscularization of the pulmonary arteries. Species that live at high altitudes, including yaks and pikas, are typically hypo-responders. In yaks there is evidence that augmented nitric oxide production is partly responsible for the low pulmonary vascular tone (Ishizaki *et al.* 2005).

In humans, the vasoconstrictor response to acute hypoxia shows considerable variation between individuals, leading Read and Fowler (1964) to refer to 'responders' and 'nonresponders'. Indeed, an attractive hypothesis is that hypoxic pulmonary vasoconstriction is vestigial in the adult and that its most important function occurs in the transition from placental to pulmonary gas exchange. Here there is a release of pulmonary vasoconstriction when the newborn baby starts to breathe air, and the circulation rapidly transforms from the fetal placental mode to the adult lung mode. Presumably this is where the primary evolutionary pressure for the phenomenon comes from.

Acclimatized lowlanders exhibit pulmonary hypertension at high altitude with a mean pulmonary arterial pressure increasing from its sea level value of about 12 mmHg to about 18 mmHg after 1 year at 4540 m (Rotta *et al.* 1956; Sime *et al.* 1974). This resting pulmonary arterial pressure increases considerably more during exercise. Figure 8.10 shows the relationship between mean pulmonary vascular pressure gradient across the lung (mean pulmonary arterial pressure minus pulmonary wedge pressure) and cardiac output in the subjects of Operation Everest II (Groves *et al.* 1987). Note that the resting values of the gradient (determined primarily by the mean pulmonary artery pressure) increased, but the most dramatic change was in the slope of the pressure gradient with respect to cardiac output. This indicates the striking increase in pulmonary vascular resistance at these great simulated altitudes.

High altitude Andean natives also show a substantial increase in mean pulmonary artery pressure during exercise. In one study, mean pulmonary artery pressure increased from 26 to 60 mmHg during exercise at an altitude of 4500 m (Sime *et al.* 1974). This was a greater increase than that found in acclimatized lowlanders.

In contrast to the dramatic effect of oxygen breathing in acute hypoxia, which causes pulmonary vascular resistance to return to its pre-hypoxic level, oxygen breathing has relatively little effect in acclimatized lowlanders and high altitude natives. For example, after the subjects had been exposed to low pressure for 2–3 weeks in Operation Everest II, 100% oxygen breathing resulted in a lower cardiac output and pulmonary artery pressure but there was no significant fall

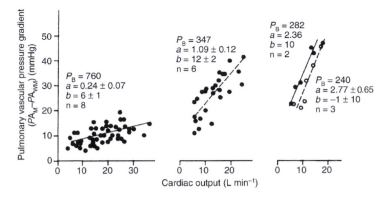

Figure 8.10 Mean pulmonary artery pressure (PA_M) minus mean pulmonary wedge pressure (PA_{WM}) plotted against cardiac output (by thermodilution) at various barometric pressures (P_B) during Operation Everest II. For the measurements at 240 mmHg, the subjects breathed an oxygen mixture to give an inspired Po_2 of 43 mmHg; ●, 282 mmHg; ○, 240 mmHg. (From Groves et al. 1987.)

in pulmonary vascular resistance (Groves et al. 1987). In interpreting this result it should be recognized that a fall in cardiac output normally results in an increase in pulmonary vascular resistance because the reduction in capillary pressure causes derecruitment of capillaries and a reduction in caliber of those which remain open (Glazier et al. 1969). Thus the fact that pulmonary vascular resistance did not change when it was expected to rise indicated that oxygen breathing probably reduced vascular resistance to some extent. Nevertheless, it is remarkable that the subjects who were hypoxic for only 2–3 weeks when the measurements were made had a substantial degree of irreversibility of the increased pulmonary vascular resistance. This implies that there were structural changes in the pulmonary blood vessels, in addition to simple contraction of vascular smooth muscle, and is consistent with more recent studies on rapid remodeling of the pulmonary circulation (Tozzi et al. 1989). In a recent paper, Smith et al. (2009) showed that the pulmonary artery response to hypoxia was dependent on the iron status. This is probably because iron is an obligate co-factor for hydroxia-inducible factor (HIF) hydroxylase, an enzyme which degrades a subunit of HIF in normoxia. Subjects were made hypoxic for 8 hours while maintaining isocapnia. Iron infusion almost abolished the rise in pulmonary artery pressure, while a chelating agent, desferrioxamine enhanced it. Also, although not commented upon by the authors, their results indicate that after only 8 hours of hypoxia, the pulmonary artery pressure fails to return to control values after 10 minutes of normoxia.

High altitude natives also show little response of their increased pulmonary vascular resistance to breathing 100% oxygen. In this case it is known that there are substantial structural changes in the lungs including a large increase in smooth muscle in the small pulmonary arteries (section 8.5.2).

A study of a small sample of Tibetans showed that they have an unusually small degree of hypoxic pulmonary vasoconstriction compared with other high altitude natives (Groves et al. 1993). Five normal male residents of Lhasa (3658 m) were studied at rest and during near-maximal ergometer exercise. The resting mean pulmonary arterial pressure and pulmonary vascular resistance were within normal values for sea level. Alveolar hypoxia resulted in a smaller rise of mean pulmonary artery pressure than in other high altitude residents of North and South America (Reeves and Grover 1975) (Fig. 8.11). Exercise increased cardiac output more than three-fold with a reduction in pulmonary vascular resistance; 100% oxygen breathing during exercise did not reduce pulmonary arterial pressure or vascular resistance. Hoit et al. (2005) studied 57 Tibetan subjects at 4300 m. They found partial pressure of nitric oxide (NO) exhaled was 23.4 mmHg, significantly lower than that of a sea level reference group. However, the rate of NO transfer out of the airway wall was seven times higher than at sea level. This suggested a higher pulmonary blood flow. The pulmonary artery systolic pressure was 31.4 mmHg (low for this altitude compared with lowlanders or Andean altitude residents) and higher NO levels were associated with higher pulmonary blood flows.

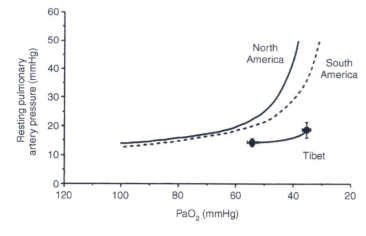

Figure 8.11 Change in mean pulmonary artery pressure during alveolar hypoxia in five Tibetans compared with high altitude residents of North and South America. (From Groves et al. 1993.)

8.5.2 Mechanisms of Hypoxic Pulmonary Vasoconstriction

The mechanism of hypoxic pulmonary vasoconstriction is not fully understood despite a great deal of research. Since the phenomenon occurs in excised isolated lungs, it clearly does not depend on central nervous connections. Furthermore, excised segments of pulmonary artery can be shown to constrict if their environment is made hypoxic (Lloyd 1965), so the response is due to local action of the hypoxia on the artery itself. It is also known that it is the P_{O_2} of the alveolar gas, not the pulmonary arterial blood, which chiefly determines the response (Duke 1954; Lloyd 1965). This can be proved by perfusing a lung with blood of a high P_{O_2} while keeping the alveolar P_{O_2} low. Under these conditions the response is well seen.

The predominant site of vasoconstriction is in the small pulmonary arteries (Kato and Staub 1966; Glazier and Murray 1971). Some studies suggest that the alveolar vessels may be partly responsible for the increased resistance, and contractile cells have been described in the interstitium of the alveolar wall, which could conceivably distort capillaries and increase their resistance (Kapanci et al. 1974). However, the fact that the pulmonary arterial pressure can increase to levels of 50 mmHg or more in subjects at high altitude without the occurrence of pulmonary edema is evidence that the main site of constriction is upstream of the pulmonary capillaries from which the fluid leaks.

Having said this, it is also true that pulmonary edema does occur at high altitude from time to time (Chapter 21) and a likely mechanism is that the hypoxic pulmonary vasoconstriction is uneven (Hultgren 1978), with the result that those capillaries which are not protected from the increased pulmonary arterial pressure develop ultrastructural damage to their walls. This results in a high permeability type of edema and this topic is considered in more detail in Chapter 21, section 21.6.5.

As indicated earlier, the exact mechanism of hypoxic pulmonary vasoconstriction is still an active area of research. Chemical mediators which have been studied in the past include catecholamines, histamine, angiotensin and prostaglandins (Fishman 1985). However, a recent study carried out in the Margherita Hut (4559 m) found that the rise in pulmonary artery pressure in their subjects did not correlate with the transpulmonary exchange of norepinephrine (Berger et al. 2011).

Goerre et al. (1995) had shown that endothelin-1 (ET-1) was raised in subjects taken rapidly to high altitude and was probably involved in the mechanism of hypoxic pulmonary hypertension. Modesti et al. (2006) investigated the role of ET-1 by giving bosantin, an ET-1 blocker, to a group of subjects who were then taken to the Margherita Hut. Their pulmonary artery pressure was significantly lower on the day after arrival than a control group taking a placebo, confirming that ET-1 is involved in the hypoxic pressor response. However, they warn that they also found impairment of diuresis and free water clearance in the bosantin group compared with controls, so it is probably not a drug to be recommended for prophylactic treatment of acute mountain sickness or HAPE.

Recently, a great deal of interest has been generated by the observation that inhaled NO reverses hypoxic pulmonary vasoconstriction. Nitric oxide is an endothelium-derived relaxing factor for blood vessels (Ignarro *et al.* 1987). It is formed from L-arginine via catalysis by endothelial nitric oxide synthase (eNOS) and is a final common pathway for a variety of biological processes (Moncada *et al.* 1991). Nitric oxide activates soluble guanylate cyclase, which leads to smooth muscle relaxation through the synthesis of cyclic GMP. Several studies suggest that voltage-gated potassium ion channels in smooth muscle cells may be involved, leading to increased intracellular concentration of calcium ions. Nitrovasodilators, such as nitroprusside and glyceryl trinitrate, which have been used clinically for many years, are thought to act by these same mechanisms.

Inhibitors of NO synthesis have been shown to augment hypoxic pulmonary vasoconstriction in isolated pulmonary artery rings (Archer *et al.* 1989), and attenuate pulmonary vasodilatation in intact lambs (Fineman *et al.* 1991). Inhaled nitric oxide reduces hypoxic pulmonary vasoconstriction in humans (Frostell *et al.* 1993) and sheep (Pison *et al.* 1993), and lowers pulmonary vascular resistance in patients with HAPE (Anand *et al.* 1998). The required inhaled concentration of NO is extremely low (about 20 ppm), and the gas is highly toxic at high concentrations. The recognition of the role of NO has opened up a new era in our understanding of hypoxic pulmonary vasoconstriction.

Vinnikov *et al.* (2010) measured exhaled NO as an index of lung levels. They found a 17% reduction in miners on their third day after ascending to the Kumtor Mine at 4000 m, in Kyrgyzstan. After 2–3 weeks there was a 30% reduction, supporting the concept that lower levels of NO are involved in the mechanism of hypoxic pulmonary hypertension. However, Donnelly *et al.* (2011), although they also found decrease in exhaled NO in lowland subjects ascending to altitude and increased pulmonary artery pressure, argued that NO was not an important factor in the mechanism of pulmonary hypertension.

The possibility that oxygen free radicals (ROS) may be generated in the lung of hypoxic subjects and result in loss of bioactive NO metabolites, was explored in a demanding study by Bailey *et al.* (2010) at the Margherita Hut (4559 m). They sampled arterial and mixed venous blood and measured cardiac output in 26 subjects at sea level and altitude. Subjects included three who had HAPE at altitude. Samples were assayed for three species of ROS, antioxidants and for a number of cytokines. Pulmonary artery pressure was estimated by echocardiography. They demonstrated the production of ROS across the lung. The level of ROS production correlated with the rise of pulmonary artery pressure. The increase in ROS may not only reduce NO bioavailability but may also have a direct effect on smooth muscle contraction through ROS signaling and Ca^{2+} release (Waypa and Schumacker 2008).

Calcium and voltage-gated potassium channels in the vascular smooth muscle have an important role in the development of vasoconstriction. This is a rapidly developing area of research and a review can be found in Remillard and Yuan (2005). Hypoxia decreases K^+ channel activity causing membrane depolarization which leads to increased Ca^{2+} influx and so to contraction of smooth muscle cells. Thus the resulting transmembrane ion flux modulates excitation–contraction coupling in the smooth muscle cells. This flux also regulates cell volume, apoptosis and proliferation which results in remodeling of the blood vessels.

Pulmonary vascular vasodilators can be used to reduce the degree of pulmonary hypertension under some conditions. Calcium channel blockers such as nifedipine reduce the pulmonary artery pressure and are useful in both the treatment and prevention of HAPE (Bärtsch *et al.* 1991b; Hackett and Roach 2001). More recently, 5-phosphodiesterase inhibitors such as sildenafil have been shown to reduce the pulmonary hypertension at high altitude both during rest and during exercise, and they may also be useful in the treatment and prophylaxis of HAPE (Zhao *et al.* 2001; Ricart *et al.* 2005; Richalet *et al.*

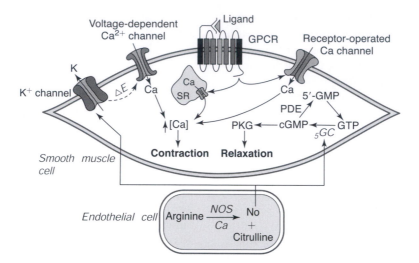

Figure 8.12 Role of ion channel function and intracellular Ca^{2+} in the regulation of pulmonary vasoconstriction. Ca^{2+} influx via voltage-dependent (VDCC) or receptor-operated (ROC) Ca^{2+} channels, and Ca^{2+} release from the endoplasmic or sarcoplasmic reticulum (SR) stores cause the rise in cytosolic free $[Ca^{2+}]$ ($[Ca^{2+}]_{cyt}$) that acts as the major trigger for pulmonary artery smooth muscle cell (PASMC) contraction. VDCC activity is modulated by a change in membrane potential (ΔE_m), which is tightly regulated by the activity of K^+ channels. In quiescent cells, normal K^+ channel activity maintains resting E_m at negative potentials. During acute hypoxia, the protein expression and function of K^+ channels are decreased and cells are depolarized (i.e. E_m becomes less negative), causing activation of VDCC, and thereby increases $[Ca^{2+}]$ in the cytosol ($[Ca^{2+}]_{cyt}$). Binding of vasoconstrictors (e.g. norepinephrine) to membrane receptors (e.g. G protein-coupled receptors, GPCR) can promote both Ca^{2+} release from the SR and Ca^{2+} influx via ROC. Hypoxia also enhances Ca^{2+} release from the SR and Ca^{2+} influx via ROC. Ca^{2+} channel blockers (e.g. nifedipine, verapamil or diltiazem), by attenuating Ca^{2+} influx in PASMC, have been used clinically to treat patients with pulmonary arterial hypertension. Nitric oxide (NO) produced in adjacent endothelial cells diffuses into PASMC to activate soluble guanylate cyclase (sGC), which catalyzes the formation of cyclic GMP (cGMP) from GTP. Catabolism of cGMP into inactive 5'-GMP is promoted by phosphodiesterases (PDE); PDE inhibitors, such as sildenafil, prevent this step and increase cytosolic cGMP concentration in PASMC. cGMP promotes and prolongs smooth muscle relaxation via a mechanism involving cGMP-dependent protein kinase (PKG). NO, which has been used therapeutically for patients with pulmonary hypertension, can also promote PASMC relaxation (a) by directly activating plasma membrane K^+ channels (shown here) to attenuate VDCC activity, (b) by directly blocking Ca^{2+} channels, and/or (c) by enhancing Ca^{2+} re-uptake into the SR, all of which result in decreased $[Ca^{2+}]_{cyt}$. Diagram and caption are courtesy of Jason Yuan.

2005a). Figure 8.12 summarizes some of the mechanisms responsible for hypoxic pulmonary vasoconstriction.

Hypoxic pulmonary vasoconstriction has the effect of directing blood flow away from hypoxic regions of lung, caused, for example, by partial obstruction of an airway. Other things being equal, this will reduce the amount of ventilation/perfusion inequality in a diseased lung and limit the depression of the arterial P_{O_2}.

This is a valuable mechanism in some patients with asthma and chronic obstructive pulmonary disease. However, the pulmonary hypertension that is seen at high altitude has no value except to cause a more uniform topographical distribution of blood flow (Dawson 1972). The improvement in ventilation/perfusion relationships resulting from this more uniform distribution of blood flow is trivial in terms of overall gas exchange (West 1962b) and we must conclude that the pulmonary hypertension of high altitude has no useful function, but in fact is deleterious because it can be responsible for the occurrence of HAPE. As stated earlier, the evolutionary pressure for the mechanism of hypoxic pulmonary vasoconstriction presumably comes from its value in the perinatal period.

8.5.3 Pulmonary hypertension and performance

The question of whether hypoxic pulmonary hypertension affects performance at altitude and might account for some of the reduction in $V_{O_{2,max}}$ was addressed in a recent study by Naeije *et al.* (2010). They studied a group of subjects at sea level in normoxia and acute hypoxia and again after trekking to the Pyramid laboratory (5050 m) in Nepal. Half the subjects were treated with the endothelin A receptor blocker sitaxsentan and the others with placebo. The drug reduced pulmonary artery pressure and this resulted in a 30% restoration of $V_{O_{2,max}}$ at sea level and by 10% at altitude. They also found a significant correlation between the reduction in pulmonary artery pressure and restoration of $V_{O_{2,max}}$. These results suggest that a brisk hypoxic pulmonary pressor response may not only be a risk factor for HAPE but also contribute to a poorer physical performance at altitude. On the other hand, a chamber study by Olfert *et al.* (2011) showed that both sildenafil and basantin increased Pa_{O_2} and could have accounted for the increase in performance. There have been other studies recently addressing this issue using drugs, which may have other effects than a reduction in pulmonary artery pressure. A fuller discussion of this topic is to be found in a 'pro–con' debate (Naeije 2011; Anholm and Foster 2011). This debate provides a good review of the whole topic but leaves the question open.

8.5.4 Remodeling

The lungs of long-term residents at high altitude show marked changes related to pulmonary hypertension (Heath and Williams 1995). Bands of smooth muscle develop in the small pulmonary

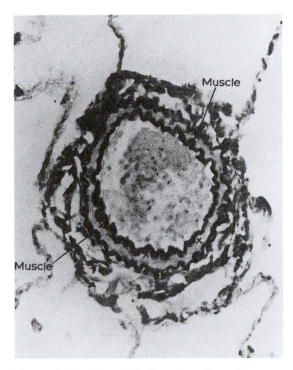

Figure 8.13 Histological section of a pulmonary arteriole from a Quechua Indian living at high altitude in the Peruvian Andes. Muscle tissue is seen between the internal and external elastic laminae. Normally there is a single elastic lamina and no muscle tissue in a vessel of this size at sea level. (Elastic van Gieson stain, ×375.) (From Heath and Williams 1995.)

arteries (arterioles) of approximately 500 μm diameter which normally have a wall consisting only of a single elastic lamina. The result is that these small vessels develop a media of circularly oriented smooth muscle bonded by internal and external elastic laminae (Fig. 8.13). These changes are associated with narrowing of the lumen and an increase in pulmonary vascular resistance. Medial hypertrophy of the parent muscular pulmonary arteries is not a common feature (Arias-Stella and Saldaña 1963), though it occurs in some individuals (Wagenvoort and Wagenvoort 1973). Occlusive intimal fibrosis apparently does not occur. However, longitudinal muscle fibers developing in the intima of pulmonary arterioles in highlanders have been described (Wagenvoort and Wagenvoort 1973). Some authors have also described an increase in mast cell density in experimental animals exposed to long-term hypoxia (Kay *et al.* 1974). This is of interest because at one stage it was thought that mediators from mast cells, for example histamine, might be involved in the vasoconstrictor response.

These structural changes are consistent with the fact that the pulmonary arterial pressure of high altitude natives falls only slightly (by 15–20%) when oxygen is breathed (Peñaloza *et al.* 1962). These authors showed that inhabitants of Cerro de Pasco (4330 m) who moved to sea level had their mean pulmonary arterial pressure halved from 24 to 12 mmHg after 2 years of residence at sea level. The fact that lowlanders who are exposed to high altitude for 2–3 weeks develop pulmonary hypertension which is not completely reversed by 100% oxygen breathing (Groves *et al.* 1987) suggests that their pulmonary blood vessels may also have developed some increased smooth muscle.

The structural changes that occur in pulmonary arteries when the pulmonary arterial pressure is raised as a result of exposing an animal to hypoxia are referred to as vascular remodeling (Riley 1991). This was studied by Meyrick and Reid (1978, 1980) who exposed rats to half the normal barometric pressure for 1–52 days. The result was an increase in pulmonary artery pressure as a result of hypoxic pulmonary vasoconstriction. After 2 days they saw the appearance of new smooth muscle in small pulmonary arteries, and after 10 days there was doubling of the thickness of the media and adventitia of the main pulmonary artery due to increased smooth muscle, collagen and elastin, and also edema. There was some recovery after 3 days of normoxia, and after 14–28 days the thickness of the media was normal. However, some increase in collagen persisted up to 70 days.

The molecular biology of the responses of the pulmonary blood vessels has been studied by several groups. Mecham *et al.* (1987) looked at the response of the pulmonary arteries of newborn calves to alveolar hypoxia. There was a two- to four-fold increase in elastin production in pulmonary arterial wall and medial smooth muscle cells. This was accompanied by a corresponding increase in elastin messenger RNA consistent with

regulation at the transcriptional level. Poiani *et al.* (1990) exposed rats to 10% oxygen for 1–14 days. Within 3 days of exposure there was increased synthesis of collagen and elastin, and an increase in mRNA for $\alpha_1(I)$ procollagen.

A particularly interesting study was done by Tozzi *et al.* (1989) who placed rat main pulmonary artery rings in Krebs–Ringer bicarbonate as explants. The investigators then applied mechanical tension equivalent to a transmural pressure of 50 mmHg for 4 hours, and found increases in collagen synthesis (incorporation of ^{14}C-proline), elastin synthesis (incorporation of ^{14}C-valine), mRNA for $\alpha_1(I)$ procollagen, and mRNA for protooncogene v-*sis*. The last may implicate platelet-derived growth factor (PDGF) or transforming growth factor (TGF)-β as a mediator. They were able to show that these changes were endothelium-dependent because they did not occur when the endothelium was removed from the arterial rings.

It is possible that this vascular remodeling is a general property of pulmonary vascular endothelium. It has been pointed out that the capillary wall has a dilemma in that it must be extremely thin for gas exchange but immensely strong to withstand the wall stresses that develop when the capillary pressure rises during heavy exercise (West and Mathieu-Costello 1992b). There is good evidence that the extracellular matrix of the blood-gas barrier, at least on the thin side, is responsible for its strength, and it is known that in mitral stenosis, where the capillary pressure rises over long periods of time, there is an increase in thickness of the extracellular matrix (Kay and Edwards 1973). Thus it may be that the capillary is continually regulating the structure of the wall in response to the capillary pressure which is sensed by the endothelium. The capillaries appear to be the most vulnerable vessels in the pulmonary circulation when the pressure rises. Thus vascular remodeling, which has been chiefly studied in larger blood vessels, may be a general property of the pulmonary vasculature, and its evolutionary advantage may be primarily to protect the walls of the capillaries.

The mechanism of capillary wall remodeling in response to increased wall stress has been the subject of several studies. Berg *et al.* (1997) exposed rabbit lungs to high levels of lung inflation because this is known to increase the wall stress of pulmonary capillaries (Fu *et al.* 1992). Increased gene expression for α_1(III) and α_2(IV) procollagens, fibronectin, basic fibroblast growth factor (bFGF), and TGF-β1 was found in peripheral lung parenchyma compared with control animals in normal states of lung inflation. However, mRNA levels for α_1(I) procollagen and vascular endothelial growth factor (VEGF) were unchanged. Parker *et al.* (1997) raised capillary transmural pressure by intermittently increasing the venous pressure in isolated perfused rat lungs. There were significant increases in gene expression for α_1(I) and α_1(III) procollagens, fibronectin and laminin compared with controls in which the venous pressure was normal. Berg *et al.* (1998) placed rats in 10% oxygen for periods from 6 hours up to 10 days. Here the hypothesis was that because the pulmonary vasoconstriction caused by alveolar hypoxia is uneven, some capillaries will be exposed to a high transmural pressure, and therefore have increased wall stress. Levels of mRNA for α_2(IV) procollagen increased six-fold after 6 hours of hypoxia, and seven-fold after 3 days of hypoxia. However, the levels decreased after 10 days of exposure. mRNA levels for PDGF-B, α_1(I) and α_3(III) procollagens and fibronectin also increased. All the above results are consistent with capillary wall remodeling in response to increased wall stress, but the overall picture is still far from clear.

The environment of the human fetus is similar in some respects to that of the high altitude dweller in that the arterial P_{O_2} is less than 30 mmHg, based on measurements on experimental animals (Itskovitz *et al.* 1987). The fetus also has pulmonary hypertension because the pulmonary artery is connected to the systemic arterial system through the patent ductus arteriosus. In keeping with this, the fetal lung shows a high degree of muscularization of the pulmonary arteries. Babies born at a high altitude show persistence of this muscularization, whereas the pulmonary arteries of those born at sea level assume the adult appearance after only a few weeks (Heath and Williams 1995).

8.5.5 Right ventricular hypertrophy

The pulmonary hypertension of high altitude causes right ventricular hypertrophy both in acclimatized lowlanders and in high altitude natives. In one study of children of 2–10 years of age it was shown that at sea level the ratio of left to right ventricular weights was about 1:8, whereas at high altitude (3700–4260 m) it was less than 1:3 (Arias-Stella and Recavarren 1962). Experimental studies on rats exposed to an altitude of 5500 m showed that they developed right ventricular hypertrophy within 5 weeks (Heath *et al.* 1973).

Data on acclimatized lowlanders are not generally available, but there is abundant indirect evidence of right ventricular hypertrophy from electrocardiographic changes (section 8.5.6). Occasionally, climbers returning from high altitude have shown evidence of right heart enlargement on chest radiograph (Pugh 1962a).

8.5.6 Electrocardiographic changes

Electrocardiographic changes are considered here because most of the changes are attributable to pulmonary hypertension. An extensive study was carried out during the 1981 American Medical Research Expedition to Everest (Karliner *et al.* 1985) when recordings were made at sea level, 5400 m, 6300 m, and again at sea level. A total of 19 subjects were studied, although complete data were not obtained from all. Resting heart rate increased from a mean of 57 at sea level to 70 at 5400 m and 80 at 6300 m (compare section 8.3.2). The amplitude of the P wave in standard lead 2 of the electrocardiogram increased by over 40% from sea level to 6300 m, consistent with right atrial enlargement. Right axis deviation of the QRS axis was seen. The mean frontal plane QRS axis increased from +64° to +78° at 5400 m and +85° at 6300 m. Three subjects showed abnormalities of right bundle branch conduction at the highest altitude and three others showed changes consistent with right ventricular hypertrophy (posterior displacement of the QRS vector in the horizontal plane). Seven subjects developed flattened T waves and four showed T-wave inversions (Fig. 8.14). All the changes

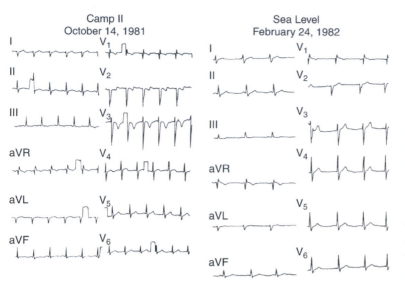

Figure 8.14 Twelve-lead electrocardiogram obtained at Camp 2 (6300 m) and about 3 months after return of the subject to sea level. Sinus tachycardia and diffuse T-wave flattening present at altitude; the T waves in leads V_2 and V_3 exhibit terminal inversion. (From Karliner et al. 1985.)

returned to normal in tracings obtained at sea level after the expedition.

Other investigators have reported similar findings in acclimatized lowlanders, though generally on smaller numbers or at lower altitudes. Milledge (1963) made measurements during the 1960–61 Silver Hut Expedition and reported data on subjects who spent several months at an altitude of 5800 m. In addition, some recordings were made as high as 7440 m in climbers who never used supplemental oxygen. He found T-wave inversions on the right pre-cordial leads in six subjects; two had left pre-cordial T-wave inversion as well. Oxygen breathing had no effect on these changes. Das *et al.* (1983) reported on over 40 subjects who were rapidly transported to either 3200 or 3771 m. There was a tendency for a rightward axis shift which, interestingly, tended to resolve in most subjects after 10 days at high altitude.

A particularly remarkable measurement was made on Ms Phantog, deputy leader of the successful 1975 Chinese ascent of Mount Everest. She lay down on the summit under the newly erected tripod while her standard lead 1 was telemetered down to base camp. However, there were no changes from sea level to 8848 m and back again (Zhongyuan *et al.* 1980). Other electrocardiographic studies at high altitude include those made by Peñaloza and Echevarria (1957), Jackson and Davies (1960), Aigner *et al.*

(1980), Kapoor (1984), Malconian *et al.* (1990), Chandrashekhar *et al.* (1992) and Halperin *et al.* (1998).

8.6 MICROCIRCULATION

Apart from the study of muscle biopsies, there have been no studies of the human microcirculation until recently. The development of sidestream dark-field (SDF) imaging and its predecessor, orthogonal polarization spectral (OPS) imaging (Groner *et al.* 1999; Goedhart *et al.* 2007) and the availability of small portable instruments allowed investigators to study subjects at altitude. Martin *et al.* (2010) conducted a study of the sublingual circulation in climbers ascending to Everest Base Camp and above. They found that hypoxia resulted in reduced microcirculatory flow index and an increase in density of vessels as compared with sea level results. They considered that these results might be due to recruitment of existing capillaries in the early stages of the expedition and possibly to angioneogenesis after prolonged altitude hypoxia. The later measurements were after 71 days at altitude. There was, of course, an increase in hematocrit at altitude but the authors considered this would have had only a minor effect. The significance of these changes is not clear. They could be beneficial in allowing a longer transit time for blood in the tissues.

Hematology

SUMMARY

Two of the best-known aspects of altitude acclimatization are the increase in red cell numbers per unit volume and the increase in hemoglobin concentration. These are achieved, initially, by a reduction in plasma volume (PV) and later by an increase in red cell mass (RCM). The mechanism for PV reduction on ascent to altitude is probably via carotid body stimulation by hypoxia, which reduces the reabsorption of sodium by the kidney via neural pathways. Hypoxia causes an increase in erythropoietin (EPO), which stimulates the bone marrow to increase red cell output. The EPO gene is induced by hypoxia through a nuclear factor, the hypoxia-inducible factor-1 alpha (HIF-1α). Although EPO levels rise within a few hours, the increase in RCM takes weeks and only reaches a steady state after some 6 months. Plasma volume is restored to near sea level values after a few weeks. The rise in hemoglobin concentration is roughly linear with altitude up to about 5500 m and is similar in acclimatized lowlanders and residents of high altitude throughout most of the world, though with wide individual variation. However, Tibetan and, possibly, Ethiopian highlanders have lower hemoglobin levels than other high altitude residents at similar altitudes. Extreme polycythemia among residents or lowlanders staying at altitude for many years is considered pathological and termed chronic mountain sickness (Chapter 22).

The effect of altitude on white cells has received little attention. Variable effects on this class of cells have been reported including a possible increase in CD16 natural killer cells and decrease in T-lymphocyte populations. Some studies suggest that leukocyte function may be altered at high altitude but a definitive link between observed changes and the perceived persistence of viral and bacterial infections at high altitude is lacking. The effects of altitude on platelets and clotting are considered in greater detail in Chapter 23.

9.1 INTRODUCTION

Following ascent to high altitude, the barometric pressure decreases, thereby leading to a decrease in the arterial partial pressure of oxygen and, as a result, a decrease in hemoglobin–oxygen saturation. Acutely, cardiac output increases and this helps to maintain oxygen delivery in the face of these changes, but over time, the primary compensatory mechanism is a rise in blood hemoglobin concentration and the subsequent increase in oxygen-carrying capacity and arterial oxygen content. This chapter examines the primary factors responsible for the rise in hemoglobin concentration, changes in plasma volume (PV), which play a large role in the initial increase in hemoglobin concentration, and changes in red cell mass (RCM), the factor responsible for the continuing rise over the following weeks to months at high altitude. The regulation of each of these factors will be discussed, as well as how the observed responses are altered by acute and chronic hypoxic exposure, exercise and other variables, and how these responses may vary between high altitude populations.

9.2 HISTORICAL PERSPECTIVE

Probably the best-known adaptation to high altitude is the increase in the number of red cells per unit volume of blood. This was recognized as long ago as 1878 when Paul Bert suggested in his book *La Pression Barométrique* (Bert 1878) that adaptation to high altitude might include an increase in the number of red cells and in the quantity of hemoglobin, responses that would allow the blood to carry more oxygen. A few years later, he examined blood from a number of domestic animals from La Paz, Bolivia (3500 m) and showed that these samples combined with 16.2–21.6 volumes of oxygen per 100 volumes of blood compared with 10–12 volumes percent in the blood of animals from lower elevations in France (West 1981).

In 1890, Viault made the first blood counts of men at high altitude. His own blood count at sea level in Lima was 5×10^6 μL^{-1} and after 3 weeks at Morococha, a mining township at 4372 m in the Andes, the value had increased to 7.1×10^6 μL^{-1}. We now know that early in altitude exposure most of this increase is due to reduced PV rather than an increase in RCM. Viault found these elevated counts present in a companion doctor from Lima and also in a number of the local Indian residents at altitude. He also noted that in a male llama the value was 16×10^6 μL^{-1}. He called the llama, 'l'animal

par excellence des grandes altitudes', although, in fact, the hemoglobin concentration of the blood is the same as in humans because the llama has very small red cells. In 1891, Viault published further observations that confirmed Bert's work on the oxygen-carrying capacity of high altitude animals. He showed in two sheep and one dog that their oxygen-carrying capacity was increased compared with similar animals in France.

Since these early reports, nearly all studies of physiologic responses to high altitude have observed this increase in red cell count, packed cell volume, or hemoglobin concentration.

9.3 OXYGEN CONTENT AND OXYGEN CARRYING CAPACITY

The increases in red cell number and hemoglobin concentration improve the oxygen-carrying capacity of the blood and, as a result, compensate for the reduction in oxygen saturation that occurs due to the decrease in the partial pressure of oxygen. The net result of these changes is that up to about 5300 m, fully acclimatized humans have the same arterial oxygen content as they do at sea level (Fig. 9.1).

While the observed response affords physiology teachers a classical example of beneficial adaptation, it is unlikely that the mechanism underlying this adaptation evolved primarily to serve humans at high altitude. The extent to which benefit can be gained by increasing hemoglobin concentration is fairly limited and indeed has been questioned as beneficial at all (Winslow *et al.* 1985; Winslow and Monge 1987, p. 203). This was nicely demonstrated by Calbet *et al.* (2002) who showed that under conditions where oxygen supply limits maximal exercise, increasing hemoglobin concentration following acclimatization does not improve maximal exercise capacity ($V_{O_{2,max}}$).

9.4 EFFECT OF ALTITUDE ON PLASMA VOLUME

As noted earlier, the initial rise in hemoglobin concentration following ascent occurs as a result

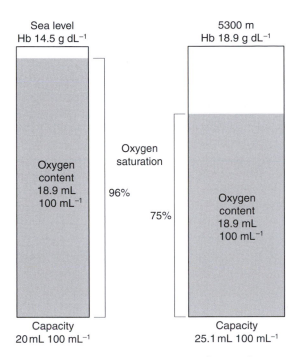

Figure 9.1 The oxygen content of arterial blood in an acclimatized subject at 5300 m and at sea level.

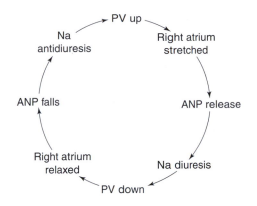

Figure 9.2 The regulation of plasma volume (PV) by atrial natriuretic peptide (ANP).

of a reduction in plasma volume. In this section, we consider how PV is regulated and how this parameter changes at altitude and in response to other variables.

9.4.1 Regulation of plasma volume

Plasma volume is primarily controlled by a feedback loop involving atrial natriuretic peptide (ANP). This hormone is released in response to increased right atrial stretch (Laragh 1985) occurring as a result of redistribution of blood volume from the periphery or by an increase in the total blood volume (i.e. PV). ANP causes sodium and water loss from the kidneys, which, in turn, reduce PV (Fig. 9.2). A series of other factors will affect this regulatory system (Fig. 9.3) including:

Hydration: Hydration and dehydration will obviously affect PV, along with all other body fluid compartments.
Vascular capacity: The vascular capacity is determined by the tone of the vessels, especially the venous capacitance vessels and vessels in the skin. Vascular tone, in turn, depends on a number of factors, such as temperature and catecholamine levels. Peripheral vasoconstriction shifts blood from the periphery to the central circulation, raising right atrial pressure and stimulating ANP release, while vasodilatation has the opposite effect. A change in vascular capacity also has a more direct effect on PV by shifting the balance of forces in the Starling equation. Vasodilatation tends to reduce the intravascular pressure, favoring inward movement of fluid at the tissue level, while vasoconstriction has the opposite effect.
Anti-diuretic hormone: Secretion of anti-diuretic hormone (ADH) will increase PV by decreasing free water loss in the kidney. ADH levels are regulated by changes in plasma osmolality. Increases in vascular volume caused by hydration cause a fall in plasma osmolality that inhibits ADH secretion. This leads to a water diuresis, which leads to an increase in plasma osmolality and a subsequent rise in ADH levels. This important feedback loop is not shown in Fig. 9.3, to avoid overloading the diagram.
Sodium status: High sodium intake can cause water retention and increase PV, particularly when intake exceeds one's ability to excrete sodium via the urine and sweat. Similar changes can be seen with sodium retention caused by stimulation of the renin–angiotensin–aldosterone system as a result of exercise or assumption of an upright posture.

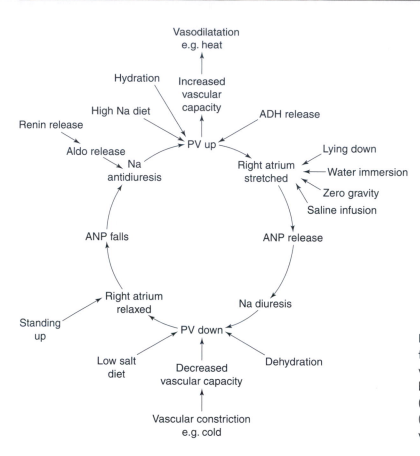

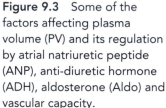

Figure 9.3 Some of the factors affecting plasma volume (PV) and its regulation by atrial natriuretic peptide (ANP), anti-diuretic hormone (ADH), aldosterone (Aldo) and vascular capacity.

Exercise and postural changes have effects on PV via other mechanisms that are discussed further below. These effects are mitigated to some extent by the rise in ANP that follows the increase in PV and the increase in right atrial stretch.

Other factors: Other factors that cause a shift of blood volume to the central circulation include assuming the supine position, lower body immersion and G-suits. Microgravity experienced by astronauts has a similar effect. Right atrial pressure is raised and ANP excretion is increased. Conversely, the upright position tends to shift volume to the lower extremities, reducing right atrial pressure and inhibiting ANP release.

9.4.2 Posture and plasma volume

The effect of posture is significant and needs to be taken into account when considering the effect of

other variables such as hypoxia or exercise on PV. Seventy percent of the blood volume is below the heart in the upright position and, of this volume, 75% is in the distensible veins. Upon standing, 500 mL of additional blood enters the legs. In individuals with intact autonomic function, this leads to a reflex tachycardia and vasoconstriction that are essential to maintain cerebral perfusion and prevent fainting. Vasoconstriction maintains the blood pressure and reduces flow, especially to the skin, muscles, kidneys and viscera.

The capillaries are exposed to the hydrostatic pressure of the column of venous blood. Upon standing, the height of the venous column is increased, leading to higher hydrostatic pressure, increased filtration of fluid out of the vascular compartment and, as a result, hemoconcentration. Numerous investigators from Thompson *et al.* (1928) onwards have confirmed these theoretical expectations. Thompson *et al.* found a reduction of plasma volume of 15% on assuming the upright position, but the magnitude of this effect is variable and is influenced by many factors, including the temperature of the environment and the subject, the state of hydration, etc.

9.4.3 Exercise and plasma volume

Exercise has an important effect on plasma volume and, therefore, hemoglobin concentration, but the effect varies according to the intensity, duration and type of exercise and can be modified by the temperatures of the environment and the subject and the posture assumed during exercise. This is because temperature and posture affect the skin blood flow and hence the distribution of cardiac output to the working muscles and other vascular beds. This, in turn, affects the capillary and venous pressures in these areas and hence the balance of forces in the Starling equation. Many studies on the effect of exercise have ignored the effect of posture and have taken control samples in a different posture from exercise samples. Another important factor that may affect PV is the high insensible fluid losses, particularly through the respiratory tract, as a result of the increased minute ventilation and decreased humidity.

Harrison (1985) reviewed the literature and, with a number of reservations, came to the conclusion that, for bicycle ergometer exercise, there is a reduction in PV soon after starting exercise. This reduction is proportional to the intensity of exercise or, more precisely, to the rise in atrial pressure. Thereafter, there is little change with continued exercise at normal room temperature but in high temperatures there is a further reduction in PV with time. However, these laboratory studies tend to look at fairly high intensity exercise (greater than 50% $V_{O_{2,max}}$) for periods of up to an hour or two.

Exercise in the mountains, on the other hand, is typically done over many hours and may go on day after day. Exercise of 8 hours or more at normal climbing rates (i.e. up to about 50% $V_{O_{2,max}}$ but often averaging much less) is associated with an increase in PV. Pugh (1969), for example, found an increase in blood volume of 7% after a 28-mile hill walk, while Williams *et al.* (1979) found PV increased progressively for 5 days of strenuous daily hill walking, eventually reaching a value 22% above the baseline value. Both these

studies were carried out under cold conditions and subjects avoided both overheating and cold stress. The changes in PV, interstitial and intracellular volumes documented in the study by Williams *et al.* are shown in Fig. 9.4. The mechanism for these exercise-induced changes in PV is probably via activation of the renin–angiotensin–aldosterone system, which results in sodium retention and thus a general expansion of the extracellular fluid (ECF) volume including the PV (Milledge *et al.* 1982).

It should also be noted that prolonged, continuous climbing can deplete the supply of fluids available and, thereby, increase the risk of dehydration and reductions in PV. In the majority of cases, however, adequate fluid supplies are available and the risk of dehydration and heat illness remains low as long as the individual is conscientious about maintaining adequate fluid intake.

9.4.4 Effect of acute hypoxia on plasma volume

Within 1–2 hours of exposure, mild-moderate degrees of acute hypoxia trigger diuretic and

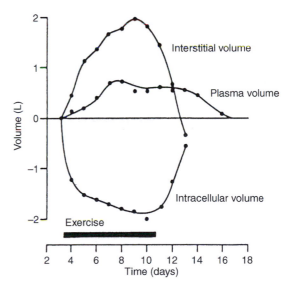

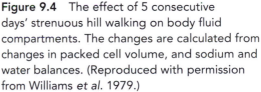

Figure 9.4 The effect of 5 consecutive days' strenuous hill walking on body fluid compartments. The changes are calculated from changes in packed cell volume, and sodium and water balances. (Reproduced with permission from Williams *et al.* 1979.)

natriuretic responses in the kidney that can last for 1–2 days, while more severe levels of acute hypoxia ($F_IO_2 < 0.10$) may actually be associated with anti-diuretic responses and sodium retention (Swenson 2001). The diuretic and natriuretic responses seen with mild-moderate exposures subsequently lead to a reduction in PV over the first several days at altitude, although the effect of hypoxia in field studies may be overshadowed in some cases by those of cold, dehydration and exercise. Singh et al. (1990), for example, found a reduction in PV from 40.4 mL kg^{-1} at sea level to 37.7 mL kg^{-1} on day 2 at 3500 m, and 37.0 mL kg^{-1} on day 12. Wolfel et al. (1991) reported similar changes in PV on ascent to 4300 m; PV fell from 48.8 mL kg^{-1} to 42.5 mL kg^{-1} on arrival at altitude and to 40.2 mL kg^{-1} by day 21. More recently, Robach et al. (2002) demonstrated a 13.6% reduction in plasma volume after 7 days at 4350 m.

Some caution must be exercised in the interpretation of these studies in the light of data from Poulson et al. (1998). They measured the change in PV of 10 subjects airlifted to the Vallot observatory (4350 m) using both the Evans' blue and the carbon monoxide methods. Twenty-four hours after arrival at altitude they found the expected reduction in PV with the carbon monoxide method (350 mL reduction) but not with the Evans' blue method (30 mL reduction). A possible explanation is that, since the Evans' blue labels albumin, and hypoxia leads to increased capillary permeability to albumin, the Evans' blue method may include this extravascular pool of albumin and thus give a falsely high result.

It should also be noted that the reported contraction in plasma volume may not apply in all circumstances. Subjects who develop acute mountain sickness, for example, may actually experience anti-diuresis and expand their PV. Vigorous exercise on the way up to altitude or following arrival can also result in expansion of the PV, as it does at sea level, via the renin–aldosterone system and expansion of the extravascular space. Withey et al. (1983), for example, found that subjects who hiked up to the Kulm Hotel on the Gornergrat (3100 m) and continued to exercise with hill walking, thereafter, had an increased PV and decreased hematocrit on the second day after ascent. In this particular situation, the effect of exercise over-rode the effect of hypoxia.

9.4.5 Effect of chronic hypoxia on plasma volume

Following the early phases of altitude exposure, there is a definite reduction in PV over the next few weeks. Pugh (1964b) found a 21% reduction in PV after 18 weeks at altitudes above 4000 m in four members of the 1960–61 Silver Hut Expedition (Fig. 9.5). During the following 7–14 weeks the PV returned towards control levels, with values being on average 10% less than control when corrected for changes in body weight. Sanchez et al. (1970) found altitude residents at Cerro de Pasco (4370 m) in Peru to have a mean PV two-thirds that of a group of students at Lima (sea level). When allowance was made for the weight difference of the groups they still had a PV 27% less in a blood volume that was 14% greater.

9.4.6 Plasma volume on return to sea level

Plasma volume is rapidly restored to baseline levels upon return to sea level. In Operation Everest III, PV was, on average, higher than before

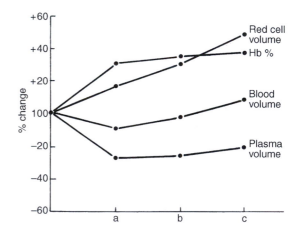

Figure 9.5 Changes in hemoglobin concentration (Hb%), red cell volume, blood volume and plasma volume in four subjects during the Silver Hut Expedition: (a) after 19 weeks at between 4000 and 5800 m; (b) after a further 3–6 weeks at 5800 m; (c) after a further 9–14 weeks at or above 5800 m. (After Pugh 1964b.)

altitude exposure after only 1–3 days back at sea level conditions (Robach *et al.* 2000), while, in the study noted earlier by Robach *et al.* (2002) PV returned to control values within 24–30 hours of returning from 4350 m to sea level. In the latter study, the observed change was attributed to decreased diuresis stemming from changes in fluid-regulating hormones such as ADH, aldosterone, ANP and renin.

9.4.7 Effect of plasma volume decrease on cardiac function and $\dot{V}O_{2,max}$

The observed decrease in PV will reduce blood volume until the RCM increases sufficiently to restore it. The possibility that this reduced blood volume might contribute to the lower maximum cardiac output and lower $\dot{V}O_{2,max}$ has been explored in two separate studies that yielded conflicting results. In Operation Everest III (Robach *et al.* 2000), subjects were examined 10–12 days after having reached an altitude of 6000 m by a progressive increase in simulated altitude in a chamber, at which time PV had decreased 26% compared to sea level values. At both sea level and high altitude, subjects received an infusion of a plasma expander to partially restore PV prior to repeat exercise testing. Infusion of the plasma expander had no effect on $\dot{V}O_{2,max}$ at sea level but did result in a 9% increase in $\dot{V}O_2$ at altitude with the greatest effect being seen in subjects with the greatest PV reduction. This result suggested that the reduced PV had some effect in reducing performance.

In a later study at Chacaltaya (5260 m) in Chile, Calbet *et al.* (2004) infused 1 liter of dextran into subjects who had been at 5260 m for 9 weeks. In contrast to Operation Everest III, this intervention had no effect on maximum cardiac output or $\dot{V}O_{2,max}$ despite the fact that maximum oxygen transport was reduced by 19% due to hemodilution. Subjects achieved the same work rate and $\dot{V}O_2$ after PV expansion by greater oxygen extraction by the working muscles. The observed differences in the effect of plasma volume expansion on performance in these two studies may relate to the fact that the subjects in the latter study had

been at high altitude for considerably longer than the subjects examined in Operation Everest III and, as a result, may already have experienced an increase in their PV prior to the dextran infusion. The results of this study do, however, add further evidence against any great advantage of a high hemoglobin concentration, [Hb].

9.5 ALTITUDE AND ERYTHROPOIESIS

Red cell mass is determined by the rate of formation of red cells (erythropoiesis) and their rate of loss. Red blood cells are generally lost by their death (their natural length of survival is about 120 days) but can also be lost as a result of hemorrhage or pathological states such as hemolytic anemia. Erythropoiesis can be impaired by bone marrow disorders or deficiencies of important cofactors necessary for hemoglobin synthesis, including iron or vitamin B12. In the absence of these problems, erythropoiesis is controlled by the level of the hormone erythropoietin (EPO).

9.5.1 EPO and its regulation

EPO is produced primarily by peritubular cells in the kidney, although 10–15% of total production occurs in the liver (Erslev 1987). The gene coding for the hormone has been cloned and expressed in cultured cells, allowing for sufficient material to be produced for clinical use, such as management of anemia in patients with chronic kidney disease. The two classical stimuli for EPO secretion are hypoxia and blood loss, both of which result in tissue hypoxia. In terms of evolutionary pressures, blood loss is probably more important than hypoxia, as blood loss is a far more common threat to survival than chronic hypoxia and erythropoiesis is far too slow a process to adequately defend against acute hypoxia.

Oxygen-sensing cells in the inner cortex and outer medulla of the kidney respond to tissue hypoxia and regulate EPO production and secretion (Semenza 2009). This was nicely demonstrated by Fisher and Langston (1967), who perfused an isolated dog kidney with hypoxic blood and noted a rise in EPO concentrations. There are several important differences between this oxygen-sensing pathway and another important oxygen-sensing system, the carotid body, which mediates the hypoxic ventilator response (HVR):

- Whereas HVR occurs within seconds following a step change in arterial P_{O_2}, there is no detectable rise in EPO concentration for over an hour following exposures to 3000–4000 m (Eckardt *et al.* 1989) and full EPO responses occur over several days (Semenza 2009).
- The oxygen-sensing cells in the kidney respond to oxygen content, unlike the carotid body, which is sensitive to reduction in P_{O_2}. As a result, anemia will lead to a rise in EPO concentrations whereas it has no effect on the carotid body and the hypoxic ventilatory response.

9.5.2 Erythropoietin, hypoxia-inducible factor-1, hypoxia and other stimuli to production

Erythropoietin is one of a number of gene products whose transcription is stimulated by hypoxia, including enzymes involved in glycolysis (aldolase A, enolase-1 glucose transporter-1, lactate dehydrogenase and phosphofructokinase) mediators of vascular tone (inducible nitric oxide synthase and heme oxygenase), and factors involved in angiogenesis (vascular endothelial growth factor). The link between hypoxia and gene induction for all these proteins are the hypoxia-inducible factors, HIF-1α and HIF-2α. First identified as a nuclear factor that bound to the hypoxia response element of the EPO gene (Semenza *et al.* 1998), HIF is normally produced and rapidly degraded in normoxia, but accumulates in hypoxia and exerts many important downstream effects on gene regulation which are described in Chapter 4 and in a recent review by Semenza (2009).

Although hypoxia is the major stimulus to EPO production, other stimuli have been investigated. Conflicting evidence has been reported regarding the effect of exercise with some studies reporting a rise in serum erythropoietin with exercise (Schwandt *et al.* 1991) and others finding no effect (Schmidt *et al.* 1991; Bodary *et al.* 1999). Roberts *et al.* (2000) investigated whether plasma volume may affect EPO production. They measured serum concentrations before and after supramaximal exercise and after 5% PV reduction by plasmapheresis. Whereas exercise resulted in a nonsignificant rise in serum EPO levels, PV reduction caused a statistically significant increase (34%) despite a small (4%) rise in hematocrit. Another stimulant to EPO production may be the plasma thiol–disulfide redox state. Using a crossover design, Hildebrandt *et al.* (2002) demonstrated that the EPO response to 2 hours of hypoxia was greater following treatment with the anti-oxidant *N*-acetyl-cysteine than following treatment with placebo.

9.5.3 Altitude and serum EPO concentration

Until about 1980, measurements of blood EPO levels were made by bioassays that could not detect the hormone until the concentration was above normal sea level values. Therefore, earlier work often relied on more indirect indices of erythropoietic activity, such as intestinal iron absorption or reticulocyte counts that did not necessarily provide an accurate sense of EPO regulation. Intestinal iron absorption, for example, has been shown to be independent of EPO and to be promoted as a direct effect of hypoxia rather than secondary to plasma iron turnover or erythropoietic activity (Raja *et al.* 1986), while the reticulocyte count rises many days following EPO secretion due to the typical time frame of red blood cell production in the marrow. Using such methods, early studies showed that following ascent, EPO concentrations rose within the first 24–48 hours (Siri *et al.* 1966; Albrecht and Little 1972).

More recently, studies using newer radioimmunoassay methods sensitive to EPO levels well below the normal range (13–37 mIU mL^{-1}) have shown that serum immunoreactive EPO concentration (SiEp) rises within 2 hours of hypoxic exposure (Eckardt *et al.* 1989), and reaches a maximum at about 24–48 hours. Thereafter, it declines to reach values not measurably different from controls after about 3 weeks (Milledge and Cotes 1985) (Fig. 9.6). Gunga *et al.* (1994) have reported similar findings at a more modest altitude of 2315 m. Even after 3 weeks above 4500 m, short-duration gains in elevation to 5500 m lead

to an increase in SiEp, which persists even after going back to lower elevation (Fig. 9.6). A similar rise in SiEP following restoration of normoxia was shown by Knaupp *et al.* (1992) who demonstrated a 50% increase in SiEP levels 240 minutes after starting a 120-minute exposure to an F_IO_2 of 0.1. The apparent rise in SiEP after descent or restoration of normoxia likely reflects the time delay necessary for gene transcription and protein production. One of the noteworthy features of the observed EPO responses is the significant degree of inter-individual variability. Richalet *et al.* (1994) studied subjects over a prolonged stay at 6540 m and documented anywhere from three-fold to 134-fold increases in SiEP values.

Even if hypoxia persists, EPO levels will fall in response to the rise in hemoglobin concentration. Wedzicha *et al.* (1985) for example, showed that in patients with polycythemia secondary to hypoxic lung disease, SiEp was within the normal range in over 50% of patients. A more recent study in mice at simulated altitude found that if the increase in [Hb] is prevented by either blood removal or treatment with the hemolytic drug, phenylhydrazine, SiEp remained elevated for the 10 days of the study whereas in control mice there was the usual fall on the second and subsequent days to levels about twice that of baseline values (Bozzini *et al.* 2005). This study suggests that the normal increase in [Hb] on ascent to altitude is sufficient to relieve, to a degree at least, the tissue hypoxia causing the rise in SiEp and provides confirmation in very controlled conditions of an incidental finding from the Sajama Expedition (Richalet *et al.* 1994) in which two female team members who showed no increase in [Hb] after 10 days at 6542 m had large increases in SiEp compared with the other subjects.

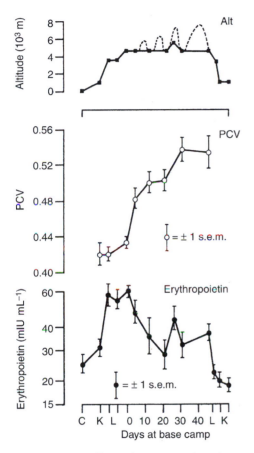

Figure 9.6 The effect of going to altitude on the serum erythropoietin concentration. The top panel shows the altitude/time profile for the eight subjects. The dotted line indicates ascent above base camp between blood samples. Note, the samples at 30 days were taken at 5500 m after four sample times at base camp (4500 m). Mean packed cell volume (PCV) is shown in the center panel and mean erythropoietin concentration in the lower panel. C, control, sea level; K, Kashgar (1200 m); L, Karakol lakes (3500 m). (Reproduced with permission from Milledge and Cotes 1985.)

INTERMITTENT HYPOXIA AND EPO CONCENTRATION

In the studies mentioned above, EPO was measured following continuous hypoxic exposures. In recent years, there has been growing interest in the concept of intermittent hypoxia as a means to improve athletic performance and also to understand the pathophysiology of diseases such as obstructive sleep apnea. Studies done to date have shown variable results regarding the effect of intermittent hypoxia on EPO regulation. Whereas some studies have shown increases in SiEP (Koistinen *et al.* 2000; Gore *et al.* 2006) other studies have shown no change in hormone levels following the intermittent hypoxic exposure (Julian *et al.* 2004; Lundby *et al.* 2005). The variability in study results may relate to the fact that the different studies typically involve widely divergent protocols for inducing intermittent hypoxia. Gore *et al.* (2006) for example, exposed subjects to a simulated altitude of 4000–5000 m for 3 hours a day, 5 days a week for a total of 4 weeks while Julian *et al.* (2004) exposed subjects to 70-minute episodes of alternating hypoxia (5 minutes) and normoxia (5 minutes) over a 4-week period.

EPO CONCENTRATION AND THE LIVE HIGH–TRAIN LOW MODEL

Changes in EPO regulation have also been examined in the context of another proposed method of improving athletic performance, the live high–train low model, in which participants either sleep or spend the bulk of their day living at either real or in simulated high altitude and then partake in training exercises at lower elevations. Using a variety of different protocols, the available studies (Stray-Gundersen *et al.* 2001; Robach *et al.* 2006; Wehrlin *et al.* 2006) have consistently shown that circulating erythropoietin levels are increased as a result of the exposure and training protocol, as are levels of soluble transferrin receptor, a marker of erythropoiesis. The studies, however, have shown inconsistent results regarding changes in exercise performance. Whereas Stray-Gundersen and Levine (2001) showed improvements in time trial performance and $V_{O_{2,max}}$ in elite runners living at 2500 m and training at 1250 m for 27 days and Wehrlin *et al.* (2006) showed improvements in $V_{O_{2,max}}$ and 5000 m running times after 24 days of living at 2500 m and training between 1000 and 1800 m, Robach *et al.* (2006) were not able to show any improvements in $V_{O_{2,max}}$ in nordic skiers who trained at 1200 m and slept 11 hours a night at elevations that rose from 2500 to 3500 m equivalent over the course of the 18-day study. Similarly, Siebenmann *et al.* (2012) showed in a placebo-controlled double-blinded design that 4 weeks of live high–train low, using 16 hours a day of normobaric

hypoxia equivalent to 3000 m, did not improve $V_{O_{2,max}}$ in normoxia and at a simulated altitude of 2500 m, and failed to improve mean power output in a simulated 26.2 km time trial.

9.5.4 Altitude and red cell mass

Because the lifespan of the red cell is unchanged at altitude (Berlin *et al.* 1954), increased erythropoiesis leads to an increase in RCM. Figure 9.5 shows the rise in red cell volume, which is quite slow but continues for a long time. After about 6 months at altitudes above 4000 m it had increased by a mean of 50% in absolute terms or 67.5% when corrected for loss of body weight. By this time the blood volume had increased over control by 7.3% or 22.8% corrected for body weight (Pugh 1964a) (Fig. 9.5). Similar changes are seen in altitude residents. Sanchez *et al.* (1970), for example, found altitude residents in the Andes to have an RCM 83% greater than sea level residents when corrected for weight difference.

9.6 ALTITUDE AND HEMOGLOBIN CONCENTRATION

9.6.1 Lowlanders going from sea level to altitude

The combined effect of changes in PV and RCM results in an increase in hemoglobin concentration [Hb]. As discussed earlier, the initial rise in [Hb] during the first few days and weeks at altitude is largely a result of reduction in PV. The [Hb] rise is roughly exponential with time, leveling out at about 6 weeks at a given altitude. RCM continues to rise after that time, but PV rises as well and, as a result, [Hb] remains approximately constant (Fig. 9.5).

Some of the clearest evidence of the changes in [Hb] over time at altitude comes from Pugh (1964c) who reviewed results from five expeditions (51 observations in 40 subjects) and concluded that the [Hb] after about 6 weeks at altitude averaged 20.5 g dL^{-1}; there was no correlation between [Hb] and performance on the mountain. Pugh also noted that the Sherpas had lower hemoglobin concentrations than the Western climbers, representing perhaps the first time that lower hemoglobin levels were described in this population. Winslow *et al.* (1984), reviewing [Hb] values from the 1981 American Everest expeditions and two previous Everest expeditions, found the range of mean values was 17.8–20.6 g dL^{-1} at altitudes of 5350–6300 m, with no correlation between altitude and [Hb] within this altitude range.

The increase in [Hb] allows more oxygen to be carried per liter of blood at any given oxygen saturation. Beyond a certain point, however, the benefits of increasing oxygen-carrying capacity may be offset by the increases in blood viscosity (discussed further below). Concern has been expressed in the past that the increase in viscosity may predispose to thrombosis at altitude but there is no systematic evidence to support either this claim or the fact that the risk of venous thromboembolism is increased at altitude (Chapter 23).

9.6.2 Residents at altitude

Figure 9.7 shows the rise in [Hb] with altitude in residents of high altitude from North and South America and Asia, with a noteworthy feature being the variability in [Hb] across the different high altitude populations. Andean subjects have been reported to have values in the region of 22 g dL^{-1} at altitudes of 4300–4500 m (Talbott and Dill 1936; Dill *et al.* 1937; Merino 1950). However, these studies may have included subjects who would now be considered to have chronic mountain sickness. More recent publications from South America that focus on healthy residents give mean values slightly lower than those earlier reported values. In a comprehensive study of hematologic parameters of high altitude residents in the Andes, for example, León-Velarde *et al.* (León-Velarde *et al.* 2000) reported mean [Hb] of 18.5 g dL^{-1} and 20.4 g dL^{-1} in adult men (40–60 years old) living at 4355 and 5500 m, respectively. Women in the same age range had mean values of 17.5 g dL^{-1} and 18.1 g dL^{-1} at the same altitudes. The authors also showed that the average [Hb] increased with increasing age at each elevation. Women had

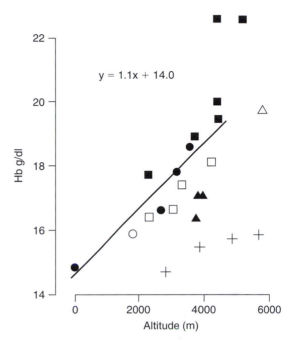

$$y = 1.1x + 14.0$$

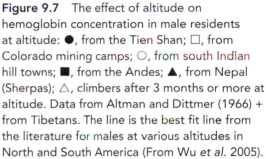

Figure 9.7 The effect of altitude on hemoglobin concentration in male residents at altitude: ●, from the Tien Shan; □, from Colorado mining camps; ○, from south Indian hill towns; ■, from the Andes; ▲, from Nepal (Sherpas); △, climbers after 3 months or more at altitude. Data from Altman and Dittmer (1966) + from Tibetans. The line is the best fit line from the literature for males at various altitudes in North and South America (From Wu *et al.* 2005).

similar values as men before puberty while older women had higher values than younger women, likely due to the absence of menstrual periods following menopause.

Other high altitude populations have been shown to have lower [Hb] than the Andean residents. Adams and Strang (1975) reported a mean of 17 g dL^{-1} in Sherpas living at 4000 m while Morpurgo *et al.* (1976) reported a mean value of 16.2 g dL^{-1} and argued that it represents greater adaptation. Beall *et al.* (1987) studied Tibetans and demonstrated a hemoglobin concentration of 18.2 g dL^{-1} in male and 16.7 g dL^{-1} in female subjects resident at an altitude of 4850–5450 m, a value substantially lower than most results from the Andes at comparable altitude. In a later study, Beall *et al.* (1998) studied highland populations at altitude in Tibet and Bolivia and found

Tibetans had significantly lower hemoglobin concentrations than the Bolivian highlanders (15.6 compared to 19.2 g dL⁻¹). The results of this study agree with those of Winslow *et al.* (1989) who compared Himalayan natives (Sherpas) to high altitude Andean natives at similar altitudes in Khundi, Nepal and Ollague (Chile) at 3700 m and reported that men's packed cell volume (PCV) values in Nepal were significantly lower than in Chile (48.4 compared with 52.2 g dL⁻¹). They also found serum EPO concentrations to be higher in the Andean population, indicating that they were functionally anemic even with the higher PCV. High altitude Ethiopian residents may have similar [Hb] to the Tibetans. Beall *et al.* (2002) examined residents at 3530 m and found mean [Hb] of 15.9 and 15 g dL⁻¹ for men and women, respectively, while in a more recent study, Hoit *et al.* (2011) reported mean [Hb] of 16.3 g dL⁻¹ and 15.3 g dL⁻¹ in Amhara men and women, respectively, living at 3700 m in elevation. Finally, Caucasian individuals living in high altitude towns in Colorado and acclimatized climbers tend to have lower hemoglobin concentration than Andeans (Fig. 9.7).

The reasons for the observed differences between these populations are not entirely clear and may be related to a variety of factors. One important factor may be the time that a given population has spent at high altitude. It is estimated that Tibetans have been resident at high altitude for at least 100 000 years, compared with about 14 000 years for Andean highlanders (Aldenderfer 2011). Support for this concept comes from a recent large study (*n* = 5887) by Wu *et al.* (2005) from north-west China and Tibet in which they compared [Hb] in Tibetans with [Hb] in lowland Han Chinese who had relocated to Tibet and remained there for many years. The rise in [Hb] with altitude in Han Chinese follows the same line as that given by a regression equation derived from the literature for North and South American populations at various altitudes. This rise is 1 g dL⁻¹ for every 1100 m increase in altitude; $y = 1.1x + 14.0$ when altitude is given in kilometers, but the [Hb] was considerably higher in this group when compared to the Tibetans, who showed only a very small rise with altitude increase from 3813 to 5200 m.

The time spent at altitude is likely providing an opportunity for selection pressures and genetic adaptation to the environment. In their study of Tibetan and Bolivian highlanders, Beall *et al.* (1998), for example, found that genetic factors accounted for a very high proportion of the phenotypic variance in hemoglobin concentration in both samples. More recent studies have provided evidence for this concept. Beall *et al.* (2011) showed that variation in genes encoding transcription factors for HIF-2α explained observed differences in [Hb] between Tibetan highlanders and ethnically similar Han Chinese who had relocated to Tibet. Two other studies published at the same time yielded similar findings and provided further strong support for the role of genetic adaptation (Simonson *et al.* 2010; Yi *et al.* 2010). These concepts are discussed in greater detail in Chapter 4.

Other factors that could explain some of the variation might include the fact that some of the groups, such as the Colorado residents move up and down in altitude more frequently than the Andeans who tend to remain on the Altiplano, or dietary factors such as the level of meat, and therefore, iron, intake in the diet, although the preponderance of evidence is now suggesting that it is the genetic factors that are the primary driving force behind the observed differences.

9.6.3 Polycythemia of high altitude

Excessive rise of [Hb] (i.e. above 22 g dL⁻¹) is generally considered to be pathological and diagnostic of chronic mountain sickness (Chapter 22). Both people native to high altitude, such as the Andean populations, and lowlanders resident at high altitude for some years, such as the Han Chinese relocated to the Tibetan plateau (Huang *et al.* 1984) are at risk of developing this condition.

9.6.4 Optimum hemoglobin concentration

The increase in [Hb] increases the oxygen-carrying capacity and oxygen content of blood and, as a result, helps compensate for a reduction in arterial P_{O_2} and oxygen saturation ($Sa_{,O_2}$). At altitudes up to about 5300 m the arterial oxygen content in acclimatized individuals is approximately equal to that at sea level (Fig. 9.1). However, increasing [Hb] results in increasing viscosity (Guyton et al. 1973). This increase in viscosity is curvilinear so that, with [Hb] above about 18 g dL^{-1}, viscosity increases rapidly. Eventually, this increased viscosity increases resistance in both systemic and pulmonary circulation, leading to reductions in pulmonary and systemic blood flow and a drop in cardiac output. With the reduction in cardiac output, oxygen delivery, the product of cardiac output and arterial oxygen content, decreases, thereby impeding oxygen supply to the tissues.

These considerations result in the concept of an optimum [Hb] below which oxygen delivery is reduced because of reduction in oxygen content, and above which it is reduced because the great increase in viscosity causes a reduction in cardiac output which more than offsets the increase in content. The major problem in calculating the optimum [Hb] is the viscosity of blood and its effect on cardiac output. Since blood is a non-Newtonian fluid (a fluid whose viscosity is not constant at all shear rates), a single value for viscosity cannot be assigned to it at any given [Hb]. The value will vary according to the way it is measured *in vitro*. *In vivo* the effect on resistance will vary according to the diameter of the vessel under consideration as well as to whether flow is streamlined or turbulent. Apparent resistance will also vary with flow. If we ignore the physics and just look at the effect of changing [Hb] on cardiac output in acute animal experiments, these may not reflect the human situation at altitude where the vascular system has time to adapt to the polycythemia. Another factor affecting the apparent viscosity is the deformability, or filterability, of the red cells. A study by Simon-Schnass and Korniszewski (1990) addressed this and concluded that altitude exposure resulted in an impaired filterability of red cells, which was prevented by the administration of vitamin E. Overall, the situation is so complex that it is clearly impossible, on theoretical grounds, to predict an optimum [Hb].

From clinical experience, it seems that the extremely high [Hb] found in chronic mountain sickness (Chapter 22) and in some patients with chronic hypoxic lung disease is deleterious. Hemodilution by venesection alone or with intravenous fluid replacement results in clinical improvement in patients with chronic mountain sickness. In such patients, reduction of PCV from 61 to 50% resulted in a decrease in pulmonary artery pressure and resistance (Weisse et al. 1975). Similarly, Winslow et al. (1985) found in Andean high altitude residents that reduction of PCV from 62 to 42% resulted in increased cardiac output and mixed venous P_{O_2}. Willison et al. (1980) found that reducing the PCV from 54 to 48% in patients resulted in an increase of cerebral blood flow from 44 to 57 mL min^{-1} 100 g^{-1} brain tissue. This would increase oxygen delivery to the brain by 15% and was accompanied by an increase in alertness. The problem of excessive erythropoiesis in chronic mountain sickness is further discussed in Chapter 22.

There is no obvious correlation between climbing performance and [Hb] within the range of values common on an expedition, at about 17–22 g dL^{-1} (Pugh 1964c). Indeed, it is usual to find that climbers who perform best are at the lower end of this range, suggesting that the optimum [Hb] at altitudes above about 5000 m is in the region of 18 g dL^{-1}. In a study of climbers at altitude by Sarnquist et al. (1986), it was found that hemodilution produced no improvement or deterioration in measured physical performance, though there was a small, significant improvement in psychomotor tests. However, the subjects studied, though having the highest PCV in the expedition, were not very polycythemic. Their PCV ranged from 57 to 60% before hemodilution. Winslow and Monge (1987, p. 203) conclude that 'Excessive polycythemia serves no useful purpose. Indeed, it is doubtful whether there is any physiologic value in "normal" polycythemia.' A study using mathematical modeling techniques (Villafuerte et al. 2004) even came to the conclusion that, at moderate altitude, at rest, a [Hb] of 14.7 was optimum, although a higher value may be better for exercise performance.

9.6.5 Effect of blood boosting on performance at sea level and altitude

At sea level there is little doubt that blood boosting (doping) by auto or hetero-infusion or by use of recombinant human EPO (rhEPO) has a significant effect in improving performance, as measured by $V_{O_{2,max}}$, and endurance. This is due to the increased oxygen-carrying capacity achieved by increasing the red cell mass by these maneuvers and hence the [Hb]. There have been numerous studies to show this improved athletic performance in middle distance running, cycling and skiing, of which, that by Ekblom et al. (1972) was probably the first. He showed that increasing the [Hb] by 13% by re-infusion of autologous blood, there was an increase in physical performance capacity (work time at a standard rate) of 23% and an increase in $V_{O_{2,max}}$ of 9%. The improvement in performance correlated with the increase in [Hb]. Buick et al. (1980) found similar results in their subjects who had genuine re-infusions but not in the group who had sham infusions thus eliminating the possibility of a psychological effect. Of course, the practice is illegal in sport. Several recent reviews of the topic (Leigh-Smith 2004; Jelkmann and Lundby 2011) summarize the history, techniques, effects and side effects of the practice as well as efforts to detect their use among elite athletes.

While the benefits of blood doping at sea level are clear and the practice is likely to persist despite efforts to combat it, the situation at altitude is not as apparent. Young et al. (1996) found no significant benefit from re-infusion of 700 mL of autologous blood in subjects at 4300 m, though mean values for $V_{O_{2,max}}$ were slightly higher on day 1 at altitude in the test subjects. In a further study by Pandolf et al. (1998), there was no significant improvement in time for a 3.2-km run in subjects infused with 700 mL of autologous blood. They suggest that the effect diminishes with increasing altitude and quote earlier work supporting that concept. More recently, Lundby and Damsgaard (2006) administered novel erythropoiesis stimulating protein (NESP) weekly over a 1-month period to healthy individuals and compared exercise performance while breathing 12.4% oxygen (altitude equivalent 4100 m) before and after the treatment. Subjects remained at sea level between exercise sessions, thereby ensuring there had been no other forms of acclimatization to high altitude. Despite a 16% increase in [Hb] and increased oxygen-carrying there were no improvements in $V_{O_{2,max}}$. They point out that, at least at altitudes above about 3500 m, it has been shown that acclimatization does not increase $V_{O_{2,max}}$ despite a rise in [Hb]. At submaximal exercise, the rise in [Hb] may well result in an increase in performance, in that endurance may be increased (Maher et al. 1974), although it is not at all clear why submaximal exercise performance is increased by acclimatization, while $V_{O_{2,max}}$ is unchanged.

Data from Robach et al. (2008) suggest that the effect of exogenously administered EPO may depend on the degree of hypoxia to which the individual is exposed. They administered rhEPO to eight healthy subjects over a 15-week period and then measured systemic and leg oxygen transport during exercise to exhaustion in normoxia and different degrees of acute hypoxia. As expected, $V_{O_{2,max}}$ increased in normoxia following rhEPO treatment. These gains persisted with exercise while breathing fractional oxygen concentrations as low as 0.134 but once the F_IO_2 was decreased to 0.115, there was no effect on systemic $V_{O_{2,max}}$ or peak leg V_{O_2}. They concluded that with severe degrees of hypoxia, $V_{O_{2,max}}$ becomes independent of arterial oxygen content, possibly as a result of central fatigue, although another consideration would be that blood flow is being diverted from the legs to support the markedly increased work of breathing.

9.6.6 Erythopoietin and hemoglobin concentration on descent from altitude

Erythropoietin levels decrease following descent back to sea level. Milledge and Cotes (1985), for example, reported that EPO levels were 66% of control values 8 and 20 hours after descent following 2 months at or above 4500 m. This is likely due to the higher [Hb] following the stay at altitude as well as the rise in arterial saturation upon descent, both of which combine to increase oxygen delivery to the renal peritubular cells responsible for EPO production.

Following descent, [Hb] declines and reaches normal sea level values after about 6 weeks (Heath and Williams 1995). While this change in [Hb] is often attributed to the decrease in EPO and subsequent decline in red blood cell production, more recent studies suggest that red blood cell destruction might also be enhanced. Rice *et al.* (2001) examined hematological parameters in high altitude residents descending to sea level and found evidence of neocytolysis, a process first observed in astronauts, in which young red blood cells are selectively hemolyzed, allowing rapid reduction in RCM. Risso *et al.* (2007) found evidence of the same phenomenon in climbers following descent to sea level after 53 days above 4500 m. Separating out the red blood cell populations into low, middle and high density subsets corresponding to young, middle-aged and old cells respectively, they found that the numbers of young and middle-aged red blood cells decreased significantly 6 days following descent, such that older, higher density red blood cells represented 97.9% of the total red blood cell population. The remaining young and middle-aged cells also acquired a senescent-like phenotype, making them more susceptible to phagocytosis. Similar to the data from Milledge and Cotes (1985), Risso *et al.* also noted a decrease in EPO relative to before acclimatization, suggesting that neocytolysis may be triggered by the fall in EPO concentration below a critical threshold.

9.7 IRON AND HEMATOLOGIC RESPONSES AT HIGH ALTITUDE

Iron is a key component of the hemoglobin molecule and adequate iron stores are likely important for ensuring appropriate hematologic responses following ascent. This was demonstrated nicely by Hannon (1967), who showed that women given iron supplementation at the time of ascent to 4260 m had larger rises in their hematocrit over a 60-day stay at that elevation than women who did not receive supplementation. The observed rise in the iron supplementation group approached that seen in the men at the same elevation.

High altitude may also affect the manner in which the body handles iron stores. Robach *et al.* (2007) examined nine healthy men over 7–9 days at 4559 m and found that acute hypoxia upregulated iron acquisition by erythroid cells and subsequently led to increases in [Hb]. Of note, there was a 35% decrease in myoglobin expression and downregulation of iron-related proteins, such as L-ferritin and transferrin receptor, in skeletal muscle, suggesting that iron was being diverted from these tissues to support red blood cell production in the marrow.

While it is unclear if iron supplementation can reverse some of the effects on skeletal muscle seen by Robach *et al.*, it may have important effects beyond the hematologic responses. Smith *et al.* (2009) administered intravenous iron hydroxide sucrose or placebo to healthy men on their third day at 4340 m and demonstrated significantly lower pulmonary artery pressures in the iron-treated group on the subsequent 4 days compared to the placebo-treated group. In a related study reported in the same paper, they performed venesection of 2 L of blood on 11 high altitude residents with chronic mountain sickness over a 1-month period and found that the iron deficiency induced by venesection was associated with a 25% increase in pulmonary artery pressure during this period. Subsequent iron supplementation did not reverse the observed effect. The mechanism underlying these findings is unclear but the results suggest iron may play a key role in a wider array of responses to hypoxia than originally suspected.

9.8 PLATELET COUNTS AND FUNCTION AT ALTITUDE

The physiological response to acute hypoxia does not seem to involve any important changes in platelet count or adhesiveness, or in clotting factors. However, there may be changes associated with acute mountain sickness, high altitude pulmonary or cerebral edema. If there are changes in clotting factors, they may represent an effect or a complication of the altitude illness rather than being essential in its genesis. These issues are considered in greater detail in Chapter 23. With regard to more chronic exposures, Vij (2009) has studied platelet counts and function in 40 healthy men during prolonged stay between 4100 and 4500 m and found that platelet counts decreased by 12% after 3 months and 31% after 13 months compared to their sea level values. Mean platelet volume increased, while there was a reduction in platelet aggregation in response to ADP, epinephrine and collagen. The clinical implications of these findings were not investigated in this study.

9.9 THE COAGULATION SYSTEM AT ALTITUDE

As discussed in more detail in Chapter 23, there has long been suspicion that high altitude exposure leads to hypercoagulability and increased risk for venous thromboembolism but, to date, there has been no consistent evidence to support this assertion. In fact, data from a recent field study by Martin et al. (2012), during which they performed thromboelastography (TEG) on health volunteers at sea level, 4250 and 5300 m, suggests that the coagulation process may even be slowed at high altitude. TEG is a functional test that examines the kinetics of clot formation and provides information on the interactions of clotting factors, platelets and fibrinogen rather than simply focusing on a single element of the coagulation process. They noted that the reaction (R) times, a measure of how long it takes for clot formation to begin and kinetic time (K), which assesses the early phases of the clot formation process were both prolonged at altitude relative to sea level values, suggesting that the blood coagulates more slowly following acute exposure to high altitude. The alpha angle, another marker of early clot formation, was decreased, providing further evidence of slowed coagulation, while the maximum altitude, a measure of clot strength was unchanged.

9.10 WHITE BLOOD CELLS

The effect of hypobaric hypoxia on white blood cell counts and function is not as clear as the situation with red blood cells. While some studies have reported no change in the total leukocyte counts (Hannon et al. 1969) others have reported a rise in the number of these cells (Simon-Schnass and Korniszewski 1990). Aside from possible changes in total white blood cell counts, there may also be changes in the distribution of white blood cells. Choukèr et al. (2005) have shown, for example, that neutrophil counts are increased during rest and exercise at 3196 m. In another field study, Facco et al. (2005) used flow cytometry to characterize the white blood cell populations in healthy female volunteers at 5050 m and found a decrease in the number of CD4$^+$ T lymphocytes, no changes in the number of B lymphocytes and an increased number of natural killer (NK) cells. The latter finding agreed with that of an earlier study performed in a decompression chamber at 380 mmHg (Klokker et al. 1993).

Anecdotal evidence over the years has suggested that viral or bacterial infections are slow to clear at high altitude raising suspicion that white blood cell function may be altered in this environment. Data supporting this claim are limited, however. Despite finding increased numbers of NK cells, Facco et al. (2005) did not find any changes in their cytotoxic activity. Faoro et al. (2011) showed that leukocyte oxygen consumption was decreased in individuals who had actively climbed to 4559 m and was accompanied by evidence of lower leukocyte mitochondrial respiration and decreased respiratory burst. This finding is similar to that of Choukèr et al. (2005) who showed that markers of neutrophil cytotoxic function, such as superoxide production, were inhibited following active ascent to 3196 m. Cytotoxic function was increased, however, following passive ascent by helicopter to the same elevation. Overall, these studies suggest there may be changes in white blood cell function at high altitude but evidence linking these changes to clinical outcomes is still lacking.

Blood-gas transport and acid–base balance

SUMMARY

The polycythemia of high altitude was covered in Chapter 9. Alterations of the oxygen affinity of hemoglobin can alter the oxygen dissociation curve at high altitude and therefore affect oxygen transport by the blood. Many animals that live in oxygen-deprived environments have high oxygen affinities of their hemoglobin. This is the case in the human fetus. It is interesting that climbers at extreme altitude increase their oxygen affinity by extreme hyperventilation which causes a marked respiratory alkalosis. The effect of the alkalosis overwhelms the small decrease in oxygen affinity caused by the increased concentration of 2,3-diphosphoglycerate in the red blood cells. The P_{50} of high altitude natives is essentially the same as the sea level value according to most studies. However, lowlanders living at high altitude for weeks tend to have a reduced P_{50}, indicating an increased oxygen affinity of hemoglobin. An increased oxygen affinity is advantageous at high altitude because it assists in the loading of oxygen by the pulmonary capillaries. The acid–base status of high altitude natives is a little controversial but many studies have found a normal arterial pH, indicating a fully compensated respiratory alkalosis. However, acclimatized lowlanders usually have a slightly alkaline pH, indicating that metabolic compensation is not complete. There is evidence that at extreme altitude, metabolic compensation for the respiratory alkalosis is slow, possibly because of chronic volume depletion caused by dehydration.

10.1 INTRODUCTION

Physiological changes in the blood play an important role in acclimatization and adaptation to high altitude. In this chapter, the main topics considered are the changes in oxygen affinity of hemoglobin, and the alterations of the acid–base status of the blood. The increase in red cell concentration of the blood was discussed in Chapter 9, where the regulation of erythropoiesis was described. Some of the consequences of an altered oxygen affinity of hemoglobin are alluded to in other chapters, especially Chapter 7 on diffusion of oxygen across the blood-gas barrier, and Chapter 13 on limiting factors at extreme altitude.

10.2 HISTORICAL

10.2.1 Oxygen dissociation curve

The honor of plotting the first oxygen and carbon dioxide dissociation curves apparently belongs to Paul Bert. In his monumental book *La Pression Barométrique* he reported the relationships between partial pressure and blood gas concentration for both oxygen and carbon dioxide as experimental animals were exposed to lower and lower barometric pressures, or as they were gradually asphyxiated by rebreathing in a closed space (Bert 1878, pp. 135–8 in the 1943 translation). However, he did not discover the S-shaped curve for oxygen because he did not reduce the Po_2 far enough.

The first oxygen dissociation curve over its whole range was published by Christian Bohr in 1885. The measurements were made on dilute solutions of hemoglobin and showed precise hyperbolas (Bohr 1885). They were clearly not compatible with the data obtained by Bert in experimental animals, although Bohr did not comment on this. Hüfner (1890) published similar curves for hemoglobin solutions and argued that a hyperbolic shape would be expected from the simple equation

$$Hb + O_2 \rightarrow HbO_2$$

An important advance was made by Bohr when he used whole blood rather than hemoglobin solutions and this led him to the discovery of the now familiar S-shaped curve. In the following year he showed, in collaboration with Hasselbalch and Krogh, that the dissociation curve was shifted to the right when the Pco_2 of the blood was increased, a phenomenon which came to be known as the Bohr effect (Bohr et al. 1904). A few years later, Barcroft found that the addition of acid displaced the dissociation curve to the right (Barcroft and Orbeli 1910), and also that an increase in temperature had the same effect (Barcroft and King 1909). Astrup and Severinghaus (1986) wrote a valuable historical review of blood gases and acid–base balance.

Soon after these important modulators of the oxygen affinity of hemoglobin were discovered, physiologists wondered about their importance at high altitude. For example, when Barcroft accompanied the first international high altitude expedition to Tenerife in 1910, he made a special study of the position of the oxygen dissociation curve, expecting it to be displaced to the left by the low arterial Pco_2. In the event, he found that the oxygen dissociation curves of some members of the expedition at 2130 and 3000 m were shifted to the right when measured at the normal sea level Pco_2 of 40 mmHg. However, when he repeated the equilibrations at the subjects' actual Pco_2 at altitude, the positions of the curves were essentially the same as at sea level (Barcroft 1911). He concluded that the decrease in carbonic acid in the blood was compensated for by an increase in some other acid, possibly lactic acid. One year later Barcroft went to Mosso's laboratory, the Capanna Regina Margherita on Monte Rosa (4559 m), and reported a slight excess acidity of the blood at that altitude (Barcroft et al. 1914).

Some 10 years later, during the 1921–22 International High Altitude Expedition to Cerro de Pasco in Peru, Barcroft and his colleagues found an increased oxygen affinity in acclimatized lowlanders as a result of the increased alkalinity of the blood. It also appeared that the increase in affinity was greater than could be explained by the change in acid–base status (Barcroft et al. 1923).

The question of oxygen affinity of hemoglobin was examined again on the International High Altitude Expedition to Chile in 1935. It was found that the 'physiological' dissociation curves (that is, measured at a subject's own Pco_2) were displaced slightly to the left of the sea level values up to about 4270 m, but above that altitude, the curves were displaced increasingly to the right of the sea level positions (Keys et al. 1936). Measurements of oxygen affinity of the hemoglobin were also made at constant pH and these showed a uniform tendency to a decreased affinity. The investigators argued that this rightward shift of the curve might be advantageous at high altitude because it would facilitate oxygen unloading to the tissues.

An important discovery was made in 1967 by two groups working independently (Benesch and Benesch 1967; Chanutin and Curnish 1967) that a fourth factor (in addition to Pco_2, pH and temperature) had an important effect on the oxygen affinity of hemoglobin. This was the concentration of 2,3-diphosphoglycerate (2,3-DPG) within the red cells. This unexpected development raised doubts about much of the earlier work where this important factor had not been controlled, and it was shown that 2,3-DPG was depleted when blood was stored. It was subsequently shown that 2,3-DPG increased at high altitude (Lenfant *et al.* 1968) and they argued that the resulting decrease in oxygen affinity, which facilitated unloading of oxygen in the tissues, was an important part of the adaptation process (Lenfant and Sullivan 1971).

Until recently, relatively little information was available on the oxygen affinity of hemoglobin at extreme altitudes. A few measurements from the Silver Hut Expedition of 1960–61 showed that lowlanders who were well acclimatized to 5800 m had an almost fully compensated respiratory alkalosis (West *et al.* 1962). Data above this altitude did not exist. It was therefore astonishing to find on the 1981 American Medical Research Expedition to Everest that climbers near the summit apparently had an extreme degree of respiratory alkalosis which greatly increased the oxygen affinity of their hemoglobin. The arterial pH of Pizzo on the Everest summit exceeded 7.7 as determined from the alveolar P_{CO_2} and base excess, both of which were measured (section 10.4.4).

10.2.2 Acid–base balance

Turning now to the early history of acid–base balance at high altitude, it is clear from the above that this overlaps considerably with a discussion of oxygen affinity of hemoglobin. However, the reaction of the blood (as it was called) at high altitude created a great deal of interest in its own right. Indeed, the acid–base status of the blood played an important role in early theories of the control of breathing at high altitude (Kellogg 1980). As long ago as 1903, Galeotti studied various experimental animals taken to Mosso's Capanna Margherita laboratory on Monte Rosa, and found that the amount of acid needed to bring their hemolyzed blood to a standard pH (determined from litmus paper) was decreased compared with sea level (Galeotti 1904). He interpreted this decrease in titratable alkalinity

to mean that there was an increase in some acid substance in the blood. It was known that hypoxia caused lactic acid production (Araki 1891) and that acid blood stimulated breathing (Zuntz *et al.* 1906). It was therefore natural to conclude that this explained the hyperventilation of high altitude, and that the P_{CO_2} fell as a consequence (Boycott and Haldane 1908). Winterstein (1911) formulated what became known as the 'reaction theory' of breathing, which stated that the effects of both hypoxia and carbon dioxide as stimulants of ventilation could be explained by the fact that they both acidified the blood.

The correct explanation of how hypoxia stimulates ventilation at high altitude had to wait for discovery of the peripheral chemoreceptors by Heymans and Heymans (1925). Meanwhile, Winterstein (1915) provided evidence against his own theory when he showed that, in acute hypoxia, the blood becomes alkaline rather than acid. A few years later, Henderson (1919) and Haldane *et al.* (1919) correctly explained the alkalinity as being secondary to the lowered P_{CO_2} caused by hyperventilation. Nevertheless, it is true that even today the control of ventilation during chronic hypoxia is a subject of intense research (Chapter 6) and interest still remains in the acid–base status of the extracellular fluid (ECF) which forms the environment of the central chemoreceptors.

10.3 OXYGEN AFFINITY OF HEMOGLOBIN

10.3.1 Basic physiology

Figure 10.1 shows the oxygen dissociation curve of human whole blood and the four factors that shift the curve to the right, that is decrease the affinity of oxygen for hemoglobin. These four factors are increases in P_{CO_2}, hydrogen ion concentration, temperature and the concentration of 2,3-DPG in the red cells. Increasing the ionic concentration of the plasma also reduces oxygen affinity.

Almost all of the change in oxygen affinity caused by P_{CO_2} can be ascribed to its effect on hydrogen ion concentration, although a change in P_{CO_2} has a small effect in its own right (Margaria

1957). The mechanism of the alteration of oxygen affinity through hydrogen ion concentration (Bohr effect) is by a change in configuration of the hemoglobin molecule which makes the

binding site less accessible to molecular oxygen as the hydrogen ion concentration is raised. The molecule exists in two forms: one in which the chemical subunits are maximally chemically bonded (T form), and another in which some bonds are ruptured and the structure is relaxed (R form). The R form has a higher affinity for oxygen because the molecule can more easily enter the region of the heme. The approximate magnitudes of the effects of change in P_{CO_2} and pH on the oxygen dissociation curve are shown in the right insets of Fig. 10.1.

An increase in temperature has a large effect on the oxygen affinity of hemoglobin, as shown in the top inset of Fig. 10.1. The temperature effect follows from thermodynamic considerations: the combination of oxygen with hemoglobin is exothermic so that an increase in temperature favors the reverse reaction, that is dissociation of the oxyhemoglobin.

The compound 2,3-DPG is a product of red cell metabolism, as shown in Fig. 10.2. An increased concentration of this material within the red cell reduces the oxygen affinity of the hemoglobin by increasing the chemical binding of the subunits and converting more hemoglobin to the low affinity T form.

A useful number to describe the oxygen affinity of hemoglobin is the P_{50}, that is the P_{O_2} when 50%

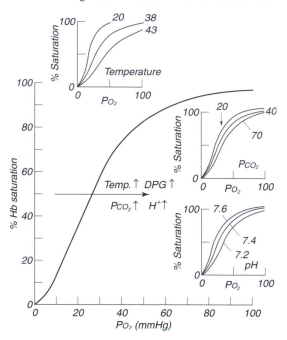

Figure 10.1 Normal oxygen dissociation curve and its displacement by increases in H$^+$, P_{CO_2}, temperature and 2,3-diphosphoglycerate (2.3-DPG). (From West 1994.)

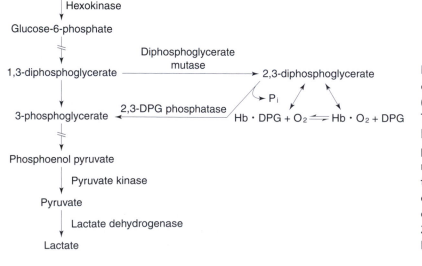

Figure 10.2 Formation of 2,3-diphosphoglycerate (2,3-DPG) in erythrocytes. The vertical chain at the left shows the glycolytic pathway in cells other than red blood cells. In red cells the enzyme DPG mutase catalyzes the conversion of much of the 1,3-DPG to 2,3-DPG. (Modified from Mines 1981.)

of the binding sites are attached to oxygen. The normal value for adult whole blood at a P_{CO_2} of 40 mmHg, pH 7.4, temperature 37°C and normal 2,3-DPG concentration is 26–27 mmHg. Human fetal blood has a P_{50} of about 19 mmHg, mainly because fetal hemoglobin has two gamma rather than two beta chains and this reduces the affinity for 2,3-DPG. An increase of 2,3-DPG within the red cell increases the P_{50} by about 0.5 mmHg mol^{-1} of 2,3-DPG. The magnitude of the Bohr effect is usually given in terms of the increase in log P_{50} per pH unit. The normal value for human blood is 0.4 at constant P_{CO_2}. Note that although historically the 'Bohr effect' referred to the change in affinity caused by P_{CO_2}, in modern usage the term is restricted to the effect of pH. The temperature effect is 0.24 for the change in log P_{50} (mmHg °C^{-1}).

Much can be learned about the effect of changes in the oxygen affinity of hemoglobin on the physiology of high altitude by modeling the oxygen transport system using computer subroutines for the oxygen and carbon dioxide dissociation curves (Bencowitz *et al.* 1982). Kelman described useful subroutines for the oxygen dissociation curve (Kelman 1966a; Kelman 1966b) and the carbon dioxide dissociation curve (Kelman 1967). The practical use of these procedures has been described (West and Wagner 1977). These procedures are able to accommodate changes in P_{CO_2}, pH, temperature and 2,3-DPG concentration, and allow the investigator to answer questions about the interactions of these variables which would otherwise be impossibly complicated.

10.3.2 Animals native to high altitude

It has been known for many years that animals that live at high altitude tend to have an increased oxygen affinity of their hemoglobin. Figure 7.7 shows part of the oxygen dissociation curves of the vicuna and llama which are native to high altitude in the South American Andes (Hall *et al.* 1936). The diagram also shows the range of dissociation curves for eight lowland animals, including humans, horse, dog, rabbit, pig, peccary,

ox and sheep. It can be seen that the hemoglobin of high altitude native animals has a substantially increased oxygen affinity. This adaptation to high altitude is of genetic origin, as is shown by the fact that a llama brought up in a zoo at sea level has the same high oxygen affinity.

High altitude birds also have high oxygen affinities for hemoglobin. Hall and his colleagues (Hall *et al.* 1936), during the 1935 International High Altitude Expedition to Chile, reported that the high altitude ostrich and huallaga have higher oxygen affinities than a group of six lowland birds including pigeon, muscovy duck, domestic goose, domestic duck, Chinese pheasant and domestic fowl. A particularly interesting example is the bar-headed goose which is known to fly over the Himalayan ranges as it migrates between its breeding grounds in Siberia and its wintering grounds in India. This remarkable bird has a blood P_{50} about 10 mmHg lower than its close relatives from moderate altitudes (Black and Tenney 1980; Scott *et al.* 2011). Diving emperor penguins also have hemoglobin with an increased oxygen affinity (Meir and Ponganis 2009). Tibetan chick embryos have a higher oxygen affinity of hemoglobin and higher red cell concentrations than lowland embryos (Zhang *et al.* 2007; Liu *et al.* 2009).

Deer mice, *Peromyscus maniculatus*, show the same relationships. A study was carried out on 10 subspecies that live at altitudes from below sea level in Death Valley in California to the high mountains of the nearby Sierra Nevada (4350 m), and it was found that there was a strong correlation between the habitat altitude and the oxygen affinity of the blood. The genetic source of this relationship was proved by moving one subspecies to another location and showing that the oxygen affinity was unchanged. Moreover, the relationship persisted in second-generation animals (Snyder *et al.* 1982). Storz *et al.* (2012) have carried out a detailed study of polymorphism in deer mice at different altitudes. By contrast, river otters living at an altitude of 2357 m have been shown to have an increased hemoglobin concentration but a normal oxygen affinity compared with those at sea level (Crait *et al.* 2012). Weber (2007) has reviewed high altitude adaptations in vertebrate hemoglobins.

10.3.3 Animals in other oxygen-deprived environments

High altitude is just one of the oxygen-deprived environments in which animals are found, and it is interesting to consider the variety of strategies that have been adopted to mitigate the problems posed by oxygen deficiency. Table 7.1 shows examples of some of the strategies that have been adopted through genetic adaptation. The change in the globin chains of hemoglobin and the subsequent alteration in the affinity for 2,3-DPG in the human fetus has already been referred to. An alteration in globin chains also occurs in the bar-headed goose. The next two groups increase the oxygen affinity of their hemoglobin by decreasing the concentration of organic phosphates. This is done with 2,3-DPG in the fetus of the dog, horse and pig, and by decreasing the concentration of adenosine triphosphate (ATP) in the trout and eel.

Some species of tadpoles that frequently live in stagnant pools have a high oxygen affinity hemoglobin, whereas the adult frogs produce a different type of hemoglobin with a lower affinity that fits their higher oxygen environment. Note also that the tadpole blood shows a smaller Bohr effect. This is useful because low oxygen and high carbon dioxide pressures are likely to occur together in stagnant water, and a large Bohr effect would be disadvantageous because it would decrease the oxygen affinity of the blood when a high affinity was most needed.

As indicated earlier, the human fetus also has a high oxygen affinity by virtue of its fetal hemoglobin. This is essential because the arterial P_{O_2} of the fetus is less than 30 mmHg. Indeed, the human fetus and the adult climber on the summit of Mount Everest have some similar features in that in both cases the arterial P_{O_2} is extremely low, and the P_{50} of the arterial blood (at the prevailing pH) is also very low (section 10.4.4).

A particularly interesting example of an unusual human hemoglobin was described by Hebbel *et al.* (1978). The authors studied a family in which two of the siblings had a mutant hemoglobin (Andrew-Minneapolis) with a P_{50} of 17.1 mmHg. They showed that the siblings with the abnormal hemoglobin tolerated exercise at an altitude of 3100 m better than the normal siblings.

The last row in Table 7.1 refers to the climber at extreme altitude who has a marked respiratory alkalosis which greatly increases the oxygen affinity of the hemoglobin. This is discussed in detail below.

10.3.4 Highlanders

Aste-Salazar and Hurtado (1944) measured the oxygen dissociation curves of 17 healthy Peruvians in Lima at sea level and 12 other permanent residents of Morococha (4550 m). These studies were subsequently extended to a total of 40 subjects in Lima and 30 in Morococha (Hurtado 1964). The mean value of the P_{50} at pH 7.4 was 24.7 mmHg at sea level and 26.9 mmHg at high altitude (Fig. 9.3). It was argued that the rightward displacement of the curve would enhance the unloading of oxygen from the peripheral capillaries.

Winslow and his colleagues (1981) reported oxygen dissociation curves on 46 native Peruvians in Morococha (4550 m, P_B 432 mmHg) and reported that at pH 7.4 the P_{50} was significantly

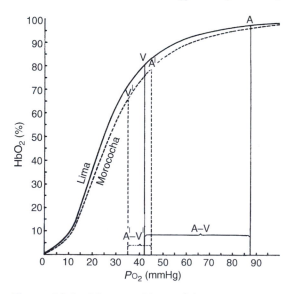

Figure 10.3 Mean positions of the oxygen dissociation curves of Peruvians in Lima (sea level) and Morococha (4540 m). Note that the high altitude natives have a slightly reduced oxygen affinity. Mean values of the P_{O_2} in arterial (A) and mixed venous (V) blood for the two groups are also shown. (From Hurtado 1964.)

higher in the high altitude population than in the sea level controls (31.2 mmHg as opposed to 29.2 mmHg, $p < 0.001$). However, these investigators also found that the acid–base status of the high altitude subjects was that of a partially compensated respiratory alkalosis with a mean plasma pH of 7.44. When the P_{50} values were corrected to the subjects' actual plasma pH, the mean value of 30.1 mmHg could no longer be distinguished from that of the sea level controls (Fig. 10.4). The conclusion was that the small increase in P_{50} resulting from the increased concentration of 2,3-DPG in the red cells was offset by the mild degree of respiratory alkalosis,

with the net result that the position of the oxygen dissociation curve was essentially the same as that in sea level controls.

In a controversial study, Morpurgo *et al.* (1976) reported that Sherpas living permanently at an altitude of 4000 m in the Nepalese Himalayas had a substantially increased oxygen affinity at standard pH. However, a subsequent study by Samaja *et al.* (1979) failed to confirm this provocative finding. Samaja *et al.* also showed that the oxygen affinity could be completely accounted for by the known effectors of hemoglobin function: pH, P_{CO_2}, 2,3-DPG and temperature.

10.3.5 Acclimatized lowlanders

Early measurements by Barcroft (1911), Barcroft *et al.* (1911), Barcroft *et al.* (1923), Keys *et al.* (1936) and Hall (1936) showed somewhat conflicting results. Possible reasons for this were clarified when the role of 2,3-DPG in the red cell was appreciated (Benesch and Benesch 1967; Chanutin and Curnish 1967). It was shown that this normal product of red cell metabolism reduced the oxygen affinity of hemoglobin, and it was then clear that many previous measurements were unreliable because of ignorance of this factor. Lenfant and his colleagues (Lenfant *et al.* 1968; Lenfant *et al.* 1969; Lenfant *et al.* 1971) showed that the concentration of 2,3-DPG was increased in lowlanders when they became acclimatized to high altitude. The primary cause of the increase in 2,3-DPG was the increase in plasma pH above the normal sea level value as a result of the respiratory alkalosis. When subjects were made acidotic with acetazolamide there was no increase in plasma pH or red cell 2,3-DPG concentration at high altitude, and the oxygen dissociation curve did not shift to the right. It was argued that the increase in 2,3-DPG was an important feature of the acclimatization process of lowlanders and of the adaptation to high altitude of highlanders (Lenfant and Sullivan 1971). Treatment with erythropoietin is known to increase 2,3-DPG levels in red cells at sea level (Birgegard and Sandhagen 2001).

Subsequent measurements on lowlanders at high altitude have confirmed these changes, although there is still some uncertainty about

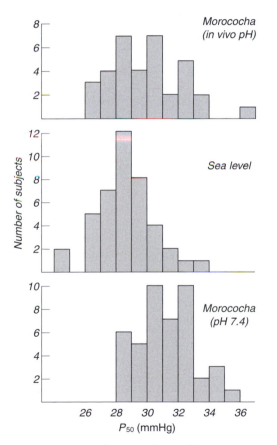

Figure 10.4 Distribution of P_{50} values at sea level and high altitude. In the top panel, values are expressed at the *in vivo* pH; in the bottom at pH 7.4. When corrected for the subjects' plasma pH, the *in vivo* P_{50} at high altitude falls in the sea level range in all but one subject. (From Winslow *et al.* 1981.)

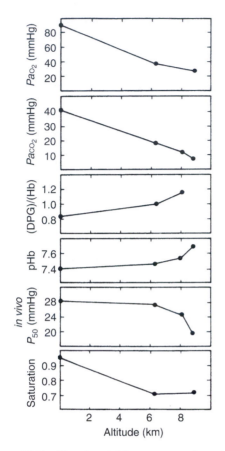

Figure 10.5 Blood variables measured on the 1981 American Medical Research Expedition to Everest at sea level, 6300 m, 8050 m and 8848 m (summit). pHb, pH blood. (From Winslow et al. 1984.)

whether acclimatized lowlanders develop complete metabolic compensation for their respiratory alkalosis (that is, whether the pH returns to 7.4). Certainly, this does not happen at extremely high altitudes. During the 1981 American Medical Research Expedition to Everest, Winslow et al. (1984) made an extensive series of measurements on acclimatized lowlanders at an altitude of 6300 m. They also obtained data on two subjects who reached the summit (8848 m). These measurements were made on venous blood samples taken at an altitude of 8050 m the morning after the summit climb. Winslow and his colleagues found that the red cell concentration of 2,3-DPG increased with altitude (Fig. 10.5) and that this was associated with a slightly increased P_{50} value when expressed

at pH 7.4. However, because the respiratory alkalosis was not fully compensated, the subjects' *in vivo* P_{50} at 6300 m (27.6 mmHg) was slightly less than at sea level (28.1 mmHg). The estimated *in vivo* P_{50} was found to become progressively lower at 8050 m (24.9 mmHg), and on the summit at 8848 m it was as low as 19.4 mmHg in one subject. Thus these data show that, at extreme altitudes, the blood oxygen dissociation curve shifts progressively leftward (increased oxygen affinity of hemoglobin) primarily because of the respiratory alkalosis. Indeed, this effect completely overwhelms the relatively small tendency for the curve to shift to the right because of the increase in red cell 2,3-DPG.

The results obtained on Operation Everest II were generally in agreement with these (Sutton *et al.* 1988) except that the P_{CO_2} values at extreme altitude were higher, and the blood pH values therefore lower. These differences can probably be explained by the smaller degree of acclimatization for reasons that are still not clear.

10.3.6 Physiological effects of changes in oxygen affinity

There have been differences of opinion on whether a decreased or an increased oxygen affinity is beneficial at high altitude. Barcroft *et al.* (1923) found a slightly increased affinity and argued that this would enhance oxygen loading in the lung. However, Aste-Salazar and Hurtado (1944) reported a slight decrease in oxygen affinity in high altitude natives at Morococha and reasoned that this would enhance oxygen unloading in peripheral capillaries (Fig. 10.3). The same argument was used by Lenfant and Sullivan (1971) when the influence of the increased red cell concentration of 2,3-DPG on the oxygen dissociation curve was appreciated. They stated that the decreased oxygen affinity would help the peripheral unloading of oxygen, and that this was one of the many features both of acclimatization of lowlanders to high altitude and of the genetic adaptation of highlanders.

However, there is now strong evidence that an increased oxygen affinity (left-shifted oxygen dissociation curve) is beneficial, especially at higher altitudes, and particularly on exercise (Bencowitz *et al.* 1982). Indeed, this should not come as a surprise when it is appreciated that many animals increase the oxygen affinity of their blood in oxygen-deprived environments by a variety of strategies (section 10.3.3 and Table 6.1). In addition, Eaton *et al.* (1974) reported that rats whose oxygen dissociation curve had been left-shifted by cyanate administration showed an increased survival when they were decompressed to a barometric pressure of 233 mmHg. The controls were rats with a normal oxygen affinity. Turek *et al.* (1978) also studied cyanate-treated rats and found that they maintained better oxygen transfer to tissues during severe hypoxia than normal animals. In addition, we have already referred to the studies of Hebbel *et al.* (1978),

who found a family with two members who had a hemoglobin with a very high affinity (Hb Andrew-Minneapolis, P_{50} 17.1 mmHg). These two members performed better during exercise at an altitude of 3100 m than two siblings with normal hemoglobin.

Theoretical studies show that a high oxygen affinity is beneficial at high altitude, especially on exercise (Turek *et al.* 1973; Bencowitz *et al.* 1982). In one study, oxygen transfer from air to tissues was modeled for a variety of altitudes and a range of oxygen uptakes (Bencowitz *et al.* 1982). The oxygen dissociation curve was shifted both to the left and right with P_{50} of 16.8 mmHg (left-shifted), 26.8 mmHg (normal) and 36.8 mmHg (right-shifted). The pulmonary diffusing capacity for oxygen was varied over a

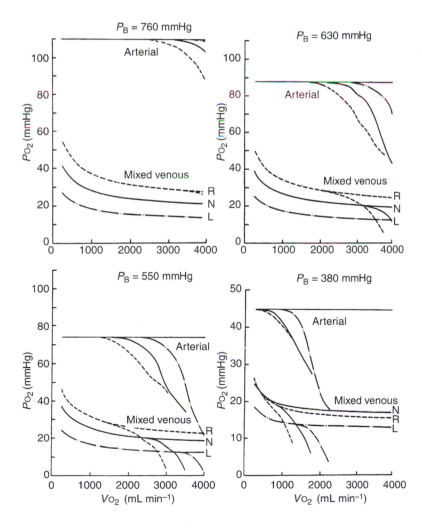

Figure 10.6 Results of a theoretical study showing changes in calculated arterial and mixed venous P_{O_2} with increasing oxygen uptake at four altitudes for three values of P_{50}. The P_{50} values are normal (N, 26.8 mmHg), right-shifted (R, 36.8 mmHg) and left-shifted (L, 16.8 mmHg). The nearly horizontal lines labeled 'mixed venous' show the P_{O_2} values for an infinitely high pulmonary oxygen diffusing capacity. The curved lines peeling away from these lines show the results of diffusion limitation. In this example, the diffusing capacity of the membrane for oxygen (DM_{O_2}) is 80 mL min^{-1} mmHg^{-1}. Note that at the highest level of exercise, and especially at high altitude, the left-shifted curve gives the highest values of P_{O_2} in mixed venous blood and therefore the tissues. (From Bencowitz *et al.* 1982.)

wide range and all the determinants of oxygen transport, including temperature, base excess, hemoglobin concentration and hematocrit, were taken into account.

The results showed that in the presence of diffusion limitation of oxygen transfer across the blood-gas barrier in the lung, a left-shifted curve resulted in the highest P_{O_2} of mixed venous blood (which was taken as an index of tissue P_{O_2}) (Fig. 10.6). In other words, in the presence of diffusion limitation, an increased oxygen affinity of hemoglobin results in a higher tissue P_{O_2}. The explanation is that the increased affinity enhances the loading of oxygen in the lung more than it interferes with unloading in peripheral capillaries. This appears to be the physiological justification for the increased oxygen affinity so frequently seen among animals that live in low oxygen environments (Table 7.1).

An analysis of the effects of changes in hemoglobin–oxygen affinity at high altitude was carried out by Samaja *et al.* (2003). They concluded that a reduction in affinity was advantageous at altitudes up to about 5000 m because it reduces the cardiac output necessary for adequate tissue oxygenation. However, at higher altitudes an increased oxygen affinity was more advantageous, in agreement with Turek *et al.* (1978) and Bencowitz *et al.* (1982). Samaja *et al.* (2003) noted that some of the experimental evidence is contradictory, and they raised the possibility of other confounding factors, such as changes in body temperature, especially differences between the muscles and lungs, changes in the Bohr effect within capillaries, heterogeneity of oxygen affinity between different red cells, possible vasodilator effects of nitric oxide carried by hemoglobin, and the effect of different red cell transit times in capillaries. Martin and his colleagues (Martin *et al.* 2009; Martin *et al.* 2010) showed increased heterogeneity of blood flow in the sublingual microcirculation of climbers at 4900 m altitude on Cho Oyu and up to 7950 m on Mount Everest. Possible factors that might be responsible include polycythemia and dehydration which could increase the hematocrit.

The role of an increased oxygen affinity was seen dramatically in a climber on the summit of Mount Everest. Despite some increase of 2,3-DPG concentration within the red cell, the extremely low P_{CO_2} of 7–8 mmHg as a result of the enormous increase in ventilation causes a dramatic degree of respiratory alkalosis with an arterial pH calculated to exceed 7.7 (West *et al.* 1983b). As a result, the *in vivo* P_{50} is about 19 mmHg, which is very similar to that of the human fetus *in utero*. The resulting striking increase in oxygen affinity of hemoglobin plays a major role in allowing the climber to survive this extremely hypoxic environment (Chapter 12).

10.4 ACID–BASE BALANCE

10.4.1 Introduction

This topic overlaps with that of the previous section, oxygen affinity of hemoglobin, because the affinity at high altitude is primarily determined by the pH of the blood together with the concentration of 2,3-DPG in the red cells. However, for convenience, available information on acid–base status is set out here.

10.4.2 During acclimatization

When a lowlander goes to high altitude, hyperventilation occurs as a result of stimulation of the peripheral chemoreceptors by the hypoxemia (Chapters 5 and 6), the arterial P_{CO_2} falls, and the arterial pH rises in accordance with the Henderson–Hasselbalch equation:

$$pH = pK + \log \frac{\left[HCO_3^- \right]}{0.03 \, P_{CO_2}}$$

where $[HCO_3^-]$ is the bicarbonate concentration in millimoles per liter and the P_{CO_2} is in mmHg. However, the kidney responds by eliminating bicarbonate ion, being prompted to do this by the decreased P_{CO_2} in the renal tubular cells. The result is a more alkaline urine because of decreased reabsorption of bicarbonate ions. The resulting decrease in plasma bicarbonate then moves the bicarbonate/P_{CO_2} ratio back towards its normal level. This is known as metabolic compensation for the respiratory alkalosis. The compensation may be complete, in which case the arterial pH returns to 7.4 or, more usually, incomplete with a steady-state pH that exceeds 7.4.

The time course of the changes in arterial pH when normal subjects are taken abruptly to high altitude has been studied by several investigators (Severinghaus *et al.* 1963; Lenfant *et al.* 1971; Dempsey *et al.* 1978). In one study, lowlanders were taken from sea level to an altitude of 4509 m (P_B 446 mmHg) in less than 5 hours, and remained there for 4 days. The arterial pH rose to a mean of about 7.47 within 24 hours and then apparently slowly declined but was still about 7.45 at the end of the 4-day period. On return to sea level the pH fell steadily to reach the normal value of 7.4 after about 48 hours (Lenfant *et al.* 1971).

In another study, four normal subjects were taken abruptly to 3800 m for 8 days. The arterial pH rapidly rose from a mean of 7.424 at sea level to 7.485 after 2 days, and remained essentially constant, being 7.484 at the end of 8 days (Severinghaus *et al.* 1963). In a further study, 11

lowlanders moved to 3200 m altitude where they remained for 10 days (Dempsey *et al.* 1978). The arterial pH rose by 0.03–0.04 unit within 2 days and then remained essentially unchanged. In all instances, the arterial P_{CO_2} continued to fall as did the plasma bicarbonate concentration. However, it appears that the return of the arterial pH to (or near to) its sea level value is very slow.

10.4.3 Highlanders

Most authors have reported a fully compensated respiratory alkalosis in high altitude natives with arterial pH values close to 7.4. Table 10.1 shows a summary of a number of published papers prepared by Winslow and Monge (1987). This is perhaps the expected finding. The body generally maintains the arterial pH within very narrow limits in health, and it seems reasonable that people who are born and live at high altitude would fully compensate for

Table 10.1   Blood-gas and pH values in high altitude natives

Altitude (m)	n	Hb[a]	Pa,o$_2$ (mmHg)	Sa,o$_2$ (%)	Pa,co$_2$ (mmHg)	pH	Source
4300	3	–	46.7	84.6	–	–	Barcroft et al. (1923)
4300	12	–	–	–	–	7.360	Aste-Salazar and Hurtado (1944)
4500	40	20.6[a]	45.1	80.1	33.3	7.370	Hurtado et al. (1956)
4515	22	19.5[a]	–	82.8	33.8	7.400	Chiodi (1957)
4300	6	56.0	–	–	32.5	7.431[b]	Monge et al. (1964)
4300	5	73.8	–	–	39.0	7.429[b]	Monge et al. (1964)
3700	–	–	–	–	3.0	7.431[b]	Monge et al. (1964)
4545	–	–	–	–	–	7.424[b]	Monge et al. (1964)
4820	–	–	–	–	–	7.426[b]	Monge et al. (1964)
3960	3	–	–	–	–		Lahiri et al. (1967)
4880	4	–	–	–	–	7.399	Lahiri et al. (1967)
4500	6	73.4	–	–	–	–	Lenfant et al. (1969)
4500	10	65.5	–	–	–	–	Lenfant et al. (1969)
4300	6	54.4	45.2	74.7	31.6	7.414	Torrance (1970)[c]
4500	4	63.3	44.1	73.3	32.2	7.405	Torrance (1970)[c]
4300	4	–	50.8	–	32.9	7.405	Rennie (1971)
4500	35	61.0	51.7	85.7	34.0	7.395	Winslow et al. (1981)

See Winslow and Monge (1987) for details and sources.
–, no data available.
[a]Hemoglobin concentration (g dL^{-1}).
[b]Plasma pH.
[c]Himalayan subjects.

their reduced $P\text{CO}_2$ by eliminating bicarbonate and restoring the pH to the normal sea level value.

However, Winslow *et al.* (1981) measured the arterial pH in 46 high altitude natives of Morococha (4550 m, P_B 432 mmHg) and reported that the mean plasma pH was 7.439 ± 0.065. In other words, these highlanders did not have a fully compensated respiratory alkalosis but their blood lay slightly on the alkaline side of normal. As pointed out in section 10.3.4, the result of this mild respiratory alkalosis was to restore the oxygen dissociation curve to the normal sea level position because there was an increase in red cell 2,3-DPG concentration which tended to move the curve to the right.

The interpretation of these results is complicated by the fact that Winslow *et al.* (1981) believed that the increased red cell concentration that is seen at high altitude had an effect on the glass electrode for measuring pH (Whittembury *et al.* 1968). If the observed pH is corrected for this effect of increased red cell concentration, the calculated plasma pH becomes 7.395, as shown in the bottom row of Table 10.1. However, no other investigators have corrected the pH in this way and the conclusion from the work of Winslow and his colleagues is that high altitude natives have a mildly uncompensated respiratory alkalosis with an arterial pH that exceeds 7.4.

10.4.4 Acclimatized lowlanders

When sufficient time is allowed for extended acclimatization to high altitude, the arterial pH returns close to the normal value of 7.4, at least up to altitudes of 3000 m. For example, during the 1935 International High Altitude Expedition to Chile, Dill and his colleagues (Dill *et al.* 1937) found that the arterial pH increased little, if at all, up to this altitude, but above 3000 m higher values of pH were found, with a mean of about 7.45 at an altitude of 5340 m. A few measurements on acclimatized subjects at an altitude of 5800 m during the 1960–61 Silver Hut Expedition indicated values of between 7.41 and 7.46 (West *et al.* 1962).

Extensive measurements were made by Winslow *et al.* (1984) during the 1981 American Medical Research Expedition to Everest. The mean arterial pH of acclimatized lowlanders living at an

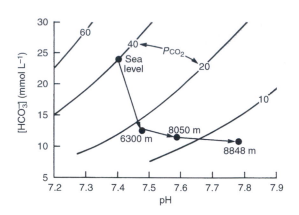
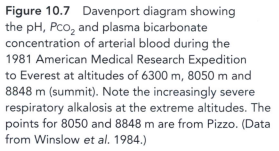

Figure 10.7   Davenport diagram showing the pH, $P\text{CO}_2$ and plasma bicarbonate concentration of arterial blood during the 1981 American Medical Research Expedition to Everest at altitudes of 6300 m, 8050 m and 8848 m (summit). Note the increasingly severe respiratory alkalosis at the extreme altitudes. The points for 8050 and 8848 m are from Pizzo. (Data from Winslow *et al.* 1984.)

altitude of 6300 m was 7.47 (Fig. 10.7). It was also possible to calculate the arterial pH at an altitude of 8050 m (Camp 5) and the Everest summit (8848 m). The calculations were made from the base excess measured on venous blood samples taken at 8050 m and measurements of alveolar $P\text{CO}_2$ on sealed samples of alveolar gas brought back to the USA. It was assumed that the arterial and alveolar $P\text{CO}_2$ values were the same, and also that base excess did not change over the 24 hours between the summit and Camp 5. As discussed in section 10.4.5, there is evidence that base excess was changing very slowly at this great altitude. The mean arterial pH of two climbers at 8050 m was 7.55, and the one subject whose alveolar $P\text{CO}_2$ was measured as 7.5 mmHg on the summit gave a calculated arterial pH of over 7.7.

These climbers were not 'acclimatized' to 8050 or 8848 m in the sense that they had spent long periods at these great altitudes. However, it is not possible to spend an extended time at an altitude such as 8000 m because high altitude deterioration occurs so rapidly. Thus the values probably represent the inevitable respiratory alkalosis which occurs in climbers who go so high.

Arterial blood samples were taken from four climbers during the Caudwell Xtreme Everest

Expedition at an altitude of 8400 m. The pH values were 7.45, 7.52, 7.55 and 7.60 (Grocott *et al.* 2009). Other measurements on these samples are discussed in Chapter 13, section 13.3.4.

Samaja *et al.* (1997) measured the pH and blood gases from arterialized earlobe blood in lowlanders and Sherpas at altitudes of 3400, 5050 and 6450 m in the Everest region. In the lowlanders the blood pH increased progressively with altitude from 7.46 to about 7.50 but, interestingly, it remained nearly constant in the Sherpas in the range of 7.45–7.46. The more marked alkalosis in the lowlanders than Sherpas was consistent with a higher P_{CO_2} in the latter group. Paradoxically, however, the P_{O_2} and O_2 saturation were the same in the two groups at all altitudes, a finding that was not fully explained.

Another study was carried out by Wagner *et al.* (2002) in which they compared the acid–base status in lowlanders and native Bolivian residents of La Paz (3600–4100 m) when both groups ascended to 5260 m. Measurements were made both at rest and maximal exercise. After 9 weeks' residence at 5260 m, the resting arterial pH in the lowlanders was 7.48. In the highlanders it was only 7.43, 2 hours after ascent. During exercise the arterial P_{CO_2} was 8 mmHg lower in the lowlanders than the highlanders, but again, as in the study of Samaja *et al.* (1997) the P_{O_2} values were the same in the two groups. The calculated diffusing capacity for oxygen was substantially higher in the highlanders than lowlanders.

10.4.5 Metabolic compensation for respiratory alkalosis

An interesting feature of the studies at extreme altitude referred to above (Winslow *et al.* 1984) is that metabolic compensation for the respiratory alkalosis appears to be extremely slow. The mean base excess measured on three subjects who were living at an altitude of 6300 m was -7.9 mmol L^{-1}. The measurements made on venous blood taken from two climbers at 8050 m gave a mean value of -7.2 mmol L^{-1}, essentially the same. The 8050 m measurements were taken several days after the climbers had left Camp 2 at 6300 m, and the data therefore suggest that metabolic compensation was proceeding extremely slowly despite the fact that the P_{CO_2} had fallen considerably. For example, the

mean P_{CO_2} at 6300 m was 18.4 mmHg, at 8050 m 11.0 mmHg and at 8848 m (summit) 7.5 mmHg. The last value was obtained from only one subject.

The reason for the very slow change in bicarbonate concentration at these great altitudes is unclear. One possible factor is chronic dehydration. Blume *et al.* (1984) measured serum osmolality at sea level, 5400 m and 6300 m in 13 subjects of the expedition and showed that the mean value rose from 290 ± 1 mmol kg^{-1} at sea level to 295 ± 2 at 5400 m, and to 302 ± 4 at 6300 m. This volume depletion occurred despite adequate fluids to drink and a reasonably normal lifestyle. An interesting feature of the fluid balance studies was that plasma arginine vasopressin (AVP) concentrations remained unchanged from sea level to 6300 m despite the hyperosmolality. A possible factor in the volume depletion was the increased insensible loss of fluid at these great altitudes as a result of hyperventilation. However, the failure of the vasopressin levels to change suggests that there was some abnormality of body fluid regulation.

It is known that the kidney is slow to correct an alkalosis in the presence of volume depletion. It appears that when given the option of correcting fluid balance or correcting acid–base balance, the kidney gives a higher priority to fluid balance. In order to correct the respiratory alkalosis, bicarbonate ion excretion must be increased (or reabsorption decreased) and this entails the loss of a cation which inevitably aggravates the hyperosmolality. This would explain the reluctance of the kidney to correct a respiratory alkalosis in the presence of volume depletion.

A different explanation was offered by Gonzalez *et al.* (1990) when they studied the slow metabolic compensation of respiratory alkalosis in a chronically hypoxic rat model. They found that the rate of metabolic compensation was indeed slower than in acute hypoxia, and they attributed this to the lower plasma bicarbonate concentration resulting from chronic hypoxia. They argued that, because proton secretion and reabsorption of bicarbonate are functions of the bicarbonate load offered to the renal proximal tubule, it is probable that the slower increase in bicarbonate excretion of the chronically hypoxic animals was ultimately the result of the lower plasma bicarbonate concentration.

Peripheral tissues

11

SUMMARY

The movement of oxygen from the peripheral capillaries to the mitochondria is the final link in the oxygen cascade. In muscle cells, the diffusion of oxygen may be facilitated by the presence of myoglobin, and it is possible that convection also occurs in the cytoplasm of some cells. There is good evidence that the P_{O_2} in the immediate vicinity of the mitochondria of many cells is very low, of the order of 1 mmHg. Many investigators believe that much of the pressure drop from the capillary to the mitochondria occurs very close to the capillary wall because of the limited surface area available for diffusion. This leads to the conclusion that the diffusion distance from the capillary wall to the mitochondria is relatively unimportant as a barrier to oxygen transport. This diffusion distance is decreased at high altitude, mainly because of the reduction in diameter of the muscle fibers. There is also an increase in myoglobin concentration and mitochondrial density at moderate altitudes. At extreme altitudes, mitochondrial volume in human skeletal muscle is decreased. Increases in the concentration of oxidative enzymes are seen at moderate altitudes, as is the case following training at sea level. The reverse occurs at extreme altitudes, where oxidative enzymes are decreased.

11.1 INTRODUCTION

The diffusion of oxygen from the peripheral capillaries to the mitochondria, and its subsequent utilization by these organelles, constitutes the final link of the oxygen cascade which begins with the inspiration of air. Despite its critical importance, many uncertainties remain concerning the changes that occur in peripheral tissues both in acclimatized lowlanders and in the adaptation of high altitude natives. An obvious reason for this paucity of knowledge is the difficulty of studying peripheral tissues in intact humans. Much of our information necessarily comes from measurements on experimental animals exposed to low barometric pressures, though some additional studies have been made on tissue biopsies in humans.

It is probable that tissue factors play an important role in the remarkable tolerance of high altitude natives to exercise at high altitude. As was pointed out in Chapter 5, people born at high altitude often have a reduced ('blunted') ventilatory response to hypoxia. At first sight this is counterproductive because it will result in a lower alveolar P_{O_2}, and therefore a lower arterial P_{O_2}, other things being equal. However, Samaja et $al.$ (1997) found that the arterial P_{O_2} and oxygen saturation (estimated from earlobe blood) were the same in a group of Caucasians and Sherpas at altitudes of 3400 m, 5050 m and 6450 m, despite the fact that the Sherpas had a higher arterial P_{CO_2}. Similar findings were reported in Bolivian highlanders who were studied at an altitude of 5260 m by Wagner *et al.* (2002) who sampled arterial blood directly. This suggests an improved efficiency of oxygen transfer in the lung, and may be linked to the higher pulmonary diffusing capacity of high altitude natives. However, even if the arterial P_{O_2} is the same in highlanders as lowlanders, the better exercise performance of the former at high altitude suggests that there are important adaptations within the tissues of which we are ignorant.

The present chapter overlaps with others to some extent. The principles of diffusion of gases through tissues were dealt with in Chapter 7, and there is a discussion in Chapter 12 of how diffusion limitation in peripheral tissues may limit oxygen delivery during exercise. This topic is also alluded to in Chapter 13 in the discussion of limiting factors at extreme altitudes.

11.2 HISTORICAL

Early physiologists interested in high altitude did not attach much importance to tissue changes. For example, Paul Bert in *La Pression Barométrique* hardly refers to the possibility of tissue acclimatization, although he deals at some length with changes in respiration and circulation. At one point he speculates with his dry wit on whether the metabolism of high altitude natives is different from that of lowlanders:

> . . . just as a Basque mountaineer furnished with a piece of bread and a few onions makes expeditions which require of the member of the Alpine Club who accompanies him the absorption of a pound of meat, so it may be that the dwellers in high places finally lessen the consumption of oxygen in their organism, while keeping at their disposal the same quantity of vital force, either for the equilibrium of temperature, or the production of work. Thus we could

explain the acclimatization of individuals, of generations, of races.

> (Bert 1878, p. 1004 in the
> 1943 translation)

Incidentally, we now know that the oxygen requirements of a given amount of work are no different at high altitude compared with sea level, or in high altitude natives compared with lowlanders. Bert goes on,

> But we should consider not only the acts of nutrition, but also the stimulation, perhaps less, which an insufficiently oxygenated blood causes in the muscles, the nerves, and the nervous centers. . . .

However, he does not carry these speculations any further.

There is a delightful section where Bert suggests that there may be changes in the blood at high altitude:

> We might ask first whether, by a harmonious compensation of which general natural history gives us many examples, either by a modification in the nature or the quantity of hemoglobin or by an increase in the number of red corpuscles, his blood has become qualified to absorb more oxygen under the same volume, and thus to return to the usual standard of the seashore.

> (Bert 1878, p. 1000 in the
> 1943 translation)

He goes on to say that this hypothesis would be very easy to test, since it had recently been shown:

> that the capacity of the blood to absorb oxygen does not change after putrefaction, nothing would be easier than to collect the venous blood of a healthy vigorous man (an acclimated European or an Indian) or of an animal, defibrinate it, and send it in a well-corked flask; it would then be sufficient to shake it vigorously in the air to judge its capacity of absorption during life.

> (Bert 1878, p. 1008 in the
> 1943 translation)

This beautiful research project handed to the research community on a silver plate was taken up by Viault (1890) with exactly the results predicted by Bert. However, this project studied a change in the blood compartment of the body rather than in the peripheral tissues with which this chapter is chiefly concerned.

Following the work of Krogh (1919, 1929) on the increase in the number of open capillaries in muscle when the oxygen demands were raised by exercise, it was natural to wonder whether increased capillarization was a feature of tissue acclimatization in response to chronic hypoxia. It was subsequently reported that capillaries in the brain, heart and liver were significantly dilated and that their number was apparently increased after hypoxic exposure (Mercker and Schneider 1949, Opitz 1951). As we shall see later, some more recent measurements confirm these findings. However, other studies show that in some situations the actual number of capillaries in muscle tissue does not increase as a result of chronic hypoxia, but the intercapillary diffusion distance lessens because the muscle fibers become smaller.

Hurtado and his co-workers (1937) reported an increase in the intracellular concentration of the oxygen-carrying pigment, myoglobin, in high altitude animals. The measurements were made on dogs born and raised in Morococha (4550 m) and the increased concentrations were found in the diaphragm, myocardium and muscles of the chest wall and leg. The controls were dogs from Lima, at sea level. Since then a number of other investigators have reported increased tissue myoglobin levels at high altitude.

An increase in mitochondrial density was shown by Ou and Tenney (1970) in the myocardium of cattle born and raised at high altitude. Changes in mitochondrial enzymes in muscle of high altitude natives were reported by Reynafarje (1962). He found alterations in the enzyme systems NADH-oxidase, NADPH-cytochrome C-reductase, NAD[P]$^+$ transhydrogenase and others. These measurements were made on muscle biopsies taken from permanent residents of Cerro de Pasco in Peru at an altitude of 4400 m. The sea level controls were residents of Lima.

11.3 DIFFUSION IN PERIPHERAL TISSUES

11.3.1 Principles

Oxygen moves from the peripheral capillaries to the mitochondria, and carbon dioxide moves in the opposite direction by the process of diffusion. Fick's law of diffusion was discussed in Chapter 6, section 6.4.1. It states that the rate of transfer of a gas through a sheet of tissue is proportional to the area of the tissue and to the difference in gas partial pressure between the two sides, and inversely proportional to the tissue thickness.

In discussing the lung, it was pointed out that the blood-gas barrier of the human lung is extremely thin, being only 0.2–0.3 μm in many places. By contrast, the diffusion distances in peripheral tissues are typically much greater. For example, the distance between open capillaries in resting muscle is of the order of 50 μm. However, during exercise, when the oxygen consumption of the muscle increases, additional capillaries open up, thus reducing the diffusion distance and increasing the capillary surface area available for diffusion. As discussed in Chapter 6, section 6.4.1, carbon dioxide diffuses about 20 times faster than oxygen through tissues because of its much higher solubility, and therefore the elimination of carbon dioxide poses less of a problem than oxygen delivery.

Early workers believed that the movement of oxygen through tissues was by simple passive diffusion. However, it is now believed that facilitated diffusion of oxygen probably occurs in muscle cells as a result of the presence of myoglobin. This heme protein has a structure which resembles hemoglobin but the dissociation curve is a hyperbola, as opposed to the S-shape of the oxygen dissociation curve of whole blood (Fig. 11.1). Another major difference is that myoglobin takes up oxygen at a much lower P_{O_2} than hemoglobin, that is, it has a very low P_{50} of about 3 mmHg. This is a necessary property if the myoglobin is to be of any use in muscle cells where the tissue P_{O_2} is very low. Scholander (1960) and Wittenberg (1959) have shown experimentally that myoglobin can facilitate oxygen diffusion.

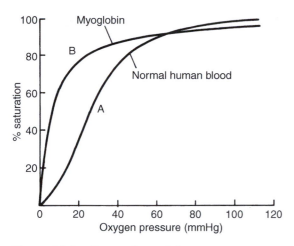

Figure 11.1 Comparison of the oxygen dissociation curves for normal human blood (curve A) and myoglobin (curve B). The P_{50} values are approximately 27 and 3 mmHg, respectively. (From Roughton 1964.)

Other modes of oxygen transport are possible within cells. Streaming movements of cytoplasm have been observed and it is conceivable that such movements, known as 'stirring', enhance the transport of oxygen by convection. Another hypothesis is that oxygen moves into some cells along invaginations of the lipid cell membrane in which it has a high solubility (Longmuir and Betts 1987).

There is good evidence that the P_{O_2} in the immediate vicinity of the mitochondria is very low in some tissues, being of the order of 1 mmHg. In fact, models of oxygen transfer in tissues often assume that the mitochondrial P_{O_2} is so low that it can be neglected in the context of the P_{O_2} of the capillary blood, which is of the order of 30–50 mmHg. In measurements of suspensions of kidney cell mitochondria *in vitro*, oxygen consumption has been shown to continue at the same rate until the P_{O_2} of the surrounding fluid falls to the region of 2 mmHg (Wilson *et al.* 1977). Measurements of P_{O_2} at the sites of oxygen utilization based on the spectral characteristics of cytochromes also indicate that the P_{O_2} is probably less than 1 mmHg (Chance 1957; Chance *et al.* 1962). In the quadriceps muscle of exercising humans, it was shown by nuclear magnetic resonance spectroscopy that partial

desaturation of myoglobin occurred at only 50% of maximal oxygen consumption implying a P_{O_2} in the myoglobin of only 2–3 mmHg (Richardson *et al.* 1995). Thus it appears that the purpose of the much higher P_{O_2} of capillary blood is to ensure an adequate pressure for diffusion of oxygen to the mitochondria and that, at the actual sites of oxygen utilization, the P_{O_2} is extremely low.

11.3.2 Tissue partial pressures

A classical model to analyze the distribution of P_{O_2} values in tissue was described by August Krogh (1919). He considered a hypothetical cylinder of tissue around a straight, thin, tubular capillary into which blood entered with a known P_{O_2}. As oxygen diffuses away from the capillary, oxygen is consumed by the tissue and the P_{O_2} falls. If simplifying assumptions are made, such as uniform consumption rate of oxygen in every part of the tissue, an equation can be written to describe the P_{O_2} profile (Krogh 1919; Piiper and Scheid 1986).

Another model is shown in Fig. 11.2 (Hill 1928). In Fig. 11.2a we see a cylinder of tissue which is supplied with oxygen by capillaries at its periphery: in (1) the balance between oxygen consumption and delivery (determined by the capillary P_{O_2}, the intercapillary distance R_c, and the oxygen consumption rate of the tissue) results in an adequate P_{O_2} throughout the cylinder; in (2) the intercapillary distance or the oxygen consumption has been increased until the P_{O_2} at one point in the tissue falls to zero. This is referred to as a critical situation. In (3) there is an anoxic region where aerobic (that is, oxygen-utilizing) metabolism is impossible. Under anoxic conditions the tissue energy requirements must be met by obligatory anaerobic glycolysis with the consequent formation of lactic acid.

The situation along the tissue cylinder is shown in Fig. 11.2b. It is assumed that the P_{O_2} in the capillaries at the periphery of the tissue cylinder falls from 100 to 20 mmHg as shown from left to right. As a consequence the P_{O_2} in the center of the tissue cylinder falls towards the venous end of the capillary. It is clear that, on the basis of this model, the most vulnerable tissue is that furthest from the capillary at its downstream end. This was

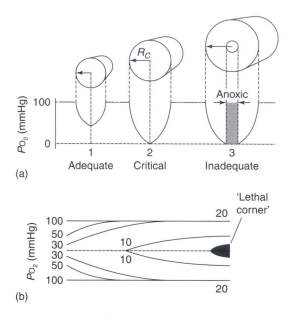

(a)

(b)

Figure 11.2 Fall in P_{O_2} between adjacent capillaries. (a) Three hypothetical cylinders of tissue are shown and oxygen is diffusing into these cylinders from capillaries at the periphery. In (2) the cylinder had a critical radius (R_c), and in (3) the radius of the cylinder is so large that there is an anoxic zone in the middle of the cylinder. (b) A section along the hypothetical cylinder of tissue. The P_{O_2} in the blood adjacent to the tissue is assumed to fall from 100 to 20 mmHg along the capillary. Lines of equal P_{O_2} are shown. Note the possibility of a 'lethal corner' in the middle of the cylinder at the venous end. (From West 1985b, modified from Hill 1928.)

cells (Potter and Groom 1983; Mathieu-Costello 1987). Although in some histological sections the capillaries of skeletal muscle appear at first sight to run chiefly parallel to the muscle fibers, this is an oversimplification. Furthermore, the density of the connections increases considerably when the muscle shortens (Mathieu-Costello 1987). Thus a more reasonable model of oxygen delivery to muscle is a syncytium of capillaries surrounding a tubular muscle cell.

Studies by Honig *et al.* (1991) have indicated that the P_{O_2} profiles shown in Fig. 11.2 may be misleading in skeletal muscle. These investigators rapidly froze working muscles of experimental animals and then measured the degree of oxygen saturation of the intracellular myoglobin using a spectrometer with a narrow light beam. The intracellular P_{O_2} was inferred from the myoglobin oxygen saturation. These data and theoretical work by the same group suggest that the major resistance to oxygen diffusion from capillary to muscle fiber mitochondria is at the capillary–fiber interface, i.e. the thin carrier-free region including plasma, endothelium and interstitium. This, in turn, necessitates a large driving force (P_{O_2} difference) at that site to deliver oxygen to the muscle fibers. Some of the results of this group are shown in Fig. 11.3 where it can be seen that most of the fall of P_{O_2} apparently occurs in the immediate vicinity of the peripheral capillary and that, throughout the muscle cell, the P_{O_2} is remarkably uniform and very low (of the order of 1–3 mmHg). This pattern results in part from the presence of myoglobin which facilitates the diffusion of oxygen within the muscle fibers.

Evidence that the P_{O_2} in human skeletal muscle is low and remains constant in the face of increasing work levels was reported by Richardson *et al.* (2001). These investigators studied oxygenation in leg muscle during knee extensor exercise of a single leg. They used magnetic resonance spectroscopy of myoglobin as a measure of tissue oxygenation exploiting the fact that the P_{50} of myoglobin is about 3.2 mmHg. They found that although the calculated P_{O_2} was relatively high up to a maximal work rate of 60%, above that the intracellular P_{O_2} fell to a relatively uniform and constant value of about 3.8 mmHg in all subjects. This ingenious technique provides

referred to as the 'lethal corner'. It is possible that this pattern of focal anoxia is responsible for some tissue damage at high altitude. For example, it may explain how some nerve cells of the brain are damaged at great altitudes causing the residual impairment of central nervous system function. This is discussed in Chapter 17.

Figure 11.2 assumes that the blood in adjacent capillaries runs in the same direction but there is evidence that this is not always the case, and that rather there is a network of capillaries with various directions of flow and many intercommunications. This concept of a network of capillaries is supported by studies emphasizing the tortuosity of capillaries around skeletal muscle

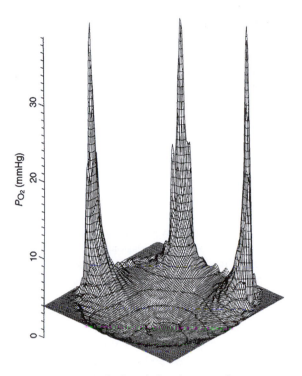

Figure 11.3 Calculated distribution of P_{O_2} around three capillaries in a heavily working red fiber of skeletal muscle. P_{O_2} contours are at intervals of 1 mmHg. There is a rapid fall of P_{O_2} in the immediate vicinity of the capillary, and within the muscle cell the P_{O_2} is relatively uniform and very low. (From Honig *et al.* 1991.)

evidence that during relatively high levels of work, the intracellular P_{O_2} in human leg muscle is very low and remains relatively constant.

11.4 CAPILLARY DENSITY

One way to improve the oxygen delivery to tissue by diffusion under conditions of oxygen deprivation, such as at high altitude, is to reduce the intercapillary distance. The technical name for the number of capillaries per unit volume of tissue is capillary volume density. It has been known since the time of Krogh (1919) that the number of open capillaries in a muscle depends on the degree of metabolic activity. During exercise, additional capillaries open up, thus reducing the diffusing distance and increasing the diffusing surface area. It has been known for many years that exercise

training increases the number of capillaries in skeletal muscle (Saltin and Gollnick 1983).

The effects of high altitude exposure on capillary volume density is complicated and the subject of continuing research. Early studies apparently showed increased vascularization of the brain, retina, skeletal muscle and liver of experimental animals exposed to low barometric pressures over several weeks (Mercker and Schneider 1949; Opitz 1951; Valdivia 1958; Cassin *et al.* 1971). Tenney and Ou (1970) measured the rate of loss of carbon monoxide from subcutaneous gas pockets in rats after 3 weeks of simulated exposure to 5600 m and concluded that there was a 50% increase in capillary number.

However, some of these studies were questioned by Banchero (1982) who argued that the results obtained by Valdivia (1958) and Cassin *et al.* (1971) might be influenced by technical errors. Many investigators now believe that although capillary volume density increases in skeletal muscles with exposure to high altitude, this is not caused by the formation of new capillaries, but by a reduction in size of the muscle fibers. This result has been found in guinea-pigs (Fig. 11.4) which were studied at sea level, in Denver at 1610 m, at 3900 m (in a species native to the Andes) and at a simulated altitude of 5100 m (Banchero 1982).

The same pattern has been described in acclimatized humans where muscle samples were obtained by biopsy. For example, Cerretelli and his co-workers obtained muscle biopsies on climbers immediately after they had spent several weeks attempting to climb Lhotse Shar (8398 m) in Nepal and showed that, although the capillary volume density was somewhat raised, the increase could be wholly accounted for by a reduction of muscle fiber size (Boutellier *et al.* 1983; Cerretelli *et al.* 1984). A similar result was found in Operation Everest II in six volunteers who were gradually decompressed to the simulated altitude of Mount Everest over a period of 40 days. Needle biopsies from the vastus lateralis muscle showed a significant (25%) decrease in cross-sectional area of type I fibers, and a 26% decrease (nonsignificant) for type II fibers. Capillary to fiber ratios were unchanged and there was a trend (nonsignificant) towards

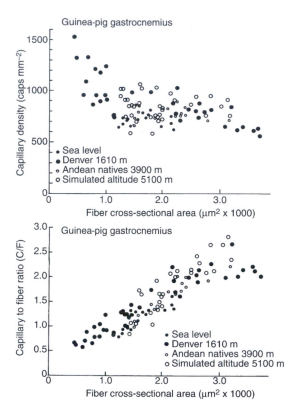

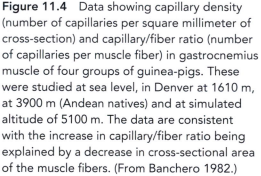

Figure 11.4 Data showing capillary density (number of capillaries per square millimeter of cross-section) and capillary/fiber ratio (number of capillaries per muscle fiber) in gastrocnemius muscle of four groups of guinea-pigs. These were studied at sea level, in Denver at 1610 m, at 3900 m (Andean natives) and at simulated altitude of 5100 m. The data are consistent with the increase in capillary/fiber ratio being explained by a decrease in cross-sectional area of the muscle fibers. (From Banchero 1982.)

an increase in capillary density (Green *et al.* 1989; MacDougall *et al.* 1991). Lundby *et al.* (2004b) showed that there was no change in the volume density of capillaries in skeletal muscle of lowlanders after acclimatization to an altitude of 4100 m. In addition, there was no increase in expression of hypoxible-inducible factor (HIF)-1α or vascular endothelial growth factor (VEGF) mRNA in biopsies of skeletal muscle.

In contrast to the studies showing that new capillaries in skeletal muscle do not develop as a result of exposure to high altitude, some recent

reports do find increased capillarization. For example, Mathieu-Costello *et al.* (1998) reported increases in the number of capillaries in flight muscles of finches at high altitude, and increased capillarity was also found in leg muscles of finches living at high altitude (Hepple *et al.* 1998). These investigators argued that whether increased capillary numbers (and mitochondrial density) occur at high altitude depends on the level of metabolic stress on the muscle, and this links with the issue of training at altitude where similar changes are seen.

Although many studies show that the number of new capillaries in skeletal muscle does not increase as a result of exposure to prolonged hypoxia, it has been suggested that there are changes in the configuration of the capillaries with increased tortuosity that would effectively increase capillary surface area and enhance gas diffusion (Appell 1978). However, this result has not been confirmed by Mathieu-Costello and Poole (Mathieu-Costello 1989; Poole and Mathieu-Costello 1990), who showed that muscle capillary tortuosity does not increase with chronic exposure to hypoxia when account is taken of sarcomere length. These investigators believe that Appell's results may be explained by failure to control the state of contraction of the muscle. It is known that the degree of capillary tortuosity increases during muscle shortening (Mathieu-Costello 1987).

Another factor that should be mentioned is increased heterogeneity of flow in capillaries as a result of an increased hematocrit. Factors that could cause this include polycythemia and dehydration of the subjects. Martin *et al.* (Martin 2009; Martin 2010) showed increased heterogeneity of flow in the sublingual microcirculation at altitudes of 4900 and 7950 m.

The lack of increase in the number of capillaries per muscle fiber at high altitude found in some studies should be contrasted with the increase in muscle capillarity which occurs with training. Longitudinal studies in humans have shown that exercise training increases muscle capillarity including both the capillary/fiber ratio and number of capillaries per square millimeter within several weeks (Andersen and Henricksson 1977; Brodal *et al.* 1977; Ingjer and Brodal 1978). Furthermore, it has been demonstrated that the increased capillary supply is proportional to the increased maximum oxygen uptake (Andersen and Henricksson 1977). The increase in number of capillaries is found in all fiber types provided that they are recruited during training (Andersen and Henricksson 1977; Nygaard and Nielsen 1978). If studies of acclimatization to high altitude involve increased levels of exercise, it is important to take account of this effect. Table 11.1 compares some of the tissue changes caused by training with those resulting from exposure to high altitude.

Recently, there has been considerable interest in the possible role of vascular endothelial growth factor at high altitude. VEGF is an endothelial cell-specific mitogen which is an important mediator of hypoxia-induced angiogenesis. Hypoxia increases transcriptional induction of VEGF and also increases post-transcriptional stabilization of VEGF mRNA. VEGF increases endothelial cell proliferation and migration, and also vascular permeability. It is known to be important in the angiogenesis of embryonic development, wound healing and tumor growth (Ferrara and Davis-Smyth 1997).

Both acute hypoxia and exercise have been shown to increase VEGF mRNA in skeletal muscle of humans (Gustafsen *et al.* 1999; Hoppeler 1999) and animals (Breen *et al.* 1996). As discussed above and shown in Table 11.1, endurance exercise training is known to increase muscle capillarity, mitochondrial density and oxidative enzyme activity, and local tissue hypoxia has been suggested as the stimulus for these changes. Therefore induction of VEGF may be the mechanism. However, whether chronic hypoxia has a similar effect on VEGF is debated. Indeed, whereas acute hypoxia increases VEGF mRNA in animal skeletal muscle, some studies show that chronic hypoxia reduces the levels below those seen in acute hypoxia. This is also true of another growth factor, TGF-β1 (Olfert *et al.* 2001).

The mechanism by which hypoxia stimulates induction of VEGF genes is through an increase in the transcriptional factor, HIF-1α. This important regulator has already been referred to in Chapters 4, 7 and 10. Its various roles in hypoxia are summarized in Fig. 4.2. In normoxia, HIF-1α is continuously formed in the cytoplasm and degraded as a result of hydroxylation by prolyl hydroxylase. However, this enzyme is inhibited in hypoxia and significant accumulation of HIF-1α occurs within 2 minutes. The HIF-1α combines with HIF-1β to form HIF-1 which moves into the nucleus to induce gene transcription. A number of genes are upregulated including *VEGF* genes resulting in angiogenesis, *EPO* genes resulting

Table 11.1 Comparison of tissue changes caused by training and those associated with exposure to high altitude

Tissue changes	Endurance training	High altitude
Capillary density in skeletal muscle	Increased due to new capillaries	Increased due to reduction in diameter of muscle fibers
Fiber diameter of skeletal muscle	May be increased	Decreased
Myoglobin concentration	No change in humans	Increased in skeletal, heart muscle
Muscle enzymes	No change in glycolytic, increase in oxidative	Similar changes at moderate altitudes; at extreme altitudes, increase in glycolytic and decrease in oxidative
Mitochondria	Increased volume density	Increased volume density in some animals at moderate altitude but reduced density in humans at extreme altitude Different intracellular distribution, e.g. loss of subsarcolemmal mitochondria in comparison to training

in erythropoiesis, and the genes for tyrosine hydroxylase which increases the sensitivity of the carotid body. HIF-1α is therefore a master switch in the general responses of the body to hypoxia. More information on hypoxia-inducible factor is found in Chapter 4.

11.5 MUSCLE FIBER SIZE

As indicated above, one way to increase capillary density and thus reduce diffusion distance within skeletal muscle is to reduce the size of the muscle fibers. There is now good evidence that this occurs during high altitude acclimatization and deterioration (Boutellier *et al.* 1983; Cerretelli *et al.* 1984; MacDougall *et al.* 1991). Figure 11.5 shows the reduction in muscle volume as measured by computed tomography in the thigh and upper arm regions of the subjects of Operation Everest II (MacDougall *et al.* 1991). This topic is discussed further in Chapters 5 and 15.

The mechanism of muscle atrophy at high altitude is not well understood. It has been suggested that one contributing factor is lack of muscular activity. Certainly, lowlanders who go to very high altitudes easily become fatigued and often spend much of their time at a reduced level of physical activity. Indeed, Tilman (1952, p. 79) once remarked that a hazard of Himalayan expeditions was bedsores!

However, reduced physical activity is unlikely to be the whole story as evidenced by the experience obtained on the 1960–61 Himalayan Scientific and Mountaineering Expedition. During several months at 5800 m, the level of physical activity was well maintained with opportunities for daily skiing and yet the expedition members suffered a relentless and progressive loss of weight which averaged 0.5–1.5 kg per week (Pugh 1964c). Moreover, estimates of energy intake were made and these were apparently more than adequate for the level of activity. It is true that appetite is reduced, and it may be that gastrointestinal absorption is impaired at high altitude (Chapter 15). However, it seems possible that there is some change in protein metabolism which results in extensive breakdown of muscle protein.

11.6 VOLUME OF MITOCHONDRIA

The muscle mitochondria are the primary sites of oxygen utilization by the body and thus constitute the final link of the oxygen cascade. In

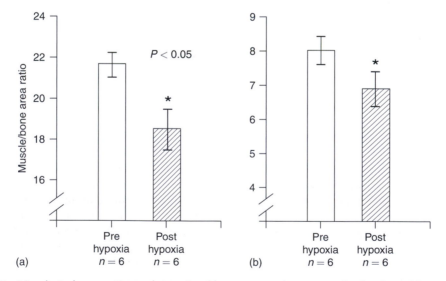

Figure 11.5   Muscle to bone ratio as determined by computed tomography for the subjects of Operation Everest II at the end of 40 days of progressive hypoxia. (a) The thigh site and (b) the upper arm. Values are means and SD. (From MacDougall *et al.* 1991.)

general, mitochondrial volume density (volume of mitochondria per unit volume of tissue) in skeletal muscle is related to maximal oxygen uptake and, for example, is greater in highly aerobic animals such as the horse compared with less active animals such as the cow (Hoppeler *et al.* 1987). It is also known that physical training increases mitochondrial volume density (Holloszy and Coyle 1984).

We might therefore expect that at high altitude where maximal oxygen uptake is reduced (Chapter 12) mitochondrial density would decrease and this is generally the case. It is known that the mitochondrial volume in human skeletal muscle decreases with exposure to very high altitude. In a study on muscle biopsies of climbers returning from two Swiss expeditions to the Himalayas, mitochondrial volume decreased by 20%. This was associated with a decrease of 10% in muscle mass. The net result was a decrease in absolute mitochondrial volume of nearly 30% (Hoppeler *et al.* 1990). A feature of the electron micrographs of muscle biopsies was the presence of poorly defined material known as lipofuscin. This substance is thought to be the consequence of lipid peroxidation related to loss of mitochondria (Howald and Hoppeler 2003). In muscle biopsies of Tibetans, low levels of mitochondrial volume density were demonstrated (Kayser *et al.* 1991) and, interestingly, low densities were also seen in second-generation Sherpas raised at low altitude (Kayser *et al.* 1996). There was no significant increase in mitochondrial volume density in biopsies of vastus lateralis in subjects of Operation Everest II (MacDougall *et al.* 1991).

Some studies in animals have given different results. In an investigation of the mitochondrial density of the myocardium of rabbits and guinea pigs from Cerro de Pasco (4330 m) in Peru, it was found that the values were the same as those at sea level (Kearney 1973). However, Ou and Tenney (1970) showed that the number of mitochondria in samples of myocardium was 40% greater in cattle born and raised at 4250 m compared with cattle at sea level. The size of individual mitochondria was found to be the same and it was argued that the increase in mitochondrial number

was advantageous because it reduced the diffusion distance of the intracellular oxygen.

It may be that these discordant results can be explained by the differences between exposure to moderate and very high altitude. The increase in mitochondrial number found by Ou and Tenney (1970) was at an altitude of 4500 m, whereas the decrease in mitochondrial volume reported by Hoppeler *et al.* (1990) was in climbers who had been to altitudes over 6000 m. Recent results from an expedition to Mount Everest are consistent with this. Ascent to the base camp, altitude 5300 m, over a period of 19 days was not associated with loss of mitochondria. However after 66 days at altitude including ascent to beyond 6400 m, mitochondrial densities fell by 21% with a loss of 73% of subsarcolemmal mitochondria. In addition, levels of transcriptional coactivator PGC-1α fell by 35%, suggesting downregulation of mitochondrial biogenesis. Sustained hypoxia also decreased expression of electron transport chain complexes I and IV and UCP3 levels. This is consistent with the fact that during subacute hypoxia, mitochondria are protected from oxidate stress. However, following sustained exposure, mitochondrial biogenesis is deactivated and uncoupling is downregulated, perhaps to improve the efficiency of ATP production (Levett *et al.* 2012). This is relevant to the discussion of high altitude acclimatization which occurs at moderate altitudes, and high altitude deterioration which occurs at extremely high altitudes, as discussed in Chapter 5. A general review of the response of skeletal muscle mitochondria to hypoxia can be found in Hoppeler *et al.* (2003).

There is an interesting difference between the mitochondrial density following exposure to high altitude on the one hand, and endurance training at sea level on the other, in their differential effects on subsarcolemmal and interfibrillar mitochondria. There is a greater loss of subsarcolemmal mitochondria at altitude, while subsarcolemmal mitochondria show a greater increase with training at sea level (Desplanches *et al.* 1993; Cerretelli and Hoppeler 1996).

11.7 MYOGLOBIN CONCENTRATION

As stated above, very early studies by Hurtado and his colleagues (1937) showed increased concentrations of myoglobin in several muscles of dogs born and raised in Morococha (4550 m) in Peru. The controls were dogs in Lima at sea level. Increased myoglobin concentrations were found in the diaphragm, adductor muscles of the leg, pectoral muscles of the chest and the myocardium.

Reynafarje (1962) measured myoglobin concentrations in the sartorius muscle of healthy humans native to Cerro de Pasco (4400 m) and in other Peruvians native to sea level. Higher concentrations of myoglobin were found in the high altitude natives (7.03 mg g^{-1}) tissue than in the sea level controls (6.07 mg g^{-1}). The result was interpreted as a true high altitude effect because it was accompanied by an increased nitrogen content of the muscle, whereas the lean body mass and body water content were the same as at sea level. This point was important because in another study (Anthony *et al.* 1959), a reported increase in myoglobin content of skeletal muscle in rats could possibly have been caused by a decrease in body weight as a result of dehydration. Other studies which have shown an increase in myoglobin as a result of acclimatization to hypoxia include those of hamster heart muscle (Clark *et al.* 1952), rat heart and diaphragm (Vaughan and Pace 1956) and various guinea-pig tissues (Tappan and Reynafarje 1957).

Moore and colleagues (2002) tested the hypothesis that myoglobin allele frequencies in Tibetans are different from those in a group of sea level residents in Texas. They found that the frequency of the myoglobin 79A allele was higher in high altitude residents compared with those at sea level, although there was no relation between frequency and altitude in Tibetans. Also, there was no association between myoglobin genotype and hemoglobin concentration. They concluded that high altitude Tibetans do not show novel polymorphism or selection for specific myoglobin alleles as a function of high altitude residence. More recent studies have shown remarkable genomic differences between Tibetans and Han Chinese and these are discussed in Chapter 4.

As discussed above, the chief value of myoglobin may be that it facilitates oxygen diffusion through muscle cells. However, it may also serve to buffer regional differences of P_{O_2} (Fig. 11.3) and act as an oxygen store for short periods of very severe oxygen deprivation. It has been shown that increased levels of exercise raise the myoglobin content of muscles in experimental animals (Lawrie 1953; Pattengale and Holloszy 1967). Animals that exhibit large oxygen uptakes in conditions of reduced oxygen availability, such as seals, typically have very large amounts of myoglobin (Castellini and Somero 1981). However, a study comparing trained and untrained human subjects (Jansson *et al.* 1982) and another study of short-term training in humans (Svedenhag *et al.* 1983) both failed to show any effect of training on muscle myoglobin concentration.

11.8 INTRACELLULAR ENZYMES

Enzymes are essential to all aspects of the metabolic pathways involved in energy production. Figure 11.6 summarizes the three main stages in energy metabolism:

1. The conversion of glucose units (from either glucose or glycogen, known as glycolysis), amino acids and fatty acids to acetyl CoA
2. The citric acid or Krebs cycle
3. The electron transport chain.

Because oxygen is not required for the glycolytic breakdown of glucose or glycogen, glycolysis represents an important though temporary source of energy under conditions of oxygen shortage or absence. By contrast, neither the Krebs cycle nor the electron transport chain can produce energy in the absence of oxygen.

There is evidence that chronic hypoxia caused by moderate or high altitude increases the concentration or activities of certain important enzymes involved in oxidative metabolism, but hypoxia does not appear to affect enzymes in the glycolytic pathway. However, it must be stressed that endurance exercise training also causes profound changes in the oxidative enzyme

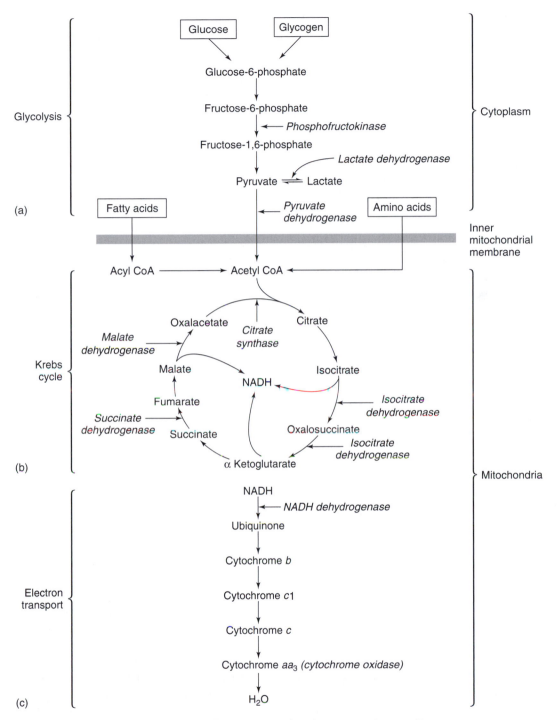

Figure 11.6   Major energy-yielding pathways in muscle. The principal controlling enzymes are indicated. Altitude or hypoxic exposure and exercise training do not affect glycolytic capacity appreciably but cause substantial increases in oxidative capacity as demonstrated by augmented mitochondrial volume in some species and activity of major enzymes of the citric acid cycle and the electron transport chain.

systems and it is difficult to maintain a given level of physical activity during exposure to chronic hypoxia. Similarly, it is also difficult to match sea level residents with residents at altitude with respect to physical activity.

One of the first studies of the enzymatic activity of human muscle at high altitude was that by Reynafarje (1962). The measurements were made on biopsies taken from the sartorius muscles of natives of Cerro de Pasco (4400 m) and these were compared with biopsies from residents of Lima at sea level. Reynafarje measured the activities of enzymes of glycolysis (lactate dehydrogenase), Krebs cycle (isocitrate dehydrogenase), and the electron transport chain (NADH and NADPH-cytochrome c-reductase and NAD[P]$^+$ transhydrogenase). In this study Reynafarje found that the activities of NADH-oxidase, NADPH-cytochrome c-reductase and NAD[P]$^+$ transhydrogenase were significantly increased in the altitude residents.

Harris *et al.* (1970) reported on the levels of succinate dehydrogenase (Krebs cycle) and lactate dehydrogenase (glycolysis) activity in myocardial homogenates from guinea-pigs, rabbits and dogs indigenous to high altitude (4380 m) and compared the measurements with those made on the same species at sea level. The investigators found a consistent increase in the activity of succinate dehydrogenase in the high altitude animals but no significant difference in lactate dehydrogenase. Ou and Tenney (1970) also found increased levels of succinate dehydrogenase and several enzymes of the electron transport chain including cytochrome oxidase, NADH-oxidase and NADH-cytochrome c-reductase in high altitude cattle.

In contrast to the effects of moderately high altitude (4000–5000 m), it appears that extreme altitude (above 6000 m) may cause a reduction in the activity of certain enzymes. The effect of exposure to extreme altitude on muscle enzyme systems has been studied by taking muscle biopsies from climbers before and after the Swiss expeditions to Lhotse Shar in 1981 (Cerretelli 1987) and Mount Everest in 1986 (Howald *et al.* 1990) and also from experimental subjects before and after prolonged decompression during Operation Everest II (Green *et al.* 1989). All of these studies reported decreased activities

of oxidative enzymes. Results on three subjects from the Lhotse Shar expedition suggest that extreme altitude reduces the activity of both Krebs cycle (succinate dehydrogenase) and glycolytic (phosphofructokinase and lactate dehydrogenase) enzymes (Cerretelli 1987). In a more comprehensive study of seven climbers from the Swiss 1986 expedition, reduced activity of enzymes of the Krebs cycle (citrate synthase, malate dehydrogenase) and electron transport chain (cytochrome oxidase) were reported (Howald *et al.* 1990). In contrast to the Lhotse Shar study, this latter study found increases in enzyme activities of glycolysis. In Operation Everest II, significant reductions were found in succinate dehydrogenase (21%), citrate synthase (37%) and hexokinase (53%) at extreme altitudes (Green *et al.* 1989).

Interestingly, the enhanced capacity for oxidative metabolism found in the face of an unchanged glycolytic potential after high altitude (below 5000 m) exposure is qualitatively similar to the changes found in skeletal muscle after endurance exercise training (Holloszy and Coyle 1984). This observation supports the notion that tissue hypoxia may be responsible for the changes in mitochondrial density and oxidative enzyme capacity under both conditions. However, as pointed out earlier, there are differences between the two stresses, for example in the intracellular distribution of mitochondria.

It has been argued that the primary importance of an augmented oxidative capacity of skeletal muscle lies not in the ability to achieve a higher maximum oxygen uptake but, rather, to sustain a given submaximal oxygen uptake with less intracellular metabolic disturbance (i.e. change of ADP and inorganic phosphate (P_i), both potent stimulators of glycolysis) (Gollnick and Saltin 1982; Holloszy and Coyle 1984; Dudley *et al.* 1987). Thus, for strenuous exercise where fatigue is associated with depletion of muscle glycogen stores, an augmented muscle oxidative capacity enables a given oxygen uptake to be sustained at lower intracellular ADP and P_i concentrations. Consequently, muscle glycogen stores would be conserved and fat oxidation would contribute proportionally more to the energetic output of the muscle, resulting in an enhanced endurance capacity (Holloszy and Coyle 1984; Dudley *et al.* 1987). In conclusion, these changes in tissue enzymes (with the exception of those at extreme altitudes) are consistent with the assumption that the muscles are improving their ability for oxidative metabolism in the face of oxygen deprivation or deficiency.

Humans who are acutely exposed to high altitude develop high blood lactate concentrations on exercise. However, after acclimatization, the lactate levels at the same altitude and exercise level are much less, a phenomenon known as the lactate paradox. Consistent with this, exercise at extreme altitudes results in very low blood lactate levels. This topic is discussed in Chapter 12.

12

Exercise

SUMMARY

In the face of the reduction in the inspired P_{O_2} encountered at high altitude, exercise in this environment makes enormous demands on the transfer of oxygen from the air to the blood in the lung and eventually to the mitochondria of the exercise muscles. Consequently, reduced exercise tolerance is one of the most obvious features of exposure to high altitude. Maximal exercise is accompanied by extremely high ventilations (measured at body temperature and pressure); these can approach 200 L min^{-1} at extreme altitudes, which is close to the maximum voluntary ventilation. Diffusion-limitation of oxygen transfer across the blood-gas barrier is also an important limiting factor. As a result, arterial P_{O_2} levels typically fall greatly as the work rate is increased. Some additional ventilation–perfusion inequality also often develops, possibly because of subclinical pulmonary edema. Maximal cardiac output is reduced at high altitude, although in acclimatized subjects, the relationship between cardiac output and work rate is the same as at sea level, and oxygen consumption for a given work rate is independent of altitude. Maximal oxygen consumption in acclimatized subjects falls from about $4–5 \text{ L min}^{-1}$ at sea level to just over 1 L min^{-1} at the Everest summit. Part of the reduction in $\dot{V}_{O_{2,max}}$ can be ascribed to diffusion limitation within the exercising muscle, as well as a limited blood flow to the muscles of locomotion because of the increased demand of the respiratory muscles. Although aerobic performance is greatly impaired at high altitude, there is no change in maximal anaerobic peak power (for example, as measured by a standing jump) unless muscle mass is reduced.

12.1 INTRODUCTION

The hypoxia of high altitude puts stress on the oxygen transfer system of the body, even at rest. If the oxygen requirements are further increased by exercise, the problems of oxygen delivery to the mitochondria of the working muscles are correspondingly exaggerated. Indeed, one of the most obvious consequences of going to high altitude is a reduction in both maximal and endurance exercise tolerance.

In this chapter, we examine the physiology of oxygen transfer from the air to the mitochondria in the face of the reduced inspired P_{O_2}. The steps in the oxygen cascade involve the convection of air in the airways to the alveoli via pulmonary ventilation, then diffusion of oxygen across the blood-gas barrier, uptake by the pulmonary capillary blood, removal from the lung by the cardiac output, again convection of the oxygenated blood to the tissues, diffusion of oxygen from the blood to the cell to the mitochondria, and then utilization of oxygen by the cellular biochemical reactions. The present chapter synthesizes information, some of which occurs in other chapters. The subject of limitation of oxygen uptake under the conditions of extreme altitude is dealt with in Chapter 13. The literature on exercise at altitude is very extensive, and the present chapter is necessarily selective. Many monographs and reviews have been published including Margaria (1967), Cerretelli and Whipp (1980), Sutton *et al.* (1983), Sutton *et al.* (1987), Cerretelli (1992), Wagner (1996) and Martin *et al.* (2010).

12.2 HISTORICAL

A reduced exercise tolerance at high altitude has been recognized since humans began to climb high mountains. For example, extreme fatigue was often reported in the early climbs of the European Alps which, in fact, led to one of the popular theories of mountain sickness. The argument ran that the normal barometric pressure was necessary to maintain the proper articulation of the head of the femur in the acetabulum of the pelvis, and that at high altitude, when the reduced barometric pressure did not assist this as it should, the muscles became fatigued as a result (Bert 1878, pp. 343–6).

Some of the earliest measurements of exercise at high altitude were made by Zuntz, Durig and their colleagues in the first few years of the twentieth century (Durig 1911; Zuntz *et al.* 1906). For example, Zuntz *et al.* showed that there was a decline in oxygen consumption, but increase in ventilation at high altitude when trekkers walked at the speed that they normally adopted

in an Alpine setting. Douglas *et al.* (1913) studied muscular exercise during walking uphill on Pikes Peak during the Anglo-American expedition of 1911. They made the important observation that a given amount of work required the same amount of oxygen consumption at 4300 m altitude as at sea level.

Vivid descriptions of the great difficulties of exercise at very high altitudes were common in the early Everest expeditions. Indeed the accounts of the 1921 reconnaissance expedition (Howard-Bury 1922), and the expeditions of 1922 (Bruce 1923) and 1924 (Norton 1925) make graphic and compelling reading even today. Typical is EF Norton's account of his climb to nearly 8600 m without supplementary oxygen in 1924 (Norton 1925). He wrote,

> Our pace was wretched. My ambition was to do 20 consecutive paces uphill without a pause to rest and pant elbow on bent knee, yet I never remember achieving it – 13 was nearer the mark.

Norton was accompanied to just below that altitude by the surgeon TH Somervell who subsequently wrote 'for every step forward and upward, 7 to 10 complete respirations were required' (Somervell 1925).

Of course, these observations were by lowlanders who were at extreme altitudes after relatively short periods of time for acclimatization. It is interesting to compare the observations of Barcroft who led an expedition at about the same time (winter of 1921–22) to Cerro de Pasco at an altitude of 4330 m in the Peruvian Andes (Barcroft *et al.* 1923). Naturally, this was at a considerably lower altitude than near the summit of Mount Everest. Nevertheless, the lowlanders were amazed at the capacity of the high altitude residents for physical work, and they were astonished at the popularity of energetic sports such as football (soccer), a phenomenon experienced by this author (RBS) while doing research on the high altitude natives of Ollague in Northern Chile in 1986. The contrast between poorly acclimatized lowlanders and native high altitude dwellers, who had been at the same altitude for perhaps generations, was very clear.

Valuable findings on exercise at high altitude were made during the 1935 International High Altitude Expedition to Chile (Keys 1936). The expedition members showed that their own maximal working capacity fell as the altitude increased in spite of acclimatization. Christensen (1937) made measurements up to an altitude of 5340 m using a bicycle ergometer and confirmed the findings of Douglas *et al.* (1913) that the efficiency of muscle exercise was independent of altitude, that is that the oxygen consumption for a given work level was the same. In addition, he showed that although exercise ventilation measured at body temperature, ambient pressure, saturated with water vapour (body temperature and pressure saturated, BTPS) was greatly increased at high altitudes, ventilation expressed at standard temperature and pressure, dry gas (STPD) was essentially independent of altitude over a wide range of altitudes and work rates.

An interesting observation was made by Edwards who documented a curious paradox about lactate levels in the blood on exercise. Generally, exhaustive exercise is accompanied by relatively high blood lactate levels, especially in unfit subjects, as the muscles outstrip their capacity for aerobic work and resort to anaerobic glycolysis. It would be natural to expect this to occur to an extreme extent at high altitude, as it does in acute hypoxia, but Edwards found the opposite. Exhaustive work at very high altitude was associated with very low levels of blood lactate (Edwards 1936). Dill and colleagues (1931) had previously seen the same phenomenon in a similar series of measurements.

The expedition members were also surprised by the tolerance of the miners for energetic physical activity at the Aucanquilcha mine, which they believed was at an altitude of 5800 m. We now know that the mine is actually higher, the altitude being 5950 m. The exercise level of the miners is indeed astonishing as they break large pieces of sulfur ore (caliche) with sledgehammers (McIntyre 1987). The miners are predominantly Bolivians who were born at moderately high altitudes and since most of them live at Amincha (altitude 4200 m), they have a considerable degree of high altitude acclimatization.

In preparation for the British Mount Everest Expedition of 1953, Pugh measured oxygen uptakes on climbers in the field near Cho Oyu in the Nepal Himalaya in 1952. These data were then used to determine the amount of oxygen to be carried by the 1953 expedition during which Pugh made further measurements of exercise physiology (Pugh 1958). He subsequently extended this program in the ambitious Himalayan Scientific and Mountaineering Expedition (Silver Hut) of 1960–61 in which several physiologists, including authors JBW and JSM, spent the winter in a prefabricated hut at an altitude of 5800 m (Pugh 1962). Further measurements of maximal oxygen consumption were carried out in the spring when the expedition moved to Mount Makalu (8481 m) and a bicycle ergometer was erected on the Makalu Col (altitude 7440 m) (Chapter 1, Fig. 1.6) (Pugh *et al.* 1964). The data assembled by Pugh and his co-workers (Fig. 12.1) were of great interest because they predicted that, near the summit of Mount Everest, the maximal oxygen uptake would be very close to the basal oxygen requirements, and therefore it seemed problematic whether man could ever reach the

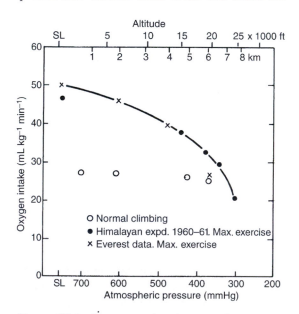

Figure 12.1 $\dot{V}o_{2,max}$ against barometric pressure in acclimatized subjects (closed circles, crosses) as reported by Pugh *et al.* (1964). Data from normal climbing rates are also shown (open circles).

summit without supplementary oxygen (West and Wagner 1980).

Additional measurements of maximal oxygen consumption were made by Cerretelli during an Italian expedition to Mount Everest in 1973 (Cerretelli 1976a). All the data were obtained at Base Camp (altitude 5350 m), but they included measurements on climbers who had been above 8000 m. One of the many interesting observations was the failure of the maximal oxygen uptake of acclimatized subjects at 5350 m to return to the sea level value when pure oxygen was breathed. The explanation of this finding, also made by Pugh and others, is still controversial but is certainly multifactorial, involving in part some deterioration of oxidative function at the tissue level, as well as a decrease in muscle power from muscle cell atrophy that has long been recognized.

The issue of whether the partial pressure of oxygen at the summit of Mount Everest was sufficient for man to reach it without supplementary oxygen was finally answered in 1978 by Reinhold Messner and Peter Habeler. However, their accounts make it clear that neither had much in reserve (Habeler 1979; Messner 1979). The intriguing question of how the body is just able to transport sufficient oxygen to the exercising muscles under these conditions of profound hypoxia is considered in detail in Chapter 13.

During the 1981 American Medical Research Expedition to Everest (AMREE), extensive measurements of maximal oxygen uptake were made in the main laboratory camp, altitude 6300 m. However, data were also obtained for exercise at higher altitudes by giving the well-acclimatized subjects inspired mixtures containing low concentrations of oxygen. For example, when the inspired P_{O_2} was only 42.5 mmHg, corresponding to that on the summit of Mount Everest, the measured maximal oxygen consumption was just over 1 L min^{-1}; whereas at sea level in the same subjects, the values were around 5 L min^{-1} (West et al. 1983a). Although this is very low and equivalent to that of someone walking slowly on the level, it is apparently just sufficient to explain how a climber can reach the summit without supplementary oxygen (Chapter 13). A further

extensive series of exercise measurements were made during Operation Everest II in the autumn of 1985 (Houston et al. 1987). The eight subjects spent 40 days in a large low-pressure chamber being gradually decompressed to the barometric pressure existing at the summit of Mount Everest, and a series of measurements of maximal exercise were made using a bicycle ergometer. The measured oxygen consumptions agreed well with those found in the field by the 1981 expedition (Sutton et al. 1988), but Operation Everest II had the great additional advantage that many invasive measurements could be made which were impracticable in the field. These included extensive measurements of pulmonary vascular pressures, muscle volume, and muscle biopsies (Sutton et al. 1987). As suggested on AMREE and OEII, there is individual variability in the response to extreme altitude which was further documented on the Caudwell Xtreme Everest expedition with unclear implications on performance (Grocott et al. 2009).

12.3 VENTILATION

12.3.1 Increase in ventilation

Exercise at high altitude is accompanied by very high levels of ventilation. Indeed, this was one of the most obvious features of climbing at extreme altitudes in the early Everest expeditions as evidenced by the quotations from Norton and Somervell in the preceding section.

Ventilation is normally expressed at body temperature, ambient pressure, and with the gas saturated with water vapour (BTPS). This is because the volumes of gas moved then correspond to the volume excursions of the chest and lungs. Ventilation can also be expressed at standard temperature and pressure for dry gas (STPD). These volumes are very much smaller at high altitude and bear no obvious relationship to the actual chest movements. However, the oxygen consumption and carbon dioxide output are traditionally expressed in these units so that the values are independent of altitude.

For a given work level, the ventilation expressed as BTPS increases at high altitude.

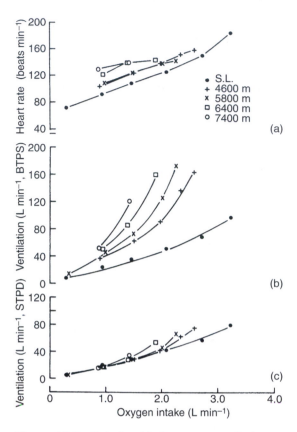

Figure 12.2 Relationship between ventilation, both BTPS and STPD, and oxygen uptake at various altitudes. Heart rate is also shown (from Pugh *et al.* 1964).

Typical results are shown in Fig. 12.2b which shows data obtained during the 1960–61 Silver Hut Expedition (Pugh *et al.* 1964). Figure 12.2c shows ventilations expressed as STPD. Here the values also tend to be somewhat higher than those measured at sea level, especially at work levels approaching the maximum for the altitude, but the differences are clearly much less than for ventilation expressed as BTPS.

Ventilation (BTPS) can reach extremely high levels as evidenced by data obtained during the 1981 AMREE at an altitude of 6300 m (P_B 351 mmHg). In eight subjects who exercised at a work rate of 1200 kg min^{-1}, the mean ventilation (BTPS) was 207 L min^{-1} with a mean respiratory frequency of 62 breaths min^{-1}. These values were for a mean oxygen consumption of 2.31 L min^{-1} and correspond to a ventilatory equivalent (V_E/V_{O_2},

i.e. the amount of expired ventilation dedicated to a given metabolic rate), almost four times greater than sea level. In spite of a lower gas density which will decrease the work of breathing a modest amount, this degree of ventilation still results in a much greater work of breathing for any given energy expenditure (Cibella *et al.* 1999; Schoene 2005). These levels of ventilation are approaching the maximal voluntary ventilation (MVV) that is the maximal amount of air that can be moved per minute by breathing in and out as rapidly and deeply as possible, usually measured over 12 s.

12.3.2 Work of breathing

When climbing at high altitude, the body must decide how to apportion its energy output between the muscles of locomotion and those of respiration which require a precise amount of perfusion to deliver oxygen. Cibella *et al.* (1999) demonstrated in subjects that, in spite of the lower gas density, there was substantially greater energy expenditure for respiration at high altitude than at sea level. The respiratory muscles in this study, therefore, required a greater proportion of cardiac output for a given workload at high than low altitude, thus depriving the locomotory muscles of perfusion, 5.5% versus 26% at low and high (5000 m) altitude, respectively. An increase in resistance of leg muscle blood flow in deference to flow to the respiratory muscles at high levels of work have been shown at low altitude (Barclay 1986, Babcock *et al.* 1995, Harms *et al.* 1997, Wetter *et al.* 1999) and can only be assumed to be greater at higher altitude where respiration is much greater. It is primarily the diaphragm which has been shown both at low and high altitude to compete for the limited blood flow (Marciniuk *et al.* 1994). Lundby *et al.* (2006) demonstrated a persistent decrease in blood flow to the lower extremities in lowlanders even after 8 weeks of acclimatization to 4100 m, suggesting this pattern as an important factor in limiting maximal exercise at very high altitudes. Part of this decrease in blood flow can be restored in this same population when hemoglobin and presumed blood viscosity are decreased with isovolumic hemodilution (Calbert *et al.* 2002).

12.3.3 Extreme altitude

It is interesting that these extremely high levels of ventilation are not seen at the highest altitudes. For example, when two subjects on the 1981 expedition were given a 14% oxygen mixture to breathe at an altitude of 6300 m (inspired P_{O_2} 42.5 mmHg) to simulate the summit of Everest, the maximal exercise ventilation was only 162 L min^{-1}. A reasonable explanation for the lower exercise ventilation is that the work rate was very much lower, being only 450 and 600 kg min^{-1} as opposed to 1200 kg min^{-1} at the altitude of 6300 m while breathing air. Another possibility is that, as mentioned above, the respiratory muscles were limited by the severe hypoxemia and a limitation of blood flow. Figure 12.3 shows maximal exercise ventilation plotted against inspired P_{O_2} (dashed line), and there is a maximal value although there are only four points on the curve. A similar pattern was found during the 1960–61 Silver Hut Expedition. For example, the maximal exercise ventilation at 5800 m had a mean value of 173 L min^{-1}. At an altitude of 6400 m, this had fallen to 161, while at an altitude of 7440 m, the value was only 122 L min^{-1}. Corresponding to the fall in maximal exercise ventilation, the $\dot{V}_{O_{2,max}}$ decreased from 1200 kg min^{-1} at 5800 m, to 900 kg min^{-1} at 6400 m, to 600 kg min^{-1} at 7400 m. These extremely high exercise ventilations are facilitated, only in part, by the reduced work of breathing as a result of the lowered density of the air at high altitude. The reduced density also results in an increased maximal voluntary ventilation (or maximum breathing capacity) as altitude is increased (Cotes 1954). For example, Cotes showed that the maximal voluntary ventilation (BTPS) increased from 158 at sea level to 197 L min^{-1} at a simulated altitude of 5180 m in a low-pressure chamber. In a further study, a mean value of 203 L min^{-1} was observed at a simulated altitude of 8250 m (Cotes 1954). The increase in MVV was compatible with the hypothesis that the work of maximum breathing remains constant at high altitude. The reduction in the work of breathing at high altitude caused by the change in gas density was also analyzed by Petit *et al.* (1963).

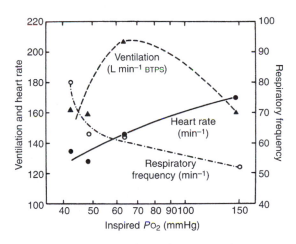

Figure 12.3   Maximal ventilation (BTPS), maximal respiratory frequency, and maximal heart rate plotted against inspired P_{O_2} on a log scale. This scale was chosen only because otherwise the high-altitude points fall very close together. Note that both maximal ventilation and heart rate fall at extreme altitudes because work levels become so low. However, respiratory frequency continues to increase (from West *et al.* 1983c). (1 Torr = 1 mmHg).

12.3.4 Oxygen breathing

Oxygen breathing reduces exercise ventilation for a given work rate at high altitude. However, as Fig. 12.4 shows, the ventilations do not return to the sea level values, but are intermediate between the high altitude and sea level values for ambient air. This observation is probably secondary to the increased sensitivity of the carotid body which is the primary organ of ventilatory acclimatization (see Chapter 5).

12.3.5 Respiratory pattern

The pattern of breathing during exercise at high altitude is characterized by very high frequencies and relatively small tidal volumes. Somervell's observation referred to in section 12.2 of 7–10 complete respirations per step is evidence for that. The highest measurements of respiratory frequency and tidal volume yet made were those on Pizzo during the 1981 Everest expedition

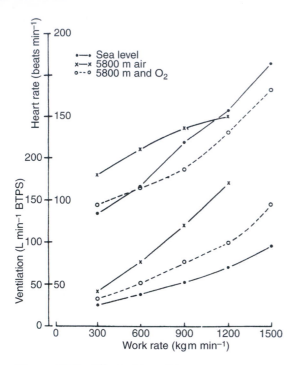

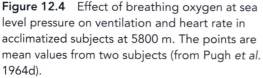

Figure 12.4 Effect of breathing oxygen at sea level pressure on ventilation and heart rate in acclimatized subjects at 5800 m. The points are mean values from two subjects (from Pugh *et al.* 1964d).

(West *et al.* 1983a). He climbed for about 7 min at an altitude of 8300 m (P_B 271 mmHg), while measuring his ventilation with a turbine flow meter, and the output was registered on a slow-running tape recorder. During the middle 4 min of this period, his mean respiratory frequency was 86 ± 2.8 (SD) breaths per minute, mean tidal volume was 1.26 L, and mean ventilation was 107 L min^{-1} at BTPS. Thus, his breathing was shallow and extremely rapid. Reference has already been made to the measurements of maximal exercise at an inspired P_{O_2} of 42.5 mmHg corresponding to that on the Everest summit which was obtained by making the subjects inspire 14% oxygen at an altitude of 6300 m. For two subjects, the mean respiratory frequency was 80 breaths min^{-1}. This tachypneic response of a low tidal volume, high frequency pattern is the body's attempt to minimize the overall work of breathing.

This pattern of breathing is consistent with the very powerful hypoxic drive via the peripheral chemoreceptors. As pointed out in Chapter 6, it is remarkable that the hypoxic drive is so strong under these conditions because the arterial P_{CO_2} is less than 10 mmHg and the arterial pH is over 7.7. A very low P_{CO_2} and high pH normally inhibit ventilation, but the overriding hyperventilatory stimulus is the marked hypoxemia.

12.4 VENTILATION–PERFUSION RELATIONSHIPS

For many years, it was believed that the only change in ventilation–perfusion relationships at high altitude was a more uniform topographical distribution of blood flow. This is caused by the increased pulmonary arterial pressure as a result of hypoxic pulmonary vasoconstriction (Chapter 8). For example, measurements with radioactive xenon have shown that the topographical differences of blood flow between apex and base of the upright lung are reduced at an altitude of 3100 m (Dawson 1972). As discussed in Chapter 13, measurements by Wagner and his co-workers (1988b) show a broadening of the distribution of ventilation–perfusion ratios during high levels of hypoxic exercise, the cause of which is still uncertain. The change in the distribution of ventilation and perfusion demonstrates an increase in blood flow to poorly ventilated lung units, seen in normal subjects who are exercising while acutely exposed to hypoxia in a low pressure chamber (Gale *et al.* 1985), exercising normal subjects who are inhaling low oxygen mixtures (Hammond *et al.* 1986), and normal subjects during a 40-day exposure to low pressure in a chamber during Operation Everest II (Wagner *et al.* 1988b). Evidence from this last study suggests that the ventilation–perfusion abnormalities are most likely to be seen in poorly acclimatized subjects after a rapid ascent. In general, the abnormalities were most marked at the most severe levels of hypoxia, and at the heaviest exercise levels.

Acclimatization does convey a modest improvement in gas exchange as noted by Wagner *et al.* (2002) and Lundby *et al.* (2004). They studied lowlanders before and after ascent and over 8 weeks at 4100 m and found an improvement in exercise Sa,o_2 that was secondary both to a modest improvement in the (A−a) Do_2, as well as ongoing ventilatory adaptation. On the other hand, litter greyhounds exposed to high altitude for five months had higher diffusion capacities than control dogs, suggesting that actual improvement in pulmonary function and gas exchange from the effect of high altitude requires that the exposure needs to be during the somatic maturation (McDonough *et al.* 2006). These findings support previous impressions in humans that actual changes in pulmonary function and gas exchange can only occur during the formative growth phase. The study by Lundby *et al.* (2004) supports the findings of improved gas exchange in lowlanders during altitude exposure which still could not achieve that of high altitude natives.

Two reasonable hypotheses to explain the impairment in gas exchange are that these changes are caused: (1) in some way by subclinical pulmonary edema which results in inequality of ventilation and/or (2) increased diffusion limitation of oxygen to the blood across the pulmonary capillaries with a greater cardiac output during exercise, which will be discussed in section 12.5. As discussed in Chapter 21, high altitude pulmonary edema is a well-known complication of going to high altitude. The likely mechanism is uneven hypoxic pulmonary vasoconstriction, which allows some capillaries to be exposed to high pressure with subsequent damage to their walls (West and Mathieu-Costello 1992). The increase in pulmonary artery pressure is exaggerated during heavy exercise (Groves *et al.* 1987).

12.5 DIFFUSION

As discussed in Chapter 7, there is strong evidence that diffusion limitation of oxygen transfer in the lung occurs during exercise at high altitude. This is the primary reason for the fall in arterial Po_2 and arterial oxygen saturation which has been consistently observed. Analysis of the situation at extreme altitude indicates that the diffusing capacity of the blood-gas barrier is one of the chief limiting factors for maximal exercise (Chapter 13).

There is no evidence that the diffusing capacity of the blood-gas barrier increases during acclimatization to high altitude in lowland subjects, whereas high altitude natives demonstrate higher diffusion capacities compared to lowlanders (Wagner *et al.* 2002). Measurements from the 1960–61 Silver Hut Expedition showed that the diffusing capacity of the blood-gas barrier for a given level of exercise was the same as at sea level (West 1962). Overall pulmonary diffusing capacity for carbon monoxide increased by 19% at an altitude of 5800 m, but this could be attributed to the more rapid rate of combination of carbon monoxide with oxygen because of the low prevailing Po_2. The volume of blood in the pulmonary capillaries as determined by measuring the diffusing capacity at two values of alveolar Po_2 showed no change or possibly a slight fall. This may have been due to hypoxic pulmonary vasoconstriction.

These results also imply that, in acclimatized subjects, the transit time for red cells in the pulmonary capillaries at a given work level is approximately the same as at sea level. The transit time of the pulmonary capillary blood is given by the pulmonary capillary blood volume divided by the cardiac output (Roughton 1945). As discussed in Chapter 8, there is good evidence that in acclimatized lowlanders at high altitude, the cardiac output for a given work level is the same as at sea level (Pugh 1964; Reeves *et al.* 1987). Thus, since both the pulmonary capillary blood volume and the cardiac output are essentially unchanged, this indicates that the transit time through the pulmonary capillaries will also be the same as at sea level, but because of the lower driving pressure for oxygen from the air to the blood, there is still not enough time for equilibration into the pulmonary capillary blood.

The effect of an increased cardiac output and transit time for blood across the pulmonary capillary on oxygen diffusion from the air to the blood and (A−a)Do_2 is discussed in detail in Chapter 7. Calbet *et al.* (2008) furthered this discussion by showing that at moderate altitude during steady-state exercise (100–120 watts) with a cardiac output of ~2 L min^{-1}, there was no widening of the (A−a)Do_2. Even at these levels of work and altitude, the model of Piiper and Scheid (1980) would have predicted some diffusion limitation. It is generally accepted though that the magnitude of the widening of the $(A-a)Do_2$ and diffusion limitation is proportional to the altitude and cardiac output.

Lovering *et al.* (2008) postulated another mechanism for high altitude exercise hypoxemia. Using saline contrast echocardiography, they studied nine males during incremental exercise to exhaustion during normoxia and hypoxia ($FIo_2 = 0.12$). Their intent was to evaluate intrapulmonary shunting possibly induced by exercise and/or hypoxia. At rest, none of the subjects under normoxia and three of the subjects during hypoxia demonstrated shunting; whereas, during exercise, eight of nine and nine of nine demonstrated shunting in normoxia and hypoxia, respectively. They hypothesized that increased pressures and/or blood flow opened up anatomically defined microvascular channels which were the location for right-to-left intrapulmonary shunting. The significance of these findings has been challenged (Hopkins *et al.* 2008). She based her skepticism on several observations. First, the detection of shunt depends on the appearance of bubbles in the left atrium. Hopkins noted that the size of bubbles that transit the pulmonary vasculature is not known nor is the importance of reaggregation of these bubbles on the left side. Second, previous quantitation of shunt by other methods has shown that, if there is any shunt at all, it has been thought to be trivial and physiologically insignificant. Third, using the multiple inert gas elimination technique (MIGET) which elegantly quantitates pulmonary gas exchange between ventilation/perfusion ratio, shunt, and diffusion at high levels of exercise, the percent shunt has never been shown to be >1.0%. Lovering *et al.* (2009) defended their findings and explained away the MIGET findings by invoking precapillary gas exchange which could affect the transit of soluble gases across the alveolar–capillary membrane and thus underestimate shunt. These anatomic shunts may be real, but are they physiologically significant? Thus, it seems that this area of hypoxic exercise physiology will remain controversial for a while.

12.6 CARDIOVASCULAR RESPONSES

These were discussed in Chapter 8. In non-acclimatized and poorly acclimatized lowlanders who go acutely to high altitude, cardiac output at rest and during exercise for a given work level is increased compared with sea level values. The same is true of heart rate.

In acclimatized lowlanders, cardiac output for a given work level returns to its sea level value as shown by Pugh (1964) during the 1960–61 Silver Hut Expedition, and more recently during Operation Everest II (Reeves *et al.* 1987). However, heart rate for a given level of exercise remains higher at altitude and therefore stroke volume is less. Maximum heart rate, on the other hand, decreases with duration of stay at high altitude, especially very high altitude (Lundby *et al.* 2001; Lundby and van Hall, 2001; Lundby *et al.* 2004; Lundby *et al.* 2006). Measurements of contractile function of the heart during Operation Everest II in exercising subjects at all altitudes showed remarkable preservation in spite of the very severe hypoxemia (Reeves *et al.* 1987). Of note though, are data which support some decrease in cardiac function that persists for a while after exposure to high altitude. Holloway *et al.* (2011) measured cardiac function in 14 subjects by using ^{31}P magnetic resonance (MR) spectroscopy of the myocardium within 4 days return from a 17-day trek to Everest Base Camp (5300 m). They found an 11% decrease in left ventricular mass, a 24% decrease in diastolic function, and decrease in PCr/ATP ratio as a reflection of myocardial oxidative capability. These changes returned to normal baseline values in months.

Pulmonary artery pressures are increased during exercise at altitude compared with sea level values at the same work level. The elevated pressures are seen in both unacclimatized (Kronenberg *et al.* 1971) and acclimatized (Groves *et al.* 1987) lowlanders, and in native highlanders (Penaloza *et al.* 1963; Lockhart *et al.* 1976). Naeije speculates that a substantial portion of the decrease in exercise performance at altitude may be secondary to impairment of right ventricular output from pulmonary hypertension (Naeije 2010). The basic cause of the pulmonary hypertension is presumably hypoxic pulmonary vasoconstriction. However, it is of considerable interest that in the subjects of Operation Everest II, the pulmonary vascular pressures did not return to normal when 100% oxygen was breathed even though the subjects had been at high altitude only 2 or 3 weeks (Groves *et al.* 1987). This indicates some structural changes (remodeling) in the pulmonary arteries in addition to hypoxic vasoconstriction even in this relatively brief time of exposure to hypobaria. Hergistad and Robbins (2009) exposed 10 subjects to 8 hours of hypoxia (end-tidal P_{O_2} 55 mmHg) and room air at low altitude and then used Doppler echocardiography to measure the maximum pressure gradient across the tricuspid valve as an index of pulmonary artery pressure. The subjects were then studied on room air at rest and at exercise of a heart rate 30 beats per minute above resting values. There was a modest but significant increase in the pressure gradient across the tricuspid valve at rest and a 35% increase during exercise after the hypoxic exposure. The cause for this increase is not known, but engenders the speculation that there is upregulation of the mediators of pulmonary vascular response that is not evanescent and/or there are rapidly developing morphologic changes in the pulmonary vasculature that affect pulmonary vascular reactivity.

Interest in the effect of increased pulmonary vascular resistance during altitude exposure on cardiac output and thus exercise performance has generated studies on pharmacologic intervention to minimize that rise. Phosphodiesterase type-5 (PDE-5) inhibitors and endothelin receptor blockers are the two leading modulators of pulmonary vascular response which have been studied the most.

Sildenafil, a PDE-5 inhibitor, potently inhibits hypoxic pulmonary vasoconstriction. Richalet *et al.* (2005a) carried out a randomized, double-blind, placebo-controlled (RDBPC) trial of sildenafil and placebo in subjects exposed for 6 days at 4350 m. Pulmonary artery pressure (PAP) rose 29% upon hypoxic exposure before medication. Sildenafil resulted in a PAP that was 6% less than sea level values, a lower alveolar–arterial oxygen difference, and a decrease in exercise performance that was less than the placebo group (Figs 12.5 and 12.6). At Everest Base Camp (approximately 5400 m),

Ghofrani *et al.* (2004) looked at the effect of acute administration of sildenafil to subjects during exercise in another RDBPC trial and found a lower PAP, a higher Sa_{O_2}, and greater work capacity than on placebo. Hsu *et al.* (2006) exposed 10 cyclists to normoxia and simulated high altitude (approximately 3874 m, $FI_{O_2} = 0.128$) on placebo and three doses (0, 50, and 100 mg) of sildenafil, and studied cardiac performance as well as time trial lengths of 10 km at sea level and 5 km during hypoxia. During hypoxia, sildenafil resulted in an increase in stroke volume and cardiac output and a mean decrease of 15% time in the time trial, but no difference with normoxia. Of interest was the finding that there were responders (39% decrease in time trial time) and non-responders (1% decrease). This latter finding is fascinating and reinforces the notion that, as in most physiologic responses, the PAP response to hypoxia is a genetically controlled mechanism that is different in each person. Faoro *et al.* (2007) studied the effect of sildenafil an exercise ($V_{O_2,max}$) oxygen saturation (Sp_{O_2}), and echocardiographic indices for pulmonary vascular hemodynamics. They studied 16 healthy subjects in a double-blind, placebo-control, cross-over study with 50 mg of sildenafil and placebo in normoxia, acute hypoxia ($FI_{O_2} = 0.1$), and after 2 weeks at 5000 m. In normoxia, the drug had no effect on any of these variables while in acute hypoxia, $V_{O_2,max}$ increased from 27 ± 5 to 32 ± 6 cc kg^{-1} min^{-1} and Sp_{O_2} from $62–68 \pm 9$%. Sildenafil did not affect these variables after 2 weeks at 5000 m. Calculated mean pulmonary artery pressures were 16 ± 3, 28 ± 5 and 32 ± 6 mmHg in the respective conditions. Pulmonary vascular resistance did decrease with sildenafil 30–50% in these hypoxic conditions. Sildenafil was studied in a double-blind, placebo-control trial in 62 subjects flown to La Paz, Bolivia, and after 4–5 days of acclimatization there (3650 m) ascended in 90 min to 5200 m. Both echocardiographically calculated PAP and scoring of acute mountain sickness (AMS) were undertaken. Calculated PAP was not different, but AMS scores were higher in the sildenafil group. It is conceivable that headache, one of the known side effects of PDE-5 inhibitors, could have been from the drug rather than AMS per se. Of interest, were the results of a study by Fischler *et al.* (2009)

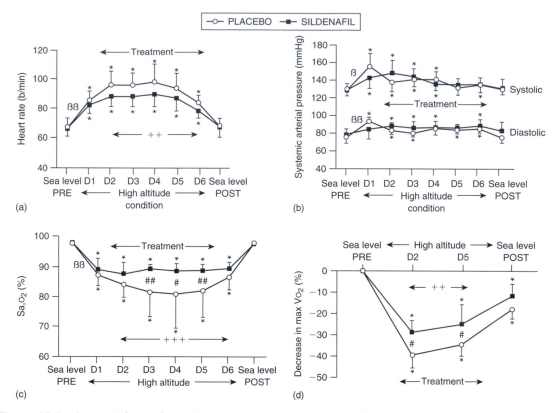

Figure 12.5 Systemic hemodynamic parameters and exercise performance. *$p < 0.05$ versus sea level pre; #$p < 0.05$, ##$p < 0.01$ sildenafil versus placebo; $p < 0.05$, $p < 0.01$ D1 versus sea level pre for the whole group; ++$p < 0.01$, +++$p < 0.001$ sildenafil versus placebo for pooled high altitude with treatment values (from Richalet *et al.* 2005).

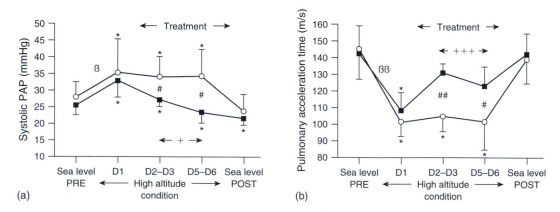

Figure 12.6 Echocardiographic evaluation of pulmonary hemodynamics. Pulmonary artery pressure (PAP). *$p < 0.05$ versus sea level pre; #$p < 0.05$, ##$p < 0.01$ sildenafil (filled squares) versus placebo (open circles); $p < 0.05$, $p < 0.01$ D1 versus sea level pre for the whole group; +$p < 0.05$, +++$p < 0.001$ sildenafil versus placebo for pooled high altitude with treatment values (from Richalet *et al.* 2005).

who studied a longer-acting PDE-5 inhibitor, tadalafil, and dexamethasone and placebo at low altitude and 4559 m altitude in high altitude pulmonary edema (HAPE)-susceptible subjects. Tadalafil did result in lower calculated PAPs and higher Sp,O_2 than placebo, but dexamethasone interestingly had even more impressive effects on these variables and resulted in less of a decrease in predicted $VO_{2,max}$, compared to sea level than tadalafil which was comparable to placebo. The mechanisms of these differences are not known.

Endothelin-1 (ET-1) is a potent endogenous pulmonary vasoconstrictor released from the pulmonary vascular endothelium. In an elegant display of the use of basic science information into the clinical arena, therapeutic agents which block the ET-1 (endothelin receptor blocker, ERB) have come into use to treat pulmonary hypertension. These agents, thus, have appropriately become a focus of studies to look at their effect on hypoxic pulmonary vasoconstriction at high altitude. Pham et al. (2010) studied resting and submaximal exercise variables with an ERB, bosentan (250 mg), in an RDBPC trial versus placebo after a 90-minute exposure to normobaric hypoxia ($FIO_2 = 0.12$). Bosentan significantly decreased the resting but not exercise calculated PAP and had no effect on arterial blood gases or cardiac output. To test the hypothesis that increased pulmonary vascular resistance (PVR) in part impairs exercise at high altitude, Faoro et al. (2009) studied subjects in an RDBPC design at weekly intervals between bosentan and placebo with echocardiography and exercise after 1 hour of breathing normoxic or hypoxic ($FIO_2 = 0.12$) gas. In the drug arm of the study, bosentan was administered for 3 days (62.5 mg the first day and 125 mg the next 2 days). Subjects became hypoxemic on the hypoxic gas, increased their PVR 5.6 ± 0.3 to 7.2 ± 0.5 mmHg L min^{-1} m^2 and decreased their $VO_{2,max}$ from 47 ± 2 to 35 ± 2 cc kg^{-1} min^{-1}. Bosentan decreased PVR to baseline measurements, restored 30% of the hypoxia-induced decrease in $VO_{2,max}$ and this correlated with PAP reduction. The effect of another ERB, sitaxsentan (100 mg per day for 7 days) on exercise and PVR was studied in 13 healthy subjects at sea level and 1 hour of acute hypoxia ($FIO_2 = 0.12$), as well as 22 healthy subjects acclimatized to 5050 m. The study was a double-blind, randomized design. PVR was decreased with drug and $VO_{2,max}$ was restored by 30% and 10% in acute and prolonged ambient hypoxia. The improvement in $VO_{2,max}$ was correlated with the change in PVR. These authors attribute part of this improvement in $VO_{2,max}$ to an increase in pulmonary blood flow from pharmacologic vasodilatation (de Bisschop et al. 2011). Not all studies have shown a physiologic benefit. Seheult et al. (2009) undertook an RDBPC trial of bosentan versus placebo started 5 days before ascent to 3800 m in eight, healthy subjects who then did a cycle ergometry time trial (TT) echocardiographically calculated PAP. There was no difference in TT or PAP, but there was a higher Sp,O_2 (85 ± 8 versus $78 \pm 6\%$) in the placebo group.

12.7 ARTERIAL BLOOD GASES

At high altitude, the resting pattern of a low arterial PO_2 and PCO_2 is also seen during exercise. Arterial PO_2 typically falls further on exercise because of diffusion limitation. In addition, at high work levels, the arterial PCO_2 often falls below the resting value, indicating that alveolar ventilation increases more than CO_2 production. The falling PCO_2 is associated with an increased respiratory exchange ratio which may rise to values over 1.2 at the highest workloads at very high altitudes (West et al. 1983a). This represents an unsteady state since the respiratory quotient of the metabolizing tissues in a sustainable energy output cannot exceed 1.0. At sea level, such an increase in respiratory exchange ratio is often associated with lactate production from exercising muscles as a result of anaerobic glycolysis. However, at very high altitude, blood lactate levels remain surprisingly low even following exhausting exercise (Edwards 1936; Cerretelli 1980; West 1986; Lundby et al. 2000).

Arterial pH is near normal in well-acclimatized subjects up to altitudes of about 5400 m, although Winslow obtained evidence that there is often a small degree of uncompensated respiratory alkalosis, even in native highlanders (Winslow et al. 1981; Winslow and Monge 1987). At higher altitudes, the arterial pH at rest tends to increase, and it exceeded 7.7 in one subject on the Everest summit (West et al. 1983b). The respiratory alkalosis is exaggerated on exercise because the arterial P_{CO_2} tends to fall and levels of blood lactate are low.

As stated in section 12.2, extensive observations that blood lactate is low in acclimatized subjects at high altitude, even during maximal work, were first made by Edwards (1936) during the 1935 International High Altitude Expedition to Chile, although Dill *et al.* (1931) had obtained some data prior to that. Figure 12.7 is redrawn from Edward's paper and shows that the levels of blood lactate during exercise at high altitude (up to 5340 m) were essentially the same as at sea level. This means that the blood lactate levels for a given work level were apparently independent of tissue P_{O_2}. The only clear exceptions to this were the points shown by the open circles which were obtained at the lowest altitude of 2810 m. The days spent at altitude are shown on the abscissa, and it is clear that in most instances these data were obtained before the subject had had time to become fully acclimatized. Since maximal work capacity declines markedly with increasing altitude, the data of Fig. 12.7 imply that maximal blood lactate falls in acclimatized subjects as altitude increases.

These results have been extended by Cerretelli (Cerretelli 1976a; Cerretelli 1976b; Cerretelli 1980) with additional measurements made at an altitude of 6300 m on the 1981 AMREE (West *et al.* 1983a). Figure 13.6 summarizes the data on resting and maximal blood lactate (West 1986) and suggests the surprising conclusion that, after maximal exercise at altitudes exceeding 7500 m, there will be no increase in lactate in the blood at all in spite of the extreme oxygen deprivation. Possible reasons for this are discussed in more detail in Chapter 13.

Of great interest has been the speculation about the actual blood gas values at extreme altitude. On AMREE in 1981, alveolar gas samplings and venous blood sampling at 8000 m the next day allowed calculations of what the presumed arterial samplings might have been on the summit (West *et al.* 1983c). Although there will be more discussion in the next chapter on extreme altitude, it is important to emphasize the effect on exercise of hypoxemia as it is related to very high altitudes, as well as the individual variation that is observed (Schoene *et al.* 1984). The hypoxic ventilatory response (HVR) and the prolonged ventilatory acclimatization, as has been discussed, is the primary defense of alveolar and thus arterial P_{O_2}. This response is reflected in a progressive decrease in P_{CO_2} from hyperventilation and the consequent respiratory alkalosis which because of the effect on the oxygen–hemoglobin dissociation curve result in a well-preserved arterial oxygen content up to

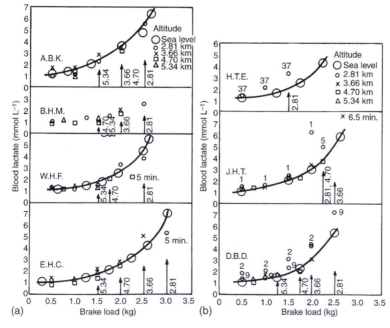

Figure 12.7 Venous blood lactate after exercise as reported by Edwards from the 1935 International High Altitude Expedition to Chile. The lines are drawn through the sea-level values. In general, lactate levels at high altitude lie on the same line, the only obvious exceptions being measurements made at the lowest altitude of 2.81 km. The small figures above these points indicate the number of days spent at that altitude and in most instances this was insufficient for acclimatization (from Edwards 1936).

7011 m (see Figure 2 in Grocott *et al.* 2009). The question then arises: if arterial oxygen content is preserved as high as 7100 m, then what is it that limits cardiac output and/or oxygen extraction and thus physical exertion?

These data (Grocott *et al.* 2009) report results of arterial blood gases drawn at 8400 m in four climbers descending from the summit of Mt Everest (8848 m). The remarkable findings were the interindividual variability of the ventilatory response which had the predictable effect, based on the alveolar air equation on $PaCO_2$ and thus PaO_2 values. $PaCO_2$ ranged from 10.3 to 15.7 mmHg which at that altitude is profound with PaO_2 from 19.1 to 29.5 mmHg. Although these investigators did not measure subjects' HVR values, these values of $PaCO_2$ are sound enough evidence that there was distinct variability. Additionally, these subjects had a very modest elevation of blood lactic acid values (~2.2 mmol L^{-1}), suggesting that glycolytic metabolism was not playing a substantial role in energy production at these altitudes. Additionally, their data also show that gas exchange, as reflected in a mean $(A−a)DO_2$ of 5.4 mmHg, in healthy individuals without clinical evidence of HAPE is well preserved.

The limitations of exercise performance at high altitude (very high to extreme) is multifactorial and will especially be discussed with respect to extreme altitude in the next chapter. Suffice it to say that preservation of arterial oxygen content even up to very high altitudes (7100 m) does not lead to exercise levels noted at lower altitudes. Part of the perfusion of the locomotory muscles is diverted to the muscles of respiration which are working many times in excess of low altitude values to preserve arterial oxygen content. Cardiac output is appropriate for a given level of energy output, but the reasons for the limitation of maximal exercise performance, especially at extreme altitude, may lie in the oxygen delivery to the active muscles and/or the limiting effect of cerebral hypoxia.

12.8 PERIPHERAL TISSUES

The changes that occur in peripheral tissues at high altitude were discussed in Chapter 11. Animal studies indicate an increase in capillary density in some tissues as a result of chronic hypoxia. However, data available from human muscle biopsies indicate that the number of capillaries remains constant in acclimatized lowlanders with no increase of mRNA expression of regulatory factors for angiogenesis (VEGF) during acclimatization to 4100 m (Lundby *et al.* 2004a). On the other hand, the average distance over which oxygen diffuses is reduced because the muscle fibers become smaller, perhaps secondary to ongoing oxidative damage with prolonged high altitude exposure (Lundby *et al.* 2004b). There are changes in intracellular enzymes, and some studies show an increase in muscle myoglobin which may enhance oxygen diffusion. Mizuno *et al.* (2008) looked at the effect of exercise versus sedentary existence at 5250 m or higher for 75 days. There was no difference on the previously noted effects of high altitude on muscle morphology or chemistry. In other words, muscle fiber size decreased; capillary number (2.1–2.2 capillaries per fiber) was not different between groups, while capillary density increased about 30%; enzymes chosen to reflect mitochondrial capacity (citrate synthase and 3/hydroxyl-CoA-dehydrogenase) did not change after the altitude exposure. However, muscle buffer capacity did increase with the altitude exposure, but not differently between the exercising and sedentary groups. Using ^{31}P-NMR spectroscopy, Edwards *et al.* (2010) studied trekkers to Everest Base Camp at 5300 m and climbers to 7950 m before and after the journey. Although resting Pi was higher in the climbers prior to the trip perhaps secondary to better conditioning, all of the other markers of mitochondrial function were preserved even after profound and prolonged altitude exposure. These findings confirm those from the earlier OEII chamber study (Green et al. 1989).

There has been considerable interest in the possible role of oxygen diffusion from capillaries to mitochondria as a factor limiting exercise at high altitude. Traditionally, many physiologists have argued that the power of working muscles at high altitude is determined by the amount of oxygen reaching them via the arterial blood. Oxygen delivery defined as the arterial oxygen concentration multiplied by the blood flow to the muscle has often been regarded as the critical variable.

Wagner and co-workers have analyzed the relationship between oxygen uptake and the P_{O_2} of muscle capillary blood on the assumption that the uptake is limited by oxygen diffusion from the capillaries to the mitochondria (Hogan et al. 1988a). Figure 12.8a shows a diagram relating oxygen uptake to the P_{O_2} of muscle venous blood, taken as an index of muscle capillary P_{O_2}. The line sloping from top left to bottom right shows the amount of oxygen being delivered to the muscle by the capillaries (Fick principle). The line from bottom left to top right shows the pressure gradient available to cause oxygen diffusion from the red cells to the mitochondria (Fick's law) assuming that the mitochondrial P_{O_2} is nearly zero. The slope of this line is the lumped 'diffusing capacity for oxygen' of the tissues. The point where the two diagonal lines cross represents the $\dot{V}_{O_{2,max}}$. Regions to the left of this indicate situations where ample oxygen is available in the blood, but the diffusing head of pressure is inadequate. Regions to the right indicate a more than adequate diffusing head of pressure, but inadequate amounts of oxygen in the blood.

Figure 12.8b shows the same diagram with another line added indicating the presumed situation at high altitude. Because the oxygen concentration of the arterial blood is low, the line representing the Fick principle is displaced downwards and to the left. The $\dot{V}_{O_{2,max}}$ is therefore lower. The diagram assumes that the 'diffusing capacity for oxygen' of the tissue is the same at sea level and at altitude. It could be argued that this is not the case if the diffusing distance is reduced by the appearance of more capillaries, or the size of muscle fibers is reduced. However, experimental evidence indicates that these factors are unimportant and that the diffusing capacity is essentially determined by the number of open capillaries (Hepple et al. 2000), congruent with the fact that most of the fall in P_{O_2} is believed to be at the capillary wall (see Chapter 11), and that the myoglobin or other mechanisms of enhanced intracellular transport make the diffusion distance unimportant.

Several pieces of evidence now support this concept. For example, a retrospective analysis of data from Operation Everest II showed that the points relating the P_{O_2} of mixed venous blood to oxygen uptake tend to lie on a straight line passing through the origin. On the assumption that the P_{O_2} of mixed venous blood reflects the P_{O_2} of the blood in the capillaries of the exercising muscles, this relationship supports the notion. Indeed, it was this observation that prompted the hypothesis.

More direct evidence comes from a prospective study in which normal subjects exercised at high

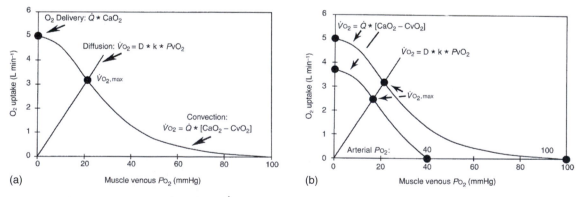

Figure 12.8 (a) Diagram to show how $\dot{V}_{O_{2,max}}$ is determined assuming that oxygen diffusion from the peripheral capillary to the mitochondria is the limiting factor. The two lines show the oxygen uptake available from the Fick principle on the one hand, and Fick's law of diffusion on the other. The $\dot{V}_{O_{2,max}}$ is given by the intersection of the two lines. See text for more details (from Wagner 1988a). (b) As panel (a), except an additional line has been added to represent the Fick equation at high altitude. This reduces the $\dot{V}_{O_{2,max}}$ as shown. See text for further details (from Wagner 1988a).

workloads breathing hypoxic mixtures, and samples of femoral venous blood were taken via an indwelling catheter (Roca *et al.* 1989). Again, a plot of the P_{O_2} of femoral venous blood against oxygen uptake for different inspired oxygen concentrations showed the points lying close to a straight line passing near to the origin. A similar plot was found when the calculated mean capillary P_{O_2} was substituted for femoral venous P_{O_2}.

Additional studies have been carried out on an isolated dog gastrocnemius preparation where the muscle was supplied with hypoxic blood and stimulated maximally. Again a good relationship was found between the P_{O_2} of the effluent blood and the maximal oxygen uptake at different levels of hypoxia (Hogan *et al.* 1988a). This preparation allowed a test of two competing hypotheses, that referred to above, and an alternative hypothesis that $\dot{V}_{O_{2,max}}$ is determined by the amount of oxygen delivered to the muscle via the blood. The test was made by supplying the isolated muscle with the same amounts of oxygen (arterial oxygen concentration × blood flow), but using different blood flows (and therefore oxygen concentrations). The results showed that $\dot{V}_{O_{2,max}}$ was more closely related to the P_{O_2} of muscle venous blood than to the oxygen delivered via the arterial blood, and therefore the results support the hypothesis of diffusion limitation (Hogan *et al.* 1988b).

The diffusion–limitation hypothesis has also been tested in more recent studies. In one, the oxygen affinity of hemoglobin was increased by feeding dogs sodium cyanate, and it was shown that for the same convective oxygen delivery (cardiac output × arterial oxygen concentration), the maximal oxygen concentration of dog muscle was reduced compared with animals in which the oxygen affinity was normal (Hogan *et al.* 1991). The converse experiment was also carried out by reducing the oxygen affinity of hemoglobin using the allosteric modifier methylpropionic acid. In this case, the dog muscle showed an increased maximal oxygen consumption at a constant blood oxygen delivery compared with an animal with a normal oxygen affinity of hemoglobin (Richardson *et al.* 1998). Therefore, there are considerable experimental data supporting the analysis shown in Fig. 12.8.

Also of note, is the fact that vascular conductance is decreased at high altitude. This response is mediated by an increased vascular tone. Lundby *et al.* (2008) infused ATP (80 μg kg body weight^{-1} min^{-1}) during exercise in eight healthy male subjects at 4559 m and studied the hemodynamics and energetics of femoral artery distribution during maximal exercise. Cardiac output was preserved; mean arterial pressure decreased. Although oxygen delivery was similar with and without ATP infusion, oxygen extraction was decreased, and thus there was a 20% decrease in leg $V_{O_{2,max}}$. The authors concluded that altitude-induced vasoconstriction does not reduce aerobic capacity, but may be important in optimally matching oxygen supply with active muscular beds. These findings support the diffusion–limitation hypothesis, as well in that the natural response of vasoconstriction seems to minimize blood flow to areas where increased flow may lead to greater diffusion limitation.

Limitations of aerobic capacity in humans are clearly related to inadequate cardiac output compared to many other mammals. The vascular capacitance is greater than the heart's ability to supply a robust volume of blood and subsequently oxygen. Calbet *et al.* (2008) looked at the effect of acute hypoxia (AH) and chronic hypoxia (CH) on cycle and knee (leg extension) ergometry. The design was intended to look at reducing the size of exercising muscle mass to see if oxygen delivery could be preserved at 5260 m (Pa_{O_2} = >55 mmHg. Their remarkable findings were that (1) cardiac output was similar in one- and two-leg maximal exercise; (2) the oxygen–hemoglobin dissociation (OHD) curve was less shifted to the right with one-leg exercise perhaps because of lower tissue temperature and higher pH; (3) improved pulmonary gas exchange. The less right-shifted OHD curve results in substantially less of a decrease if Ca_{O_2} which provides better oxygenation of tissues throughout the body. The authors also hypothesize that if a lower proportion of the total cardiac output is needed for one-leg exercise, then other tissues of the body would be better perfused. They feel that this is particularly important with respect to cerebral blood flow and oxygenation.

12.9 ROLE OF PERIPHERAL MUSCLE AND CENTRAL FATIGUE IN PHYSICAL PERFORMANCE

The roles of cerebral oxygenation per se versus central perception of muscle fatigue in limiting exercise under hypoxic conditions are not fully understood. Accounts from climbers at extreme altitude who remember their vision becoming narrow or dark when they go one step further beyond a certain level of exertion suggest that cerebral oxygen delivery is being limited either from cerebral vasoconstriction with marked hyperventilation or more profound hypoxemia from exertion. Experiments to study this hypothesis in a controlled fashion are difficult or perhaps self-evident.

There has been increasing interest in the effect of peripheral muscle fatigue conveyed to the brain via metaboreceptive (group III/IV) afferent fibers from exercising muscles and the subsequent central motor output to the muscles. The theory goes that these inhibitory signals prevent premature fatigue or over-stress mechanical failure. A number of studies have tested this hypothesis in both the normoxic and acute hypoxic environment without any work yet published looking at the effect of acclimatization on central motor output. The present studies are still very intriguing.

Amann et al. (2006) tested the effect of hypoxia ($FIO_2 = 0.15$) and normoxia on peripheral muscle fatigue in eight cyclists. They used magnetic femoral nerve stimulation (MFNS) immediately and 2.5 minutes after constant heavy workloads (314 watts). The degree of fatigue was greater after the hypoxic ride. Romer et al. (2007) studied nine male cyclists to exhaustion under normoxic and hypoxic ($FIO_2 = 0.13$, $SpO_2 = 76 \pm 1\%$) conditions and looked at peripheral muscle fatigue with nerve stimulation. Time to exhaustion was reduced by two-thirds under hypoxic conditions, but peripheral fatigue was not different in the two groups. These findings and those of Katayama et al. (2007) suggest that hypoxia plays a role in performance in spite of similar levels of fatigue. Amann et al. (2006) used four repeated time trials of 5 km in trained cyclists with four levels of oxygenation from modest hypoxemic ($FIO_2 = 0.15$) to hyperoxic levels which resulted in CaO_2 from 17.6 to 24.4 cc O_2 dL^{-1}. Quadricep fatigue was gauged by change in force output before and after exercise by MFNS, and central neural drive by quadriceps electromyograms. Higher oxygenation resulted in 43% increase in central nerve output, 30% greater power output and 12% better time trial times. There was, however, no difference in peripheral muscle fatigue. The authors interpreted their results to mean that there is an effect of hypoxemia on central motor output that reaches a threshold so as not to exceed a critical muscle fatigue.

Amann et al. (2007) extended this work and studied eight cyclists to exhaustion under normoxic and two levels of hypoxia ($FIO_2 = 0.15$ and 0.10, with SpO_2 ~82 and 67%, respectively). They found that supplemental O_2 prolonged the more severe hypoxic ride, but not the normoxic or moderate hypoxic ride. The hypoxic rides were quite reduced (278 ± 16 and 125 ± 6 s, respectively) compared to the normoxic ride (656 ± 82 s). They used MFNS and quadriceps twitch to assess fatigue and found that muscle fatigue was less in the more hypoxic session. The authors interpreted these findings as being consistent with the more profound hypoxemia transitioning from a peripheral muscle fatigue to an inhibitory effect on central motor output which limits performance. There is controversy about the issue of a decrease in central motor drive initiated by the afferent signals from the peripheral muscles (Amann and Secher 2010; Marcora 2010), but further work which can isolate the afferent signals more specifically might be able to clarify and substantiate this line of thought.

12.10 *ACE* GENE AND ALTITUDE PERFORMANCE

Recently, there has been great interest in the polymorphism of the angiotensin converting enzyme (*ACE*) gene and deletions or insertions of the I and D alleles. *ACE* constricts microvascular tone. Insertion of the I-allele leads to inhibition of *ACE*, while deletion of the D allele leads to increased *ACE* activity and vasomotor tone.

Most (Montgomery *et al.* 1999; Myerson *et al.* 1999; Woods 2000), but not all studies (Rankinen *et al.* 2000a; Rankinen *et al.* 2000b) show a strong association of the endurance athletic performance and insertion of the I-allele in the *ACE* gene, resulting in an inhibition of the microvasoconstrictive response in the tissues. Some studies have shown a similar association between the insertion of the I-allele and performance at very high altitudes (Montgomery *et al.* 1998; Tsianos 2005). This same configuration is also linked with a greater hyperventilatory response to hypoxic exercise (Patel *et al.* 2003). The implications of these findings are not clear, but suggest that a better understanding of the genetic signal of physiologic responses is on the horizon.

More recent work by Thompson *et al.* (2007) found a correlation of the *ACE* genes and success at extreme altitude. They tested 141 mountaineers who had been above 8000 m and found that those with the I-allele as opposed to the D allele achieved significantly higher altitudes (8559 ± 565 and 8079 ± 947 m, respectively), while those with ID genotypes achieved intermediate altitudes (8107 ± 653 m), $p < 0.007$. The role of regulation of microvascular tone as mediated by genetic control is still in the early phase of understanding and will provide important insights as the mechanisms are unraveled.

12.11 MAXIMAL OXYGEN UPTAKE AT HIGH ALTITUDE

Many investigators have documented the fall in maximal oxygen uptake at high altitude since the early studies of Zuntz *et al.* (1906), and the results of Pugh and his co-workers are shown in Fig. 12.1. Figure 12.9 shows data from a number of studies collated by Cerretelli (1980). Note that, even at the very modest altitude of 2500 m, there is already an average decrease of $\dot{V}_{O_{2,max}}$ of 5–10% as compared to sea level. Cerretelli pointed out that these data do not show any consistent differences between subjects exposed to acute hypoxia and those who have had the advantage of acclimatization to high altitude. This conclusion goes against the experience of many climbers who feel that they can work harder at high altitude

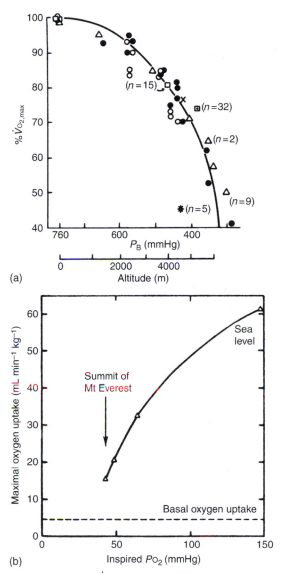

Figure 12.9 (a) $\dot{V}_{O_{2,max}}$ as a percentage of the sea-level value plotted against barometric pressure and altitude. (open circles, triangles), acute hypoxia; (closed circles), chronic hypoxia; (crosses), high-altitude natives. See original text for complete explanation of symbols (from Cerretelli 1980). (b) Maximal oxygen uptake against inspired P_{O_2} as measured on the 1981 American Medical Research Expedition to Everest. The lowest point was obtained by giving well-acclimatized subjects at an altitude of 6300 m an inspired gas mixture containing 14% oxygen. The inspired P_{O_2} was 42.5 mmHg which is equivalent to that on the Everest summit. Compare Fig. 12.2 (modified from West *et al.* 1983a) (1 Torr = 1 mmHg).

after acclimatization, and the conclusion cannot presumably be true at the most extreme altitudes where acute exposure to the prevailing barometric pressure (for example, on the summit of Mount Everest) results in loss of consciousness within a few minutes in most unacclimatized individuals. It is of interest that some, but not all, elite high altitude climbers have only moderately high levels of maximal oxygen consumption at sea level (Oelz *et al.* 1986).

These data on maximal oxygen uptake were extended by the 1981 AMREE studies, where measurements were made at an altitude of 6300 m on subjects breathing ambient air, but also breathing 16 and 14% oxygen (West *et al.* 1983a). The last gave an inspired P_{O_2} of 42.5 mmHg equivalent to that on the Everest summit. The results are shown in Fig. 12.10, where it can be seen that in these subjects who were well acclimatized to very high altitude, the $\dot{V}_{O_{2,max}}$ fell to 15.3 mL min^{-1} kg^{-1} O_2 which was equivalent to 1.07 L min^{-1}. Thus at the highest point on Earth, the maximal oxygen uptake is reduced to between 20 and 25% of the sea level value. As pointed out in Chapter 13, this oxygen uptake is equivalent to that seen when a subject walks slowly on the level, but nevertheless is apparently sufficient to explain how Messner and Habeler were able to reach the Everest summit without supplementary oxygen in 1978. Indeed Messner's statement that the last 100 m took more than an hour to climb fits with this measured oxygen uptake (Messner 1979).

Measurements of $\dot{V}_{O_{2,max}}$ at various altitudes were also made during Operation Everest II and the data are almost superimposable on those shown in Fig. 12.9b at the highest altitudes (Sutton et al. 1987). This is interesting because the subjects of Operation Everest II were probably not as well acclimatized to the extreme altitudes as the members of the 1981 expedition, as judged from their alveolar gas composition and other measurements (West 1993). The values for $\dot{V}_{O_{2,max}}$ at any given altitude as determined by the 1981 Everest expedition (Fig. 12.9b) are higher than those earlier reported by Pugh *et al.* (1964) based on measurements made during the Silver Hut Expedition and previous measurements on Mount Everest. This can be explained by the higher level of fitness of subjects on the 1981 expedition. For example, several of

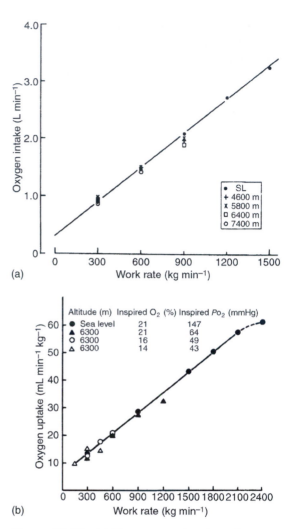

Figure 12.10   (a) Oxygen uptake plotted against work rate at various altitudes during the Silver Hut Expedition showing that the relationship remains essentially the same as at sea level (from Pugh *et al.* 1964). (b) Similar plot as in panel (a), but showing the much higher work rates at sea level obtained during the 1981 American Medical Research Expedition to Everest (from West *et al.* 1983a) (1 Torr = 1 mmHg).

the AMREE members were competitive marathon runners with very high maximum aerobic capacities as measured at sea level.

Several studies since the early measurements of Douglas *et al.* (1913) have shown that the relationship between oxygen uptake and work rate (or power) is independent of altitude. Figure 12.10a shows a comparison of data from the 1960–61 Himalayan Scientific and Mountaineering Expedition, and Fig. 12.10b from the 1981 Everest expedition. The message of the two plots is the same, but note the much higher work rates at sea level recorded prior to the 1981 expedition which is further evidence of the high level of athletic ability of these subjects.

As indicated earlier, breathing pure oxygen at high altitude does not return the $\dot{V}o_{2,max}$ to the sea level value as shown by Cerretelli (1976a) and others. The reason is unclear; the opposite might be expected since the subjects acclimatized to high altitude have higher blood hemoglobin levels. However, against this are the results of a more recent study showing that when erythrocytes were infused into lowlanders after 1 or 9 days at an altitude of 4300 m, there was no improvement in the decreased $\dot{V}o_{2,max}$ (Young et al. 1996). It has been suggested that the reduced $\dot{V}o_{2,max}$ is caused by the loss of muscle mass at high altitude, and that if $\dot{V}o_{2,max}$ were related to lean body mass, the reduction would not be found. As discussed in Chapter 10, the diameter of muscle fibers decreases during acclimatization. Another possibility is that the increased red blood cell concentration causes uneven blood flow and sludging in peripheral capillaries and this interferes with oxygen unloading.

Does a period of acclimatization at high altitude improve $\dot{V}o_{2,max}$ at sea level? Again the answer is not clear. Cerretelli (1976a) measured $\dot{V}o_{2,max}$ in a group of subjects at sea level shortly before they were exposed to an altitude of 5350 m for 10–12 weeks, and again at sea level about 4 weeks after return from altitude. Although there was an approximately 11% increase in hemoglobin concentration, this was not accompanied by a statistically significant rise in $\dot{V}o_{2,max}$. On the other hand, more recent studies involving the reinjection of a subject's own red cells in order to raise the hematocrit have shown a small but significant increase in $\dot{V}o_{2,max}$ at sea level (Spriet et al. 1986). This result would suggest that a period at medium altitude (certainly lower than 5350 m) may improve exercise tolerance at sea level. Perhaps the reduction of muscle fiber size at very high altitudes is the explanation for the failure to see an increase in $\dot{V}o_{2,max}$ after acclimatization at very high altitude. As noted above, erythrocyte infusions into lowlanders exposed to an altitude of 4300 m for 1 or 9 days did not improve the $\dot{V}o_{2,max}$ at that altitude (Young et al. 1996).

It should be pointed out that the $\dot{V}o_{2,max}$ determined at any particular altitude is something of an artificial measurement because climbers, for example, do not ordinarily exercise at that intensity. Pugh (1958) showed that climbers typically select an oxygen uptake of one-half to three-quarters of their maximum for normal climbing at altitudes up to 6000 m. Actual values of oxygen uptake measured by Pugh during normal climbing are included in Fig. 12.1.

12.12 ANAEROBIC PERFORMANCE AT HIGH ALTITUDE

Reference has already been made to the paradoxically low levels of blood lactate following exhaustive exercise at extreme altitude (section 13.3.5, Fig. 13.6). This phenomenon may be related to the reduced plasma bicarbonate concentration which interferes with buffering of hydrogen ion as discussed in Chapter 13. Cerretelli (1992) has shown that the rate of increase of $\dot{V}o_2$ when exercise is suddenly begun was slower in subjects after return from the 1981 Swiss Lhotse Expedition compared with before departure. This finding may be related to changes in anaerobic performance. However, it was also shown that maximal anaerobic (alactic) 'peak' power, as measured by a standing jump, was not affected by exposure of up to 3 weeks at 5200 m. Thereafter it tended to fall along with the reduction of muscle mass.

12.13 CONCLUSION

Many factors come to play in limiting exercise at high altitude. Although Cao_2 is preserved up to 7100 m, something limits cardiac output and thus exercise performance. Perhaps the factors which limit exercise are many and are doled out in different doses at different altitudes. For instance, it seems reasonable to invoke the effect of profound hypoxemia on cerebral function at extreme altitudes as being a primary factor with afferent signals from the exercising muscle as being less important in these environments; whereas, at moderate to very high altitudes, cerebral oxygenation may be preserved yet the described effect of hypoxic exercise feeds back to the brain which mobilizes an inhibitory signal at a critical threshold. Regardless of the dose of these effects, there may be a peripheral signal which acts to protect the body from injury. Further discussion is forthcoming in the subsequent chapter focused primarily on the extremes of altitude and exertion.

13

Limiting factors at extreme altitude

SUMMARY

The fact that some humans can just reach the summit of Mount Everest, the highest point on Earth, without breathing supplementary oxygen is an extraordinary coincidence. Several experimental and theoretical studies in the early part of the twentieth century predicted that this would not be possible, and therefore it was of great interest when Messner and Habeler realized the feat in 1978. A critical factor is the higher barometric pressure in the great mountain ranges at latitudes near the equator than that predicted by the standard atmosphere. Another critical factor is the extreme hyperventilation that the successful climbers generate, thus forcing their alveolar P_{CO_2} below 10 mmHg and consequently defending their alveolar P_{O_2} at viable levels. Also important is the marked respiratory alkalosis that increases the oxygen affinity of hemoglobin and thus assists in the loading of oxygen by the pulmonary capillaries. Even so, the maximal oxygen consumption on the summit of Everest is only just above 1 L min^{-1}, and the arterial P_{O_2} is less than 30 mmHg during physical work. The analysis of the physiological conditions near the Everest summit explains why tragedies occur when unexpected circumstances arise, such as a deterioration in the weather. The fact that normal humans can survive the extreme derangement of blood gases which is necessary for these climbs to extreme altitudes is a graphic reminder of the resilience of the human organism.

13.1 INTRODUCTION

It is a remarkable coincidence that when humans are well acclimatized to high altitude, they can just reach the highest point on Earth without breathing supplementary oxygen. This feat was first realized in 1978 and many physiologists and physicians interested in high altitude had previously predicted that it would not be possible (West 1998). It was truly the end of an era when Messner and Habeler reached the summit of Mount Everest on 8 May 1978.

This chapter examines the profound physiological changes that are necessary for humans to survive and do small amounts of work at extreme altitudes, such as the summit of Mount Everest. It includes an analysis of the factors that limit performance at these great altitudes and shows that such ascents are possible only if both the physiological make up of the climber and physical factors, such as barometric pressure, are right.

13.2 HISTORICAL

13.2.1 Sixteenth to nineteenth centuries

It has been known for many centuries that very high altitude has a deleterious effect on the human body and that the amount of work that a person can do becomes more and more limited as the altitude increases. One of the first descriptions of the disabling effects of high altitude was given by the Jesuit missionary Joseph de Acosta who accompanied the early Spanish conquistadores to Peru in the sixteenth century. He described how, as he traveled over a high mountain, he 'was suddenly surprised with so mortal and strange a pang, that I was ready to fall from the top to the ground.' His dramatic description was first published in 1590 (Acosta 1590).

In the eighteenth century, climbers in the European Alps reported a variety of disagreeable sensations which now seem to us greatly exaggerated. For example, the physicist de Saussure, who was the third person to reach the summit of Mont Blanc, reported during the climb:

> When I began this ascent, I was quite out of breath from the rarity of the air … The kind of fatigue which results from the rarity of the air is absolutely unconquerable; when it is at its height, the most terrible danger would not make you take a single step further.

When he was near the summit he complained of extreme exhaustion:

> This need of rest was absolutely unconquerable; if I tried to overcome it, my legs refused to move, I felt the beginning of a faint, and was seized by dizziness. …

On the summit itself he reported:

> When I had to get to work to set out the instruments and observe them, I was constantly forced to interrupt my work and devote myself to breathing.
>
> de Saussure, 1786–7

These dramatic complaints at an altitude of only 4807 m or less reflect a combination of almost no acclimatization and the fear of the unknown.

In the nineteenth century, numerous ascents were made of higher mountains, including those in the Andes, and there were abundant accounts of the disabling effects of extreme altitude. In 1879, Whymper made the first ascent of Chimborazo and described how, at an altitude of 5079 m (16 664 ft), he was incapacitated by the thin air:

> … in about an hour I found myself lying on my back, along with both the Carrels [his guides], placed hors de combat, and incapable of making the least exertion. … We were unable to satisfy our desire for air, except by breathing with open mouths. … Besides having our normal rate of breathing largely accelerated, we found it impossible to sustain life without every now and then giving spasmodic gulps, just like fishes when taken out of water.
>
> Whymper, 1892

However, Whymper and his two guides gradually recovered their strength and in fact his lively account shows that he was aware of the beneficial effects of high altitude acclimatization.

In the latter part of the nineteenth century, there was considerable interest in the highest altitude that could be tolerated by climbers. Thomas W Hinchliff, President of the (British) Alpine Club (1875–77), wrote an account of his travels around the world and described his feelings as he looked at the view from Santiago in Chile.

> Lover of mountains as I am, and familiar with such summits as those of Mont Blanc, Monte Rosa, and other Alpine heights, I could not repress a strange feeling as I looked at Tupungato and Aconcagua, and reflected that endless successions of men must in all probability be forever debarred from their lofty crests. … Those who, like Major Godwin Austen, have had all the advantages of experience and acclimatization to aid them in attacks upon the higher Himalayas, agree that 21 500 ft (6553 m) is near the

limit at which man ceases to be capable of the slightest further exertion.

Hinchliff, 1876

13.2.2 Twentieth century

In 1909, the Duke of Abruzzi attempted an ascent of K2 in the Karakoram Mountains, and although his party was unsuccessful in reaching the summit, they attained the remarkable altitude of 7500 m without supplementary oxygen. According to the Duke's biographer, one of the reasons given for this expedition was 'to see how high man can go' (de Fillippi 1912), and certainly the climb had a dramatic effect on both the mountaineering and the medical communities interested in high altitude tolerance. In contrast to the florid accounts of paralyzing fatigue and breathlessness given by de Saussure, Whymper and others at much lower altitudes, the Duke made light of the physiological problems associated with this great altitude. However, as we saw earlier (Chapter 7), his feat prompted heated arguments among physiologists about whether the lungs actively secreted oxygen at this previously unheard-of altitude.

Ten years later, a milestone in the history of the physiology of extreme altitude was provided by the British physiologist, Alexander M Kellas, whose contributions were largely overlooked until recently. Kellas was lecturer in chemistry at the Middlesex Hospital Medical School in London during the first two decades of the twentieth century, but, despite this full-time faculty position, managed to make eight expeditions to the Himalayas, and probably spent more time above 6100 m than anyone else. In 1919, he wrote an extensive paper entitled, 'A consideration of the possibility of ascending Mount Everest,' which was not published until 2001 (Kellas 2001). In this, he analyzed the physiology of a climber near the Everest summit, including a discussion of the summit altitude, barometric pressure, alveolar P_{O_2}, arterial oxygen saturation, maximal oxygen consumption and maximal ascent rate. On the basis of his study, he concluded that:

Mount Everest could be ascended by a man of excellent physical and mental constitution in first-rate training, without

adventitious aids [supplementary oxygen] if the physical difficulties of the mountain are not too great.

The importance of this study was not so much that he reached the correct conclusion. He had so few data that many of his calculations were erroneous. However, Kellas asked all the right questions and he can claim the distinction of being the first physiologist to seriously analyze the limiting factors at the highest point on Earth (West 1987). It was not until almost 60 years later that all his predictions were fulfilled. For a biography of Kellas, see Mitchell and Rodway (2011).

Kellas was a member of the first official reconnaissance expedition to Everest in 1921, but tragically he died during the approach march just as the expedition had its first view of the mountain they came to climb. Three years later, EF Norton, who was a member of the third Everest expedition, reached a height of about 8589 m on the north side of Everest without supplementary oxygen. He was accompanied to just below that altitude by Dr TH Somervell, who collected alveolar gas samples at an altitude of 7010 m, though unfortunately these were stored in rubber bladders through which the carbon dioxide rapidly diffused (Somervell 1925). Somervell also referred to the extreme breathlessness at that altitude, stating that 'for every step forward and upward, 7 to 10 complete respirations were required.'

The summit of Everest was finally attained in 1953 by Hillary and Tenzing (Hunt 1953). Naturally, this was a landmark event in the physiology of extreme altitude, but the fact that the two climbers used supplementary oxygen still did not answer the question of whether it was possible to reach the summit breathing air. Hillary did remove his oxygen mask on the summit for about 10 minutes and at the end of the time reported:

I realized that I was becoming rather clumsy-fingered and slow-moving, so I quickly replaced my oxygen set and experienced once more the stimulating effect of even a few litres of oxygen.

Nevertheless, the fact that he could survive for a few minutes without additional oxygen came as a surprise to some physicians who had predicted that he would lose consciousness.

However, there was a precedent for surviving for this period on the summit in the experiment Operation Everest I, carried out by Houston and Riley in 1945. As briefly described in Chapter 1, four volunteers spent 34 days in a low pressure chamber and two were able to tolerate 20 minutes without supplementary oxygen on the 'summit.' In fact, the equivalent altitude was even higher because the standard atmosphere pressure was inadvertently used (section 13.3.2).

Additional information on whether there was enough oxygen in the air to allow a climber to reach the Everest summit while breathing air was obtained by Pugh and his colleagues during the 1960–61 Silver Hut Expedition (Pugh *et al.* 1964). Measurements of maximal oxygen consumption were made using a bicycle ergometer on a group of physiologists who wintered at an altitude of 5800 m and who were therefore extremely well acclimatized to this altitude. Figure 13.1 (lower curve) shows the

results of measurements made up to an altitude of 7440 m. Note that extrapolation of the line to a barometric pressure of 250 mmHg on the Everest summit suggested that almost all the oxygen available would be required for the basal oxygen uptake. (For details of the extrapolation procedure, refer to West and Wagner 1980.) Thus, these results strongly suggested that a climber who could reach the Everest summit without supplementary oxygen would be very near the limit of human tolerance.

This ultimate climbing achievement occurred when Reinhold Messner and Peter Habeler reached the summit of Everest without supplementary oxygen in May 1978. Messner's account (Messner 1979) makes it clear that he had very little in reserve:

> After every few steps, we huddle over our ice axes, mouths agape, struggling for sufficient breath. … As we get higher it becomes necessary to lie down to recover our breath. … Breathing becomes such a strenuous business that we scarcely have strength to go on.

And when he eventually reaches the summit:

> In my state of spiritual abstraction, I no longer belong to myself and to my eyesight. I am nothing more than a single, narrow gasping lung, floating over the mists and the summits.

The long period of 25 years between the first ascent of Everest in 1953 and this first 'oxygenless' ascent also suggests that we are near the limit of human tolerance. Again, as indicated earlier, Norton ascended to within 300 m of the Everest summit as early as 1924 without oxygen, but it was not until 1978 that climbers reached the top without supplementary oxygen. Thus the last 300 m took 54 years!

Since that historic climb, Messner has further confirmed his outstanding tolerance to the extreme hypoxia of great altitudes. In 1980, he became the first man to ascend Everest alone without supplementary oxygen (Messner 1981), and in 1986 he became the first man to climb all 14 of the 8000 m peaks without supplementary oxygen. These accomplishments assure him a place not only in the history of mountaineering

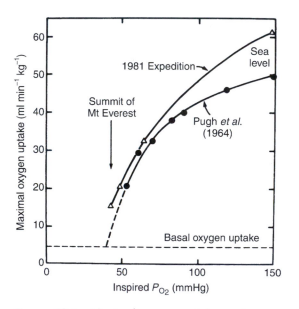

Figure 13.1 Maximal oxygen uptake against inspired P_{O_2}. The lower line shows data from Pugh *et al.* (1964) suggesting that all the oxygen available at the Everest summit would be required for basal oxygen uptake. However, as the upper line shows, the 1981 American Medical Research Expedition to Everest (AMREE) measured an oxygen uptake of just over 1 L min^{-1} for an inspired P_{O_2} of 43 mmHg (from West *et al.* 1983c).

but also in the history of the physiology of extreme altitude.

13.3 PHYSIOLOGY OF EXTREME ALTITUDE

13.3.1 Introduction

This section is devoted to human performance at altitudes over 8000 m. There was renewed interest in this topic when Messner and Habeler climbed Everest without supplementary oxygen in 1978 but, as indicated above, the issue of whether humans would be able to tolerate the highest altitude on Earth was raised early in this century, notably by Kellas in 1919.

The following analysis is based primarily on data from four studies. The first was the 1960–61 Silver Hut Expedition, during which data were obtained on maximal oxygen consumptions as high as 7440 m (P_B 300 mmHg) and alveolar gas samples were taken as high as 7830 m (P_B 288 mmHg). These measurements were extended to the Everest summit by the 1981 American Medical Research Expedition to Everest (AMREE), where measurements on the summit included barometric pressure, alveolar gas samples and electrocardiograms, with additional measurements made between the summit and the highest camp situated at 8050 m (P_B 284 mmHg). The third and fourth studies were Operation Everest II and III (COMEX '97) in 1985 and 1997 when several volunteers were gradually decompressed over a period of 31–40 days in low pressure chambers. Although the degree of acclimatization was not as great as in field studies, much valuable data was obtained.

13.3.2 Barometric pressure

Barometric pressure is a critical variable in physiological performance at extreme altitude because it determines the inspired P_{O_2}. This is the first link in the chain of the oxygen cascade from the atmosphere to the mitochondria. As pointed out in Chapter 2, there has been considerable confusion in the past about the relationships between barometric pressure and altitude on high mountains such as the Himalayan chain. The resulting errors are particularly important at extreme altitude where maximal oxygen consumption is exquisitely sensitive to barometric pressure. It is remarkable that Paul Bert gave nearly the correct value of barometric pressure for the Everest summit in Appendix I of his classic book *La Pression Barométrique* (Bert 1878). His figure of 248 mmHg was based on an extrapolation of measurements made by Jourdanet and others at various locations including the Andes (Jourdanet 1875).

However, when the standard atmosphere was introduced and used extensively by aviation physiologists in the 1930s and 1940s, it was erroneously applied to Mount Everest, giving a value of 236 mmHg, which is much too low. Nevertheless, this figure was used by several high altitude physiologists. For example, during Operation Everest I when four naval recruits were gradually decompressed to what was thought to be the simulated altitude of Mount Everest, they were exposed to a pressure of 236 mmHg and their alveolar P_{O_2} fell to as low as 21 mmHg (Riley and Houston 1951)! As the next section shows, this is about 14 mmHg less than that of a well-acclimatized climber on the summit of Mount Everest.

As described in Chapter 2, Dr Christopher Pizzo measured a barometric pressure of 253 mmHg on the Everest summit on October 24, 1981. This was about 2 mmHg higher than that expected from the mean barometric pressure for that month based on extensive weather balloon data (see Fig. 2.4 in Chapter 2). The discrepancy can be accounted for by normal variation and the high pressure system which made the weather ideal for climbing. The reading of 253 mmHg was within 1 mmHg of the pressure predicted for an altitude of 8848 m from radiosonde balloons released in New Delhi, India, on the same day (West *et al.* 1983a). Several direct measurements on the summit since 1981 have given similar values (see section 2.2.6 in Chapter 2).

Measurements of $\dot{V}_{O_{2,max}}$ on AMREE (West *et al.* 1983c) and Operation Everest II (Sutton *et al.* 1988), as well as the analysis described in section 13.4 show that exercise performance at these extreme altitudes is exquisitely sensitive to barometric pressure. For example on AMREE, a decrease in inspired P_{O_2} of only 1 mmHg resulted in a fall of $\dot{V}_{O_{2,max}}$ by about 63 mL min^{-1} (West 1999a). This is partly because the lung is working very low on the oxygen dissociation curve where the slope is steep. As a consequence, a fall of barometric pressure of as little as 3 mmHg (less than twice the daily standard deviation) will apparently cause a reduction of maximal oxygen uptake of about 4%. This means that even the daily variations of barometric pressure caused by weather may affect physical performance.

Seasonal variations of barometric pressure can be expected to have a marked effect on maximal oxygen uptake. As Fig. 2.2 shows (Chapter 2), mean barometric pressure falls from nearly 255 mmHg in the summer months to only 243 mmHg in mid-winter. This decrease is predicted to reduce maximal oxygen uptake by some 15%. It is noteworthy that Mount Everest has only once been climbed during winter without supplementary oxygen (in December 1987), despite several attempts, and although the very cold temperatures and high winds are naturally a factor, the reduced barometric pressure must certainly contribute (section 2.2.8 in Chapter 2).

As pointed out in Chapter 2, the location of Mount Everest at 28°N latitude is fortunate because the barometric pressure at its summit is considerably higher than would be the case if it were at a higher latitude. As an example, if Mount McKinley (Denali) were 8848 m high, its barometric pressure for May and October (preferred climbing months for Everest) would be only 223 mmHg. It would apparently be impossible to reach the summit without supplementary oxygen under these conditions.

A similar argument would apply if the barometric pressure on the Everest summit were only 236 mmHg, as predicted from the standard atmosphere model. The reduction of pressure by 17 mmHg below that measured by Pizzo would reduce the maximal oxygen consumption by over 20%, according to the analysis presented in the present chapter. It seems very probable that climbing Everest without supplementary oxygen under these conditions would be impossible. Thus the higher pressure that Everest enjoys because of its near equatorial latitude makes it just possible for humans to reach the highest point on Earth.

13.3.3 Alveolar gas composition

On ascent to high altitude, the alveolar P_{O_2} falls because of the reduction in the inspired P_{O_2}. At the same time, alveolar P_{CO_2} falls because of increasing hyperventilation. As described in Chapter 6, Rahn and Otis (1949) clarified the differences between unacclimatized and fully acclimatized subjects at high altitude by plotting their alveolar gas P_{O_2} and P_{CO_2} values on an oxygen–carbon dioxide diagram (Fig. 6.6 in Chapter 6). There are apparently differences between the results obtained in the field, that is on expeditions to high altitude, on the one hand, and simulated ascents in a low pressure chamber on the other. The field studies will be discussed first followed by those using simulated ascents.

Figure 13.2 shows alveolar P_{CO_2} plotted against barometric pressure at extreme altitude from field studies. The closed circles show data reported by Greene (1934), Warren (1939), Pugh (1957) and Gill et al. (1962). The triangles show data obtained on the AMREE (West et al. 1983b). It can be seen that alveolar P_{CO_2} declines approximately

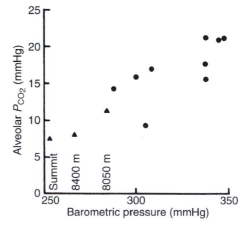

Figure 13.2   Alveolar P_{CO_2} against barometric pressure at extreme altitudes. Triangles show the means of measurements on the American Medical Research Expedition to Everest (AMREE). Circles are results from previous investigators at barometric pressures below 350 mmHg (Table 13.1) (from West et al. 1983b).

linearly as barometric pressure falls and that the pressure on the summit of Mount Everest is about 7–8 mmHg. The measurements made on the summit itself had high respiratory exchange ratio (R) values, for reasons which are not clear. However, the data obtained at the slightly lower altitude of 8400 m (P_B 267 mmHg) had a mean R value of 0.82 with a P_{CO_2} of 8.0 mmHg, which means we can be confident of the very low values at this great altitude.

Figure 13.3 shows the line drawn by Rahn and Otis (1949) for fully acclimatized subjects (lower line on Fig. 5.4 in Chapter 5) together with additional data obtained at barometric pressures below 350 mmHg (Table 13.1). Note that the AMREE data (triangles) fit well with the extrapolation of the line. This method of plotting the data shows that as well-acclimatized humans go to higher and higher altitudes, the P_{O_2} falls because of the decreasing inspired P_{O_2}, and the P_{CO_2} falls because of the increasing hyperventilation. However, above an altitude of about 7000 m (P_B 325 mmHg), the alveolar P_{O_2} becomes essentially constant at a value of about 35–37 mmHg. More recent measurements of alveolar P_{O_2} up to an altitude of 8000 m by Peacock and Jones (1997) are in good agreement

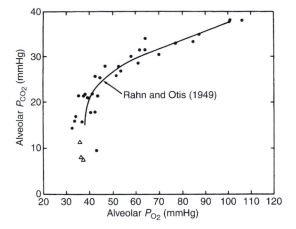

Figure 13.3   Oxygen–carbon dioxide diagram showing alveolar gas values collated by Rahn and Otis (1949) (circles) together with values obtained at extreme altitudes by the American Medical Research Expedition to Everest (AMREE) (triangles) (from West et al. 1983b).

with these data. This means that successful climbers are able to defend their alveolar P_{O_2} by the process of extreme hyperventilation. In other words, they insulate the P_{O_2} of their alveolar gas from the falling value in the atmosphere around

Table 13.1   Alveolar P_{O_2} and P_{CO_2} in acclimatized subjects at barometric pressures below 350 mmHg

Source	Barometric pressure	P_{O_2}	P_{CO_2}	Respiratory exchange ratio (R)
Greene (1934)	337	40.7	17.7	0.87
	305	43.0	9.2	0.79
Warren (1939)	337[a]	37.0	15.6	0.60
Pugh (1957)	347	39.3	21.0	0.87
	337	35.5	21.3	0.87
	308	34.1	16.9	0.77
Gill et al. (1962)	344	38.1	20.7	0.82
	300	33.7	15.8	0.78
	288	32.8	14.3	0.77
West et al. (1983b)	284	36.1	11.0	0.78
	267	36.7	8.0	0.82
	253	37.6	7.5	1.49

All pressure values are given in mmHg.
[a]Barometric pressure estimated from curve of Zuntz et al. (1906).

them. This appears to be the most important feature of acclimatization at extreme altitude.

Not everyone can generate the enormous increase in ventilation required for the very low P_{CO_2} values shown in Figs 13.2 and 13.3. This explains why climbers with a large hypoxic ventilatory response usually tolerate extreme altitude better than those with a more modest response (Schoene *et al.* 1984). Indeed, experience on the AMREE showed that individuals who had a low hypoxic ventilatory response were not able to remain at the higher camps (West 1985a).

The pattern of alveolar gas values shown in Fig. 13.3 is only obtained if sufficient time is allowed for full respiratory acclimatization. Figure 13.4 compares the results found in unacclimatized and fully acclimatized subjects at high altitude (Figs 5.4 in Chapter 5 and 13.3) with alveolar gas data reported from two low pressure chamber experiments in which the simulated rate of ascent

was much faster. It can be seen that in Operation Everest I (Riley and Houston 1951), the subjects reached the simulated summit after only 31 days and at the extreme altitudes the data fell close to the region predicted by the line for unacclimatized humans. In Operation Everest II (Malconian *et al.* 1993), the ascent was a little slower, with the first simulated summit excursion occurring after 36 days. However, the alveolar gas values at extreme altitudes still deviated considerably from those found in fully acclimatized subjects. Little information is available about the time required for full respiratory acclimatization at extreme altitudes, say over 8000 m, but Fig. 13.4 suggests that 36 days is inadequate, whereas 77 days clearly is much better. However, it may be that other factors, such as the level of physical activity, are also important.

13.3.4 Arterial blood composition

Until recently, no one had attempted to sample arterial blood at extreme altitude because of the obvious technical difficulties, although a possible procedure had been suggested (Catron *et al.* 2006). A landmark advance was made during the Caudwell Xtreme Everest Expedition (CXEE) when four arterial samples were collected at an altitude of 8400 m, barometric pressure 272 mmHg (Grocott *et al.* 2009). A small tent was erected on the 'balcony' about 450 m below the Everest summit during the descent, and samples were taken from the right femoral artery of four climbers. They used supplementary oxygen for climbing, but this was removed before the samples were taken. The blood samples were placed in an ice-water slurry and rapidly transported down to 6400 m, where the analyses were made using a Siemens blood gas analyzer which was modified for use at high altitude.

Table 13.2 shows the results for the P_{O_2}, P_{CO_2} and pH and some other variables. Figure 13.5 shows the P_{O_2} and P_{CO_2} values plotted on an O_2–CO_2 diagram together with the mean results from two low pressure chamber experiments, Operation Everest II and III. More information on these is given later in the chapter. The chamber

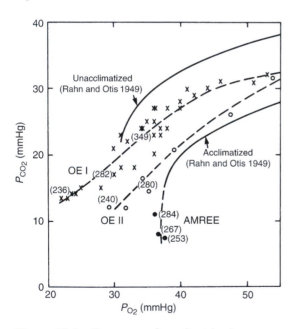

Figure 13.4 Oxygen–carbon dioxide diagram showing the two lines described by Rahn and Otis (1949) for unacclimatized and acclimatized subjects at high altitude (compare Figure 5.4 in Chapter 5). In addition, data from Operation Everest I (OEI) and Operation Everest II (OEII) are included. Note that the OEI subjects were poorly acclimatized at extreme altitudes, whereas the OEII had intermediate values (from West 1998a).

Table 13.2 Arterial blood values at altitude 8400 m, P_B 272 mmHg, from CXEE (Grocott *et al.* 2009)

Subject No.	1	2	3	4
Po_2 mmHg	29.5	19.1	21.0	28.7
Pco_2 mmHg	12.3	15.7	15.0	10.3
pH	7.55	7.45	7.52	7.60
Bicarbonate (mmol/liter)	10.5	10.67	11.97	9.87
Base excess of blood (mmol/liter)	−6.3	−9.16	−6.39	−5.71
Lactate concentration (mmol/liter)	2.0	2.0	2.9	1.8
O_2 saturation %	68.1	34.4	43.7	69.7
Hemoglobin (g/dl)	20.2	18.7	18.8	19.4

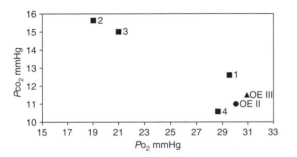

Figure 13.5 Arterial Po_2 and Pco_2 for four subjects from the Caudwell Xtreme Everest Expedition taken at an altitude of 8400 m, P_B 272 mmHg (Grocott *et al.* 2009). Also shown are the means of the summit measurements from Operation Everest II and III.

data were obtained at a barometric pressure of 253 mmHg corresponding to the Everest summit so that slightly lower values for Po_2 and Pco_2 might be expected.

Figure 13.5 shows that two of the subjects on CXEE had Po_2 and Pco_2 values that fit well with those from OEII and OEII. However, the results from the other two subjects were far removed, and the reasons for this are not clear (West 2009). Possibly these two subjects had low hypoxic ventilatory responses. Not shown in the figure are the calculated values from one subject from AMREE on the summit. His Po_2 was 28 mmHg which fits well with the other data, but his Pco_2 was 7–8 mmHg which is substantially lower. This might be related to his exceptionally high ventilatory response to hypoxia.

Incidentally, the altitude of 8400 m and barometric pressure of 272 mmHg do not match

previous measurements on Everest discussed in Chapter 2. They give an altitude of 8309 m for that pressure. Perhaps the altitude was incorrectly estimated or the barometer was reading low. A barometer reading on the summit would have clarified this, but unfortunately that was not recorded.

13.3.5 Acid–base status

BASE EXCESS

Relatively little is known about acid–base changes at extreme altitude, despite the importance of this topic. Some data are available from two well-acclimatized subjects of the AMREE, based on blood samples removed during the morning after they had reached the summit. Venous blood samples taken at the highest camp (8050 m; P_B 267 mmHg) showed a mean base excess of −7.2 mmol L^{-1}. This was a considerably higher base excess than expected (in other words, the base deficit was less than predicted) and the result was an extremely high arterial pH of over 7.7 calculated for the Everest summit (West *et al.* 1983b). This calculation is based on the measured alveolar Pco_2 and base excess. It assumes that there was no change in base excess in the previous 24 hours and that a climber resting on the summit had a negligible blood lactate concentration (see below). In addition, the measured alveolar Pco_2 of 7.5 mmHg is assumed to apply to the arterial blood.

A remarkable feature of these base excess values is that they were essentially unchanged from those measured in 14 subjects living for several weeks at Camp 2 (6300 m, P_B 351 mmHg) where the mean value was -8.7 ± 1.7 mmol L^{-1} (Winslow *et al.* 1984). This suggests that base excess was changing extremely slowly above an altitude of 6300 m. The reason for this is not known, but may be related to the chronic volume depletion which was observed in climbers living at 6300 m. At this altitude, the serum osmolality was 302 ± 4 mmol kg^{-1}, which was significantly higher ($p < 0.01$) than in the same subjects at sea level, where the value was 290 ± 1 mmol kg^{-1} (Blume *et al.* 1984). It is known that the kidney gives a higher priority to correcting dehydration than acid–base disturbances, and in order to excrete more bicarbonate to reduce the base excess, it would be necessary to lose corresponding cations, which would aggravate the volume depletion. This may be the basis for the slow renal bicarbonate excretion.

These acid–base changes may be part of the explanation of why climbers can spend only a relatively short time at extreme altitudes, say above 8000 m. It was pointed out in Chapter 7 that the marked respiratory alkalosis which increases the oxygen affinity of the hemoglobin at extreme altitude is beneficial because it accelerates the loading of oxygen by the pulmonary capillaries. If a climber remains at extreme altitude for several days, presumably there is some renal excretion of bicarbonate (though this appears to be slow) and the resulting metabolic compensation would move the pH back towards 7.4. Thus, the advantage of a left-shifted dissociation curve would tend to be lost.

One way to counter this disadvantage during a climb of Mount Everest would be to put in the high camps and then return to Base Camp at a lower altitude for several days. This period at medium altitude would then allow the body to adjust again to this more moderate oxygen deprivation and enable the blood pH to stabilize nearer its normal value. The final summit assault would then be as rapid as possible to take advantage of the nearly uncompensated respiratory alkalosis. In fact, this was the pattern adopted by Messner and Habeler in their first ascent of Mount Everest without supplementary oxygen in 1978 and is now used by most climbers.

THE LACTATE PARADOX

Humans acutely exposed to high altitude develop very high blood lactate concentrations during heavy exercise. However, after acclimatization, the same subjects have much lower lactates at the same altitude and work level. This is known as the lactate paradox. It was first described by Edwards (1936) during the International High Altitude Expedition to Chile in 1935. He showed that blood lactate remains very low in acclimatized subjects at high altitude even during maximal work. Figure 13.5 shows data on resting and maximal blood lactate obtained by Cerretelli (1980). Also shown are measurements made at 6300 m after maximal exercise at the rate of 900 kg min^{-1}, that is, an oxygen uptake of 1.75 L min^{-1} (West 1986c). The mean value after exercise at 6300 m was only 3.0 mmol L^{-1} despite an arterial P_{O_2} of less than 35 mmHg and therefore extreme tissue hypoxia. Note that extrapolation of the line relating maximal blood lactate concentration to altitude suggests that after maximal exercise at altitudes exceeding 7500 m, there will be no increase in lactate in the blood at all despite the extreme oxygen deprivation. This is indeed a paradox since it has often been observed that lactate release occurs during tissue hypoxia and the tissue P_{O_2} must be extremely low under these conditions.

The blood lactate concentrations after maximal exercise were appreciably higher on Operation Everest II (Sutton *et al.* 1988). For example, at an inspired P_{O_2} of 63 mmHg, the mean lactate concentration following maximal exercise was 4.7 mmol L^{-1}, that is about 56% higher than on the AMREE for the same inspired P_{O_2}. Moreover, the 'summit' measurements on Operation Everest II gave a blood lactate concentration of 3.4 mmol L^{-1}, a higher value than that found at only 6300 m on the AMREE (Fig. 13.6). It is known that the low lactate concentrations following maximal exercise at high altitude come about as a result of high altitude acclimatization because acute hypoxia causes very high lactate levels. Presumably therefore the higher values seen on Operation Everest II compared with the AMREE and other field studies can be explained by the lesser degree of acclimatization.

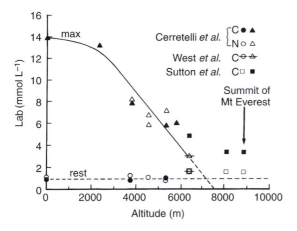

Figure 13.6 Maximal blood lactate (Lab) as a function of altitude. Most of the data are redrawn from Cerretelli (1980). The filled circles and triangles show data for acclimatized Caucasians (C); the open circles and triangles are for high altitude natives (N). The data for 6300 m are from the American Medical Research Expedition to Everest (AMREE) for acclimatized lowlanders (from West 1986). The points marked Sutton *et al.* are from Operation Everest II (Sutton *et al.* 1988).

The reasons for the low blood lactate levels following maximal exercise in well-acclimatized subjects as opposed to poorly acclimatized subjects at high altitude are still unclear. The topic was extensively discussed in a Point–Counterpoint feature in the June 2007 issue of *Journal of Applied Physiology* (**102**, 2398–410) following initial statements on whether the paradox exists (van Hall 2007; West 2007). The discussion includes a large number of references which the interested reader should consult. One hypothesis is that on acute exposure to hypoxia, sympathetic stimulation leads to augmented muscle lactate production and blood lactate concentration through a beta-adrenergic mechanism. By contrast, chronic hypoxia causes beta-adrenergic adaptation and the result is a reduced lactate response after acclimatization (Kayser 1996). However, studies on unacclimatized and acclimatized subjects at 4300 m altitude have not supported this hypothesis (Brooks *et al.* 1998). Another hypothesis is that the bicarbonate depletion that

occurs as a result of acclimatization interferes with the buffering of released lactate and hydrogen ions, and the consequent fall in local pH inhibits the enzyme phosphofructokinase in the glycolytic cycle and thus puts a brake on glycolysis (Fig. 11.7 in Chapter 11). It is known that the activity of phosphofructokinase is reduced as the pH is lowered. Certainly, Cerretelli has shown that the changes in blood hydrogen ion concentration as a result of increases in blood lactate are higher in acclimatized than unacclimatized subjects (Cerretelli 1980). However, many other factors affect blood lactate and the issue is far from settled.

13.3.6 Cardiac output

Intuitively, it would be reasonable to expect an increased cardiac output for a given work level at extreme altitude compared with sea level. It is known that cardiac output increases as a result of acute hypoxia (Chapter 8). Furthermore, the oxygen concentration of the arterial blood is extremely low at very high altitude, and an increase in cardiac output would be expected to help to compensate for the reduced oxygen delivery. Paradoxically, however, the relationship between cardiac output and oxygen uptake in acclimatized subjects at an altitude of 5800 m is essentially the same as at sea level (Fig. 8.2 in Chapter 8) and this apparently holds true even at extreme altitudes, although data are sparse. Reeves *et al.* (1987) showed that the sea level relationship was maintained down to a barometric pressure of 282 mmHg, and almost maintained at an inspired P_{O_2} equivalent to the summit of Mount Everest, though at that extreme altitude the cardiac output appeared to be slightly higher (Fig. 8.3 in Chapter 8). Possibly this apparent paradox is related to the fact that when the cardiac output is increased under these very hypoxic conditions, there is increasing diffusion limitation of oxygen transfer, both in the lung and in the muscle. In a theoretical study, Wagner (1996) showed that increasing cardiac output for the conditions on the Everest summit did not improve calculated $\dot{V}_{O_2,max}$ because of diffusion limitation (Fig. 8.5 in Chapter 8).

13.3.7 Pulmonary diffusing capacity

As discussed in Chapter 7, oxygen transfer during exercise at high altitude is, in part, diffusion limited, and all calculations suggest that this limitation will be exaggerated at the extreme altitudes near the summit of Mount Everest. However, very few data on diffusing capacity at high altitude are available. Available measurements at an altitude of 5800 m (P_B 380 mmHg) indicate that the diffusing capacity for carbon monoxide during exercise is essentially unchanged from the sea level value, except for the expected increase caused by the faster rate of combination of carbon monoxide with hemoglobin under the prevailing hypoxic conditions (West 1962a). These data suggest that the diffusing capacity of the pulmonary membrane itself is unaltered by acclimatization. A recent study of lowlanders who trekked into the Everest Base Camp, altitude 5400 m, and spent 2 weeks there reported a substantial increase in diffusing capacity for carbon monoxide (Agostoni *et al.* 2011), but this seems to be at variance with most previous studies.

Measurements of the diffusing capacity for carbon monoxide at different alveolar P_O_2 values allow calculation of the pulmonary capillary blood volume. Again, in measurements made at 5800 m, there appeared to be little change in capillary blood volume, although there was a suggestion that it was slightly lower, possibly as a result of hypoxic pulmonary vasoconstriction (West 1962a). If we accept the conclusion that capillary blood volume is unchanged, and that the cardiac output/oxygen consumption relationship is the same as at sea level (section 13.3.5), this implies that capillary transit time in the lung is normal since this is given by capillary blood volume divided by cardiac output (Roughton 1945).

Using these data, it is possible to calculate the changes in P_O_2 along the pulmonary capillary for a climber at rest on the summit of Mount Everest (Fig. 7.5 in Chapter 7). This shows that the rate of oxygenation is extremely slow and that the end-capillary P_O_2 is much lower than the alveolar value, indicating severe diffusion limitation of oxygen transfer. This topic is discussed further in section 7.7 in Chapter 7.

13.3.8 P_O_2 of venous blood

During maximal exercise at extreme altitude, the extraction of oxygen by the peripheral tissues results in very low values of venous P_O_2 in the exercising muscles. This in turn reduces the P_O_2 of mixed venous blood. In order to analyze the relationships between the many variables and determine what limits exercise performance at extreme altitude, one possible assumption is that the body will not tolerate a P_O_2 of mixed venous blood below a certain value, for example 15 mmHg (West and Wagner 1980; West 1983). This assumption received strong support from Operation Everest II, where direct measurements of the P_O_2 in mixed venous blood gave similar values (Sutton *et al.* 1988). For example, on the 'summit' during 60 W of exercise, the P_O_2 of mixed venous blood had a mean value of 14.8 mmHg, and at 120 W, which was the highest work level, the mean P_O_2 was 13.8 mmHg.

13.3.9 Heat loss by hyperventilation

Matthews (1932) argued that tolerance to extreme altitude might be limited by the high rate of heat loss from the lungs as a result of the extreme hyperventilation. However, subsequent experience has not borne this out. Calculations of net heat loss are complex because the upper respiratory tract acts as a heat exchanger. During expiration, expired gas warms the respiratory tract, and this heat is then available to warm the cold inspired gas. Climbers who have reached the summit of Mount Everest without supplementary oxygen have not been affected by cold beyond the extent expected from the very low temperatures of the environment. When Pizzo reached the summit to take his alveolar gas samples during the course of the AMREE, he became overheated during the climb and photographs taken on the summit when he was breathing air show that he was not even wearing his down jacket, which he carried with him in his backpack (West 1985a, facing p. 51).

13.3.10 Oxygen cost of ventilation

A climber at extreme altitude has considerable hyperventilation at rest, and even more during moderate exercise. An alveolar P_{CO_2} of 7–8 mmHg was measured on the Everest summit and, since it is known that the carbon dioxide production both at rest and for a given work level is independent of altitude, we can conclude that the alveolar ventilation on the summit was at least five times the resting value. Even small amounts of physical activity will greatly increase this. If we take the normal resting ventilation to be 7–8 L min^{-1}, this means that the resting ventilation on the summit is at least 40 L min^{-1}.

Cibella *et al.* (1999) studied the oxygen cost of ventilation in four normal subjects during exercise at sea level and after a one-month sojourn at 5050 m. From simultaneous measurements of esophageal pressure and lung volume, the mechanical power (work rate) of breathing was determined. As expected, maximal exercise ventilation and maximal power of breathing were higher at high altitude than at sea level, whereas maximal oxygen uptake was reduced in all subjects at high altitude. Interestingly, in three subjects the relationship between mechanical power of breathing and minute ventilation was the same at sea level and high altitude, whereas in only one individual was it lower at high altitude for a given ventilation. It might have been expected that the mechanical power of breathing would be reduced at high altitude in all subjects because of the reduced density of the air.

Assuming a mechanical efficiency of 5%, the oxygen cost of breathing at high altitude and sea level amounted to 26 and 5.5% of $\dot{V}o_{2,max}$, respectively. The authors concluded that, at high altitude, the mechanical power of breathing may substantially limit the ability to do external work. They also calculated what they called the 'critical ventilation,' that is the ventilation at which the mechanical power of breathing was so high that increasing ventilation above this level did not provide additional oxygen for external work. At the altitude of 5050 m, the maximal exercise ventilation exceeded the critical ventilation even when the efficiency was assumed to be as high as 20% (Fig. 13.7).

13.3.11 Studies using low pressure chambers

A question that is frequently asked is why perform field studies, for example on Mount Everest, when the low pressure conditions can be simulated in a high altitude chamber. Three extensive studies have been carried out in this way and they have certainly produced important information on how humans respond to low pressure. However, for some unclear reason, the results from low pressure chambers are different from field studies.

OPERATION EVEREST I

This was carried out in 1944 under the leadership of Charles Houston and Richard Riley at the US Naval School of Aviation Medicine in Pensacola, Florida (Riley and Houston 1951). Four Navy volunteers were placed in a small chamber for a period of 35 days and the pressure was gradually reduced to that believed to occur on the summit of Mount Everest. However, as indicated earlier, the standard atmosphere was used and the chamber pressure was reduced to as low as 234 mmHg which actually corresponds to an altitude of about 9400 m, some 550 m above the Everest summit. The small chamber measured only about 3.0 × 3.0 × 2.1 m and contained four bunks. After 29 days, the pressure was reduced to that at the 'summit' and two of the subjects were able to tolerate the severe hypoxia at rest during air breathing, while the other two needed oxygen. During these studies, alveolar P_{O_2} values in the low 20s were measured (Riley and Houston 1951, Table 2). These are presumably the lowest values of alveolar P_{O_2} ever recorded for periods of several minutes. As indicated earlier (Fig. 13.4), the subjects of Operation Everest I showed almost no acclimatization at the extreme altitudes as judged from their alveolar gas values.

OPERATION EVEREST II

This took place in 1985 and again was spearheaded by Charles Houston (Houston *et al.* 1987). A sophisticated low pressure chamber at the US Army Research Institute of Environmental

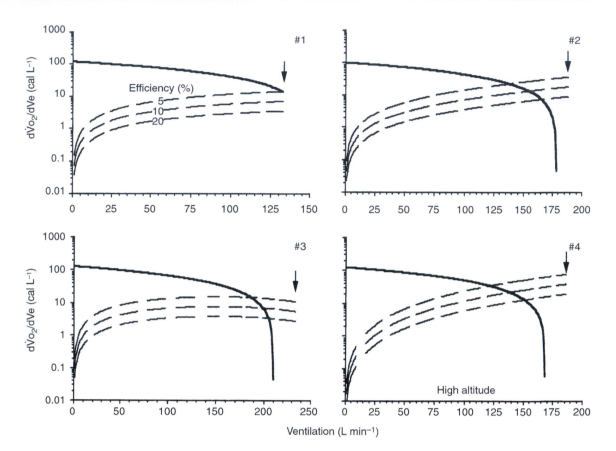

Figure 13.7   Increase in oxygen consumption divided by the increase in ventilation for four subjects at an altitude of 5050 m. The solid line shows the relationship for total oxygen consumption; the dashed lines show the relationship for the oxygen consumption of the respiratory muscles, assuming mechanical efficiencies of 5, 10 and 20%. Arrows show the maximal exercise ventilation. The intersection of the solid and dashed lines shows the critical ventilation above which no increase in external work was possible because the oxygen consumption of the respiratory muscles was so high. In three of the subjects, the maximum ventilation exceeded the critical ventilation for all assumed mechanical efficiencies, though in one of the subjects this was only the case for an efficiency of 5% (from Cibella *et al.* 1999).

Medicine in Natick, Massachusetts was used, and eight subjects aged 21–29 years spent 40 days and nights in the chamber. The subjects were gradually decompressed over a period of about 35 days followed by excursions to the 'summit' where the inspired P_{O_2} was 43 mmHg, which this time was the correct value. Not all the subjects made it to the 'summit', but nevertheless very valuable physiological information was obtained. An advantage of a chamber study over a field study is that much more invasive procedures can be carried out because if a subject becomes sick he can rapidly be removed to a medical facility.

Some of the most important studies were on the pulmonary circulation, and these were referred to in Chapter 8. Cardiac catheterization was carried out using a Swan–Ganz catheter at barometric pressures of 760, 347, 282 and 240 mmHg. For the last measurement, the oxygen concentration in the chamber was 22% giving an inspired P_{O_2} of 43 mmHg. The mean pulmonary arterial pressure at rest at sea level was 15 ± 0.9 mmHg, but this increased to 34 ± 3 mmHg at a barometric pressure of 282 mmHg (Groves *et al.* 1987). At the same time, the pulmonary vascular resistance increased from 1.2 to 4.3 mmHg L^{-1} min^{-1}. When the subjects performed maximal exercise, the increases in mean pulmonary artery pressure were even more remarkable, rising from 33 ± 1 mmHg at sea level to 54 ± 2 mmHg at a barometric pressure of 282 mmHg (Fig. 7.10 in Chapter 7). However, the pulmonary arterial wedge pressure was unchanged with the increase in simulated altitude.

Cardiac output was measured and shown to have the same relationship with oxygen consumption as at sea level (Fig. 8.3 in Chapter 8), confirming earlier measurements made on the Silver Hut Expedition (Pugh 1964). However, heart rate as a function of work level was higher as altitude increased. A particularly interesting finding was that when the subjects breathed 100% oxygen at the high altitudes, pulmonary vascular resistance did not return to the sea level values. This indicated a substantial degree of irreversibility in pulmonary vascular resistance after 2 or 3 weeks of hypoxia indicating vascular remodeling as discussed in Chapter 8.

Additional information was found in the area of pulmonary gas exchange where it was possible to use the multiple inert gas elimination technique to separate the effects of ventilation–perfusion inequality from those of diffusion limitation. These studies were referred to in Chapter 7. Diffusion limitation of oxygen transfer across the blood-gas barrier occurred at oxygen uptakes greater than 3 L min^{-1} at sea level, and at less than 1 L min^{-1} on the 'summit.' This is a graphic demonstration of diffusion limitation at extreme altitude. A new finding was the increasing ventilation–perfusion inequality from rest to exercise at all altitudes. There was indirect evidence that this may have been caused by interstitial pulmonary edema. Table 13.3 summarizes the arterial blood gases during rest and maximal exercise on Operation Everest II.

Another invasive study that would be difficult to perform in the field was the analysis of skeletal muscle taken by needle biopsies. Skeletal muscle volume was also inferred from computed tomography scans of the arms and legs. Muscle area decreased by about 14% during the 'ascent.' The biopsies showed that this could be accounted for by a significant decrease in the cross-sectional area of both type I and type II fibers. As a result, there was an apparent increase in capillary volume density although this was not significant. Muscle enzymes were also measured and showed that at the highest altitude of 282 mmHg where biopsies were taken, there were significant reductions in succinic dehydrogenase, citrate synthetase and hexokinase compared with measurements made after returning to sea level. Finally, the biopsies showed significant reductions in muscle lactate concentrations at the higher altitudes consistent with the low blood lactate concentrations referred to in section 13.3.4.

Table 13.3 Barometric pressures, equivalent altitudes, and arterial blood gases during rest and maximal exercise on Operation Everest II (from Houston *et al.* 1987. and Sutton *et al.* 1988)

Barometric pressure (mmHg)	Inspired P_{O_2} (mmHg)	Altitude on Mount Everest (m)	Rest P_{O_2} (mmHg)	P_{CO_2} (mmHg)	pH	Maximum exercise P_{O_2} (mmHg)	P_{CO_2} (mmHg)	pH
760	149	0	99	34	7.43	87	35	7.30
429	80	4825	52	25	7.46	42	20	7.42
347	63	6482	41	20	7.50	34	17	7.44
282	49	8043	37	13	7.53	33	11	7.49
253*	43	8848	30	11	7.56	28	10	7.52

*Actual chamber pressure was 240 mmHg but because of oxygen contamination of the chamber air, the oxygen concentration was 22%. Therefore the inspired P_{O_2} was 43 mmHg corresponding to a barometric pressure of 253 mmHg for 21% oxygen. From west (1996a).

OPERATION EVEREST III

This low pressure chamber experiment in 1997 was carried out at the COMEX facility in Toulouse, France, and had a number of similarities with Operation Everest II (Richalet *et al.* 1999). However, an innovative feature was that the eight volunteers pre-acclimatized in the Vallot Observatory (4350 m) for several days before spending a total of 31 days in the low pressure chamber, ultimately reaching the 'summit' barometric pressure of 253 mmHg. The arterial blood-gas values were similar to those found on Operation Everest II (Table 13.3) with a 'summit' arterial P_{O_2} of 31 mmHg, P_{CO_2} of 12 mmHg and pH of 7.58. The fact that the P_{CO_2} was higher than on AMREE in both of the chamber studies is consistent with a lesser degree of acclimatizing (compare Fig. 13.4). Body weight fell by an average of 5.4 kg, again in line with Operation Everest II and AMREE. Cardiovascular measurements largely confirmed those made on Operation Everest II (Boussuges *et al.* 2000). An interesting new finding was transient neurological disorders which were attributed to gas emboli, and there were also marked changes in mood of some of the subjects (Nicholas *et al.* 2000).

13.4 WHAT LIMITS EXERCISE PERFORMANCE AT EXTREME ALTITUDE?

13.4.1 Concept of limitation

The oxygen cascade from the atmosphere to the mitochondria includes the processes of convective and diffusive ventilation of oxygen to the alveoli, diffusion of oxygen across the blood-gas barrier, uptake of oxygen by the hemoglobin in the pulmonary capillaries, convective flow of the blood to the peripheral capillaries, unloading of the oxygen from the hemoglobin, diffusion to the mitochondria and utilization of oxygen by the electron transport system. How can we determine to what extent each of these factors is limiting exercise at extreme altitude?

One approach is to use the analogy of a turbine that is fed by water flowing through a pipe which has a series of constrictions in it. Clearly, all sections of the pipe limit the flow of water to some extent. However, a useful description of the extent to which flow is limited by any particular section of the pipe can be found by calculating the percentage change in total flow for a given (say 5%) change in diameter at that point. In carrying out this calculation, we assume that all other factors remain unchanged. Such an analysis can only be carried out if the whole system is modeled using a computer.

13.4.2 Limitations to oxygen uptake on the summit of Mount Everest

The model analysis described above has been carried out for a hypothetical subject exercising on the summit of Mount Everest (West 1983). Some assumptions and extrapolations are necessary because so few data have yet been obtained at these great altitudes. In general, the physiological variables were those set out in section 13.3 and Table 13.4 summarizes these.

Table 13.4 Key variables for the analysis of factors limiting oxygen uptake on the summit of Mount Everest

Key variables Measured	
Barometric pressure	253 mmHg
Alveolar P_{CO_2}	7.5 mmHg
Hemoglobin concentration	18.4 g dL^{-1}
P_{50} at pH 7.4	29.6 mmHg
Base excess	27.2 mmol L^{-1}
Assumed	
Respiratory exchange ratio	1.0
Cardiac output/ oxygen uptake	Same as sea level
Maximal DM_{O_2}[a]	100 mL min^{-1} mmHg^{-1}
Capillary transit time	0.75 s
Minimum P_{O_2} in mixed venous blood	15 mmHg

[a]DM_{O_2}, diffusing capacity of the membrane for oxygen.

The whole oxygen transport system was modeled using numerical procedures previously described (West and Wagner 1977; West and Wagner, 1980). The details of a model analysis like this are not important because of uncertainties in the assumptions. However, some interesting predictions emerge (Fig. 13.8).

The most important variable affecting the maximal oxygen consumption ($\dot{V}_{O_2,max}$) is the barometric pressure. In this analysis, a 5% increase in pressure increased the $\dot{V}_{O_2,max}$ by over 20% when all other variables were held constant. Other important variables were the alveolar ventilation and the membrane diffusing capacity of the lung. The first increased the $\dot{V}_{O_2,max}$ by raising the alveolar P_{O_2}, whereas the second improved the arterial P_{O_2} because of the marked diffusion limitation of oxygen across the blood-gas barrier. An increase in oxygen affinity for hemoglobin as a result of increasing respiratory alkalosis also improved $\dot{V}_{O_2,max}$. In this analysis, an increase in cardiac output was also beneficial but in another theoretical analysis which took account of diffusion limitation of oxygen transfer in the exercising muscles, this improvement was not seen (Fig. 8.5 in Chapter 8).

The chief conclusions from the analysis are as follows:

1. A climber attempting an ascent of Mount Everest without supplementary oxygen should ideally choose a day with a relatively high barometric pressure. Indeed, this appears to be the most critical variable. Fortunately, climbers generally try to make a summit assault when the weather is fine and usually this means a high pressure. Note, however, that this factor makes a winter ascent of Mount Everest without supplementary oxygen particularly difficult.
2. The climber should not have a low hypoxic ventilatory response because a high ventilation is critical in maintaining an adequate alveolar P_{O_2}.
3. It is advantageous to have a high oxygen diffusing capacity at a moderate work level.
4. The climber should have as high a base excess as possible. Presumably one way to ensure this is to avoid prolonged stays at extreme altitudes.

13.4.3 How high can humans climb without supplementary oxygen?

We have seen that the $\dot{V}_{O_2,max}$ in acclimatized subjects with an inspired P_{O_2} of 43 mmHg, equivalent to that on the Everest summit, is only a little over 1 L min^{-1}. This oxygen uptake is equivalent to walking slowly on level ground. Clearly, humans at the highest point on Earth are very close to the limit of hypoxic tolerance.

Nevertheless, people often ask how much higher humans could climb without supplementary oxygen. The answer from the available data is very little. For example, as indicated earlier, a reduction of barometric pressure by 17 mmHg from 253 to 236 mmHg (the value for the Everest summit given by the standard atmosphere), would reduce the $\dot{V}_{O_2,max}$ by about 21% (West 1999a). It seems unlikely that the mountain could be climbed under these conditions emphasizing again that it is only the equatorial bulge in barometric pressure (Figs 2.3 and 2.5 in Chapter 2) which allows humans to reach the highest mountain top without supplementary oxygen.

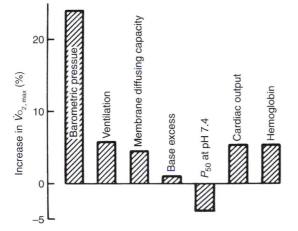

Figure 13.8 Sensitivity of calculated maximal oxygen consumption ($\dot{V}_{2,max}$) to changes in variables for a climber on the summit of Mount Everest. The initial conditions are those shown in Table 13.4, and each variable was increased by 5% leaving all the others constant. See text for details. (From West 1983.)

14

Sleep

SUMMARY

Sleep is very commonly impaired at high altitude. Typically, people complain that they wake frequently, have unpleasant dreams and do not feel refreshed in the morning. Polysomnographic studies confirm the increased frequency of arousals while electroencephalography shows changes in sleep architecture, usually with a great reduction in time spent in rapid eye movement (REM) sleep. Periodic breathing is almost universal at high altitude, and is accompanied by apneic periods lasting as long as 10–15 s. Periodic breathing likely occurs as a result of strong hypoxic ventilatory drive and may worsen as ventilatory acclimatization occurs during prolonged stays at high altitude. High altitude natives who have a blunted ventilatory response to hypoxia show less or no periodic breathing compared with lowlanders at high altitude. The severe arterial hypoxemia that follows the long apneic periods may reduce the arterial P_{O_2} to its lowest levels of the 24-h period. Acetazolamide reduces the time spent in periodic breathing, and improves the arterial oxygen saturation during sleep, while benzodiazepines and gamma aminobutyric acid receptor agents, such as temazepam, zolpidem and zaleplon, have also been shown to improve sleep quality. Oxygen enrichment of room air at high altitude results in fewer apneas, less time spent in periodic breathing, and an improved subjective assessment of sleep quality but intermittent hypoxic exposure prior to high altitude travel has not convincingly been demonstrated to improve sleep quality at high altitude. Patients with obstructive sleep apnea at sea level will likely still experience obstructive events at high altitude as well as an increased frequency of central apneas.

14.1 INTRODUCTION

Everyone who has been to high altitude knows that sleeping is often impaired. This ubiquitous problem affects the skier or trekker who sleeps at altitudes of 2500–3000 m, as well as the well-acclimatized climber who spends time as high as 8000 m. Common complaints include difficulty falling asleep, frequent awakenings, and persistent feelings of fatigue upon awakening in the morning. Vivid dreams and racing thoughts are other common features for many people. Underlying these subjective complaints are important changes in sleep physiology including changes in sleep architecture and the control of breathing. Alterations in the latter frequently lead to periodic breathing, a major contributor to altered sleep quality at high altitude that has been recognized as a problem since the nineteenth century. This common problem, which can cause severe degrees of hypoxemia following apneic periods at extreme altitudes (West *et al.* 1986) may be one of the factors that influences tolerance to very great altitudes and sheds light on the control of breathing under these special conditions.

This chapter considers the physiology of sleep at high altitude in greater detail, including sleep architecture, control of breathing and the periodic breathing phenomenon noted above. Consideration is also given to pharmacologic and non-pharmacologic measures to improve sleep quality in this environment as well as changes that may occur in patients with sleep-disordered breathing at sea level who travel to higher elevations. The material considered here overlaps somewhat with that of Chapter 6 on the control of ventilation, as well as some of the material in Chapter 8 on cardiovascular responses because of heart rate alterations that occur during periodic breathing.

14.2 HISTORICAL

14.2.1 Quality of sleep

There have been a number of anecdotal references to the poor quality of sleep at high altitude. Barcroft gave a particularly colorful description when he recounted his experiences during the glass chamber experiment carried out at Cambridge, UK (Barcroft *et al.* 1920). On that occasion he spent 6 days in a closed chamber in which the concentration of oxygen was regulated so that the initial equivalent altitude was 3048 m and the final altitude 4877 m. He wrote:

> In the glass case experiment I had the opportunity of judging a little more exactly of anoxaemic sleeplessness than is usually the case. A committee of undergraduate pupils of mine made up their minds that I was never to be left alone, two of them therefore sat up each night outside the case lest help of any sort should be required. I used to ask them in the morning how I had slept, and each morning except perhaps the last they said I had slept well. My own view

of the matter was quite otherwise. I thought I had been awake half the night and was unrefreshed in the morning. I was conscious of their moving about and looking in through the glass to see whether or not I was awake. I used to count my pulse at intervals. The two opinions can only be reconciled on the hypothesis that whilst I spent most of the night in sleep, the slumber was very light and fitful with incessant dreams. Even some low degree of consciousness which fell short of wakefulness. At Cerro it was the same: measured in hours we slept well, but the quality of the sleep in most cases was of an inferior order. The night seemed long and we woke unrefreshed.

(Barcroft 1925, p. 166)

Barcroft's impression that despite a normal sleep time sleep is less refreshing than normal due to the increased frequency of awakenings has proven to be accurate over time as more recent studies have subsequently confirmed this finding (Reite *et al.* 1975; Zielinski *et al.* 2000).

14.2.2 Periodic breathing

Various references to the uneven pattern of breathing during sleep at high altitude were made during the nineteenth century. One was by the eminent English physicist Tyndall, one of the most ardent Alpine mountaineers in the middle of the century about whom Paul Bert once commented, 'every year sees him planting his alpenstock on some new summit' (Bert 1878). During Tyndall's first ascent of Mont Blanc in 1857, he became very fatigued and laid down to rest. He subsequently wrote:

> I stretched myself upon a composite couch of snow and granite, and immediately fell asleep. My friend, however, soon aroused me. 'You quite frighten me' he said, 'I listened for some minutes and have not heard you breathe once.'

On renewing the ascent, Tyndall complained of palpitations.

> At each pause my heart throbbed audibly, as I leaned upon my staff, and the subsidence

of this action was always the signal for further advance.

(Tyndall 1860)

Another early comment on periodic breathing was made by Egli-Sinclair (1894) in an article on mountain sickness. He noted that, at an altitude of 4400 m, respiration

> had the Stokes character, that is, it seemed regular during a certain time, after which a few rapid and profound breaths were drawn, a total suspension of a few seconds then following.

Here he was referring to the Irish physician, Dr William Stokes, who described the pattern of breathing which

> consists in the occurrence of a series of inspirations, increasing to a maximum and then declining in force and length until a state of apparent apnoea is established.

(Stokes 1854)

Another Irish physician, John Cheyne, had described the same pattern in 1818 (Cheyne 1818) and so the breathing pattern became known as Cheyne–Stokes breathing, although Ward (1973) pointed out that John Hunter had given a lucid and succinct description of the same condition in 1781 (Hunter 1781).

The first extensive studies of periodic breathing at high altitude were made by Angelo Mosso, Professor of Physiology at the University of Turin, Italy, who, as mentioned earlier, was one of the first people to use the Capanna Regina Margherita on the Monte Rosa (4559 m) for scientific work. He measured the breathing movements by means of a lever that rested on the chest. An example of one of his measurements on his brother, Ugolino Mosso, is shown in Fig. 14.1a. The periods of apnea lasted about 12 s. Note that, in this instance, the first breath after the apneic period was the largest. A more typical pattern is that shown in Fig. 14.1b, which was measured on Francioli, keeper of the Regina Margherita hut. In this instance the waxing and waning of breathing movements are clearly seen and the periods of apnea are shorter (Mosso 1898).

A curious feature of Mosso's measurements was that he concluded that ventilation was actually decreased at high altitude, apparently because he converted his readings to standard conditions (0°C and 1000 mmHg in his case) rather than BTPS (body temperature and pressure saturated). Interestingly, Paul Bert also believed that hyperventilation did not occur at high altitude (Bert 1878, p. 106 in the 1943 translation). He wrote

> What is really certain is that . . . a dweller in lofty altitudes, does not even try to struggle against the decrease of oxygen in his arterial blood by speeding up his respirations excessively, as was first supposed. The observations of Dr. Jourdanet are conclusive.

Bert probably reached this conclusion because he worked exclusively with low pressure chambers that only allowed short-term observations. It was

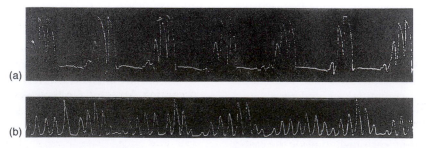

Figure 14.1 Earliest tracings showing periodic breathing at an altitude of 4560 m: (a) a record from Ugolino Mosso, brother of Angelo Mosso. Note the apneic periods of approximately 12 s; (b) a tracing from Francioli, keeper of the Regina Margherita hut. Note the waxing and waning of respiration. (From Mosso 1898.)

not until Mosso worked in the Capanna Regina Margherita a few years later that measurements were easily made on subjects exposed to high altitude for several days although, as indicated above, he also concluded ventilation was decreased.

Mosso realized that the alveolar P_{CO_2} was reduced in people living in the Capanna Regina Margherita at 4559 m, but instead of attributing this to increased ventilation, he argued that the low pressure at high altitude extracted carbon dioxide from the blood just as does a mercury pump in a blood-gas analysis apparatus. Barcroft (1925) could not follow Mosso's argument and remarked:

> I speak with all deference, but Mosso seems to me to have overlooked the fact that the body is exposed to what is practically a vacuum of carbon dioxide, whether it be at the Capanna Margherita or in his own laboratory at Turin.

Mosso introduced the term 'acapnia' to refer to the reduction of P_{CO_2} and believed that this was an important factor in the development of acute mountain sickness (AMS). Indeed, it may well be that the symptoms of this condition are related in part to the respiratory alkalosis. However, Barcroft (1925) pointed out that Mosso's theory was not supported by the experience at the Alta Vista hut (3350 m) on Tenerife during the First International High Altitude Expedition of 1910. Barcroft had an almost normal alveolar P_{CO_2} (38 mmHg) but was incapacitated by the altitude, whereas Douglas, whose P_{CO_2} was only 32 mmHg, was 'perfectly free from all symptoms'. Thus hypoxia (which was more severe in Barcroft because he did not increase his ventilation) rather than the low P_{CO_2} was implicated in the etiology of mountain sickness.

14.3 PHYSIOLOGY OF SLEEP

Sleep can be defined as a state of unconsciousness from which the subject can be aroused by sensory or other stimuli. As such it can be distinguished from deep anesthesia and disease states that cause coma, though these have some features in common with true sleep. Two major types of sleep are recognized.

14.3.1 Slow wave sleep

This is often called non-REM or NREM (non-rapid eye movement) sleep, or sometimes normal sleep. It is characterized by decreased activity of the reticular activating system, and is called slow wave sleep (SWS) because of the predominance of slow delta waves in the electroencephalogram (EEG). These slow waves have a high voltage and occur at a rate of 1 or $2\,s^{-1}$. In the early stages of sleep, the alpha rhythm (8–13 Hz), which is always present during wakefulness, becomes more obvious. In addition, sleep spindles (14–16 Hz) may appear. These features can be used to divide SWS into four stages (I–IV). The delta waves probably originate in the cortex of the brain when it is not driven from below because of the reduced level of activity of the reticular activating system. SWS is dreamless, very restful and associated with a decreased peripheral vascular tone, blood pressure, respiratory rate and basal metabolic rate.

14.3.2 REM sleep

This is called REM sleep because, although the eyes remain closed, there are rapid horizontal eye movements. In a normal night of sleep, bouts of REM sleep lasting 5–20 min usually appear on the average about every 90 min. The first such period occurs 80–100 min after the subject falls asleep and then more frequently through the night. The EEG tracing resembles the waking state, but the person is actually more difficult to arouse than during NREM sleep. REM sleep is usually associated with active dreaming. Muscle tone throughout the body is greatly depressed, but there may be occasional muscular twitching and limb jerking. The heart rate and respiration usually become irregular. Thus, in this type of sleep, the brain is quite active but the activity is not channeled in the proper direction for the person to be aware of his or her surroundings.

14.3.3 Control of breathing during sleep

In general, minute ventilation is depressed during sleep compared to the awake state as are the ventilatory responses to hypoxia and carbon dioxide. The hypercapnic ventilatory response appear to be reduced in both NREM and REM sleep (Bulow 1963; Douglas *et al.* 1982b) but there is more uncertainty about the hypoxic ventilatory response; some studies indicate that it is increased in NREM sleep (Pappenheimer 1977; Phillipson *et al.* 1978) while other studies suggest it is decreased in all sleep stages including REM sleep (Berthon-Jones and Sullivan 1982; Douglas *et al.* 1982a; Douglas *et al.* 1982b). While these observed changes in minute ventilation and the ventilatory responses to chemical stimuli are often attributed to loss of the wakefulness drive to breathe during sleep (Douglas 2000; Orem and Kubin 2000) important changes in neurochemical regulation of breathing, including enhanced gamma aminobutyric acid (GABA) activity, also play a significant role (Joseph *et al.* 2002). The decrease in minute ventilation is also due in part to changes in upper airway patency during sleep that occur as a result of both mechanical factors, as well as changes in neurochemical control of pharyngeal motor neurons responsible for maintaining upper airway tone (Dempsey *et al.* 2010).

14.3.4 Alterations in normal sleep patterns

Alterations in the normal sleep patterns described above through sleep deprivation or fragmentation impair mental function, the higher brain functions being the most susceptible. There are similarities between the behavior of sleep-deprived subjects and people at high altitude whose brains are affected by hypoxia. In both instances, mental activities that are 'mechanical' in nature, such as tabulating a set of data, can be accurately accomplished, whereas activities that require problem solving and initiative are seriously affected (Chapter 17). It may be that some of the impairment of central nervous system (CNS) function in individuals living at high altitude can

be ascribed to the poor quality of sleep, but the direct effects of hypoxia on the brain also clearly play a role.

14.4 CHARACTERISTICS OF SLEEP AT HIGH ALTITUDE

In this section, we consider how sleep is affected by hypobaric hypoxia with the discussion focused largely on changes reported in adults. The limited information available about sleep in children at high altitude is considered in Chapter 27.

14.4.1 Increased frequency of arousals

People at high altitude often report that they wake more frequently during the night than at sea level. This phenomenon has been confirmed in several careful studies (Reite *et al.* 1975; Weil *et al.* 1978; Salvaggio *et al.* 1998; Zielinski *et al.* 2000) using continuous recordings of the EEG, electromyography (EMG) and eye movements, during which arousal was recognized by the occurrence of EMG activation, eye movements and alpha wave activity on the EEG. In one study, for example, an average of 36 arousals per night occurred at an altitude of 4300 m compared with 20 at sea level (Weil *et al.* 1978). An example of frequent arousals is shown in Fig. 14.2. Administration of the drug acetazolamide, which is known to stimulate ventilation at high altitude, reduced the frequency of arousals.

Some investigators believe that the arousals are caused in some way by periodic breathing and there is some evidence that arousals are more frequent when the strength of periodic breathing is high. It is easy to imagine that the strenuous muscular activity required to generate large breaths after a prolonged period of apnea could contribute to an arousal. A common nightmare at high altitude is that the tent has been covered with snow by an avalanche and the subject wakes violently feeling suffocated and very short of breath. This may be associated with the air hunger caused by long apneic periods during periodic breathing. Periodic breathing cannot be

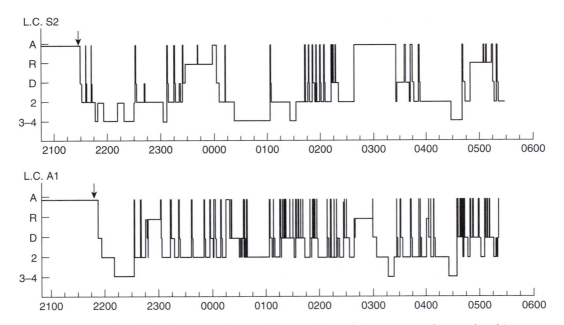

Figure 14.2   Example of the change in sleep architecture in a subject measured at sea level (upper tracing) and on the first night at an altitude of 4300 m (lower tracing). Time is on the horizontal axis and sleep stages are shown on the vertical axis. A, awake; R, REM; D, stage I; 2, stage II; 3–4, stages III and IV. At altitude there was greatly increased sleep fragmentation and a reduction in slow wave sleep. (From Reite *et al.* 1975.)

solely responsible for the increased frequency of arousals at high altitude, however, as arousals also occur in individuals who do not develop periodic breathing (Reite *et al.* 1975; Wickramasinghe and Anholm 1999).

14.4.2 Changes of sleep state

Multiple EEG studies have provided objective evidence of changes in sleep architecture at high altitude that support climbers' subjective conclusions that sleep at high altitude is often of poor quality, and not as refreshing as sleep at sea level. One of the earliest studies in this regard was performed by Joern *et al.* (1970) who evaluated changes in sleep architecture near the South Pole where the barometric pressure is reduced because of the actual altitude and also the very high latitude (see Chapter 2, section 2.2.4). They reported a near absence of sleep stages III and IV coupled with an approximately 50% reduction in REM sleep. Although the light–dark cycle was atypical compared to other sleep settings, their

findings have been confirmed at more moderate latitudes.

Several years later, Reite *et al.* (1975) studied sleep patterns in subjects following a rapid ascent to Pikes Peak (4300 m). They found a similar shift from deeper to lighter sleep stages and a great reduction in REM sleep. Periodic breathing was common but disappeared during REM sleep. The changes in the pattern of sleep and respiration were greatest on the first night at high altitude and then declined thereafter.

Subsequent studies have generally confirmed the findings that time spent in light sleep (stages I and II of NREM) is increased, while the time spent in deep sleep (stages III and IV of NREM) is decreased. The data regarding the time spent in REM sleep has been conflicting however, with some studies reporting that it is virtually abolished (Pappenheimer 1977; Megirian *et al.* 1980) and other studies reporting either a decrease (Anholm *et al.*, 1992; Goldenberg *et al.* 1992) or no change in the time spent in this stage (Normand *et al.* 1990; Zielinski *et al.* 2000; Johnson *et al.* 2010a).

14.4.3 Changes in control of breathing

Few studies have examined the impact of high altitude on the hypercapnic and hypoxic ventilatory responses during sleep. In one of the few studies on this issue, White *et al.* (1987) monitored hypercapnic ventilatory responses in six healthy men on nights 1, 4 and 7 at 4300 m and found that the response was diminished to similar degrees seen at sea level during both NREM and REM sleep. They also observed that minute ventilation fell from wakefulness to NREM and REM sleep with the bulk of the decrease being attributable to a decrease in tidal volume. Minute ventilation did increase over time at altitude, largely due to increases in respiratory rate.

14.5 PERIODIC BREATHING

14.5.1 Characteristics

Early records of chest movements during periodic breathing are shown in Fig. 14.1. This pattern has now been confirmed in many studies carried out at various altitudes from sea level up to 8050 m (Douglas and Haldane 1909; Douglas *et al.* 1913; Weil *et al.* 1978; Sutton *et al.* 1979; Berssenbrugge *et al.* 1983; Lahiri *et al.* 1983; West *et al.* 1986; Johnson *et al.* 2010a).

A typical pattern recorded at an altitude of 6300 m (P_B 351 mmHg) in a well-acclimatized lowlander using modern equipment is shown in Fig. 14.3 (West *et al.* 1986). Note that the tidal volume waxed and waned during each burst of breathing, with apneic periods of about 8 s. Arterial oxygen saturation as measured by ear oximeter fluctuated with the same frequency as the periodic breathing. There was a phase difference in these changes, however, with the highest arterial oxygen saturation (inverted scale) occurring at approximately the end of the apneic period. This can be accounted for by the circulation time from the lung capillaries to the ear where the oxygen saturation was measured. Heart rate was measured from the electrocardiogram (ECG) and showed marked fluctuations with the same frequency as the periodic breathing. Note that the highest heart rate appeared at the end of the burst of ventilation.

Beyond the fact that periodic breathing is common among lowlanders who ascend to high altitude there are several important features of this phenomenon. The first feature is that it persists for a considerable period of time at high altitude. In the study from which Fig.14.3 is taken (West *et al.* 1986), all eight subjects showed obvious periodic breathing during the several weeks over which the measurements were made at 6300 m. More recently, Bloch *et al.* (2010) studied nocturnal breathing patterns in 34 mountaineers

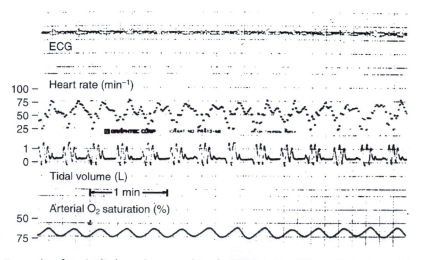

Figure 14.3   Example of periodic breathing at altitude 6300 m (P_B 351 mmHg). (From West *et al.* 1986.)

during ascent and descent from Muztagh Ata (7546 m) and found not only a persistence of periodic breathing over a several-week period but also that climbers spent a greater time in periodic breathing upon returning to base camp at the end of their climb when compared to their stay at base camp during the ascent. Despite persistence of periodic breathing over time at high altitude, overall sleep quality seems to improve with acclimatization (Nussbaumer-Ochsner *et al.* 2012b).

The second important feature is that the percentage of time occupied by periodic breathing increases with altitude. For example, Waggener *et al.* (1984) reported that periodic breathing with apnea occupied 24% of the time at 2440 m, and that the percentage increased to 40% at 4270 m. This increase in proportion of time is consistent with a theoretical model discussed below (Khoo *et al.* 1982) and has been documented in other studies (Insalaco *et al.* 2000; Bloch *et al.* 2010; Johnson *et al.* 2010a).

Multiple studies have shown that periodic breathing is very common during NREM sleep at high altitude and may even occur during the drowsy period that precedes sleep onset (Reite *et al.* 1975; Berssenbrugge *et al.* 1983). It typically does not occur during REM sleep at moderate altitudes, although periodicity may still occur during REM sleep at high elevations (Wickramasinghe and Anholm 1999).

There is also evidence that cycle length decreases with increasing altitude (Waggener *et al.* 1984). Studies done at sea level indicate a cycle period of about 30 s (Douglas and Haldane 1909; Specht and Fruhmann 1972; Lugaresi *et al.* 1978) whereas subjects in the American Medical Research Expedition to Everest (AMREE) study had a mean cycle period of only 20.5 s, a value similar to that measured in a companion study at 5400 m (Lahiri *et al.* 1983). Further evidence for the decrease in cycle length is provided in Fig. 14.4, which shows a plot of cycle time against altitude for several experimental studies and the theoretical model developed by Khoo *et al.* (1982), although it should be noted that the cycle lengths seen in the AMREE study were somewhat greater than that predicted by the model.

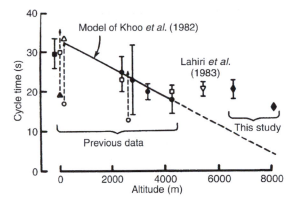

Figure 14.4 Variation of cycle time of periodic breathing with altitude. Points marked 'Previous data' were originally published as Figure 8 in the paper by Khoo *et al.* (1982), the solid line being results predicted by their model (d). Vertical broken lines indicate differences caused by scaling between neonates and adults. For sources of data see Khoo *et al.* (1982). 'This study' refers to West *et al.* (1986). (From West *et al.* 1986.)

Another important feature of periodic breathing is the fact that the duration of time spent in this pattern does not appear to be affected by acclimatization, particularly at higher elevations. An excellent example of this phenomenon is provided by Bloch *et al.* (2010) in the Muztagh Ata study discussed above. Subjects in this study spent a greater percentage of the night in periodic breathing upon returning to base camp (4497 m) at the end of the expedition than they did on their initial stay at this elevation. The reason for the persistence or increase in periodic breathing at high elevations is not clear but may be related to ventilatory acclimatization and its effect on the loop gain phenomenon that contributes strongly to periodic breathing (discussed further below).

Periodic breathing may also be accompanied by cyclical changes in heart rate although cardiac rhythm disturbances are uncommon. The heart rate changes are demonstrated nicely in the sleep tracing in Fig. 14.3 obtained at 6300 m (West *et al.* 1986). A similar pattern was seen in all subjects in this study with the maximum heart rate appearing shortly after the peak of the hyperpnea. Insalaco *et al.* (2000) reported similar cyclical changes in heart rate, as well as systemic blood pressure, although they noted that heart rate peaked before the end of the hyperpneic period and before the decline in systemic blood pressure. Further evidence regarding heart rate changes comes from data collected from four subjects, at an altitude of 8050 m (P_B 282 mmHg) on Mount Everest. Breathing movements were not recorded directly because of the very remote location of the camp but continuous ECG tracings obtained during the night using a Holter-type monitor demonstrated variations in heart rate similar to those described by Guilleminault *et al.* (1984). Figure 14.5 shows data from one of the subjects who demonstrated extremely regular cyclic regulation of heart rate for periods as long as 40 minutes.

The percentage of time spent in periodic breathing decreases with descent to lower elevation and can also be decreased with the addition of supplemental oxygen. Lahiri and Barnard (1983), for example, showed that administration of oxygen leads to an immediate increase in the apneic period from about 10 to 17 s, followed by

shortening and then elimination of the apneas (Fig. 14.6). Periodicity is not totally eliminated but is diminished in intensity. The changes can be partly explained by the reduction in respiratory drive from the peripheral chemoreceptors when the arterial P_{O_2} was raised. Addition of carbon dioxide to the inspired gas did not totally abolish the periodic breathing, although it did eliminate the periods of apnea. Withdrawal of carbon dioxide from the inspired gas was followed by a prompt reappearance of apnea, suggesting a dominant role for the peripheral chemoreceptors.

14.5.2 Mechanism

In contrast to obstructive sleep apnea, in which recurrent episodes of upper airway obstruction are responsible for the development of apneic periods, it is clear that periodic breathing at high altitude is of central nervous system origin. This is supported by

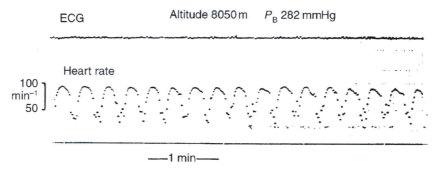

Figure 14.5   Cyclic variation of heart rate caused by periodic breathing in a climber at 8050 m altitude. P_B = 282 mmHg. (From West *et al.* 1986.)

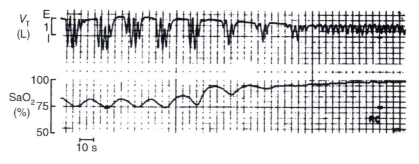

Figure 14.6   Effect of increasing the inspired P_{O_2} on periodic breathing in a lowlander during sleep at 5400 m. Note that adding oxygen to the inspired gas raised the arterial oxygen saturation, eliminated the apneic periods, and reduced the strength of periodic breathing. V_T, tidal volume; Sa_{O_2}, arterial oxygen saturation; E, expiration, I, inspiration. (From Lahiri and Barnard 1983.)

the absence of rib cage and abdominal movements as determined from an inductance plethysmograph, a device used for detecting changes in circumference of the chest and abdomen.

Control theory can be used to better understand the central mechanisms responsible for periodic breathing (Khoo *et al.* 1982; Cherniack and Longobardo 2006). Control systems are marked by two key features: a 'disturbance' (e.g. a change in alveolar ventilation) followed by a 'corrective action' which tends to suppress the disturbance. In the case of an increase in alveolar ventilation (caused by a sigh, for example) the corrective action would be a lowering of P_{CO_2}, which would tend to reduce ventilation by its action on central and peripheral chemoreceptors and thus constitute negative feedback. Sustained oscillatory behavior will occur in such a system when two requirements are met. First, the magnitude of the corrective action must exceed that of the disturbance, this ratio being known as the loop gain. Second, the corrective action must be presented 180° out of phase with the disturbance, so that what would otherwise inhibit the change in ventilation now augments it. This sustained oscillatory behavior occurs when the loop gain exceeds unity at a phase difference of 180°.

Control theory predicts that the higher the loop gain at a phase angle of 180°, the more likely periodic breathing is to occur, the more marked the pattern of periodic breathing, and the shorter the cycle length of the periodic breathing. The main factor increasing loop gain in acclimatized lowlanders at high altitude is the increased chemoreceptor gain, particularly the response to severe hypoxia (Chapter 6).

Evidence for the role of hypoxic and hypercapnic ventilatory responses was provided by Matsuyama *et al.* (1989) who performed measurements on nine Japanese climbers participating in an expedition to the Kunlun mountains (7167 m) in China and found a significant correlation between the degree of periodic breathing during sleep and both the hypoxic ventilatory response and hypercapnic ventilatory response measured at sea level. Although all climbers showed desaturation during sleep, there was a negative correlation between the degree of desaturation and the hypoxic ventilation response (HVR). The authors

concluded that the high HVR helped to maintain the arterial oxygenation during sleep, and was, therefore, advantageous.

Further evidence for the role played by the strength of hypoxic ventilatory responses is provided by the observed differences in the incidence of periodic breathing between acclimatized lowlanders and high altitude natives (Lahiri *et al.* 1983). Figure 14.7 shows the relationship between the frequency of apnea during sleep at 5400 m and the hypoxic ventilatory response in these two groups. Because native highlanders often have a blunted hypoxic ventilatory response (Severinghaus *et al.* 1966a; Milledge and Lahiri 1967), the loop gain of the control system is reduced and the factors promoting periodicity are weak. Lahiri *et al.* (1983) have argued that this represents an important feature of the true adaptation of native highlanders, such as Sherpas, to high altitude.

Another contributing factor may be the hyperventilation that develops over time at high altitude, which increases the rate of wash-out of carbon dioxide and wash-in of oxygen in the lungs. This fits with the observation in the study by Bloch *et al.* (2010) in which climbers on Muztagh Ata (7546 m) spent more time in

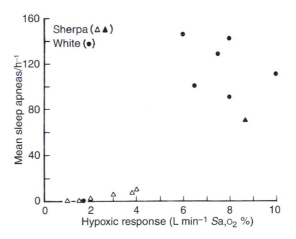

Figure 14.7 Relationship between frequency of sleep apnea and ventilatory response to hypoxia (awake). ●, acclimatized lowlanders; Δ, high altitude Sherpas; ▲, lower altitude Sherpa. One lowlander did not have periods of apnea, and the low altitude Sherpa showed periodic breathing. (From Lahiri and Barnard 1983.)

periodic breathing at base camp later in the expedition than they did earlier in the expedition. The rise in minute ventilation that occurred as a result of acclimatization during their time on the mountain served to increase the loop gain in this control system.

According to control theory, disturbances such as arousals should play an important role in the genesis of periodic breathing. However, Khoo et al. (1996) looked at the relationship between arousals and the initiation of periodic breathing in healthy volunteers at simulated altitudes of 4572, 6100 and 7620 m. They found that although arousals promoted the development of periodic breathing with apnea in some instances, they were not necessary for the initiation of periodic breathing in all circumstances.

14.5.3 Gas exchange

Periodic breathing causes marked fluctuations in the arterial Po_2 and oxygen saturation with the severity of hypoxemia being a function of both the duration of apnea and the altitude at which the individual is sleeping. Obesity may contribute to further hypoxemia beyond that observed in non-obese individuals (Ge et al. 2005). Figures 14.3 and 14.6 show the typical pattern fluctuations in arterial oxygen saturation as recorded by ear oximeter.

In the study of nocturnal periodic breathing carried out at an altitude of 6300 m during the 1981 AMREE expedition, the mean fluctuation in arterial oxygen saturation between subjects was approximately 10% (West et al. 1986). In order to determine the proportion of the time during which the arterial oxygen saturation fell below a particular value, the analysis described by Slutsky and Strohl (1980) was carried out. This showed that the arterial oxygen saturation below which the subjects spent 50% of their time varied from a minimal value of 64.5% to a maximum of 74.5% with a mean of 68.8%.

Since it is not usually feasible to sample arterial blood over prolonged periods of time, most investigations rely on ear or finger oximetry to monitor oxygen saturation. However, based on spot measurements of arterial Po_2 it was calculated that the maximum and minimum values of saturation of 73.0 and 63.4% from the AMREE study corresponded to arterial Po_2 values of approximately 39 and 33 mmHg, respectively. The conclusion was that the minimal arterial Po_2 during sleep was approximately 6 mmHg lower than the resting daytime value, a substantial difference when individuals reside on the steep part of the oxygen dissociation curve. These values are likely the lowest arterial Po_2 values seen over the course of the day at high altitude. Even though arterial Po_2 does fall considerably below the resting value at high work rates seen during climbing, for example, climbers generally do not work at more than two-thirds of their maximal power (Pugh 1958; Chapter 11, section 11.9). As a result, it is unlikely that the Po_2 values experienced with exercise are lower than those seen with periodic breathing during sleep.

The effects of arterial hypoxemia may be exaggerated by the increase in cardiac output that occurs when the arterial Po_2 is near its lowest value. As Figs 14.3 and 14.6 show, the lowest arterial oxygen saturation typically occurs just after the peak of ventilation during the periodic breathing cycle. If venous return and, therefore, cardiac output are enhanced during this hyperpneic phase, this would lead to enhanced delivery of this poorly oxygenated blood. Thus it may be that the phasing of arterial Po_2 and cardiac output aggravate the resulting impairment of oxygen delivery.

An important question is whether the severe arterial hypoxemia seen during periodic breathing affects tolerance to extreme altitude. As shown in Fig. 14.7 there is a correlation between the strength of the hypoxic ventilatory response and the magnitude of periodic breathing, as would be expected from the control theory discussed above. One would expect, therefore, that those with the strongest hypoxic ventilatory responses might have the most severe nocturnal hypoxemia and might adapt poorly to high altitude. This concern may not be borne out, however, as Schoene et al. (1984) demonstrated that climbers with strong hypoxic ventilatory responses performed better at extreme altitude than those with weaker responses. This might be explained by the better ability of these climbers to hyperventilate and defend their alveolar P_{O_2} during the daytime (Chapter 13). However, it is clear that some elite mountain climbers have, in fact, a relatively low hypoxic ventilatory response (Milledge *et al.* 1983c; Schoene *et al.* 1987). Their tolerance of extreme altitude may relate to the fact that they maintain a higher arterial P_{O_2} during the night.

14.6 IMPROVING SLEEP AT HIGH ALTITUDE

14.6.1 Pharmacologic options

Because of the poor quality of sleep at high altitude and the role periodic breathing plays in this problem, there has been considerable interest in the use of drugs to decrease periodic breathing and improve sleep quality at high altitude. Multiple studies have demonstrated that acetazolamide significantly decreases the amount of time spent in periodic breathing and improves arterial oxygen saturation (Hackett *et al.* 1987a; Weil *et al.* 1978; Sutton *et al.* 1979; Fischer *et al.* 2004) (Fig. 14.8). In addition to the effects on periodic breathing, acetazolamide decreases the incidence of acute mountain sickness, a benefit not seen with other agents such as theophylline that also decrease the incidence of periodic breathing (Fischer *et al.* 2004).

Other drugs beyond these respiratory stimulants have also been studied in an attempt to improve the quality of sleep at high altitude. Several studies, for example, have reported improvements in subjective and objective measures of sleep quality with use of 10 mg of the benzodiazepine temazepam (Dubowitz 1998; Nickol *et al.* 2006). Röggla *et al.* (2000) did report an increased P_{CO_2} and decreased P_{O_2} measured from earlobe blood during temazepam use, but these assessments were made only 1 hour following administration in unacclimatized subjects and may not reflect the utility and safety of the medication over an entire night of sleep or with a longer duration of stay at high altitude. The non-benzodiazepine hypnotics or gamma aminobutyric acid receptor agents, zolpidem and zaleplon, have also been shown to improve sleep quality and sleep architecture, including increased slow wave and stage IV sleep and total sleep time, although there is no evidence

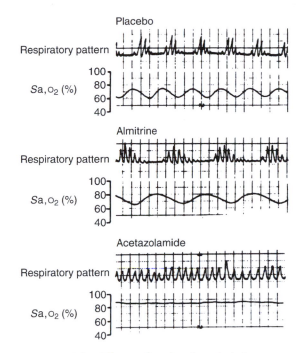

Figure 14.8 Effects of a placebo, almitrine and acetazolamide on periodic breathing and arterial oxygen saturation (Sa,O_2) at an altitude of 4400 m. Note that acetazolamide abolished the apneic periods whereas almitrine exaggerated them. (From Hackett *et al.* 1987.)

these agents have any effect on the incidence of periodic breathing (Beaumont *et al.* 1996; Beaumont *et al.* 2004; Beaumont *et al.* 2007). The sedative-hypnotic eszopiclone has not been studied at high altitude, but given that it has the same mechanism of action as zolpidem and zaleplon, one would expect it to be safe and effective at altitude as well (Luks 2008).

Despite evidence that all of the medications noted above improve some facet of sleep at high altitude, several important questions remain unanswered. The optimal doses of the various sleep aids remain unclear, as does the utility and safety of combination therapy or the relative efficacy of the various agents when used as monotherapy (Luks 2008). Finally, whether or not to even initiate pharmacologic therapy is an open question. Because sleep quality improves with acclimatization despite persistence of periodic breathing (Nussbaumer-Ochsner *et al.* 2012b), one could make the argument that unless the sleep problems interfere with an important activity or work the following day, it is better to forgo initiation of these medications.

14.6.2 Non-pharmacologic measures

Adding oxygen to the ventilation of a room shows promise as a way of combating the hypoxia of high altitude, particularly for people who commute to high altitude to work (see Chapter 28 where the technology is discussed). Luks *et al.* (1998) carried out a randomized, double-blind trial at an altitude of 3800 m to determine whether oxygen enrichment of room air to 24% at night improved sleep quality and performance and well-being the following day. They found that, with oxygen enrichment, the subjects had significantly fewer apneas and spent significantly less time in periodic breathing with apneas than when they slept in ambient air (Fig. 14.9). Sleeping in the oxygen-enriched environment also improved subjective assessments of sleep quality and acute mountain sickness scores upon awakening but no changes

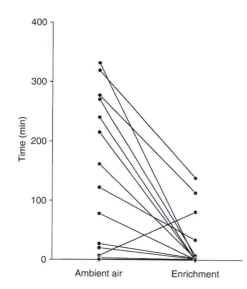

Figure 14.9 Comparison of the time spent by 18 subjects in periodic breathing with apneas during sleep in ambient air, compared with an atmosphere of 24% oxygen at an altitude of 3800 m. The paired differences were significant ($p < 0.01$). (From Luks *et al.* 1998.)

were noted during performance on psychometric testing. Using a similar study protocol, Barash *et al.* (2001) also noted improvements in sleep architecture during oxygen-enriched sleep including greater time in slow wave sleep. A finding of particular interest in the study by Luks *et al.* (1998) was that subjects who slept in the oxygen-enriched atmosphere had a significantly greater increase in arterial oxygen saturation (measured in ambient air outside the sleeping chambers) from evening to morning compared to sleeping in ambient air. McElroy *et al.* (2000) confirmed this finding in a subsequent study and suggested it was likely due to a lower incidence of subclinical pulmonary edema rather than an effect of room oxygen enrichment on ventilatory control, as no changes were observed in hypoxic or hypercapnic ventilatory responses between the different treatments. Most recreational skiers and trekkers do not travel to the altitudes described in these studies but still report significant sleep disturbances at lower elevations between 2000 and 3000 m. Oxygen enrichment of room air is feasible for resorts at such elevations (West 2002b) and can be expected to greatly improve the quality of sleep.

Continuous positive airway pressure (CPAP) is a commonly used therapy for obstructive and central sleep apnea patients at sea level, but its role in improving sleep at high altitude has not been studied. Johnson *et al.* (2010b) have documented improvements in nocturnal oxygen saturation and acute mountain sickness scores in normal individuals sleeping at 3800 m with non-invasive positive pressure ventilation (NIPPV) but did not make any objective or subjective measurements of sleep quality.

Various forms of intermittent hypoxic exposure (IHE) prior to a planned ascent have also been considered as a means to improve sleep at high altitude. Exposure to the equivalent of 4300 m for 3 hours per day over a 7-day period was not associated with improvements in oxygen saturation during sleep, sleep quality or sleep quantity during a subsequent exposure to the same elevation (Jones *et al.* 2008), while seven consecutive nights of sleep in normobaric hypoxia led to improvements in mean sleep oxygen saturation and fewer awakenings but no changes in the number of desaturation events or duration of wakefulness upon subsequent exposure to a terrestrial altitude of 4300 m (Fulco *et al.* 2011). The time spent in periodic breathing was not examined in either study. One reason for the lack of clear benefit from IHE may relate to the fact that IHE enhances ventilatory acclimatization and, as a result, may worsen the loop gain phenomenon that contributes to the periodic breathing problems that play a large role in poor sleep quality.

14.7 OBSTRUCTIVE SLEEP APNEA PATIENTS AT HIGH ALTITUDE

In addition to the issues described above, it is useful to consider what happens to sleep at high altitude in those individuals with known sleep disorders at sea level. A question of particular importance is whether obstructive sleep apnea patients will experience the same or fewer obstructive events during a high altitude sojourn when not using CPAP compared to what they normally experience at home. Burgess *et al.* (2006) reported a fall in the obstructive respiratory disturbance index in five men with moderate obstructive sleep apnea (baseline apnea hypopnea index 25.5 ± 14.4 per hour) exposed to 2750 m that was accompanied by a significant rise in the central respiratory distress index. This study was done in normobaric hypoxia, however, and subsequent field studies involving exposure to hypobaric hypoxia have shown that despite the fall in barometric pressure and air density at high altitude, the number of obstructive events remained relatively stable. The total number of apneas increased, however, as these individuals experienced a greater number of central events (Nussbaumer-Ochsner *et al.* 2010; Nussbaumer-Ochsner *et al.* 2012a). Use of acetazolamide decreased the number of central events but had no significant effect on the number of obstructive events in these patients.

The results of these studies suggest that CPAP therapy may still be necessary for obstructive sleep apnea patients traveling to high altitude. A question that remains unanswered, however, is whether the barometric pressure changes at high altitude will affect the level of CPAP necessary to control their obstructive apneas at high altitude. Older machines lacking pressure compensating features may not deliver the set pressure at high altitude (Fromm *et al.* 1995) and adjustment may be necessary. Patz *et al.* (2010) used more recent generation auto-titrating CPAP devices to track CPAP requirements in seven high altitude residents traveling to lower elevation and found no significant changes in the pressures used to prevent obstructive events, but it is difficult to draw firm conclusions from this study due to the low number of subjects and the fact that these were mountain residents traveling to sea level rather than sea level residents traveling to high altitude, a more clinically relevant issue.

Nutrition, metabolism and intestinal function

SUMMARY

Loss of appetite and loss of weight are common at altitude. Initially these may be due to acute mountain sickness (AMS). At heights below about 4500 m appetite returns after a few days but at more extreme altitudes anorexia persists and may get worse. Weight loss on an altitude trip can have many causes. On trek, initial weight loss may be the shedding of excess fat caused by a sedentary lifestyle. Intestinal infections can cause diarrhea and weight loss. High on the mountain, unavailability of food and liquid can be the cause but even in the absence of these factors weight loss is seen, as it is in long-term chamber studies.

In considering energy balance at altitude, basal metabolic rate is increased 10–17% at 4000–6000 m and possibly more at extreme altitudes. Exercise increases energy needs, though the reduction in maximum work rate would be expected to reduce the energy requirement of climbing. However, the use of new techniques has given values of energy expenditure when climbing at extreme altitudes that are at least as high as in the European Alps, if not higher, so

daily energy needs are high while intake is often reduced because of anorexia. This anorexia may be mediated by the hormones such as leptin, ghrelin or cholecystokinin.

Weight loss results in a change of body composition; fat tends to be lost preferentially at low elevations but muscle at higher altitudes.

Apart from calorie imbalance, there is some evidence that at altitudes above about 5500 m there may be malabsorption of food and an increase in intestinal permeability. This effect of hypoxia on the gut will increase the weight loss. However, almost certainly, the main cause of weight loss is calorie imbalance due to anorexia.

Diet is important on treks and expeditions. There are good physiological reasons to advise a high carbohydrate, low fat diet and many, though not all climbers seem to favor this. However, palatability is more important than composition in combating the loss of appetite. Taste is dulled and most find that they want more highly flavored, spicy foods. A craving for fresh rather than preserved food develops. Fluids remain acceptable and many calories can be taken in sweet milky drinks. Supplements such as vitamins and minerals are probably not necessary if a balanced diet is taken, with the possible exception of iron supplements for pre-menopausal women.

Hydration is important at altitude in maintaining performance and fluid may only be available by melting ice or snow. Fluid is lost in expired gas though this has been overstated in the past, because the fluid conserving effect of the upper airways has been ignored. Insensible sweating (in the dry air of altitude) is probably more important.

15.1 INTRODUCTION

Anorexia and weight loss are well-known features of life at high altitude, especially extreme altitudes. The mechanism of this anorexia is not known. During the first few days after a rapid ascent, anorexia may be part of the symptomatology of acute mountain sickness (AMS), but after this, when all other symptoms of AMS are gone, anorexia may remain. Studies have suggested that the anorexia of AMS may be mediated by the hormone leptin (Techop *et al.* 1998) though others have suggested this not to be the case (Zaccaria *et al.* 2004). Other appetite hormones may be involved, such as cholecystokinin (Bailey *et al.* 2000). This continuing anorexia is not common below about 5000 m but is almost universal above 6000 m and becomes worse at even higher altitudes, though the severity varies considerably between individuals.

Weight loss is also common, though not inevitable, even at extreme altitudes and is largely due to the reduced energy intake consequent on the anorexia, but the possibility that other factors may contribute, such as malabsorption, is reviewed in this chapter. This chapter also considers diet at altitude and the evidence for the value of a high carbohydrate diet.

15.2 ENERGY BALANCE AT ALTITUDE

15.2.1 Energy output

Energy expenditure can be divided into three components:

- Basal metabolism during sleep and lying or sitting quietly
- Energy expenditure during periods of activity
- Food-induced energy expenditure.

The metabolic rate during basal conditions is the basal metabolic rate (BMR) while during activity, the active metabolic rate may be increased up to many times the BMR during maximal exercise. Mountaineers hardly ever use maximal work rate in climbing. Their preferred up-hill climbing rate is typically about 50% of maximum (Pugh *et al.* 1964) and this occupies only a part of the total time out 'climbing'; the rest being resting, walking down hill, etc. Any periods of intense activity are usually of short duration so that under normal conditions it is the BMR that is the largest component of daily energy expenditure. This is determined mainly by body size or more exactly the fat-free mass. Food-induced energy expenditure is the energy required to digest the food eaten and is about 10% of the energy intake on a normal mixed diet.

BASAL METABOLIC RATE AT ALTITUDE

Nair *et al.* (1971) found that after a week at 3300 m the BMR was elevated by about 12%. Exposure to cold as well as hypoxia (in a second group of subjects) made no difference to this effect compared with hypoxia alone. By week 2, BMR was back to control values and was below control by week 3. Cold exposure at this time resulted in elevation of BMR to above sea level values by week 5 and it remained elevated a week after return to sea level. Butterfield *et al.* (1992) found BMR to be elevated by 27% on day 2 at Pikes Peak (4300 m) in Colorado. The BMR then decreased over the next few days to plateau at 117% compared with sea level by day 10. The metabolism of a group of fit women was studied at 4300 m by Mawson *et al.* (2000). The BMR was elevated after 3 days at altitude but had returned to sea level values by day 6. However, the energy requirements remained 6% elevated above control values giving rise to an apparent 'energy requirement excess' of about 670 MJ day^{-1} while at high altitude. They also found that the phase of the menstrual cycle had no effect on energy requirement at altitude. Lippl *et al.* (2010) found BMR to be elevated by 15% in 20 obese subjects after 14 days at an altitude of 2650 m.

After acclimatization, BMR measured at 5800 m was found to be elevated by about 10% in subjects who had been at altitude for 82–113 days (Gill and Pugh 1964). It is likely that BMR rises again if subjects climb to altitudes to which they are not acclimatized and we have no data on BMR at altitudes above 6000 m when weight loss becomes even more rapid, but its elevation might well be a factor.

Basal metabolic rate was found to be high at altitude in altitude residents (Ladakhis and Sherpas) compared with lowlanders and with predicted values (Gill and Pugh 1964; Nair *et al.* 1971). This elevation of BMR remained even when allowance was made for the fact that these people generally have less fat in their body composition. Picon-Reategui (1961) also reported elevated BMR in Andean miners at 4540 m. The mechanism for this rise in BMR is uncertain. Fecal and urinary excretion of energy nitrogen and volatile acids are not altered in the early days at altitude (Butterfield *et al.* 1992). There is an increase in sympathetic activity at this time (section 16.6) and the finding that this increase in metabolic rate can be inhibited by a beta-blocker (Moore *et al.* 1987) suggests it is a likely factor. Increased thyroid activity may also play a part, especially in the longer-term elevation of BMR (section 16.7).

ACTIVITY ENERGY EXPENDITURE AT ALTITUDE

Work, in absolute terms, requires the same oxygen intake at altitude as at sea level until near-maximum work rate is reached (Pugh *et al.* 1964; West *et al.* 1983c; Wolfel *et al.* 1991; Levett *et al.* 2011). At altitude the maximum work rate is reduced (Chapter 12) and all activity seems disproportionately fatiguing. At 8000 m, even rolling over in a sleeping bag demands a great effort. Thus, energy expenditure for normal activities of daily living might be expected to be reduced at extreme altitude. Another fact of life at extreme altitudes is that often the only warm place is a sleeping bag and much of the 24 hours

of the day is spent lying down. However, the increased work of breathing has the opposite effect, as does the increase in BMR, so that the daily energy expenditure is probably about the same as, or slightly above that at sea level (see below). At intermediate altitudes (2500–4500 m), although maximum work rate is reduced, energy expenditure on normal daily activities of short duration is probably not much altered. For longer-term work such as hill climbing, much will depend upon the degree of acclimatization and fitness. Pugh *et al.* (1964) found V_{O_2} intake on climbers climbing at their 'preferred' rate to decline very little up to about 5000 m (Fig. 12.1). However, the overall requirement for energy to maintain body weight increased from 13.22 MJ at sea level to 15.64 MJ a day at 4300 m due to the increase in BMR (Butterworth *et al.* 1992).

Before about 1990 it had been impossible to measure energy expenditure over long periods, but a doubly labeled water technique was then developed which made this possible, though expensive. Water is labeled with both deuterium and ^{18}O. The deuterium is eliminated as water while the oxygen is eliminated as both water and carbon dioxide. Thus carbon dioxide production can be calculated from the different elimination rates (Schoeller and van Santen 1982; Coward 1991). Using this technique, Westerterp *et al.* (1992) found average daily energy expenditure in the Alps (2500–4800 m) to be 15.7 MJ and on Mount Everest (5300–8848 m) it was not significantly different at 13.6 MJ. Very similar daily results were obtained in the 1992 British Winter Everest Expedition of 11.7–15.4 MJ (Travis *et al.* 1993). Pulfrey and Jones (1996), using the same technique at altitudes of 5900–8046 m, found the very high mean values of 19.4 MJ day^{-1} and a negative energy balance of 5.1 MJ day^{-1}. Reynolds *et al.* (1999) found the same high mean value of 20.6 MJ day^{-1} above base camp with a dietary intake of only 10.5 MJ , giving a deficit of 10 MJ day^{-1}! On the other hand, in a chamber experiment simulating an ascent of Everest over 31 days (Operation Everest III), there was a small reduction in energy expenditure from a mean of 13.6 in normoxia to 13.3 and 12.1 MJ day^{-1} in the early and late phases of the study (Westerterp *et al.* 2000). This suggests that hypoxia per se does not elevate BMR sufficiently to balance the effect of reduced daily activity in hypoxic subjects confined to a chamber, whereas on a mountaineering expedition high energy outputs and large calorie deficits can be expected.

15.2.2 Energy intake and caloric balance

Up to about 4500 m, people who have acclimatized have normal appetites and normal food intake (Consolazio *et al.* 1968). Above 6000 m, most climbers experience anorexia. This tends to become more pronounced the longer one stays at these altitudes. Climbers complain about the food available and feel that the preserved nature of food increases the anorexia and reduces their intake. There are few data on actual calorie intake under these circumstances. Those that there are, rely on diary cards and estimates of portion size. On Cho Oyu in Nepal in 1952 food eaten at between 5250 and 6750 m was only about 13.4 MJ a day compared with 17.6 MJ on the march out, and on Everest in 1953, above 7250 m, the intake was only about 6.3 MJ (Pugh and Band 1953). On the Silver Hut Expedition (1960–61), in four climbers at 5800 m whose living conditions were excellent and where a good variety and quantity of food was available, a daily intake of 12.6–13.4 MJ day^{-1} was estimated (Pugh 1962a). Boyer and Blume (1984) reported that on the American Medical Expedition to Everest (AMREE) in 1981, over 3 days, four subjects had a mean intake of 9.34 MJ at 6300 m compared with 12.5 MJ at sea level. Dinmore *et al.* (1994) found intakes similar during the march in (1500–2000 m) and above 5500 m (10.8 and 10.3 MJ). However, Westerterp *et al.* (1992) and Travis *et al.* (1993) estimated intakes high on Everest of 7.5 MJ and 8.6 MJ, respectively, indicating the expected reduction in intake above 6300 m.

Clearly, high on major mountains (above 6000 m), when actively climbing, it is not possible to maintain caloric balance even when acclimatized. Westerterp *et al.* (1994) on Mount Sajama (6542 m) in Bolivia found an energy deficit of 3.5MJ day^{-1} in 10 subjects camped on the summit for 21 days. The average weight loss was 4.9 kg (1.6 kg week^{-1}), 74% of it being due to loss of fat. In Everest climbers studied by Westerterp *et al.* (1992) there was a daily negative balance of 5.7 MJ. Clearly, more studies using the labeled water technique are needed to answer the question of whether acclimatized subjects can maintain energy balance at intermediate altitudes (4500–6000 m) when semi-sedentary.

15.3 WEIGHT LOSS ON ALTITUDE EXPEDITIONS

15.3.1 Weight loss on the march out

Most climbing and trekking groups experience weight loss in the initial 1–3 weeks of an expedition, even when walking below 3000 m. This is probably due to the change in lifestyle for most subjects from an urban semi-sedentary existence to the more active lifestyle of walking 16 km (10 miles) a day with some considerable ascents and descents. In addition, gastrointestinal infections are common.

Boyer and Blume (1984) found that 13 AMREE members, during the march out to the Everest region, lost an average of 2 kg (range 0–6 kg). Those with the highest percentage of body fat to start with lost most weight, the correlation being significant; 70% of this weight loss was due to loss of fat. Two subjects with less than 13% of body fat lost no weight. Dinmore *et al.* (1994) similarly found an average loss of 1.3 kg during the first week of trekking but only a further 0.5 kg in the next week.

Weight loss during this phase of an expedition or trek can be considered as shedding unnecessary fat.

15.3.2 Weight loss at altitude

ANOREXIA

On first arrival at altitude, AMS may cause anorexia and vomiting with resultant weight loss, though usually the duration is not long enough to do this. Also, fluid may be retained and subjects with AMS often gain weight (Hackett *et al.* 1982). Consolazio *et al.* (1972) found a small gain in weight on the first day at altitude followed by a loss of weight of about 1 kg over the next 5 days at 4300 m.

The mechanism of the anorexia as a symptom of AMS is not clear. A few humoral factors which are known to affect appetite or satiety have been investigated.

LEPTIN

Leptin is a hormone which suppresses appetite. The leptin gene is induced by HIF-1 (hypoxia-inducible factors). In subjects taken to 4559 m by helicopter, Tschop *et al.* (1998) found that the leptin levels were raised and in those who complained of anorexia levels were higher than those with no loss of appetite (Fig. 15.1). This work suggested that leptin might be involved in the mechanism of appetite loss at altitude, but some more recent studies have found a

reduction of leptin levels at altitude (Bailey *et al.* 2004; Vats *et al.* 2004; Zaccaria *et al.* 2004). Kelly *et al.* (2010) found a reduced leptin response to a 75-g dose of glucose in acute hypoxia compared to normoxia in a laboratory study. Zaccaria *et al.* (2004) found no correlation between leptin levels and AMS scores in the first few days after arrival at 5050 m. However, two further studies did find an increase (Shukla *et al.* 2005; Lippl *et al.* 2010). The latter study was in obese subjects at an altitude of 2600 m. The increase was maintained for 4 weeks after descent to low altitude. Smith *et al.* (2001) found no change at altitudes of 4000, 4750 and 5300 m. Leptin release is influenced by a number of factors other than hypoxia and these may be confounding factors in some field studies. As a recent review article summarizes, 'Exposure to altitude is usually accompanied by increased activity levels, weight loss, altered hydration, cold exposure, sympathetic activation and altered sleep patterns, all of which are potential modulators of leptin' (Sierra-Johnson *et al.* 2008).

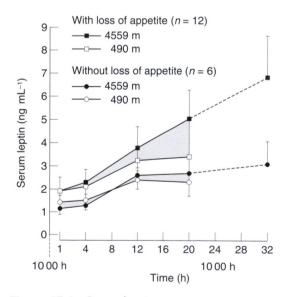

Figure 15.1   Serum leptin concentrations at 490 and 4559 m (Capanna Margherita) in 18 subjects with and without loss of appetite. The increase in leptin from low to high altitude (area between curves) was significant for subjects with loss of appetite ($p = 0.008$) but not for those with no appetite loss ($p = 0.35$). (From Tschop *et al.* (1998) with permission.)

CHOLECYSTOKININ, GHRELIN AND NEURO-PEPTIDE Y

Apart from leptin there is now a whole list of new hormones, neurotransmitters and receptors which are thought to influence appetite. A few of these have been assayed in subjects going to altitude. Cholecystokinin induces a sense of satiety. It is increased by exercise. Bailey *et al.* (2000) found significantly elevated resting cholecystokinin levels in subjects who had AMS on arrival at 5100 m compared with those without AMS. Ghrelin is an appetite-stimulating peptide produced in the stomach (Wren *et al.* 2001). Shukla *et al.* (2005) found ghrelin levels to be reduced by 30% in subjects at an altitude of 4300 m compared with baseline levels. Neuropeptide Y (NPY) is another peptide affecting appetite but Vats *et al.* (2004) found no significant change in NPY levels in subjects at 3600 and 4580 m. These results should be considered as preliminary and clearly more work is needed to try to elucidate the mechanisms involved in the loss of appetite in both AMS before acclimatization and, at higher altitudes, the increasing aversion to food after acclimatization.

ADIPONECTIN AND ACYLATION-STIMULATING PROTEIN

Adiponectin is, like leptin, an adipose tissue secreted hormone, with effects on glucose metabolism and possibly appetite. Two recent studies have measured this hormone (among others) in human subjects at altitude. Barnholt et al. (2006) measured levels in two groups of subjects on Pikes Peak (4300 m). One group ate a diet adequate to maintain their weight. The other had a restricted diet and lost weight. They found no change in levels of adiponectin in either group. Smith et al. (2011) studied climbers on an expedition to Huyana Potosi (6088 m) in Bolivia. They collected samples at sea level and at altitudes up to 5300 m. They found increased levels of adiponectin at altitude.

Acylation-stimulating protein, also produced in adipose tissue, may play a role in weight loss. It regulates the storage of triglycerides in fat cells. Smith et al. (2011) found levels to be significantly increased at altitude.

GASTROINTESTINAL BLOOD FLOW

Eating increases gastrointestinal blood flow. If at altitude this response is blunted, it might cause anorexia. This possibility was tested in a study by Kalson et al. (2010) who used ultrasound to measure velocity and vessel diameter of the hepatic portal vein in 12 subjects before and after a meal at sea level and various altitudes up to 3767 m. They found increased flow at altitude but the increase in post-prandial blood flow was still maintained. This suggests that inadequate increase in blood flow to the gut is not a cause of altitude anorexia.

WEIGHT LOSS AFTER ACCLIMATIZATION

After acclimatization, weight loss is usually seen only above about 5000 m. Dinmore et al. (1994) found an average loss of 3.9 kg during 2 weeks' climbing above 5000 m. On the 1992 British Winter Everest Expedition a mean weight loss of 5 kg was observed above 5400 m out of a total loss of 7.8 kg (Travis et al. 1993). Figure 15.2 shows the crucial effect of altitude on body weight on one well-acclimatized subject.

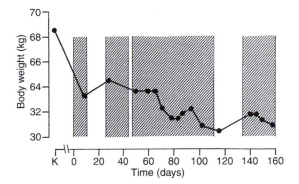

Figure 15.2 Record of body weight of one subject during the Silver Hut Expedition 1960–61. After the march out from Kathmandu (K) and the initial period of preparation, he was in residence at 5800 m (hatched areas) or at base camp at 4500 m. Note the loss of weight at 5800 m but weight gain during two breaks at 4500 m.

The combined effects of the march out and early residence at the Silver Hut, at 5800 m, produced a weight loss of 5.3 kg. Thereafter, during time spent at the Silver Hut the subject lost weight steadily at a weekly rate of just under 400 g a week but, on two occasions, on descent to altitudes of 4000–4500 m, he began to gain weight. Most subjects in the Silver Hut lost between 0.5 and 1.5 kg week^{-1} (Pugh 1962a).

Rai et al. (1975) found no weight loss in their subjects living at 3500–4700 m, even though they were working quite hard at road building and digging. Indeed, on a high fat diet (232 g daily) they actually gained an average of 1.4 kg during 3 weeks at 4700 m. Butterfield et al. (1992) also found that it was possible to attenuate weight loss at 4300 m by increasing dietary intake in proportion to the increase in BMR. However, at advanced base camp (6300 m) in the Western Cwm on Everest most subjects lost weight. Boyer and Blume (1984) documented this weight loss as an average of 4 kg (range 0–8 kg) over a mean of 47 days in 13 subjects. Again, there was considerable individual variation in the amount of weight lost which correlated with initial percentage of body fat. Boyer and Blume also found that Sherpas, who averaged only half as much body fat as the Western climbers, lost no weight during the time spent above base camp, mostly at or above 6300 m (see also section 15.9).

A possible reason for differences in weight loss response to altitude is the athletic fitness of subjects. Westerterp (2001), in a review of the limits to sustainable human metabolic rate, points out that whereas normal, healthy, untrained men, at sea level, can sustain a physical activity level (PAL) of about 1.5 times their average daily metabolic rate, trained endurance athletes can sustain a PAL of 3.0–4.5 without losing weight! This they do by increasing their food intake enormously, especially of carbohydrates. In the case of Scandinavian athletes studied, this was by frequent meals and the use of high energy carbohydrate drinks. An alternative strategy seems to be used by Sherpas and Nepali porters, accustomed to long-term high energy expenditure. For logistical reasons they can only eat two meals a day (they have to stop, light a fire and cook) but Westerners are impressed at the huge quantities of rice or tsampa that they can put away at a sitting.

Women seem to lose less weight than men do. Hannon et al. (1976) found their female subjects lost an average of only 1.8% of body weight during 7 days at 4300 m whereas studies, previously reported, of men at this altitude had found losses of 3.5 and 5.0%. Collier et al. (1997b) found changes in body mass index at Everest Base Camp (5340 m) over a median of 15 days: 22 men lost 110 g m^{-2} day^{-1} compared with 20 g m^{-2} day^{-1} in eight women, a significant difference ($p = 0.03$). The seven male climbers who climbed to between 7100 and 8848 m, using oxygen at extreme altitude, all lost weight, averaging 150 g m^{-2} day^{-1}. The one female climber who spent 4 nights above 8000 m without supplementary oxygen lost no weight between leaving and arriving back at base camp!

15.3.3 Weight loss in chamber experiments

It could be argued that some of the weight loss on expeditions is due to cold, limited food supplies and the increased energy expenditure of climbing. This may often be the case, although not so in a number of the studies quoted above. Chamber studies avoid this potential criticism; most are of too short a duration to be relevant, but Operation

Everest I and II, studies of 40 days' duration, showed that, despite good environmental conditions of temperature, humidity and diet ad libitum, subjects lost weight (Rose et al. 1988). In Operation Everest II the six subjects lost an average of 7.4 kg during the 38 days of observations as they ascended the simulated height of the summit of Everest. Energy intake fell by 43% and, interestingly, the subjects chose a diet that resulted in a reduction of carbohydrate from 62 to 53% of the total diet. The authors considered that the weight loss could not be accounted for totally by the reduction in intake and considered that malabsorption or increase in energy expenditure due to increased BMR must be invoked (section 15.2.1). The exercise taken in this chamber study would probably be less than on a climbing expedition. On Operation Everest III (Comex '97) there was a similar loss of weight, averaging 5 kg during the 31-day chamber study taking eight subjects to the simulated height of the Everest summit. Intake was reduced by 4.2 MJ day^{-1} due to subjects feeling satiated sooner (Westerterp-Plantenga 1999).

15.4 BODY COMPOSITION AND WEIGHT LOSS

Assuming much of the weight loss is due to negative energy balance, a simplistic view would be that the body would use up fat stores first and then start using protein from the lean body mass, principally the muscles. However, even with a most carefully controlled diet aimed at fat reduction, it is never possible to lose fat exclusively and retain all the lean body mass (Garrow 1987). The best that can be achieved is that, of the weight lost, 75% is fat and 25% lean body tissue. This compares with the situation during a complete fast when fat and lean body tissues are lost in roughly equal proportions (Forbes and Drenick 1979).

Boyer and Blume (1984) used skin-fold measurements to estimate body fat. There are uncertainties about the absolute results of this method, but relative changes probably can be reliable. They found that of the average 2 kg loss during the march out to base camp, 70% was due to loss of fat, which is a figure close to the most efficient muscle sparing regimen available. However, above 5400 m, mainly at or above 6300 m, of the 4 kg average weight loss only 27% was due to loss of fat and 73% due to loss of lean body tissue, despite the fact that subjects still had at least 10% of their body weight as fat. This percentage loss of muscle, greater than that seen in starvation, suggests that at this altitude hypoxia may be interfering with protein metabolism (section 15.5).

In the Operation Everest II study (Rose *et al.* 1988) there was loss of 2.5 kg of fat (1.6% body weight) and 4.9 kg of lean body tissue. Computed tomographic examination of the thigh showed a 17% loss of muscle and a 34% loss of subcutaneous fat. Although loss of muscle mass must be a disadvantage, one beneficial effect is to increase the density of muscle capillaries. This is because the loss of muscle mass is achieved by reducing fiber diameter rather than number, with the number of capillaries per fiber remaining constant. Thus the intercapillary distance decreases with an improvement in oxygenation of the muscles (Chapter 11). Evidence in support of this speculation is found in the work of Oelz *et al.* (1986), who studied muscle biopsies from six elite climbers at sea level some months after return from altitude. It was found that their muscle fibers were smaller and the capillary density greater than controls. Another explanation for the loss of muscle mass is that with decreased overall activity at altitude there is some disuse atrophy which would similarly reduce muscle fiber diameter. These two explanations are not mutually exclusive. Results of muscle biopsy studies during Operation Everest II (MacDougall *et al.* 1991) showed similar histological changes in muscle fiber size. (Chapter 11 contains a fuller discussion of changes in muscle histology.)

15.5 INTESTINAL ABSORPTION AND HYPOXIA

In view of the continued weight loss at altitudes above 5000 m with, in some cases, adequate intake and reduced energy output, the possibility of malabsorption and malutilization of food must be considered. Pugh (1962a) reported that members of the Silver Hut Expedition noted that stools tended to be greasy and bulky, suggesting possible steatorrhea due to malabsorption of fat.

As mentioned in section 15.3.2, weight loss is not a feature of living at altitudes below about 5000 m, and the fact that most altitude research is conducted below this level may explain why so little work has been carried out on the topic of intestinal absorption. Other reasons for the neglect of this field may be that the methods involved are either too sophisticated for easy use in the field (e.g. absorption of radioactive materials), or are unattractive to investigators (e.g. fecal collection, liquidization and aliquot sampling, etc.). Finally, few altitude physiologists have a background in gastroenterology.

15.5.1 Carbohydrate absorption and hypoxia

Milledge (1972) studied patients who were hypoxic either because of congenital heart disease or chronic obstructive lung disease. Xylose absorption decreased with decreasing arterial oxygen saturation (Fig. 15.3).

On relieving the hypoxia by surgery in the cardiac cases, or by 13 hours of supplementary oxygen breathing in the respiratory cases, there was improvement in xylose absorption in all

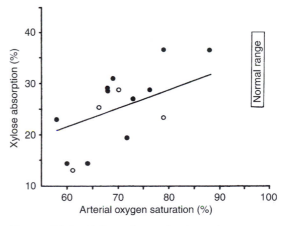

Figure 15.3 Xylose absorption in patients hypoxic because of either congenital cyanotic heart disease (solid symbols), or chronic respiratory disease (open symbols), plotted against their arterial oxygen saturation.

patients. The xylose absorption test has a rather uncertain lower normal limit, especially in a population in which intestinal parasitic infection is common (the study was carried out in southern India). However, the results suggest that below an arterial saturation of about 70%, absorption was impaired (Fig. 15.3); improvement on relief of hypoxia supports this view.

Pritchard and Lane (1974) did not find malabsorption in 26 patients with chronic obstructive lung disease. However, the lowest arterial Po_2 was 48 mmHg, equivalent to about 78% saturation. Chesner et al. (1987) found no malabsorption of xylose in 11 subjects up to 4846 m. However, 60-minute plasma xylose concentrations were reduced in subjects who ascended to 5600 m, confirming that absorption is not affected until hypoxia is severe. Boyer and Blume (1984), who studied subjects at 6300 m, found xylose absorption decreased by 24% in six out of seven subjects, compared with sea level controls.

However, absorption measured by xylose has the drawback that the result is influenced by factors such as gastric emptying time, absorption area, intestinal transit and renal function. Dinmore et al. (1994) used a double carbohydrate test; the two nonmetabolized carbohydrates used undergo different forms of mediated absorption but are otherwise subject to the same external influences which cancel out when results are expressed as a ratio (Menzies 1984). D-xylose is absorbed by passive mediated transport, whereas 3-O-methyl-D-glucose is absorbed by active mediated, sodium-dependent transport. Dinmore et al. found that at 6300 m there was 34% decrease in D-xylose (Fig. 15.4) and a 15% decrease in 3-O-methyl-D-glucose absorption. The ratio was consistently decreased at altitude and in a subsequent study the 60-minute serum xylose/3-O-methyl-D-glucose ratio was 17% lower at 5400 m than at sea level (Travis et al. 1993). These more sophisticated studies therefore support the hypothesis that at these high altitudes carbohydrate absorption is impaired.

15.5.2 Fat absorption and hypoxia

Rai et al. (1975) found no malabsorption for fat at 4700 m, neither did Chesner et al. (1987)

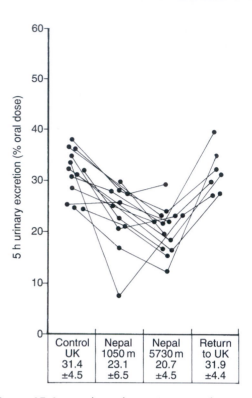

Figure 15.4 D-xylose absorption tested in a group of climbers at sea level (UK), at altitudes indicated in Nepal and after return to the UK (with mean and SD values at each location). (Data from Dinmore et al. (1994).)

at 3100 m and 4800 m. Imray et al. (1992), using the ^{14}C-triolein breath test, found no malabsorption of fat at 5500 m on Aconcagua in Argentina, and Butterfield et al. (1992) found no increase in fecal excretion of volatile fatty acids at 4300 m. However, Boyer and Blume (1984) found fat absorption decreased by 49% at 6300 m compared with sea level results in three acclimatized subjects.

15.5.3 Protein absorption and hypoxia

Kayser et al. (1992) measured protein absorption using urinary and fecal ^{15}N excretion after ingestion of ^{15}N-labeled soya protein. They found no reduction in absorption in subjects after 3 weeks at 5000 m.

15.5.4 Summary: malabsorption at altitude

There is no evidence of malabsorption up to an altitude of about 5000 m and this has been confirmed by measurements of fecal energy excretion which have shown that 96% of energy intake is assimilated (Kayser *et al.* 1992), a normal sea level value for subjects on a Western low residue diet. This test of overall food digestibility is measured over a 3-day period; the total energy values of both food and feces are measured in a bomb calorimeter and the energy of the food digested expressed as a percentage of the food eaten. Above 5000 m there may be malabsorption of carbohydrate, fat and protein although the evidence is not compelling. There is always the possibility that intestinal infections, at the time of the study or in the previous few days or weeks, may have caused some malabsorption since many of these field studies were undertaken in countries where such infections are all too common. Westerterp *et al.* (1994) on Mount Sajama (6542 m) found that gross energy digestibility decreased to 85%, indicating some malabsorption, though most of the weight loss was attributable to low food intake. On the other hand, in Operation Everest III, Westerterp *et al.* (2000) found a normal energy digestibility of 94% at 7000 m simulated altitude.

It now seems likely that malabsorption, due to hypoxia, if it exists, is only a minor factor in the weight loss seen at altitude which is predominantly due to a negative energy balance.

15.6 PROTEIN METABOLISM AT ALTITUDE

The obvious muscle wasting seen especially in climbers returning from extreme altitude prompts the question of whether hypoxia affects protein metabolism directly. There are very few data on this topic in humans.

Consolazio *et al.* (1968) studied protein balance at altitude and found no difference between subjects there and at sea level, but the altitude station was Pikes Peak (4300 m), below the crucial height at which continued weight loss is observed.

Rennie *et al.* (1983) studied the effect of acute hypoxia in a chamber (equivalent altitude 4550 m) on leucine metabolism in forearm muscles. They found that acute hypoxia resulted in a net loss of amino acids from the muscles, probably due to a fall in muscle protein synthesis. If this finding can be extrapolated to the situation of chronic hypoxia at altitudes of above 5000–6000 m (where hypoxia in acclimatized subjects would be similar to that in the above study), then it provides a further contributing factor to the loss of muscle mass described above. It has been suggested that protein or branched-chain amino acid (BCAA) supplementation might be helpful in reducing the muscle loss. Bigard and colleagues (1996b) gave one group of skiers BCAA supplementation while participating in six sessions of ski mountaineering at altitudes of 2500–4100 m. They found that they did no better than a control group given 98% carbohydrate supplement with respect to changes in body composition or performance of isometric contraction. However, body weight loss was possibly less in the BCAA group. In another study (Bigard *et al.* 1996a) they found that adding protein to the diet of growing rats did not affect the depression of muscle growth caused by altitude.

A study of 8–9-year-old children resident at altitude (La Paz, 3600 m) by San Miguel *et al.* (2002) found that protein absorption or utilization was significantly reduced as compared with a group of children at low altitude. The high altitude group had only oxidized 19% of the casein after 6 hours, compared with 25% in the low altitude group ($p < 0.02$). The method used was ingestion of ^{13}C-labeled leucine incorporated into casein. Expired $^{13}CO_2$ was then analyzed. However, this method does not distinguish between reduced absorption and increased utilization of protein.

15.7 WATER BALANCE AT ALTITUDE

There is no doubt that dehydration was common among early high altitude climbers, and one of Pugh's contributions to the success of the 1953 Everest Expedition was his insistence on the importance of planning for adequate fluid intake of climbers high on the mountain. Pugh writes:

> For men climbing seven hours a day [at altitude] 3–5 litres of fluid, in the form of beverages and soup, were required in order to maintain a urine output of 1.5 l/day. This high fluid requirement was partly explained by the high rate of fluid loss from the lungs associated with increased ventilation and the dry cold air, and partly by sweating.
>
> (Pugh 1964a)

(But see section 15.7.1 below.) Since then all those involved with advice to trekkers and mountaineers have emphasized the importance of adequate hydration. Dehydration certainly impairs performance and it has been suggested that it may be a risk factor for AMS (see Chapter 19). While not denying the importance of hydration, it is possible to overstate the case and be too enthusiastic about pushing fluids, especially electrolyte-free water which can lead to hyponatremia. Cases have been described in hot environments (Backer *et al.* 1993, four cases), in a cold environment (Zafren 1998) and in the mountains (Basnyat *et al.* 2000a). At altitude this condition is easily misdiagnosed as AMS.

Water balance is the difference between intake and output of water. Water intake may well be restricted because of unavailability of water especially at high altitude where it can only be obtained by melting snow or ice; hence the need to plan for adequate fuel to achieve adequate fluid intake. Water is also derived from metabolism of food as well as the water content of food, so if food intake is reduced at altitude, as it often is, that will increase the requirement for fluids. The sensation of thirst is probably dulled by hypoxia. This has been shown in rats to be the case (Jones *et al.* 1981).

Fluid output is the sum of fluid loss in urine and feces and insensible loss (Jones *et al.* 1981). The latter consists of loss by sweat and respiratory loss. There may be considerable sweat loss. Although the air is cold, climbers are dressed for it and the solar load may be high because of the reduced filtering effect of air and the effect of reflection of heat from snow. Because the air is

so dry, sweat evaporates very efficiently, and the climber is unaware that he is sweating, perhaps profusely. Of course, in really cold conditions sweat loss may be minimal. The effect of altitude hypoxia alone on insensible water loss was found to be unchanged from control conditions in the chamber study Operation Everest III (Westerterp *et al.* 2000).

15.7.1 Respiratory water loss and its calculation

As mentioned, it has been assumed that hyperventilating in the cold dry air of high altitude must result in considerable respiratory water loss. Respiratory water loss is the loss in the expired gas minus any water in the inspired air. The latter depends upon the temperature and relative humidity. At sea level typical indoor conditions of 22°C and 50% humidity the inspired water vapor pressure ($PI,_{H_2O}$) is 10 mmHg and each liter of inspired air contains 10.6 mg of water. At altitude both temperature and humidity are low and the water content of the air is close to zero. On inspiration air is warmed and wetted so that by the time the gas reaches the alveoli it is fully saturated and warmed to body temperature. The $PI,_{H_2O}$ is 47 mmHg and the water content 49.7 mg L^{-1}. On the assumption that expired gas is at body temperature and fully saturated there would be an estimated net loss of 49.7 mg of water for each liter expired, when dry air is breathed, or 39.1 mg L^{-1} under typical indoor conditions. At rest, assuming a ventilation of 6 L min^{-1}, the loss would be 234.7 mg min^{-1} or 338 mL day^{-1} and if the air was completely dry, 298.1 mg min^{-1} or 429 mL day^{-1}.

Exercise, by increasing the minute ventilation, will increase this figure. From studies of daylong (8 hours) hill walking at altitudes up to 1000 m, total 24-hour oxygen consumptions of 596 and 928 L have been reported for rest and exercise days, respectively (Williams *et al.* 1979). This represents a total ventilation of about 14 900 and 23 200 L in 24 hours and respiratory loss of 584 and 909 mL water.

At altitude, the increased ventilation and dry air will increase these figures. With a barometric pressure at half an atmosphere (about 5800 m) the acclimatized subject roughly doubles his ventilation both at rest and at sub-maximal work rates so that on these assumptions the 24-hour respiratory losses work out at 859 mL on rest days and 1.718 L on climbing days. If we consider a climber spending a day climbing above 8000 m and assume an average minute ventilation over the 24 hours of 40 L min^{-1} (an extreme value), the water loss would be 2.863 L.

However, it has been known for many years (though often forgotten and rediscovered) that the temperature of expired gas is below body temperature and probably is not fully saturated with water at even this lower temperature (Loewy and Gerhartz 1914; Burch 1945; Webb 1951; Ferrus *et al.* 1984). Therefore the actual respiratory water loss will be less than figures calculated using our starting assumptions.

As cold dry air is inhaled the mucosal surfaces are cooled and partially dried. During expiration the temperature of the initial portion of the expirate, the dead-space gas, is well below body temperature and less than fully saturated. The next portion of the expirate leaving the alveoli is fully saturated and at body temperature. It warms and wets the mucosal surfaces of the upper airways but is itself cooled and loses water to the airways surface. The final portion of the expirate may or may not be expired at body temperature, fully saturated, depending on the inspired gas conditions and respiratory factors. In either case the total, mixed expirate will be well below body temperature and not fully saturated.

Ferrus *et al.* (1984) have studied a number of factors which affect the temperature and water saturation of mixed expired gas. These include:

- Temperature of inspired air
- Partial pressure of inspired water
- Respiratory frequency
- Tidal volume
- Density of inspired gas.

They found that the mass of water per liter of expired gas was affected by all the above, although tidal volume and gas density have only a small effect. They proposed an equation linking them which allows a calculation of how much

respiratory loss is saved by this mechanism under a variety of conditions. The lower the inspired temperature and the higher the respiratory frequency (and ventilation) the greater the saving in respiratory water loss. Thus if we consider the extreme case (above) of the climber above 8000 m with a calculated respiratory water loss of almost 3 L, and apply the Ferrus equation, we find the loss reduced to just under a liter, a saving of 65%. For full details of such calculations and their effect of respiratory water loss see Milledge (1992).

In conclusion, water loss in the expired gas is not great. Under extreme conditions of exercise at extreme altitude, when minute ventilation is very high and when water loss is greatest, the conservation of water has its greatest effect. This is due to the expirate being at a lower than body temperature and less than fully saturated. Even assuming an average ventilation of 40 L min^{-1} for 24 hours in dry air at $-15°C$, the respiratory water loss is calculated to be less than 1 liter suggesting that water loss due to sweating is more important than respiratory loss.

15.8 DIET FOR HIGH ALTITUDE

Views on diets (not only at altitude) are strongly held, often the strength of opinion being inversely related to the strength of scientific evidence.

15.8.1 High carbohydrate diet

There is sometimes a preference among climbers for a high carbohydrate, low fat diet at altitude and there are good physiological reasons for this. Figure 15.5 shows the basis for advising a high carbohydrate diet, which moves the respiratory quotient (RQ) from 0.7, if one uses fat exclusively for energy, to 1.0 when carbohydrate (or protein) is used.

The result of such a change of RQ is that for any given PA,CO_2 the PA,O_2 is increased. In the case illustrated in Fig. 15.5, the subject is considered to be at 5800 m when the barometric pressure is half that at sea level and the PI,O_2 is 70 mmHg. PA,CO_2 is assumed to be 23 mmHg. With an RQ of 0.7 the PA,O_2 would be 37.2 mmHg, whereas with an RQ

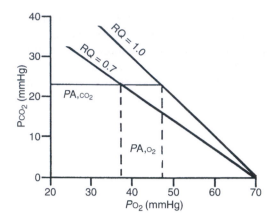

Figure 15.5 Oxygen–carbon dioxide diagram showing the effect of the respiratory quotient (RQ) on alveolar P_{O_2} at a given P_{A,O_2}. By changing from an RQ of 0.7 (the RQ when utilizing fat) to 1.0 (the RQ when using carbohydrate) the P_{A,O_2} is increased from 37.2 to 47.0 mmHg.

of 1.0 it would be 47 mmHg; this is an important gain in arterial oxygen saturation. This represents the extreme case of a switch from pure fat to pure carbohydrate utilization, but even a partial switch in this direction would be helpful to the climber at extreme altitudes.

Consolazio *et al.* (1969) compared a normal with a high carbohydrate diet in two groups of subjects at 4300 m. The performance of the group on a high carbohydrate diet was superior in that they had a greater endurance for heavy work, though $\dot{V}_{O_{2,max}}$ was not significantly better. Also, the symptoms of AMS were less in the high carbohydrate group.

A laboratory study confirms this suggestion. Subjects were given either water or a glucose solution after a period of monitored normoxia. They were then monitored during hypoxia ($F_{I_{O_2}}$ 12.8%). CO_2 production and ventilation was increased and the $S_{A_{O_2}}$ was increased by 4% (Golja *et al.* 2008).

In a recent field study (Oliver *et al.* 2012), on a trek to 5192 m, 41 subjects were given either a carbohydrate energy drink supplement or placebo. In the carbohydrate supplement group, those who achieved the target intake of 3.5 g kg^{-1} showed an 18% reduction in perceived exertion on a timed trial at 5192 m and completed the trial in a time 17% faster than the placebo group.

Another reason for recommending a high carbohydrate diet is that it has been suggested that the body becomes more dependent upon glucose as a fuel at altitude after acclimatization (Brooks *et al.* 1991; Roberts *et al.* 1996). Lundby and van Hall (2002) addressed this question in subjects acutely exposed to an altitude of 4100 m and after 4 weeks' acclimatization to this altitude. When the same absolute rates of exercise were compared there was a shift towards more glucose and less free fatty acid use but this change disappeared when the same relative work rates were compared. It could be argued that, in practice, climbers at altitude are often exercising at higher relative rates than they would adopt at sea level, though lower than the same absolute work rate. Hence they would be shifting to more glucose utilization.

15.8.2 Low fat diet

Many climbers find fatty foods become distasteful at altitude, in contrast to the preference shown by Arctic and Antarctic travelers. Tilman, who was experienced in both Arctic and mountain travel, writes:

> If you do succeed in getting outside a richly concentrated food like pemmican a great effort of will is required to keep it down – absolute quiescence in a prone position and a little sugar are useful aids. Eating a large mug of pemmican soup at 27,200 feet as Peter Lloyd and I did in '38 is, I think, an unparalleled feat and shows what can be done by dogged greed
>
> (Tilman 1975)

There are good physiological reasons for a low fat diet at altitude: the effect of fat as an energy source on the RQ (as discussed above) and the possible effect of fat malabsorption on the absorption of sugars and amino acids. This fat intolerance is unfortunate because fat provides more calories weight for weight than carbohydrate or proteins.

In conclusion, the main problem of nutrition at high altitude is the deficit in energy intake due to loss of appetite. Any diet that helps climbers take in more calories is beneficial and should be encouraged.

15.8.3 Other dietary constituents

IRON

Since the red cell mass is increased at altitude it has been suggested that extra iron should be taken. Unless there is pre-existing iron deficiency the iron stores of the body and the iron content of a normal diet will be adequate. However, in pre-menopausal women there may be a degree of deficient iron stores and the addition of iron may be indicated (Richalet *et al.* 1994). A rapid response to hypoxia is an increase in intestinal iron absorption from the gut before any change in plasma iron turnover, at least in rats and mice (Hathorn 1971; Raja *et al.* 1986). Thus the iron stores of the body are replenished even before they begin to be depleted.

VITAMINS

It is common for expedition and trekking parties to take added vitamins, but although such dietary supplements probably do no harm, there is no evidence that they are needed provided that a normal, balanced diet is taken.

15.8.4 Fresh food, flavor and variety

The appetite becomes jaded at high altitude and the most common complaints on expeditions are about the drab sameness of the flavor of preserved foods. More experienced climbers tend to adopt a policy of eating local fresh foods, supplemented by the minimum of imported preserved foods. The sense of taste seems to be dulled at altitude, and Western food tastes insipid. The addition of strong flavors, such as curries and herbs, is increasingly appreciated. There is great individual variation in likes and dislikes, even more than at sea level. The wise quartermaster of an expedition will attempt to meet this by providing as wide a variety of foods and flavors as possible. However, the task is unenviable since, whatever the quartermaster provides, fellow expedition members will yearn for what is unavailable.

15.9 NUTRITION AND METABOLISM IN HIGH ALTITUDE RESIDENTS

Little work has been done on nutrition in peoples native to high altitude. There is the impression that Sherpas do better than lowland climbers with respect to weight loss, and Boyer and Blume (1984), as mentioned in section 15.3.2, documented this. There were caretakers who lived at the Aucanquilcha mine in Chile (5950 m) for 1–2 years, but have now left. Presumably they did not lose weight in the relentless way we did in the Silver Hut (5800 m), though it must be added that only a subset of miners is able to stay at this altitude indefinitely (West 1998, p. 227).

Holden *et al.* (1995) studied the cardiac metabolism of Quecha (Andean natives) and found they relied on glucose as a fuel to a greater extent than lowlanders. Hochachka *et al.* (1996) studied the metabolism of Sherpas under normoxic and hypoxic conditions. They too found that, compared to lowlanders, the Sherpas made greater use of carbohydrate substrates for cardiac function and less use of free fatty acids. This metabolic organization is advantageous in hypoxic conditions because the adenosine triphosphate yield per molecule of oxygen is 25–60% greater with glucose than with free fatty acids.

16

Endocrine and renal systems at altitude

SUMMARY

The chronic hypoxia of altitude has an effect on many endocrine systems. Among those most studied are hormones that affect the salt and water balance of the body and are involved in cardiovascular function. Exercise affects many hormonal systems and is an important activity at altitude; both altitude and exercise, therefore, need to be considered. The possible role of certain hormones in the mechanism of acute mountain sickness (AMS) has to be addressed by comparing levels in subjects with and without AMS.

Levels of anti-diuretic hormone (ADH) are not affected by altitude or exercise. Previously it seemed that AMS was not associated with changes in ADH except in cases with severe nausea when levels are elevated. However, a more recent study suggests that in AMS-resistant subjects there is a reduction in ADH levels within an hour of exposure leading to a water diuresis while AMS-susceptible subjects have a rise in ADH and water retention. After full acclimatization and at more extreme altitudes there is high osmolality with inappropriately low levels of ADH. The change

in response of ADH to osmolality with altitude acclimatization appears to be both in the slope and intercept of the response line.

The renin–angiotensin–aldosterone system is activated by exercise and, in the case of the long continued exercise involved in mountaineering, can produce sodium and some water retention. Altitude in the absence of exercise results in lower levels of aldosterone, but exercise involved with ascent to altitude results in raised levels of aldosterone.

On first arrival at altitude, corticosteroids are elevated by adrenocorticotropic hormone (ACTH) then decline to baseline levels over 5–7 days. Even in subjects who have spent some weeks above 6000 m, corticosteroid levels are normal, but one report of subjects who spent months at this altitude did show high levels.

The sympathoadrenal system is stimulated during the first few days at altitude with high levels of urinary catecholamines. These decline with acclimatization in line with the changes in resting heart rate.

Thyroid function is enhanced in humans at altitude, unlike in animals in which it is depressed by hypoxia. Because of this and the increased sympathetic activity, basal metabolic rate (BMR) is increased on going to altitude and remains elevated after acclimatization.

Insulin sensitivity is reduced on first arrival at altitude but with acclimatization insulin sensitivity becomes enhanced.

Plasma endothelin levels are raised by hypoxia in line with the raised pulmonary artery pressure and are high in high altitude pulmonary edema (HAPE) patients and subjects susceptible to HAPE.

Glucagon, growth hormone, bradykinin and the sex hormones are little affected by hypoxia except that the exercise response to growth hormone is enhanced and sex hormones tend to be decreased.

The hormone erythropoietin is discussed in Chapter 9, sections 9.2 and 9.4.

Renal function is remarkably little affected by altitude. At extreme altitude, above 6500 m, renal compensation for further respiratory alkalosis seems to be incomplete. There is an increase in microproteinuria, especially on first going to altitude, which is greater in subjects with AMS.

16.1 INTRODUCTION

Endocrinology comprises many systems controlling a great variety of bodily functions and the effect of altitude has been studied on only a fraction of these. The areas studied reflect the interests of scientists going to altitude. Thus hormones that play a part in fluid and electrolyte balance have been widely studied because of their possible relevance to acute mountain sickness (AMS) and its complications, as have thyroid hormones because of their effect on metabolic rate. Another factor in the selection of systems for study has, of course, been the availability and ease of relevant assays. This chapter surveys the principal systems studied to date, but clearly there are great areas of endocrinology in which the effects of acute and chronic hypoxia have yet to be explored.

The study of endocrinology at altitude is perfectly feasible, but attention to details of sampling, such as time of day, subject's posture, diet and exercise is required, as it is in studies at sea level.

16.2 ANTI-DIURETIC HORMONE

Anti-diuretic hormone (ADH), also known as vasopressin, is secreted by the posterior pituitary in response to a rise in plasma osmolality. It has the effect of increasing the reabsorption of water in the renal collecting ducts thus reducing the urine volume. In some animals it has an effect on the arterioles resulting in hypertension, hence its alternative name, but this effect is minimal in humans.

There is considerable evidence that ascent to altitude is associated with changes in body fluid compartments both in those with AMS and in asymptomatic subjects. Not surprisingly, therefore, investigators have studied the role of ADH in both the normal (healthy) response to hypoxia and AMS. Reports on the effect of hypoxia on ADH have given conflicting results.

16.2.1 Exercise and ADH

Williams *et al.* (1979) studied exercise in the absence of hypoxia. They studied the effect of daylong hill walking over 7 consecutive days and found no alteration in ADH concentration, despite the fact that their subjects developed peripheral (exercise) edema associated with sodium retention (section 16.3.3).

16.2.2 Acute hypoxia and ADH

Forsling and Milledge (1977) found that breathing 10–10.5% oxygen for 4 hours had no effect on ADH levels in samples taken at intervals of from 3 minutes to 4 hours of hypoxia. In a chamber experiment, where subjects were taken to an equivalent altitude of 4000 m for 14 hours, there was no significant change in ADH plasma concentration until subjects began to feel nauseated, when levels rose markedly (Forsling and Milledge 1980). Claybaugh *et al.* (1982) took subjects to various equivalent altitudes in a chamber and found an initial increase of urinary ADH at 8–12 hours of hypoxia with subsequent return to sea level values. In two subjects with AMS there was a rise in urinary excretion of ADH at 2–4 hours of hypoxia. De Angelis et al. (1996) studied 26 young pilots in a chamber at an altitude of 5000 m equivalent for 3 hours. They found a significant increase in ADH as a result of this quite severe hypoxic stress.

Loeppky et al. (2005a) studied 51 men in a chamber at 4880 m equivalent altitude over 8–12 hours and measured fluid balance, various hormones and AMS scores. They found that those with the most severe AMS compared to those with the least, had significant fluid retention with lower urine output. ADH rose in those with AMS and fell in those with little or no AMS. Thus perhaps the physiological response to acute hypoxia is a water diuresis stimulated by a fall in ADH level while those subjects who fail to lower their ADH are likely to get AMS.

Bocqueraz et al. (2004), in a chamber study of cyclists at an altitude equivalent to approximately 4200 m, found no change in ADH during 60 minutes of exercise at 50 and 75% of $V_{O_{2,max}}$.

16.2.3 Chronic hypoxia and ADH

Studies conducted in the field include one by Singh et al. (1974), who measured a number of hormones in a group of subjects who had a history of high altitude pulmonary edema (HAPE). In those who remained free of symptoms on going to altitude, there was no change in ADH concentration. In subjects who became sick, there was a tendency to higher levels but this was mainly seen after a few days at altitude and was not statistically significant. Harber et al. (1981) found no significant change in urinary ADH concentration on going to altitudes up to 5400 m; nor was there any relationship with AMS. Even in a fatal case of high altitude cerebral edema there was no significant rise in ADH. Cosby et al. (1988) found higher levels of ADH in five skiers with HAPE compared with controls at the same altitude, but the difference did not reach statistical significance. Ramirez et al. (1992) found no change in ADH with altitude.

Hackett et al. (1978) found normal levels in trekkers at 4300 m, including those with and without symptoms of AMS; the only exceptions were higher concentrations in two cases of HAPE.

The conclusion from this work would seem to be that hypoxia per se has no significant effect on ADH concentration. High values may be associated with AMS, but not all cases have high values (Claybaugh et al. 1982). Where high concentrations are found they may be an effect of AMS rather than its cause.

However, a recent large chamber study produced evidence that the ADH response to hypoxia may be important in the mechanism of AMS (Loeppky et al. 2005). These workers studied 51 subjects in a chamber at 4880 m equivalent altitude for 8–12 hours and then compared the 16 subjects most affected and 16 least affected by AMS. The non-AMS subjects showed a drop in ADH at 1 hour whereas the AMS group showed a small rise. Thereafter both groups showed a rise, the non-AMS back to baseline and the AMS to almost double baseline values. Free water clearance showed reciprocal changes. The diuresis in the non-AMS group was clearly shown and it was a water diuresis, the sodium excretion being unchanged as were levels of atrial natriuretic peptide and aldosterone. Thus the diuresis was ADH driven (a reduction in ADH level) and, by the end of the altitude exposure, resulted in a cumulative free water balance of 955 mL in the AMS group and 534 mL in the non-AMS. The water balance results were even more distinct. The AMS group had a positive balance of 1197 mL while the non-AMS had a negative balance of 724 mL, a difference of almost 2 L (p = 0.002). This suggests that the early diuresis which is ADH driven is crucial in the physiological response to hypoxia and the resistance to AMS.

This early water diuresis was also found by Hildebrandt et al. (2000) in a 90-minute chamber experiment where the effect of hypoxia (12% O_2) was studied with either iso- or poikilocapnia. It was found with both forms of hypoxia, and was not related to the hypoxic ventilatory response. Swenson et al. (1995) had earlier shown that the later sodium diuresis was correlated with hypoxic ventilatory response.

16.2.4 Responses of ADH to increased plasma osmolality

Blume *et al.* (1984) presented evidence of inappropriately low secretion of ADH at altitude. They studied 13 subjects after some weeks at 5400 m and 6300 m on Everest during the American Medical Research Expedition to Everest (AMREE) in 1981 and found ADH concentration unchanged from sea level despite a significant increase in plasma osmolality with increasing altitude. At 6300 m the serum osmolality was 302 mosm kg^{-1} compared with 290 mosm kg^{-1} at sea level (normal value 280–295 mosm kg^{-1}). An overnight dehydration test at sea level which might produce this degree of hyperosmolality would result in ADH concentrations of about 7 µUmL^{-1}, whereas subjects on Everest had a mean value of only 0.9 µUmL^{-1}; 12-hour urinary ADH showed the same lack of response. Sodium, potassium, calcium and phosphate concentrations were all modestly increased compared with sea level values. A study by Ramirez *et al.* (1992) confirmed these observations. They increased osmolality by intravenous sodium, loading a group of subjects at sea level and at altitude (3000 m). At sea level there was the expected rise in ADH but at altitude there was no significant rise. Thus, at altitude, there seems to be a failure of the osmoregulatory

mechanism. This is the converse of the clinical syndrome of inappropriate ADH secretion often associated with small cell carcinoma of the lung (Bayliss 1987). In such cases serum sodium concentration and osmolality are low but ADH secretion is inappropriately high. A later study (Ramirez *et al.* 1998) found evidence of reduced sensitivity of the kidney to ADH in acclimatized individuals and that infusion of exogenous ADH caused an increase of urinary arginine vasopressin (AVP)-sensitive water channel (aquaporin-2).

A study by Maresh *et al.* (2004) explored the response in ADH secretion to a water deprivation test at sea level, on acute altitude exposure (2 days) and more chronic exposure (20 days) on Pikes Peak (4300 m). Similar to other studies they found higher plasma osmolality at altitude but no change in baseline levels of ADH. With water deprivation the rise in ADH was greater at altitude, and more so on day 20 than at day 2 of their altitude stay, and the osmolality threshold which stimulated ADH release appeared to rise. This is shown in Fig. 16.1.

An 8-day study by Bestle *et al.* (2002) at the Capanna Margherita (4559 m) using a hypertonic saline loading test found the AVP response unchanged from sea level though they too found the set point of plasma osmolality to AVP level elevated at altitude.

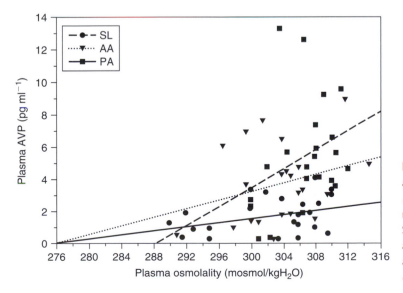

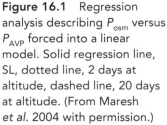

Figure 16.1   Regression analysis describing P_{osm} versus P_{AVP} forced into a linear model. Solid regression line, SL, dotted line, 2 days at altitude, dashed line, 20 days at altitude. (From Maresh *et al.* 2004 with permission.)

Those failing to achieve this may be at risk of AMS, HAPE or HACE (high altitude cerebral edema). After acclimatization the set point for plasma osmolality is reset to a higher level and the response to ADH may be increased.

16.3 RENIN–ANGIOTENSIN–ALDOSTERONE SYSTEM

This system is depicted in Fig. 16.2. Renin is released in response to a number of stimuli, including posture, exercise and, possibly, hypoxia. The mechanism common to these stimuli is sympathetic activation, and both circulating catecholamine and direct sympathetic nervous stimulation result in release of renin from the juxtaglomerular apparatus of the kidney.

Renin has no biological activity but acts on its circulating substrate (angiotensinogen), cleaving it to produce the octapeptide angiotensin I, which is also devoid of activity. Angiotensin converting enzyme (ACE), found on the luminal surface of endothelial cells, converts angiotensin I to angiotensin II by cleaving the final two amino acids. The principal site of conversion is in the rich capillary network of the lung, where nearly 90% of angiotensin I is converted to angiotensin II in a single passage. Angiotensin II is a powerful vasopressor and also acts on the cells of the adrenal cortex via a receptor mechanism to release aldosterone. Aldosterone acts on the renal tubules, promoting the reabsorption of sodium. In this way the system is important in the salt and water economy of the body, which is why it has been intensively studied at altitude.

16.3.1 Aldosterone and altitude

Indirect evidence of the effect of altitude on aldosterone activity was first provided by Williams (1961), who brought back samples of saliva from the Karakoram. The ratio of sodium to potassium in these samples indicated suppression of aldosterone at altitude. This has been confirmed by direct measurements of either plasma aldosterone concentration or urinary metabolites (Tuffley *et al.* 1970; Hogan *et al.* 1973; Frayser *et al.* 1975; Pines *et al.* 1977; Sutton *et al.* 1977; Keynes *et al.* 1982; Ramirez *et al.* 1992; Antezana *et al.* 1995; Zaccaria *et al.* 1998). In one study the secretion rate was shown to be reduced (Slater *et al.* 1969). Milledge *et al.* (1983a) studied the time course of the effect of altitude over a 6-week stay at or above 4500 m. After initial suppression, aldosterone concentration rose to control values after 12–20 days. All these studies were made on resting subjects. In subjects who had been above 6000 m for more than 10 weeks and had expanded fluid compartments (blood volume 85% above normal), the aldosterone concentration was twice normal (Anand *et al.* 1993). These subjects were probably in incipient right heart failure due to high altitude pulmonary hypertension, previously known as subacute mountain sickness (Chapter 22).

16.3.2 Renin activity and altitude

The effect of altitude on plasma renin activity (PRA) has been studied by a number of groups with conflicting results. Some have found a rise (Slater *et al.* 1969; Tuffley *et al.* 1970; Frayser *et al.* 1975) and others a fall (Hogan *et al.* 1973; Maher *et al.* 1975a; Keynes *et al.* 1982; Antezana *et al.* 1995; Zaccaria *et al.* 1998) and one group no change (Sutton *et al.* 1977). However, most studies have shown a reduced response of aldosterone to renin. This is obvious where PRA has increased and aldosterone has decreased but even where both have declined, the reduction in aldosterone has usually been greater.

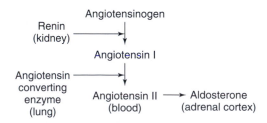

Figure 16.2   Renin–angiotensin–aldosterone system. Renin and angiotensin converting enzyme (ACE) act as enzymes hydrolyzing angiotensinogen and angiotensin I to angiotensin II. The latter stimulates release of aldosterone from adrenocortical cells by a receptor mechanism.

It is not clear why these different studies produced different results. One possibility is that subjects, though sampled at rest, may have been more active in some studies, resulting in a rise in PRA. However, this is unlikely in view of the fact that one study showing a rise in PRA was conducted in a chamber (Tuffley *et al.* 1970) and in another, samples were taken before getting up in the morning after subjects had been flown to altitude in a helicopter (Slater *et al.* 1969). The main stimulus to renin release is thought to be sympathetic drive and this certainly occurs with exercise but is probably also induced by altitude hypoxia alone if sufficiently severe (section 16.4), although with great individual variation.

16.3.3 Exercise and the renin–aldosterone system

Since exercise frequently accompanies ascent to altitude, the effect of exercise needs to be considered in relation to the effect of altitude. Exercise stimulates renin release via activation of the sympathoadrenal system. The effect can be blocked by beta-blockers (Bonelli *et al.* 1977; Bouissou *et al.* 1989). After intense short-term exercise (3 × 300 m sprints in 10 minutes), PRA, angiotensin II and aldosterone concentration were elevated at 30 minutes but measurable elevation was still present up to 6 hours later (Kosunen and Pakarinen 1976). The rise in PRA is also proportional to the intensity of the work, both at sea level and at altitude (Maher *et al.* 1975a).

Mountaineers are more concerned with daylong exercise, often continuing for a number of days. Williams *et al.* (1979) showed that this form of exercise resulted in marked sodium retention after 7 days and suggested that this was due to activation of the renin–aldosterone system. There was a mean cumulative retention of 358 mmol of sodium with a modest retention of 650 mL of water. Since plasma sodium concentration did not change significantly it was argued that the extracellular space must have been expanded by 2.68 L (of which 0.68 L was in the plasma volume), mainly at the expense of the intracellular volume. These calculated changes are shown in Fig. 16.3. This increase in extracellular fluid (ECF)

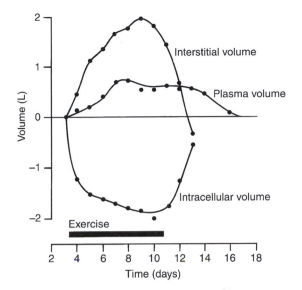

Figure 16.3   Calculated changes in body fluid compartments with exercise at sea level. (From Williams *et al.* 1979.)

is the probable cause of the dependent edema frequently found after exercise of this sort.

The same group (Milledge *et al.* 1982) studied the effect of five consecutive days' hill walking on the renin–aldosterone system and on sodium and water balance, and confirmed the suggestion, from the previous study, that the sodium retention was associated with activation of the renin–aldosterone system. There was elevation of PRA and aldosterone at the conclusion of each day's exercise. Values were back to control on day 2 after stopping exercise. The effect of exercise and altitude was studied by repeating the same protocol, but on the first exercise day subjects climbed to 3100 m and stayed there for 5 days, exercising for 8 hours each day. The results were very similar to sea level results in terms of changes in fluid and sodium balance and hematocrit. Renin and aldosterone also increased, but the aldosterone response to the renin rise was blunted (see section 16.3.5; Milledge *et al.* 1983d).

16.3.4 Control of aldosterone release

The control of aldosterone release via renin and angiotensin has been mentioned above and is shown in Fig. 16.2, but ACTH and the sodium status of the subject also control aldosterone concentration. Salt depletion increases aldosterone release whereas salt loading inhibits it. Anderson *et al.* (1986) have shown that atrial natriuretic peptide (ANP) infusion inhibits the response of aldosterone to angiotensin II.

16.3.5 Effect of altitude on the aldosterone response to renin

Milledge and Catley (1982) showed that, if after 1 hour of exercise the inspired oxygen was reduced, renin activity increased while aldosterone levels decreased, indicating that the aldosterone response to renin became blunted. In the chronic situation of hill walking or climbing at altitude compared with sea level the same phenomenon is seen. This is shown in Fig. 16.4, which shows data from three studies, at sea level, at 3100 m and on Mount Everest. This blunting has been confirmed by Shigeoka *et al.* (1985), who found the response completely abolished by hypoxia, by Lawrence *et al.* (1990), and, in acute hypoxia, by De Angelis *et al.* (1996). Antezana *et al.* (1995) also found the response in lowlanders to be blunted in La Paz (3600 m). Andean highlanders with polycythemia showed a reduced response but highlanders

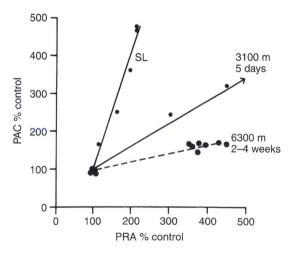

Figure 16.4 Plasma aldosterone concentration (PAC) response to plasma renin activity (PRA) from a sea level (SL) study and from two separate altitude studies. (From Milledge *et al.* 1983b.)

without polycythemia had a normal response at this altitude.

Aldosterone secretion is stimulated by ACTH as well as by angiotensin II. Ramirez *et al.* (1988) found this effect to be reduced in subjects at altitude whereas the ACTH-induced secretion of cortisol was unaffected. ANP has been found to inhibit aldosterone release (Elliott and Goodfriend 1986). It is therefore possible that the rise in ANP on going to altitude (section 16.4.4) may be a factor in blunting this response at rest (Lawrence *et al.* 1990) and on exercise (Lawrence and Shenker 1991).

16.4 ATRIAL NATRIURETIC PEPTIDE, AND BRAIN NATRIURETIC PEPTIDE, ADRENOMEDULLIN

16.4.1 ANP release and actions

Atrial natriuretic peptide is secreted by the atria of the heart in response to stretching. Atrial stretch is usually caused by an increase in atrial pressure. However, in the case of cardiac tamponade the pressure is high but the atrial wall is not stretched. As the tamponade is relieved the pressure falls and the atrium dilates. It has been found that relief of tamponade results in a rise in ANP plasma levels, indicating that stretch rather than pressure is the stimulus for ANP synthesis and release (Au *et al.* 1990).

Among its actions, ANP has the effect of increasing sodium excretion by the kidneys and thus of promoting a natriuresis and diuresis (Morice *et al.* 1988). This provides a homeostatic mechanism for salt and water. If the plasma volume is increased, the raised atrial pressure results in atrial stretch and secretion of ANP, diuresis follows and vascular pressures and volume return to normal. This system is further considered in relation to the regulation of plasma volume in Chapter 9, section 9.2.2.

Atrial natriuretic peptide probably also has a role as a vasodilator, countering the pressor effect of hypoxia on the pulmonary artery. It has been shown to have this effect in a dose-dependent manner in the isolated rat lung (Stewart *et al.* 1991b) and in the pig (Adnot *et al.* 1988). Liu *et al.* (1989) infused ANP (20 mg min^{-1} for 10 minutes) into four patients with HAPE and showed a reduction in pulmonary artery pressure for 1 hour after the infusion. A recent study by Chen *et al.* (2006) using ANP knock-out mice (Nappa$-/-$) found that chronic hypoxia resulted in greater remodeling of pulmonary arteries in the knock-out mice than in wild-type controls.

16.4.2 ANP and hypoxia

Since the first edition of this book 23 years ago, there have been numerous reports of the effect of hypoxia on the plasma levels of ANP at rest and on exercise. Ten minutes of severe hypoxia on isolated rat and rabbit heart with constant flow perfusion caused a four-fold increase in ANP released (Baertschi *et al.* 1986). The same group found increases in ANP blood levels in the whole animal made hypoxic under anesthesia. There was great variability in the response, which correlated with the baseline central venous pressure, but not with any other measured variables.

In healthy volunteers, Kawashima *et al.* (1989) studied the effect of 10 minutes of hypoxia at two levels: 15% oxygen breathing produced no change, but 10% oxygen breathing increased ANP levels by 15% accompanied by an increase in pulmonary artery pressure. Vonmoos *et al.* (1990) found that 60 minutes of 12% oxygen breathing produced a small but significant elevation of ANP. Lawrence *et al.* (1990) found that the same hypoxic stimulus produced a 50% increase in ANP levels in subjects on a low salt diet and whose endogenous cortisol was suppressed with dexamethasone. Conversely, Ramirez *et al.* (1992) did not find a significant rise in ANP levels with either acute (60 minutes) or chronic hypoxia at 3000 m, although the ANP response to a sodium load was greater at altitude. Antezana *et al.* (1995) found a reduction in ANP levels in lowlanders at 3600 m compared with sea level and highlanders had significantly lower ANP than lowlanders at altitude.

16.4.3 Exercise and ANP: normoxia

Somers *et al.* (1986) found that a progressive exercise test to maximum exercise resulted in an almost four-fold increase in plasma ANP with a decline to baseline after 1 hour at rest. Similar results have been found for short-term exercise by Schmidt *et al.* (1990) and by Lawrence and Shenker (1991). Hill walking exercise for 5 days also resulted in elevated ANP levels to about twice baseline values (Milledge *et al.* 1991b). It is interesting to note that during this type of exercise, sodium is retained despite elevated ANP levels.

16.4.4 Exercise and ANP: hypoxia

Mountaineers and trekkers going to altitude normally have the double stimulus of exercise and hypoxia. Schmidt *et al.* (1990) studied exercise while breathing air or reduced oxygen (PI,O_2 92 mmHg). With both maximal and sub-maximal exercise the ANP response to exercise was reduced under hypoxic conditions. In contrast, Lawrence and Shenker (1991), using less severe hypoxia (16% inspired oxygen) and exercise such as to give a heart rate of 70–75% of maximum for 30 minutes, found that hypoxia enhanced the ANP response. A third study, using a decompression chamber to give a simulated altitude of 3000 m and a progressive exercise test to maximum, showed a reduced response (Vuolteenaho *et al.* 1992). The reasons for these differing results are not apparent.

Milledge *et al.* (1989) reported levels of plasma ANP in 15 subjects before and after ascent on foot from 3100 m to 4300 m. Values tended to be higher at altitude but were significantly so only in the 4 a.m. sample on the second altitude day, there being no difference on day 1 at altitude or in the 9 a.m. sample on either day. Bärtsch *et al.* (1991a) found in blood samples taken on the morning after the ascent to 4559 m on foot no increase in ANP levels in a group of nine climbers who did not have AMS. Five subjects who did become sick had elevated levels. These subjects had a history of HAPE and were shown by echocardiography to have increased atrial diameters at altitude. The increase in ANP is probably secondary to developing high pulmonary artery pressures. Kawashima *et al.* (1992) showed that in subjects susceptible to high altitude pulmonary edema, breathing 10% oxygen resulted in a greater rise in ANP levels than in controls, and that the rise correlated with the rise in pulmonary artery pressure.

Later in altitude exposure the effect of maximum exercise in raising ANP levels is reduced (Robach *et al.* 2000) but then so is maximum work rate.

16.4.5 ANP, AMS and HAPE

An important motive for the study of the effect of altitude hypoxia on ANP has been the hypothesis that it may play a part in the genesis of AMS. Milledge *et al.* (1989) did not find any correlation between levels of ANP on the morning after arrival at altitude and the AMS symptom score. However, Bärtsch *et al.* (1988) found subjects with AMS and Cosby *et al.* (1988) in subjects with HAPE, to have higher levels than subjects without AMS or HAPE. If the rise in ANP in AMS sufferers is related to high pulmonary arterial pressure, elevation would be expected mainly in AMS with pulmonary edema and not in the milder, non-HAPE cases. In the first-mentioned study there was no clinical evidence of pulmonary edema. The finding of raised ANP in HAPE cases may be due to their pulmonary hypertension, which may cause right atrial stretch. Recent animal studies show that ANP is protective of lung vascular leak (lipopolysaccharide induced) in ANP knock-out mice (Birukova *et al.* 2010).

16.4.6 ANP and chronic mountain sickness

Antezana *et al.* (1995) have reported higher levels of ANP in patients with chronic mountain sickness (CMS) than in controls in Andean highlanders. In this study, pulmonary artery pressure was assessed by Doppler ultrasound and found to be raised. Ge *et al.* (2001) also found raised levels of ANP in patients with CMS (Han Chinese and Tibetans). There was a significant correlation between the hemoglobin concentration, [Hb], and ANP.

In conclusion, it seems that although both exercise and hypoxia cause an elevation of ANP, the combined stimulus does not result in very high levels at altitude. Despite its name, ANP is not a powerful natriuretic hormone. Levels of ANP are elevated in conditions where the pulmonary artery pressure is raised, including HAPE and polycythemia, and this rise is presumably secondary to the raised pressure causing some atrial enlargement. The rise in ANP is probably beneficial in that it tends to reduce the pressure by its vasodilatory function.

16.4.7 Brain natriuretic peptide

Brain natriuretic peptide (BNP) is a hormone related to ANP but having been more recently discovered, has been less studied. It was first discovered in porcine brain, hence the name, but is now understood to be mainly derived from heart muscle (Hall 2005). It has diuretic and natriuretic effects like ANP (though mild) and is released, as proBNP, from heart muscle in response to stretch. proBMP is then cleaved to form the active BNP. It also has the effect of reducing renin and aldosterone levels (Hall 2005). It further has the effect of reducing hypoxic pulmonary hypertension.

Two field studies (Toshner *et al.* 2008; Feddersen *et al.* 2009) have measured proBNP in subjects after ascent to altitude, the first to 5200 m in Bolivia and the second to 5050 m. Both studies found no significant increase in proBNP (or ANP). Toshner *et al.* point out that their findings support the view that ventricular function is well preserved at altitude. Feddersen *et al.* also measured nocturnal urine volumes, which they found to be increased, as expected, on going to altitude but that these did not correlate with proBNP levels. They conclude that BNP is not involved in altitude diuresis. However, Woods *et al.* (2011), in subjects trekking to Island Peak to an altitude of 5150 m found that BNP levels were often raised after the exercise of trekking, especially in those with AMS. The incidence of AMS was significantly higher in those with a BNP response at 5150 m than in those showing no response. The same team reported a follow-up study from a trek going to Kala Patthar (5643 m) (Woods *et al.* 2012a). They showed that after exercise (trekking) BNP and proBNP levels increased with altitude, that levels were still elevated after a night's rest and that those with the greater BNP response had significantly more AMS than those with less or no response. They also measured total body water (TBW). In those with severe AMS at 5150 m, there was an apparent net gain in TBW between Katmandu and 5050 m of 1.88 L and a loss of 1.49 L in those without severe AMS, although this was not significant (p = 0.067).

16.4.8 Adrenomedullin

Adrenomedullin (AM) has many biological effects including, in the kidneys, increased renal blood flow, urine output, and urinary Na^+ excretion in a dose-dependent manner when infused in animals (Hinson *et al.* 2000). It is expressed in many tissues in response to hypoxia via hypoxia-inducible factor (HIF)-1 induction (Cormier-Regarde al. 1998).

Toepfer *et al.* (1998) reported raised levels of plasma AM in subjects (all of whom had AMS) on the first and second days after arrival at the Margherita Hut (4560 m). Haditch *et al.* (2007) studied 33 subjects trekking to 5150 m (the Pyramid laboratory). Measurements were made at 150, 3440 and 5050 m. They showed that urinary AM correlated significantly with nocturnal diuresis and sodium excretion, while plasma AM, although raised at altitude, did not. Their data suggest that renal AM production is involved in the water and sodium diuresis of early altitude acclimatization. The place of this hormone in relation to both altitude diuresis and hypoxic pulmonary hypertension clearly needs more study.

16.5 CORTICOSTEROIDS AND ALTITUDE

On ascent to altitude, there is stimulation of the adrenal cortex by ACTH and cortisol is secreted. Early work documented this as a rise in 17-hydroxycorticosteroids (17-OHCSs) during the first few days at altitude, which decreased to control values by days 5–7 (MacKinnon *et al.* 1963; Moncloa *et al.* 1965). This has been confirmed by measurement of plasma cortisol by Frayser *et al.* (1975) and Sutton *et al.* (1977), who showed that with the elevation of plasma cortisol there was a decrease in its normal diurnal variation on the first day of altitude exposure. Richalet *et al.* (1989), in a chamber experiment, also found elevation

of plasma cortisol with re-establishment of the diurnal variation after the first altitude day. Many of the subjects of these studies, taken rapidly to an altitude of 4300–5300 m, suffered from AMS, but even those free of symptoms showed this transitory rise in cortisol or its urinary metabolite. It is assumed that this is a nonspecific stress response. A paper by Barnholt *et al.* (2006) reporting a study from Pikes Peak (4300 m) confirmed these earlier findings and also found no difference between a group who had a restricted calorie diet (and lost weight) and one on a diet adequate to maintain body weight. Both groups had cortisol levels elevated throughout the 21 days at altitude.

A recent study by Woods *et al.* (2012b) of 47 trekkers reported changes in salivary cortisol from Kathmandu (1300 m) to 5100 m on the trail to Everest Base Camp in morning and post-trek afternoon samples. This modest form of exercise resulted in a small rise in cortisol at all altitudes. Interestingly, they found a fall in levels with increasing altitude in both pre-exercise (morning) and post-exercise samples except at the highest point of 5100 m. Their cortisol levels, both pre- and post-exercise were higher than all other points and only there, did they find significant correlation of cortisol post-exercise with arterial oxygen saturation ($Sa,o_2\%$). There was no correlation with AMS scores.

16.5.1 Case report

An interesting case report shows that there is a clinical lesson to be learnt. A 58-year-old man, who had had his pituitary removed 10 years earlier for an adenoma, went trekking in Nepal. On arrival at Menang (3535 m) he complained of fatigue, abdominal pain, nausea and vomiting, but no headache. He was on regular medication with cortisone 25 mg daily and had taken his treatment. Twenty-four hours later he had deteriorated and was unable to stand. He was treated with dexamethasone 5 mg i.v., 5 mg i.m. and oral rehydration, and his cortisone dose was quadrupled. Within 24 hours all symptoms had disappeared, and the next day he successfully crossed the Thorong La (5450 m) (Westendorp *et al.* 1993). Clearly, the lesson is that subjects on corticosteroid replacement therapy should increase their dosage on going to altitude. The authors point out that this does not apply to thyroid replacement therapy since thyroid-stimulating hormone (TSH) is not increased by hypoxia.

16.5.2 Corticosteroids at altitude

The effect of prolonged stay at more extreme altitude was studied by Siri *et al.* (1969). They brought back urine samples from the 1963 Everest expedition from climbers staying at 5400 and 6500 m. The 17-OHCS levels were not significantly different from sea level values. They also demonstrated a normal response to injected ACTH. Mordes *et al.* (1983) collected samples from subjects who had been at 5400 and 6300 m for some weeks and found no change from sea level values in either morning or evening cortisol concentrations.

In animals studied after chronic hypoxia there was some hyperplasia of the adrenal cortex and of the corticotrophic cells in the pituitary. No such morphological changes have been found in humans with long-standing chronic bronchitis (Gosney 1986). However, in subjects who had spent more than 10 weeks above 6000 m, the cortisol level was found to be three times normal (Anand *et al.* 1993). Marinelli *et al.* (1994) studied athletes taking part in a marathon race from 3860 m to 5100 m and down to finish at 3400 m. Cortisol levels were similar at altitude before the race but were greatly elevated at the end.

In people resident at the moderate altitude of 2600 m in Colombia, Ramirez *et al.* (1995) found an enhanced response to corticotrophin releasing hormone, with higher levels of both ACTH and β-endorphin after stimulation than in sea level control subjects. This was true for a number of trophic hormones (sections 16.7.1 and 16.9.2).

16.6 SYMPATHOADRENAL SYSTEM

16.6.1 Acute hypoxia

Acute hypoxia increases heart rate at rest and on exercise (Maher *et al.* 1975b). This is presumed to be due to increased sympathetic activity stimulating

the β-adrenergic receptors on heart muscle cell membrane. Within 4 hours of arrival at altitude there is an increase in arterial epinephrine, at rest, due to hypoxia stimulating release from the adrenal medulla (Mazzeo and Reeves 2003). Bouissou *et al.* (1989) also found a 32% increase in norepinephrine after 48 hours at altitude. Levels of epinephrine reach a peak on about days 2–4 and then decline as hypoxia is relieved by increasing ventilation and [Hb] over the next 7–14 days (Mazzeo and Reeves 2003). Norepinephrine is released by sympathetic nerves and about 10–20% spills over into the circulation. This is measured as plasma norepinephrine and, in contrast to epinephrine, values rise only slowly, in line with increasing ventilation, reaching a plateau after 10–14 days at altitude. Exercise results in a further rise in epinephrine depending on the work rate and degree of hypoxia. The two stimuli, hypoxia and exercise, are additive for epinephrine. Norepinephrine levels also rise with exercise depending upon the workload but if workloads relative to $V_{O_{2,max}}$ are compared, the rise at altitude is similar to that seen at sea level (Mazzeo and Reeves 2003). Recently, Berger *et al.* (2011) found that central venous and arterial epinephrine positively correlated with systolic blood pressure, heart rate and pulmonary blood flow. They also found that the rise in pulmonary artery pressure and resistance is largely independent of the sympathetic nervous system. This may be due to the opposing effects of stimulation of β_2 receptors by norepinephrine causing vasodilatation and epinephrine α-adrenergic receptors causing vasoconstriction. Of course, the main cause for pulmonary hypertension at altitude is alveolar hypoxia.

16.6.2 Chronic hypoxia

Cunningham *et al.* (1965) reported elevated plasma and 24-hour urinary catecholamines during 17 days at 4559 m on Monte Rosa. There was no significant change in epinephrine but the increase in norepinephrine was greater on day 12 at altitude. Pace *et al.* (1964) found similar results at 3850 m, with urinary norepinephrine excretion rising slowly during 14 days at altitude without change in urinary epinephrine secretion. Maher *et al.* (1975b) found increased urinary catecholamines at 4300 m. Levels were increased on day 1 compared with sea level and further increased on day 11. On exercise, both light and severe, the effect of chronic hypoxia compared with acute was to increase levels still further. Hoon *et al.* (1977) found no significant change in urinary catecholamine secretion in a total of 76 subjects who had no symptoms of AMS. However, in 29 symptomatic subjects there was a small but significant rise on the first day at altitude, which was maintained through to day 10 at altitude. Mazzeo *et al.* (1991) found that at rest norepinephrine and epinephrine levels were higher at altitude than at sea level. With sub-maximal exercise, norepinephrine rose to higher values than expected at sea level, whereas epinephrine levels did not rise, though values remained above those at sea level. In Operation Everest II at extreme altitude (282 mmHg) after 40 days in the chamber, resting plasma norepinephrine was raised but epinephrine was reduced. On maximum exercise, values for both catecholamines fell with increasing altitude (Young *et al.* 1989).

In subjects who had spent more than 10 weeks above 6000 m the plasma norepinephrine concentration was found to be almost three times normal (Anand *et al.* 1993). Gosney *et al.* (1991) studied the adrenal and pituitary glands of five lifelong residents of La Paz who had lived at 3600–3800 m and compared their glands with those of controls from sea level. The adrenal glands were significantly bigger, by about 50%. The pituitary glands were not larger but contained more corticotrophs. They surmised that greater amounts of ACTH were required to maintain adrenal function, perhaps because of hypoxic inhibition of adrenocortical sensitivity. However, Ramirez *et al.* (1988) found no such inhibition.

Calbet (2003) studied nine subjects during 9 weeks' stay at 5260 m and found an increase in arterial blood pressure (measured directly) with increased plasma epinephrine and norepinephrine. He showed that blood norepinephrine spillover from the leg was increased compared with sea level values. This increase in sympathetic nervous activity was after arterial oxygen content had been restored by the normal rise in [Hb] with time at altitude. Hansen and Sander (2003),

on the same expedition, measured sympathetic activity directly by peroneal microneurography after 4 weeks at altitude. They found activity to be about three times sea level values. They also studied the effect of oxygen breathing and a saline infusion (to reduce baroreflex deactivation). These interventions had only minor effect on sympathetic activity. Three days after returning to sea level sympathetic activity was still significantly higher than pre-expedition values as were results for blood pressure and heart rate.

Bogaard *et al.* (2002) studied the effect of blocking either the sympathetic or parasympathetic arms of the autonomic system in a group of subjects at 3800 m on the heart rate and cardiac output on exercise. Propranolol had the expected effect of reducing heart rate and glycopyrrolate increased the maximum heart rate to sea level values. However, interestingly, neither medication had any effect on maximum cardiac output, $V_{O_{2,max}}$, or work rate at altitude, though, of course, these values were lower than sea level. Mazzeo *et al.* (2003) showed that blocking the α-adrenergic system in a group of female subjects at 4300 m resulted in increased norepinephrine levels compared with unblocked controls both at rest and exercise.

Women appear to have the same sympathoadrenal response to altitude as men and there is no difference related to the menstrual cycle (Mazzeo and Reeves 2003). However, it is worth noting that this elevated response may be a factor in the increased incidence of pre-eclampsia in pregnant women at altitude.

16.6.3 Adrenergic response and acclimatization

Acute hypoxia causes an increase in heart rate and cardiac output. However, after several days at altitude the heart rate and cardiac output fall back towards sea level values. On exercise the maximum heart rate is limited to well below the sea level maximum, being typically 140–150 beats min^{-1} at 5800 m compared with 180–200 beats min^{-1} at sea level (Chapter 8). This reduction in maximal heart rate and cardiac output takes place at a time when the plasma and urinary catecholamines are higher than at sea level.

Evidently, the heart's response to sympathetic stimulation becomes blunted. This has been demonstrated by Maher *et al.* (1975b), who showed in dogs that the cardio-acceleratory effect of an infusion of isoproterenol was reduced after 10 days' altitude acclimatization. Workers from the same institution (Maher *et al.* 1978) found in cardiac muscle of acclimatized goats that there was a two-fold rise of the enzyme O-methyltransferase. This enzyme inactivates cardiac norepinephrine, and its induction during acclimatization may account for the blunting of the adrenergic response to exercise. Another possibility is that there may be downregulation, that is, a reduction in the density of adrenergic receptors on the heart muscle. Voelkel *et al.* (1981) have shown this to be the case in rats kept for 5 weeks at a simulated altitude of 4250 m. These two possible mechanisms are not mutually exclusive. Sherpa high altitude residents do not suffer this heart rate limitation on maximal exercise. Their heart rates can go up to 190–198 beats min^{-1} at 4880 m (Lahiri *et al.* 1967).

16.6.4 Autonomic system response and AMS

Duplain and colleagues (1999a) studied eight climbers who were susceptible to HAPE measuring their sympathetic activity directly with intraneural electrodes and compared them to seven subjects resistant to HAPE. Measurements were made at low altitude breathing a hypoxic gas mixture and at high altitude (4599 m). In both situations the HAPE-susceptible subjects had significantly higher sympathetic activity than resistant subjects. This increased activity at altitude preceded the onset of lung edema. Also, taking both groups together, there was a direct, significant relationship between sympathetic nerve activity and pulmonary artery pressure.

Loeppky *et al.* (2003) carried out a chamber study measuring autonomic responses by heart rate variability and plasma catecholamines. There were significantly higher levels of catecholamines and higher low/higher frequency ratios in AMS subjects indicating greater sympathetic activity. These differences became greater with time (over

6–12 hours). They also found lower temperature in their AMS subjects which they attributed to greater vasodilatation despite greater sympathetic activity.

Lanfranchi *et al.* (2005) studied 41 mountaineers at the Capanna Margherita (4559 m) using spectral analysis of the R–R interval and blood pressure variability as a measure of autonomic system activity. Seventeen subjects had AMS. Measurements were repeated at low altitude 3 months later, breathing air and a hypoxic gas mixture. They found evidence of autonomic dysfunction in subjects with AMS at altitude and claimed that AMS-prone subjects could be identified as those showing marked low-frequency component of systolic blood pressure variability in the field. However, the short-term, acute hypoxia test at sea level did not show a difference between those who were AMS prone and those who were resistant.

16.6.5 Sympathoadrenal response: summary

Acute hypoxia has no effect on epinephrine levels in the blood or urine but there is a modest rise in norepinephrine levels. In the first few days at altitude there is increased sympathetic and parasympathetic activity. This increased sympathetic activity results in increased heart rate but does not affect cardiac output. The increase in sympathetic activity is more marked in subjects with AMS and HAPE. The response of the heart to adrenergic stimulation becomes blunted after a week or 10 days at altitude and this is probably due to downregulation of receptors and induction of the enzyme responsible for catecholamine metabolism. After prolonged altitude exposure the enhanced sympathoadrenal activity continues for some days after return to normoxia.

16.7 THYROID FUNCTION AND THE ALTITUDE ENVIRONMENT

Hypothalamic–pituitary–thyroid axis function is affected by hypoxia and possibly by cold. The effect of cold on thyroid function is considered in Chapter 24. Iodine is essential for synthesis of thyroid hormone and is deficient in the soil and water of some mountainous regions, so that thyroid function in residents of these regions is affected.

16.7.1 Thyroid function and hypoxia

The response of the hypophyseal–thyroid axis to hypoxia seems to be quite different in humans compared with animals. In animals, hypoxia results in depression of thyroid function (Heath and Williams 1995, pp. 265–6). In the pituitary gland the number of thyrotrophs – cells that secrete TSH – is reduced, suggesting a decreased output of TSH (Gosney 1986). In humans, however, thyroid activity is increased at altitude. Surks (1966) found elevated levels of thyroxine-binding globulin (TBG) and free thyroxine (T_4) in the first 2 weeks at altitude (4300 m), with a peak at 9 days. Kotchen et al. (1973), in a 3-day chamber experiment (3650 m equivalent), found T_4 elevated (free and bound) but TSH to be unchanged, suggesting a shift of T_4 from extravascular to intravascular compartments rather than increased pituitary activity. Westendorp et al. (1993) also found no increase in TSH in response to a 1-hour acute hypoxia equivalent of 4115 m.

These results have been confirmed in a number of field studies (Rastogi et al. 1977; Stock et al. 1978b) which showed levels returning towards control in the third week at altitude. Sawhney and Malhotra (1991) studied both acclimatized lowlanders and high altitude natives, and found levels of triiodothyronine (T_3) and T_4 to be higher than sea level residents. T_4 concentration in red cells was decreased at high altitude but there was no change in levels of reverse T_3 (rT_3), TBG, and T_4 binding capacity of TBG and thyroxine-binding prealbumin. They also found no change in TSH. In L-eltroxine-treated men they still found a rise in T_3 and T_4, suggesting the rise to be independent of pituitary stimulation.

Exercise increases T_3 and T_4 to a greater extent at altitude than at sea level (Stock et al. 1978b). At higher altitudes of 5400 and 6300 m, Mordes et al. (1983) showed elevated resting T_3, free T_4 and T_3 in subjects who had been at altitude for some weeks. In these subjects TSH was also elevated, in contrast to the finding at lower altitudes.

Barnholt et al. (2006) in a three-arm, 3 weeks' trial, studied endocrine responses to altitude and weight loss. A control group at sea level had a calorie-deficient diet, the other two groups were at altitude (4300 m), one group had a diet adequate to maintain body weight and the other a deficient diet to lose weight. This weight control was achieved. The results: both altitude groups showed no change in TSH whilst the sea level group showed a rise in TSH followed by a decline. Free T_3 showed a rise in the first few days at altitude followed by a fall, the weight loss group having higher values. The sea level group showed a modest decline in free T_3 values as they lost weight. These results confirm earlier work on thyroid hormones and indicate that the altitude effect tends to override the effect of weight loss due to calorie deficiency.

Benso et al. (2007) studied nine climbers who had returned to base camp after climbing Everest. They had, of course, lost weight (mean 5 kg). None of the climbers suffered from AMS. They found significant increases in free T_4, decreases in free T_3 and no change in TSH. This pattern suggests low T_3 syndrome (non-thyroidal illness syndrome). Richalet et al. (2010) studied the effect of altitude (3–4 days at the Observatoire Vallot, 4350 m) on the hormonal response to a number of hypothalamic factors including TSH. They found that the response to injected TSH was not significantly different from that at sea level.

16.7.2 Basal metabolic rate

The basal metabolic rate is elevated during the first 2 weeks at moderate altitude and correlates with the free T_4 (Stock et al. 1978a). At higher altitudes (above 5500 m) it remains elevated for months (Gill and Pugh 1964), as does T_4 (Mordes et al. 1983). Mordes et al. (1983) also found evidence of impaired conversion of T_4 to T_3 at 6300 m. Perhaps there is a change in the set point for the pituitary negative feedback system, resulting in higher levels of TSH. They also found that the response of the pituitary to an injection of thyrotrophin-releasing hormone was enhanced at

6300 m compared with sea level. A similar finding has been reported by Ramirez et al. (1995) in resident highlanders at only 2600 m.

16.7.3 Iodine deficiency, goiter and altitude

The frequency of goiter in mountainous areas is well known and is discussed in Chapter 18. In England, it was known as 'Derbyshire neck' and it was equally well known in the Pyrenees, the Alps, the Andes and the Himalayas, but it is not confined to the mountains.

The association of iodine deficiency and mountainous areas is mainly due to the geological factors causing iodine deficiency in the soil and hence in the diet, but altitude hypoxia stimulates thyroid function (Chapter 17, section 17.7.1). Thus the effect of iodine deficiency will result in more exaggerated hyperplasia, which contributes to the extremely high rate of goiter in resident populations at altitude in the past. The incidence is now very much reduced in many areas due to measures to increase iodine intake, particularly by adding iodine to dietary salt.

16.8 CONTROL OF BLOOD GLUCOSE AT ALTITUDE

16.8.1 Acute hypoxia

On acute exposure to hypoxia there is a rise in fasting blood glucose of about 1.7 mmol L^{-1}, followed by a fall towards control values by the end of a week. At the same time insulin levels are elevated (Williams 1975). This is presumably part of the nonspecific stress response indicated by the concurrent rise in plasma cortisol levels (Chapter 16, section 16.5).

16.8.2 Chronic hypoxia

In subjects acclimatized to high altitude, fasting blood glucose was found to be lower than at sea level by some workers (Blume and Pace 1967; Stock et al. 1978b; Blume 1984) but unchanged by others (Sawhney et al. 1986). Singh et al.

(1974) found a persistently raised glucose level after 10 months at altitude. Resting insulin levels have also been found to be reduced (Stock et al. 1978b).

Glucose loading increases both blood glucose and insulin levels at altitude as it does at sea level, but the rise in both was found to be less than at sea level in two studies (Stock et al. 1978b; Blume 1984) but greater in one (Sawhney et al. 1986). There are a number of explanations for this blunted response. Glucose may be absorbed less rapidly, though this is probably only true above about 5500 m (Chapter 15, section 15.5). Liver glycogen synthesis may be enhanced at altitude and some evidence for this has been found in rats injected with labeled glucose at altitude (Blume and Pace 1971). There may be increased target organ sensitivity to insulin, presumably by upregulation of insulin receptors on target cells. This is a feature of athletic training and may well happen as part of altitude acclimatization. A study by Lee and colleagues (2003) in healthy subjects found that as little as 3 days' sedentary living at 2400 m resulted in an improvement in the oral glucose tolerance test. That is a faster decline of glucose levels after a similar rise in response to glucose loading, suggesting increased insulin sensitivity.

The effect of the action of insulin at altitude was investigated by Larsen and colleagues (1997) using a euglycemic clamp technique in a group of men, at sea level and on days 2 and 7 of altitude exposure at 4559 m. They found that insulin action decreased markedly on day 2 but had improved somewhat by day 7 at altitude. More recently, Braun et al. (2001) studied a group of women at an altitude of 4300 m over 12 days. They found the same pattern of initial decrease in insulin sensitivity followed by enhanced sensitivity with acclimatization. They also investigated whether the reduced insulin sensitivity was due to adrenaline secretion early in altitude exposure by using an α-adrenergic antagonist. They concluded that this was not the case. De Glisezinski et al. (1999) studied lipolysis in subcutaneous fat biopsies in subjects exposed to prolonged simulated altitude exposure in a chamber (Operation Everest III). They found that the anti-lipolytic activity of insulin was significantly decreased.

K. Moore *et al.* (2001), in a group of trekkers attempting Kilimanjaro (5895 m), found that insulin requirements reduced from a mean of 67 to 12 units day^{-1}. This may have been partly due to AMS and reduction in food intake. However, in mountaineers with type 1 diabetes, the insulin requirements during a climb of Cho Oyu (8201 m) increased from a mean of 38 to 51 units day^{-1} (Pavan *et al.* 2004). Of course, insulin requirements depend upon many factors apart from insulin sensitivity. For a discussion of the problems faced by patients with diabetes see Chapter 25.

Braun *et al.* (1998) studied the glucose response to a standard meal in women at sea level and at 4300 m in the presence of estrogen (E) and estrogen plus progesterone (E+P). The peak of glucose was lower and returned to baseline more slowly at altitude than at sea level although the insulin levels were the same. The response was also lower in E than E+P at sea level but the difference at altitude was not significant. It would seem that at altitude the relative concentration of ovarian hormones does not appear to be important in glucose control.

16.9 ENDOTHELIN

16.9.1 Endothelin family

The endothelins are a family of peptides produced by a wide variety of cells affecting mainly blood vessels. Endothelin-1 (ET-1), clinically the most important member of the family, is the most potent vasoconstrictor yet discovered with about 100 times the activity of norepinephrine. Other members of the family identified are ET-2 and ET-3, which are more localized to certain organs. All three peptides bind to the same two receptors, A and B, though with differing binding affinities. Synthetic inhibitors of these receptors are now available and their use has served to elucidate some of the actions of these peptides. ET-1 is produced by the endothelium and as much as 75% of the production is exported from the side of the cell opposite to the vessel lumen, where it acts on the adjacent smooth muscle without contributing to the plasma pool. In this way

it perhaps should be considered as mainly a paracrine, rather than an endocrine, hormone. However, plasma levels probably do reflect the output of ET-1 and parallel the severity of the condition in, for instance, congestive cardiac failure. A good clinical review has been published by Levin (1995), and Holm (1997) has provided a more pharmacological review.

16.9.2 Altitude and endothelin

Horio *et al.* (1991) showed that ET-1 in rats increased with increasing hypoxia. Since then there have been a number of studies in humans at altitude. Cargill *et al.* (1995) found that 30 minutes of acute hypoxia ($Sa_{,O_2}$ 75–80%) raised plasma ET-1 levels to about 2.5 times baseline. A group of hypoxic patients with cor pulmonale had similar levels. Similar results were found by Ferri *et al.* (1995) in patients with chronic obstructive lung disorder (COLD). They also found that ET-1 levels correlated with pulmonary artery pressure. Morganti *et al.* (1995) studied 10 subjects on a 2-day ascent of Monte Rosa (4559 m) and eight subjects in the Everest region at 5050 m. They found plasma ET-1 rose progressively with increasing altitude, the level correlating with the fall in $Sa_{,O_2}$. There was no correlation with blood pressure or hematocrit. Richalet *et al.* (1995) studied 10 subjects on Sajama (6542 m) and found modest increases in ET-1 at both rest and exercise. Levels were highest after 1 week and decreased slightly after 3 weeks' altitude exposure.

Blauw *et al.* (1995) studied the effect of hypoxia and ET-1 infusion on forearm blood flow. Forearm blood flow was not changed by hypoxia, but the ET-1 plasma increased significantly. They concluded that hypoxia causes release of ET-1 from the pulmonary circulation but that this does not influence peripheral vascular tone. Cruden *et al.* (1998) measured both ET-1 and big ET-1 in a group of mountaineers. Both were increased on ascent to altitudes above 2500 m, indicating that the increase in ET-1 was due to increased production and not decreased elimination. After 3 weeks at altitude, levels had returned to baseline values. Exercise had no effect on endothelin levels. In a separate study, they also found increases in both ET-1 and big ET-1 with cold exposure (Cruden *et al.* 1999).

16.9.3 Endothelin and HAPE

A Japanese group (Droma *et al.* 1996a) reported detailed findings on a single case of HAPE with pulmonary hypertension and found ET-1 levels elevated on admission. The levels reverted to normal as the patient recovered and pulmonary artery pressure fell. The same team (Droma *et al.* 1996b) studied a group of HAPE-susceptible subjects. Their subjects had a greater hypoxic vascular response than controls but no significant change in ET-1 levels with a hypoxic challenge. However, the hypoxia was only of 5 minutes' duration (10% oxygen).

Sartori *et al.* (1999b) studied a group of 16 mountaineers prone to HAPE, comparing them with a group resistant to HAPE. At altitude (4559 m) the HAPE-prone group had ET-1 plasma levels 33% higher than the HAPE-resistant group. There was a significant direct relationship between changes in ET-1 levels and pulmonary artery pressure from low to high altitude. In a recent study, Modesti *et al.* (2006) carried out a double-blind trial of the ET-1 antagonist bosentan in subjects at 4559 m. In the treated group the pulmonary artery pressure was significantly reduced compared with the placebo group and their Sa,O_2 was mildly increased. However, their urinary volume and free water clearance was reduced suggesting that ET-1 may also be involved in the diuresis of early acclimatization.

Berger *et al.* (2009) studied the transpulmonary concentration of ET-1 in 34 subjects at low and high altitude (4559 m). At low altitude there was a net loss (clearance) of ET-1. At high altitude levels were greatly increased and there was a net gain (production) of ET-1. Both the actual levels and the concentration v-a difference correlated with the pulmonary artery pressure.

Low birth weight of babies is a feature of obstetrics at altitude (Chapter 18) and a recent study suggests that ET-1 with nitric oxide (NO) levels may be a factor in the mechanism of this feature of life for residents of high altitude. Julian *et al.* (2008) studied blood flow in uterine arteries

(UA) of mothers in Denver (1600 m) and in Leadville (3100 m). They also measured ET-1 and NO metabolites (NO_x) in venous blood. They found that birth weight correlated with UA blood flow, in both groups. The higher the ratio of ET-1/NO_x, the more vasoconstriction of UA and the lower the blood flow to the uterus. This ratio, in both groups was found to correlate with birth weights of the babies. However, in the low altitude mothers, ET-1/NO_x ratios were clustered at the low end of the range, while the high altitude mothers' ratios were spread out to higher ratios, suggesting that increased ET-1 and/or decreased NO production resulted in lower uterine blood flows and smaller babies at altitude.

In conclusion, it seems likely that ET-1 plays a part in the mechanism of hypoxic pulmonary vasoconstriction and possibly in altitude diuresis. The augmented release of ET-1 in HAPE-susceptible subjects suggests that it may have a role in the mechanism of HAPE. It may also be a factor in the phenomenon of low birth weight babies at altitude.

16.10 ALTITUDE AND OTHER HORMONES

16.10.1 Bradykinin

The levels of bradykinin, a potent vasodilator, were found not to be changed by acute hypoxia by Ashack *et al.* (1985) but Mason *et al.* (2009) found a reduction in levels in a group of miners after 2 weeks at 3800 m. Wang, P. *et al.* (2010) found no association between alleles of the bradykinin receptor-B2 gene and AMS.

16.10.2 Growth hormone

Levels are unchanged in most subjects but were found to be increased five-fold in two subjects who had lost 15 kg in body weight (Blume 1984). Although acute hypoxia causes no change in growth hormone levels, exercise under acute hypoxic conditions causes a 20-fold increase in this hormone, whereas normoxic exercise causes only a modest rise (Sutton 1977; Raynaud *et al.*

1981). Ramirez *et al.* (1995) studied residents at Pasto, Colombia (2600 m), and found that response of growth hormone to stimulation with growth hormone releasing hormone was greatly enhanced compared with lowland control subjects. On the other hand, the *in vitro* lipolytic response to growth hormone (and parathormone) was significantly decreased in biopsies of subcutaneous fat in subjects exposed to simulated altitude in a chamber (Operation Everest III) (de Gliszinski *et al.* 1999). Benso *et al.* (2007), in a study of climbers arriving back at Everest Base Camp after climbing the peak, found a significant increase in growth hormone. They had lost weight (mean 5 kg) during the climb.

16.10.3 Testosterone, luteinizing hormone, follicle-stimulating hormone and prolactin

Sawhney *et al.* (1985) studied levels of testosterone, luteinizing hormone (LH), follicle-stimulating hormone (FSH) and prolactin in lowland men after ascent to 3500 m. On day 1 at altitude there were no significant changes from sea level values, although LH and testosterone levels were already falling. By day 7, LH and testosterone levels were significantly reduced and remained so to day 18; by then prolactin levels were significantly elevated. After 7 days at sea level all values had reverted to control except for some residual depression in LH levels. These results are in accord with previous work (Guerra-Garcia 1971) which found urinary testosterone excretion to be reduced by 50% on day 3 at 4300 m. Sawhney *et al.* (1985) also found a negative correlation between prolactin and testosterone levels at altitude but no correlation with LH levels. They suggested that the reduction in testosterone is due to an increase in prolactin secretion rather than to a reduction in LH or a direct effect of hypoxia on the testes.

In a separate experiment at sea level, Sawhney *et al.* (1985) showed a reduction in LH levels in response to daily cold exposure after 1 and 5 days, and suggested that the reduction in LH found at altitude might be due to cold rather than hypoxia. However, low levels of LH have been found in hypoxia due to chronic lung disease in hospital patients with no cold exposure (Semple 1986); these patients also had low testosterone levels which correlated with their Pa,O_2.

Semple (1986) found normal testosterone levels in patients who were hypoxic because of congenital cardiac defects, presumably because of lifelong adaptation to hypoxemia. He suggests that an alternative mechanism may be that testosterone depression is a response to dips in oxygen saturation at night, due to sleep apnea in patients with chronic obstructive lung disease, and a result of periodic breathing in lowlanders at altitude. In high altitude residents, Bangham and Hackett (1978) found reduced levels of LH after 10 days but no changes in levels of FSH, testosterone or prolactin.

Testosterone is increased in exercise and Bouissou *et al.* (1986) studied the effect of acute hypoxia (14% oxygen, equivalent to 3000 m) on this response. They found that, when the exercise was expressed as a percentage of maximum exercise, there was no effect of acute hypoxia. This is also true for the acute hypoxic effect on the exercise-induced rises of lactate, epinephrine and norepinephrine. Barnholt *et al.* (2006) in their study, on Pikes Peak (4300 m), of calorie restriction or adequate diet to maintain weight, found that testosterone levels rose in both groups in the first 48 hours of altitude exposure, remained elevated in the adequate diet group but fell to below control values in the calorie restricted group who lost weight. Benso *et al.* (2007), in a study of climbers arriving back at Everest Base Camp after climbing the peak and losing weight (mean 5 kg), also found a significant decrease in testosterone levels. Clearly many factors common on mountains affect testosterone levels; hypoxia and exercise raise and calorie deficit lower levels.

16.11 MALE REPRODUCTIVE FUNCTION AT ALTITUDE

The effect of altitude on male reproductive function at altitude has been little studied. Donayre *et al.* (2003) found in nine subjects decreased sperm count, increased abnormal forms and decreased motility during a 4-week stay at an altitude of 4267 m and 15 days after return to sea level. Okumura *et al.* (2003) studied three members of an expedition to the Karakoram where heights of 7100 m were reached. They did not carry out measurements at altitude but extended the study to results at 1 month, 3 months and 2 years after return to sea level. The sperm count was reduced at 1 and 3 months and had recovered at 2 years. There was also an increase in abnormally shaped sperm, which recovered by 3 months. In this study, testosterone was low at 1 and 3 months but had recovered by 2 years after return from altitude. These results have recently been confirmed by Verratti *et al.* (2008) who found complete recovery of sperm count and sperm abnormalities 6 months after return to sea level.

16.12 RENAL FUNCTION AT ALTITUDE

16.12.1 General function

The kidney is remarkably resistant to altitude hypoxia. This is not surprising since it is designed to suffer quite severe reductions in blood flow, and therefore oxygen delivery, during exercise. At 5800 m, after 24-hour dehydration, the kidney concentrates urine normally and eliminates a water load as well as it does at sea level. It also responds to ingestion of bicarbonate or ammonium chloride (metabolic alkalosis or acidosis) by producing appropriate changes in pH (Ward, reported by Pugh 1962a). Olsen *et al.* (1993) found a 10% reduction in effective renal plasma flow (ERPF) but normal glomerular filtration rate and sodium clearance in eight normal subjects at 4350 m. Dopamine infusion had less effect on ERPF than at sea level, presumably because of increased adrenergic activity (norepinephrine was increased). The diuretic effect of dopamine was reduced, possibly because of an altitude effect on distal tubular function. High altitude residents at 4300 m showed no evidence of deficient renal oxygenation (Rennie *et al.* 1971a).

However (as discussed in Chapter 10, section 10.4.5), at extreme altitude (above 6500 m) the renal compensation for respiratory alkalosis is slow and incomplete; that is, the blood bicarbonate

is very little further reduced and the blood pH becomes very alkaline as the P_{CO_2} is reduced by extreme hyperventilation. Whether this represents a degree of renal failure is debatable, since it results in a shift of the oxygen dissociation curve to the left (because of the alkaline pH), which is beneficial for oxygen transport at extreme altitude (Chapter 10, section 10.3.6). A study by Hackett *et al.* (1985) showed that in acclimatized subjects at 6300 m acetazolamide still resulted in the excretion of bicarbonate producing further base deficit. Exercise performance was not increased and, indeed, in two out of four subjects it was decreased.

There is also fluid volume depletion at altitude and it is known that the kidney gives a higher priority to correcting dehydration than acid–base disturbances. In order to excrete more bicarbonate to reduce the base excess, it would be necessary to lose corresponding cations, which would aggravate the volume depletion. This may be the basis for the slow renal bicarbonate excretion at extreme altitude.

Recently, Brito *et al.* (2007) studied renal function in a group of healthy army personnel who regularly commuted to an altitude of 3550 m from sea level and had been doing so for at least 12 years. Some of them were found to have a mild decrease of glomerular filtration rate (34% under 90 mL min^{-1} and 8% under 80 mL min^{-1} of creatinine clearance).

The diuresis of early acclimatization has been considered in the sections on anti-diuretic hormone (section 16.2) and endothelin (section 16.9). This diuresis is an important feature of acclimatization and is thought to help prevent AMS.

16.12.2 Proteinuria at altitude

Rennie and Joseph (1970) showed that proteinuria became apparent on ascent to altitude. Values rose from 290 to 578 mg mmol^{-1} as their subjects climbed to 5800 m in 12 days. There was a time lag of 1–3 days between peak altitude and peak proteinuria. Figure 16.5 shows that there is a good correlation between the degree of proteinuria and altitude, provided allowance is made for a 24-hour time lag between ascent and its effect on the kidney.

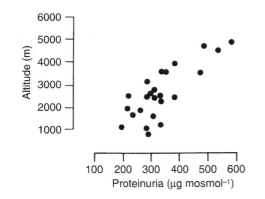

Figure 16.5 Proteinuria at altitude, the altitude being that of the subjects 24 hours before urine sampling. (After Rennie 1973.)

In another study, Rennie *et al.* (1972) found no effect of acclimatization on proteinuria but Pines (1978) found less proteinuria on repeat ascents to the same altitude, and also that subjects with AMS had the greatest proteinuria. High altitude residents excrete more protein in the urine than subjects of the same race at sea level (Rennie *et al.* 1971b).

Patients with cyanotic heart disease who are chronically hypoxic from birth also have increased proteinuria, the severity being directly related to the degree of polycythemia (and hypoxia) (Rennie 1973); it is also found in patients with chronic obstructive lung disease (Wilkinson *et al.* 1993).

The mechanism for altitude proteinuria may be either a reduction in tubular reabsorption of protein or increased glomerular permeability to protein, or both.

A study from La Paz, Bolivia, in patients with chronic mountain sickness also found significant proteinuria which was improved on treatment with an ACE inhibitor. Twenty-four-hour protein excretion fell from 359 to 248 mg. The hematocrit (Hct) fell as well from 63.5 to 56.8% (Plata *et al.* 2002). Another study from the Andes (Jefferson *et al.* 2002) also found significant proteinuria in CMS patients. There were high levels of urate (and a high incidence of gout) as well, which they attribute mainly to high levels of generation of uric acid, although a relative impairment of renal excretion might also contribute.

17

Central nervous system

SUMMARY

The central nervous system is exquisitely sensitive to hypoxia, so it is not surprising that impairment of neuropsychological function occurs at high altitude. Brain oxygenation is a function of both the arterial P_{O_2} and cerebral blood flow. The latter is regulated in part by the arterial blood gases. Hypoxemia causes cerebral vasodilatation while a reduced arterial P_{CO_2} results in cerebral vasoconstriction. Therefore, these are conflicting factors at high altitude. Some impairment of neuropsychological function, for example slow learning of complex mental tasks, can be demonstrated at altitudes of less than 2000 m. At higher altitudes many aspects of neuropsychological function have been shown to be impaired including reaction time, hand–eye coordination, and higher functions such as memory and language expression. Several studies have documented residual impairment of neuropsychological function after ascents to very high altitude. An interesting finding is that climbers with a high hypoxic ventilatory response tend to have the most severe residual impairment, possibly because the associated reduced arterial P_{CO_2} causes cerebral vasoconstriction and

therefore diminished oxygen delivery, and more severe cerebral hypoxia. Oxygen enrichment of room air improves neuropsychological function at an altitude of 5000 m and therefore improves performance in people who commute to work in mines and telescopes.

17.1 INTRODUCTION

Of all the parts of the body, the central nervous system (CNS) is the most vulnerable to hypoxia. It is not surprising, therefore, that people who go to high altitude often have changes in neuropsychological function, including special senses such as vision, higher functions such as memory, and affective behavior such as mood. Such changes have been observed in individuals acutely exposed to hypoxia, in lowlanders sojourning at high altitude, and in high altitude natives.

In addition to the changes in neuropsychological function seen in individuals at high altitude, there is evidence of persistent defects of CNS function upon return to sea level after periods of severe hypoxia at high altitude. These findings are of special interest now because increasing numbers of climbers choose to climb at great altitudes without supplementary oxygen. Many people are concerned about the increase in morbidity and mortality on expeditions to extreme altitude and irrational decisions made by severely hypoxemic climbers probably play an important role. A review of human mental performance at high altitude, and the biology of the hypoxic brain is available (Raichle and Hornbein 2001).

17.2 HISTORICAL

Changes in mood and behavior at high altitude have been recognized from the early days of climbing high mountains. However, the most extreme effects of hypoxia on the CNS were seen by the early balloonists where partial paralysis, difficulties with vision, mood changes, and even loss of consciousness are well documented. For example, during the famous flight of the balloon *Zenith* by Tissandier and his two companions (Tissandier 1875), we read:

> towards 7500 meters, the numbness one experiences is extraordinary . . . One does not suffer at all; on the contrary. One experiences inner joy, as if it were an effect of the inundating flood of light. One becomes indifferent. . . .

This lack of appreciation of the dangers of acute hypoxia is well known to aircraft pilots and is the reason why there are stringent regulations on using oxygen above certain altitudes in spite of the fact that the pilot may not feel that he needs it.

Some balloonists developed paralysis as described during the balloon ascent by Glaisher and Coxwell in 1862 (Glaisher *et al.* 1871). At the highest altitude, Glaisher collapsed unconscious in the basket, and it was left to Coxwell to vent the hydrogen from the balloon to bring it down. However, Coxwell had apparently lost the use of his hands and instead had to seize the cord that controlled the valve with his teeth and dip his head two or three times. Incidentally, this flight also underscored the rapid recovery from severe acute hypoxia. When the balloon landed, Glaisher stated that he felt 'no inconvenience', and they both walked between 7 and 8 miles to the nearest village because they had come down in a remote

country area. Actually, paralysis is not frequently seen in acute hypoxia and indeed it has been suggested that Coxwell may have been suffering from decompression sickness (Doherty 2003).

When climbers began to reach great altitudes, neuropsychological disturbances were frequently reported. For example, there were several descriptions of bizarre changes in perception and mood on the early expeditions to Mount Everest. During the 1933 Everest expedition, Smythe gave a dramatic description of a hallucination when he saw pulsating cloud-like objects in the sky (Ruttledge 1933). Smythe also reported a strong feeling that he was accompanied by a second person; he even divided food to give half to his non-existent companion. On occasions, the changes in CNS function suggest attacks of transient cerebral ischemia. For example, the very experienced mountaineer Shipton had a remarkable period of aphasia at an altitude of about 7000 m on the same expedition (Shipton 1943). He reported that:

> if I wished to say 'give me a cup of tea', I would say something entirely different – maybe 'tram-car, cat, put' . . . I was perfectly clear-headed . . . but my tongue just refused to perform the required movements. . . .

In the last few years, there has been increasing interest in the neuropsychological effects of high altitude. For example, the Polish climber and psychiatrist Ryn found a range of psychiatric disturbances in mountaineers who had ascended to over 5500 m (Ryn 1971). He also reported that symptoms similar to an organic brain syndrome persisted for several weeks after the expedition. Some climbers had electroencephalogram abnormalities after climbs to great altitudes. Studies made during the war between China and India in the early 1960s, when Indian troops were rapidly airlifted to high altitude, showed residual changes in psychomotor function on return to sea level (Sharma *et al.* 1975; Sharma *et al.* 1976). Townes *et al.* (1984) made measurements on members of the American Medical Research Expedition to Everest (AMREE) after they had returned to sea level following about 3 months at altitudes of 5400–8848 m and found residual abnormalities of neuropsychological performance.

Similar results were found on Operation Everest II, including the additional interesting observation that climbers with the highest hypoxic ventilatory response were more severely affected (Hornbein *et al.* 1989). The authors postulated that in spite of the less severe hypoxemia in the individuals with the higher ventilatory responses, the resultant more profound hypocapnia may have caused a relatively greater vasoconstriction and therefore lower blood flow and thus oxygen delivery to the brain. The findings in the more controlled Operation Everest II chamber study were similar to those in the field study on Mount Everest (AMREE 1981), and the results were combined for the Hornbein (1989) publication. There have been steady improvements in the techniques of neuropsychological testing and it is becoming clear that minor changes in function are extremely common at high altitude, and that some residual impairment often remains in some climbers who return to sea level from great altitudes.

17.3 MECHANISMS OF ACTION OF HYPOXIA

17.3.1 Hypoxia and nerve cells

In spite of a great deal of research over the last few decades, a clear understanding of the effect of hypoxia on the brain remains elusive (see Siesjo 1992a; Siesjo 1992b; Haddad and Jiang 1993; Hossmann 1999; Raichle and Hornbein 2001 for recent reviews).

There are three consistent findings from years of research on the effect of hypoxia on the brain. First, whole human brain oxygen consumption remains constant during hypoxia, even severe levels. In order to maintain this equilibrium, a commensurate increase in blood flow has to occur. Second, in spite of no change in oxygen consumption, hypoxia accelerates glucose utilization and lactate production suggesting an increase in glycolytic flux by nerve cells, but utilization is depressed during severe hypoxemia while oxygen consumption remains the same. In clinical states of severe ischemia, the hippocampus, white matter, superior colliculus and lateral geniculates appear particularly sensitive to levels of oxygen. The increase in brain lactate levels in early stages of hypoxia is counter-balanced by an increase in bicarbonate which results in a near normal pH. Third, brain tissue concentrations of ATP, ADP and AMP as markers of the energy state of the tissue remain close to normal even during severe hypoxia, comparable to elevations above 8000 m. While the brain is very sensitive to a decrease in oxygen supply, as evidenced by the changes in blood flow and glucose metabolism, examples from nature demonstrate some species' phenomenal resistance to profound hypoxia, such as the turtle (Perez-Pinon *et al.* 1992), the harbor seal (Kerem and Elsner 1973) and high altitude birds (Faraci 1986; Faraci and Fedde 1986).

IONIC CHANGES IN BRAIN WITH HYPOXIA

Altered ion homeostasis during hypoxia clearly occurs though whether the ionic changes are primary, or whether they are due to altered oxidative or neurotransmitter metabolism, is unclear. Hypoxia interferes with calcium homeostasis. For example, very low oxygen levels diminish calcium uptake at synapses. One hypothesis is that the decrease of calcium in the endoplasmic reticulum is a critical factor in cerebral dysfunction in hypoxic environments (Paschen 1966). Intracellular levels of potassium are increased during severe hypoxia. There is accumulation of free radicals which causes further injury, particularly to the capillaries. Neurotransmitter metabolism is thought to be sensitive to hypoxia although there is conflicting evidence about which transmitter or metabolic step is most sensitive. There is evidence that acetylcholine synthesis by brain is oxygen-dependent as is the biosynthesis of amino acid neurotransmitters. Brain catecholamine concentrations are apparently decreased by hypoxia though the mechanism is unclear. Much of the experimental work has been done on ischemia, and the relationship of the changes to those caused by pure hypoxia is controversial, but it is clear that ischemia is a far more important condition than hypoxia alone in causing brain damage although hypoxia accentuates ischemic injury in rat brains (Miyamoto *et al.* 2000).

VASCULAR ENDOTHELIAL GROWTH FACTOR AND HYPOXIA

As mentioned in Chapter 20, certain factors, such as hypoxia-induced vascular endothelial growth factor are known to induce fluid leak from capillaries in the brain (Fischer *et al.* 1999; Schoch *et al.* 2002), an effect known to occur with acute hypoxic exposure. The mechanism of the stimulation of vascular endothelial growth factor (VEGF) has been unraveled in the last few years, and the beneficial effects to the brain in terms of improvement of oxygen delivery have been fascinating to observe.

The response of the brain to chronic hypoxia and ischemia is one of survival which takes the forms of angiogenesis and neuroprotection, respectively. The initiation of these events depends on the stimulation of the transcription factor, hypoxia-inducible factor 1 (HIF-1) (Semenza 2000). The alpha portion of the heterodimer is the one which acts as an immediate transcription factor for a number of growth factors, one of which is VEGF (see Chapter 4). HIF-1α is present in many tissues and responds immediately and transiently to hypoxia and/or ischemia. HIF-1α targets mRNA genes and stimulates the induction of the *VEGF* gene which, along with the synergistic effect of glycolytic metabolism, induces angiogenesis in the insulted cerebral tissue (Bergeron *et al.* 2000; Marti *et al.* 2000).

With several weeks of exposure to hypoxia, rats demonstrate an immediate and sustained increase in HIF-1α (Chavez *et al.* 2000) which stimulates VEGF. This together with other growth factors results in angiogenesis and vascular remodeling such that there is an increase in capillary density and improvement and maintenance of oxygen delivery (Boero *et al.* 1999; Dor *et al.* 2001; Pichiule and LaManna 2002; LaManna *et al.* 2004). Good reviews about this area of research are available (Semenza 2000; LaManna *et al.* 2004; Xu and LaManna 2006). This body of work is an impressive example of the quest to understand down to the genetic level the adaptation to hypoxia which minimizes the decrease in availability of oxygen whether it be from high altitude or disease.

Another fascinating area of investigation recently has been the discovery of the neuroprotective effect of various growth factors, especially erythropoietin, under the conditions of ischemia and/or hypoxia. HIF-1α plays an important role in initiating this process (Bergeron *et al.* 2000; Semenza 2000; Kerendi *et al.* 2005; and see Chapter 8). It is the transcription factor for erythropoietin which has been found to minimize cerebral damage (Sirén *et al.* 2001; Bernaudin *et al.* 2002; Wen *et al.* 2002). Some investigators have hypothesized that 'preconditioning' by sublethal exposure to hypoxia might protect the brain from subsequent damage from ischemic and hypoxic exposure. Hypoxia stimulates HIF-1α which is rapidly inactivated by proline hydroxylation. Inhibition of this proteosome is being investigated as a therapeutic intervention in stroke therapy (Ratan *et al.* 2004). This line of research may have profound implications in clinical medicine, especially in the area of cerebrovascular disease.

HYPOXIA AND THE ELECTROENCEPHALOGRAM

The effects of hypoxia on brain synapses and membrane polarization interfere with the normal electrical activity of the brain and alter the EEG (electroencephalogram). In cats in which the arterial P_{O_2} is gradually reduced from 80 to 20 mmHg, the EEG amplitude initially increases slightly and then slow waves and sharp spikes appear. Subsequently, the slow waves decrease in amplitude and then disappear. Later these small spikes become sporadic, and finally the EEG flattens. The initial activation which is followed by depression may be due to the effect of hypoxia on the reticular activating system. Since acute exposure to high altitude results in increased cortical activity on the EEG, high altitude exposure may increase susceptibility to seizures by decreasing the threshold for the initiation of epileptic discharge (Basynat 2000a; Daleau *et al.* 2006). However, this theory is disputed by many who advise patients with seizure disorders who wish to go to high altitude.

EVOKED POTENTIALS AND HYPOXIA

Evoked potentials are also altered by hypoxia. Brainstem auditory response is abolished by low levels of oxygen. Visually evoked potentials are initially increased and then abolished as the level of oxygen is reduced.

HISTOLOGICAL CHANGES

Histological changes in the brain result from severe hypoxia. The changes are indistinguishable from those due to hypotension and the greatest changes are seen in the cortex and basal ganglia. Microvacuolization of neuronal perikaryon occurs first, the H1 zone (Sommer sector) of the hippocampus being the most vulnerable region.

17.3.2 Cerebral blood flow

The levels of arterial P_{O_2} and P_{CO_2} have important effects on cerebral blood flow and since these levels are greatly altered by going to high altitude, the results are important (Xu and LaManna 2006). Arterial hypoxemia dilates cerebral blood vessels and greatly increases cerebral blood flow. Figure 17.1 shows typical results found in anesthetized normocapnic rats. It can be seen that cerebral blood flow was little changed until the arterial P_{O_2} fell below 60 mmHg but with lower

levels of P_{O_2} there was a dramatic increase in cerebral blood flow. Note that at an arterial P_{O_2} of 25 mmHg, cerebral blood flow was approximately five times the normoxic level. As indicated in Chapter 13, the arterial P_{O_2} of a climber resting on the summit of Mount Everest is between 25 and 30 mmHg.

The results shown in Fig. 17.1 were obtained in mechanically ventilated animals where P_{CO_2} was kept constant at the normoxic level. However, in conscious animals and humans, the hyperventilation caused by the hypoxemia will cause a reduction in arterial P_{CO_2} and an increase in pH which will cause cerebral vasoconstriction. Therefore the results shown in Fig. 17.1 cannot be applied directly to the climber at extreme altitude.

A reduction in arterial P_{CO_2} has a strong vasoconstrictor effect on cerebral blood vessels and consequently reduces cerebral flood flow. Figure 17.2 shows typical results in mechanically ventilated anesthetized dogs which were made hypocapnic by increasing the ventilation, or hypercapnic by adding carbon dioxide to the inspired gas. In every instance the arterial P_{O_2} was maintained at approximately the normal level.

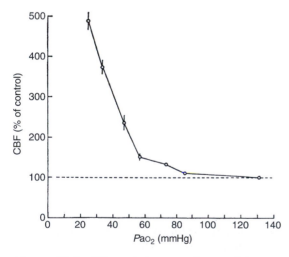

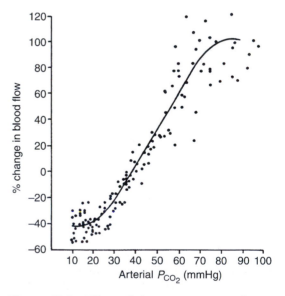

Figure 17.1 Effect of changes of arterial P_{O_2} on cerebral blood flow (CBF) in anesthetized rats. The arterial P_{CO_2} was maintained normal. Note the very sharp rise in blood flow as the arterial P_{O_2} was reduced below 50 mmHg. (From Borgström *et al.* 1975.)

Figure 17.2 Effect of alterations in arterial P_{CO_2} on cerebral cortical blood flow in anesthetized dogs. The zero reference line for blood flow is at an arterial P_{CO_2} of 40 mmHg. Animals were normoxic and normotensive. (From Harper and Glass 1965.)

Note that when the arterial P_{CO_2} fell to about 15 mmHg, cerebral blood flow was reduced by about 40% (Harper and Glass 1965).

In humans at high altitude, the two effects of hypoxemia and hypocapnia will clearly have opposing effects on the cerebral circulation. However, in some studies, they have been found to balance each other so that after 3 weeks' exposure to high altitude, cerebral blood flow returns to low altitude baseline levels (Møller et al. 2002).

There have not been systematic studies of cerebral blood flow in humans at various altitudes partly because of the difficulties of measurement. However, Severinghaus et al. (1966) measured cerebral blood flow in seven normal subjects by a nitrous oxide method at sea level and after 6–12 hours and 3–5 days at an altitude of 3810 m. The blood flow increased by an average of 24% at 6–12 hours, and by 13% at 3–5 days at altitude. Acute correction of the hypoxia restored the cerebral blood flow to normal. Extrapolation of additional data suggested that if the P_{CO_2} had not been reduced at high altitude, the cerebral blood flow would have been 60% above the control. An interesting feature of the data obtained by Severinghaus et al. (1966) is that the subsequent analysis shows that oxygen delivery to the brain (as calculated from cerebral blood flow multiplied by arterial oxygen concentration) was held essentially constant (Wolff 2000). However, there is no known receptor that responds to oxygen delivery.

Indirect evidence about cerebral blood flow in humans can be obtained by measuring blood flow velocity in the internal carotid artery by Doppler ultrasound. Huang et al. (1987) measured flow velocities in the internal carotid and vertebral arteries in six subjects within 2–4 hours of arrival on Pikes Peak (4300 m), and found that the velocities in both arteries were slightly increased above sea level values; 18–44 hours later, a peak increase of 20% was observed. However, over days 4–12, velocities declined to values similar to those at sea level. In the further study by the same group (Huang et al. 1991) the effect of prolonged exercise (45 minutes at approximately 100 W) on blood flow velocity in the internal carotid artery was studied at sea level and at 4300 m. The velocities at sea level and high altitude were similar. In a low-pressure chamber study, Reeves et al. (1985) measured blood flow velocity in the internal carotid artery of 12 subjects at Denver (1600 m) and repeatedly up to 7 hours at a simulated altitude of 4800 m. Their hypothesis was that an increase in blood flow velocity might be associated with the development of high altitude headache, but no correlation was found. Other studies by Doppler ultrasound have shown no correlation between cerebral blood flow and acute mountain sickness (Baumgartner et al. 1999), or cerebral blood flow and susceptibility to high altitude pulmonary edema (Berre et al. 1999). On the other hand, Jansen et al. (1999) reported that subjects with acute mountain sickness had higher cerebral blood flows than normals, and also a greater hemodynamic response to hyperventilation.

Huang et al. (1992) measured blood flow velocity in the internal carotid arteries of 15 native Tibetans and 11 Han Chinese residents of Lhasa (3658 m) both at rest and during exercise. There were no differences at rest and during submaximal exercise. However at peak exercise, the Tibetans showed an increase in flow velocity and cerebral oxygen delivery whereas the Hans did not. Frayser et al. (1970) measured the mean circulation time through the retina following fluorescein injection and found that the circulation time decreased from a mean of 4.9 seconds at base camp to 3.4 seconds at an altitude of 5330 m. This is consistent with an increase in cerebral blood flow.

Another possible factor at high altitude which could influence cerebral blood flow is an increased viscosity of the blood caused by polycythemia. It is known that a blood flow of less than half the normal value can occur in severe polycythemia vera (Kety 1950) and that cerebral blood flow is significantly increased in severe anemia (Heyman et al. 1952; Robin and Gardner 1953). Tomiyama et al. (2000) reduced and increased blood viscosity in rats by hemodilution or transfusion, respectively, and measured cerebral blood flow during hypoxia and hypercapnia. They found that cerebral blood flow correlated with viscosity with the most profound effect being a decrease in the animals with the highest viscosity. Some drugs, including caffeine, reduce cerebral blood flow.

17.4 CENTRAL NERVOUS SYSTEM FUNCTION AT HIGH ALTITUDE

17.4.1 Moderate altitudes

There is general agreement that CNS function is impaired at altitudes over about 4500 m but an interesting question is the lowest altitude at which minor alterations in function occur. This question frequently arises in the aviation industry because it is relevant to selecting the cabin pressure of commercial aircraft. Most high flying commercial aircraft are pressurized to maintain the cabin pressure at or below an equivalent altitude of about 2500 m. This ceiling was accepted after considering the penalty of extra weight and expense which would have to be paid in order to reduce it further. However, there is some evidence that at a pressure equivalent to an altitude of 2440 m, subjects are slower to learn complex mental tasks than at sea level. The cabin pressure of newer aircraft such as the Boeing 787 and Airbus 380 has been increased to the equivalent altitude of 1800 m.

It has been reported that at the lower altitude of only 1524 m, eight subjects were slower to learn complex tasks than a matched group breathing an enriched oxygen mixture (Denison *et al.* 1966). The tests involved recognizing the posture of man-like figures having different orientations and presented in random sequence on a screen. However, other studies have not confirmed these findings. For example, Paul and Fraser (1994) using similar tests, involving the learning of new tasks, found no impairment at altitude equivalent to 1524, 2438 and 3048 m.

Interesting problems concerning CNS function at moderate altitudes occur in relation to the operation of optical and infrared telescopes on mountain summits (see also Chapter 28). The reduction in the absorption of optical and infrared radiation because of the reduced thickness of the Earth's atmosphere at high altitude makes high mountains ideal locations for astronomical observatories. For example, several telescopes are located on the summit of Mauna Kea, altitude 4200 m, on the island of Hawaii.

The barometric pressure on the summit of Mauna Kea is only about 468 mmHg, giving a moist inspired P_{O_2} of 88 mmHg. The telescope operators frequently live at sea level and ascend rapidly by car to the summit. Forster (1986) measured arterial blood gases on 27 telescope personnel on the first day of reaching 4200 m and reported a mean arterial P_{O_2} of 42 mmHg, P_{CO_2} 29 mmHg and pH 7.49. After 5 days, during which time the nights were spent in dormitories at an altitude of 3000 m, the arterial blood gases at 4200 m showed a mean P_{O_2} of 44 mmHg, P_{CO_2} 27 mmHg and pH of 7.48 (see Figure 7.2).

A number of psychometric measurements showed no change on ascending to 4200 m, though performance of the digit symbol backwards test did deteriorate on the first day. At the end of 5 days, however, the scores had returned to sea level values. Numerate memory and psychomotor ability were also reported to be impaired in commuters to Mauna Kea. Several features of acute mountain sickness were noted in shift workers, particularly on their first day at the summit. Headache was the most disabling symptom but others included insomnia, lethargy, poor concentration and poor memory.

17.4.2 High altitudes

A classical series of studies were carried out by McFarland (1937a, 1937b, 1938a, 1938b) in connection with the International High Altitude Expedition to Chile which took place in 1935. In his first study, McFarland reported on the psychophysiological effects of sudden ascents to 5000 m in unpressurized aircraft and compared the results with ascents by train and car to villages as high as 4700 m in Chile. The measurements showed that the rate of ascent was an important variable, with the rapid increase in altitude by aircraft being the most damaging. Both simple and complex psychological functions were significantly impaired at high altitudes including arithmetical tests, writing ability, and the appearance and disappearance time of after-images following exposure of the eye to a bright light. There were increased memory errors, errors in perseverance, and reductions in auditory threshold and words apprehended.

In a second study of sensory and motor responses during acclimatization, when measurements were obtained at altitudes as high as 5330 and 6100 m, significant reductions in audition, vision, and eye–hand coordination were seen. Measurements were made at several altitudes but, in general, impairment of function was not significant below an altitude of 5330 m. Again, members of the expedition with the longest periods of acclimatization appeared to suffer less deterioration.

In a further study, mental and psychosomatic tests were also administered at the same altitudes and these showed deterioration. Tests involving the quickness of recognizing the meaning of words, mental flexibility or tendency to perseveration, and immediate memory showed significant impairment. It was noted that complex mental work could be carried out if the subjects increased their concentration but, in general, there was increased distractibility and lethargy which tended to reduce the ability to concentrate.

In a final series of measurements, sensory and circulatory responses were measured on sulfur miners residing permanently at an altitude of 5330 m at Aucanquilcha. They were compared with a group of workmen at sea level who were similar in age and race, and also with members of the expedition. It was found that the miners at high altitude were slower in simple and choice reaction times and less acute in auditory sensitivity than the workmen at sea level. However, McFarland and his colleagues were impressed by the evidence for circulatory and respiratory adaptation in these permanent residents at an altitude of 5330 m.

Additional studies on the deleterious effects of acute hypoxia on visual perception have been carried out, partly because of the importance of this topic in aviation. For example, Kobrick (1975) documented impaired response times in the detection of flash stimuli at equivalent altitudes of sea level, 4000 m, 4600 m and 5200 m during acute exposure in a low-pressure chamber. The effects of hypoxia on other peripheral stimuli have also been studied (Kobrick 1972).

A special opportunity to study the central nervous system effects of high altitude occurred during the India–China border war in the early 1960s when large numbers of Indian troops were rapidly taken to an altitude of 4000 m and remained there for as long as 2 years. Sharma *et al.* (1975) measured psychomotor efficiency in 25 young Indians ranging in age from 21 to 30 years. Psychomotor performance including speed and accuracy was determined by administering an eye–hand coordination test in which a stylus was moved in a narrow groove so that it did not touch the sides. The tests were performed at sea level and at an altitude of 4000 m after periods of 1, 10, 13, 18 and 24 months. Figure 17.3 shows how overall psychomotor efficiency declined over the first 10 months of altitude exposure but then recovered somewhat over the ensuing 13 months.

Overall psychomotor efficiency as shown in Fig. 17.3 includes both the speed and accuracy scores from the test. Figure 17.4 shows a breakdown of the accuracy and speed of this test of psychomotor performance. Note that the accuracy of the measurement increased substantially after the 10-month period but there was little improvement in speed. This result is consistent with the impression given by many people who have worked at high altitude, namely that thought processes are slowed, but if one concentrates hard enough, accurate procedures can be carried out.

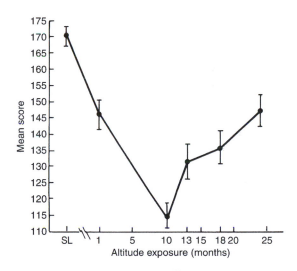

Figure 17.3 Psychomotor efficiency in young adults rapidly taken to an altitude of 4000 m where they remained for 2 years. Psychomotor efficiency was calculated using an eye–hand coordination test which included speed and accuracy. Note the deterioration in psychomotor efficiency over the first 10 months, which then gradually improved. (From Sharma *et al.* 1975.)

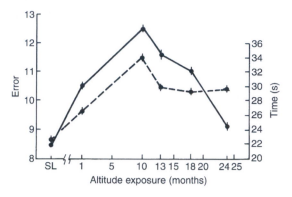

Figure 17.4 Same data as in Fig. 17.3 except that psychomotor efficiency is broken down into accuracy and speed of eye–hand coordination. Note that the accuracy of the measurement increased after 10 months but there was relatively little improvement in speed. (From Sharma *et al.* 1975.)

In a related study, Sharma and Malhotra (1976) compared the performance of three groups of Indians drawn from the Corkha, Madrasi and Rajput areas after 10 months' stay at altitude of 4000 m. There were no differences in the scores for eye–hand coordination and social interaction at altitudes for the three ethnic groups. However, the Corkhas showed a better toleration of altitude stress as evidenced by the effects on concentration, anxiety and depression.

In a study of 20 male soldiers exposed to a simulated altitude of 4700 m for 5–7 hours, the relationships between symptoms and signs of acute mountain sickness, mood and psychometric performance were studied (Shukitt-Hale *et al.* 1991). It was found that evidence of acute mountain sickness was best correlated with symptoms, then mood changes, and least with performance.

Cognitive and emotional changes at simulated high altitude were studied by Pavlicek *et al.* (2005) in 21 men exposed to altitudes up to 4500 m for short periods in a low pressure chamber. They found that both cognitive and affective functions mediated by the frontal lobe were preserved.

An unusual opportunity for studying the effects of very high altitude on mental performance of lowlanders was offered by the 1960–61 Silver Hut Expedition when several normal subjects spent up to 3 months at an altitude of 5800 m. Mental efficiency was tested by asking the subjects to sort playing cards into bins using specially designed equipment which recorded events on magnetic tape (Gill *et al.* 1964). It was found that the efficiency of sorting cards was less at the high altitude than at sea level. The inefficiency took the form of a delay in placing the cards into the correct bins rather than errors of sorting. Again, these results reinforce the common notion that accurate work can be done at high altitude, but it takes longer, and more effort in concentration is required. Cahoon (1972) also showed a reduced efficiency of card sorting in eight normal subjects exposed to a simulated altitude of 4600 m for 48 hours.

During the 1981 AMREE, a series of psychometric tests were carried out prior to the expedition, at the base camp (5400 m), at the main laboratory camp (6300 m) and immediately after and 1 year after the expedition (Townes *et al.* 1984). The main emphasis was on a comparison of CNS function before and after exposure to extreme altitude, and only a few of the measurements made at high altitude were reported. However, finger-tapping speed decreased significantly over the course of the expedition. Mean taps of the right hand were 53.7 (pre-test), 52.6 (5400 m altitude), 50.8 (6300 m altitude), 48.1 (on subjects returning to 6300 m altitude from 8000 m) and 45.4 (immediately after the expedition). It is not clear from these results whether the reduction in finger-tapping speed was a function of altitude, time at high altitude, or both.

Hainsworth *et al.* (2007) have reviewed the function of the autonomic nervous system in lowlanders who ascend to high altitude and also in high altitude residents. There are discussions of heart rate, myocardial contractility and systemic blood pressure in lowlanders. These topics are also addressed in Chapter 8. Hainsworth *et al.* also discuss the possible role of the autonomic nervous system in chronic mountain sickness.

17.4.3 Electroencephalogram

Ryn (1970, 1971) reported EEG abnormalities in 11 of 30 climbers who had been over 5500 m altitude. The predominant abnormality was a decreased frequency of alpha waves and a diminution of their amplitude. He also reported paroxysmal and focal pathology in EEG records performed at high altitude.

Zhongyuan and his colleagues (1983) also reported changes in the EEG at altitudes above 5000 m in members of a Chinese expedition to Mount Everest. There was a reduced amplitude of the alpha rhythm but in this instance there was an increase in its frequency. The EEG changes were less than those observed during acute hypoxia of the same degree in a low-pressure chamber prior to the expedition. Apparently, members of the expedition who tolerated the acute hypoxia well tended to show fewer EEG changes on the mountain itself.

Nevison carried out an extensive series of EEG measurements during the Silver Hut expedition of 1960–61. Although the results were not written up in the open literature, he apparently found no abnormalities in subjects living at 5800 m. Also, the EEG appearances were not altered by hyperventilation or 100% oxygen breathing.

17.5 RESIDUAL CENTRAL NERVOUS SYSTEM IMPAIRMENT FOLLOWING RETURN FROM HIGH ALTITUDE

In view of the known vulnerability of the CNS to hypoxia, it is hardly surprising that neurobehavioral abnormalities can be demonstrated at high altitudes. However, there has been great interest in the demonstration of residual impairment of CNS function following return to sea level.

An extensive study was carried out by Townes *et al.* (1984), referred to in section 17.4.2. The subjects were 21 members of the 1981 AMREE, and all were males between 25 and 52 years of age with a mean age of 36.4 years. The general level of education was high with 15 subjects having either an MD or PhD degree. Prior to the expedition, the following psychological tests were administered at the San Diego Veterans Administration Hospital: Halstead–Reitan battery (Reitan and Davison 1974), repeatable cognitive–perceptual–motor battery (Lewis and Rennick 1979), selective reminding test (Buschke 1973) and the Wechsler memory scale (Russell 1975). These same measurements were repeated immediately after the expedition in Kathmandu, Nepal. At an expedition meeting held in Colorado 1 year later, the following tests were re-administered:

Halstead–Wepman aphasia screening test, B trials and the finger-tapping test from the Halstead–Reitan battery, the digit vigilance task from the repeatable battery, and a verbal passage from the Wechsler memory scale.

Table 17.1 shows the significant changes found between pre-expedition, post-expedition and follow-up performance on the neuropsychological tests. It can be seen that verbal learning and memory declined significantly from the beginning to the end of the expedition as measured by the Wechsler memory scale. In the Halstead–Wepman aphasia screening test, the number of expressive language errors increased significantly between pre-test and post-test after the expedition. The number of aphasic errors was significantly related to the altitude attained by the subject.

As indicated in section 17.4.2, finger-tapping speed decreased significantly over the course of the expedition. This was measured by requiring the subject to tap a lever as rapidly as possible over a period of 10 seconds. For a test to be acceptable, five measurements on each hand gave a difference of less than five taps between trials. Before the expedition all subjects reached this criterion. However, at Kathmandu immediately after the expedition, 15 of 20 subjects could not sustain motor speed, and 13 of 16 subjects could not do so 1 year later.

These findings are of great interest because they provide strong objective evidence for CNS deterioration as a result of exposure to high altitude, a subject which has been debated vigorously in the past. However, other authors have reported similar or consistent findings. Ryn (1970, 1971) also found persistent abnormalities in a group of 20 male and 10 female Polish climbers several weeks after a Himalayan expedition. Half of the male climbers who ascended over 5500 m experienced symptoms similar to the acute organic brain syndrome, and for several weeks after the expedition they had changes in affect and impaired memory. Eleven of the 30 climbers had EEG abnormalities immediately after the climb. Psychological testing (Bender, Benton and Graham–Kendall tests) were reported to be normal in 13 persons, borderline in 12 persons, and indicative of organic pathology in five chambers.

Table 17.1 Wilcoxon signed-rank tests comparing performance before, immediately after (in Kathmandu), and 1 year after expedition to Mount Everest

Performance	Results (means ± SE)			Paired responses		
	Before	After	Follow up	Before and after	After and follow up	Before and follow up
Improved performance						
Tactual performance test (right hand)	4.68 ± 1.56	3.86 ± 1.46		2.72*		
Category test	24.29 ± 15.46	11.05 ± 8.39		3.48+		
Decline in performance						
Finger tapping test						
Right hand	53.71 ± 4.07	45.40 ± 6.18	48.40 ± 6.60	3.39+	1.32	2.20‡
Left hand	47.65 ± 4.60	42.45 ± 5.96	41.73 ± 5.23	2.30‡	0.66	2.93*
Criterion right	1.00 ± 0	0.14 ± 0.36	0.27 ± 0.46	3.06*	0.73	2.67*
Criterion left	1.00 ± 0	0.14 ± 0.36	0.13 ± 0.35	2.93‡	0.54	2.93*
Wechsler memory scale						
Short-term verbal recall	18.12 ± 1.90	15.90 ± 2.15	17.13 ± 2.20	2.60*	2.12‡	0.98
Trials to criterion	1.24 ± 0.44	2.40 ± 1.54	2.27 ± 0.70	2.37‡	0	2.67*
Long-term verbal recall	16.35 ± 2.91	12.70 ± 3.78	14.50 ± 2.85	2.32‡	2.75	0.94
Aphasia screening test	0.59 ± 0.79	1.25 ± 1.25	0.47 ± 0.52	2.22‡	2.31‡	0.47

*p 0.01; +p 0.001; ‡p 0.05.
From Townes et al. 1984.

Persistent cognitive impairment was described in five world-class climbers who had reached summits over 8500 m without supplementary oxygen (Regard *et al.* 1989). The abnormalities were in the ability to concentrate, short-term memory and cognitive flexibility (the ability to shift from one learned concept to another).

In a brief report, Cavaletti *et al.* (1987) showed residual impairment of memory in seven climbers who returned to sea level after ascending to 7075 m on Mount Satopanth without supplementary oxygen. The measurements were made before leaving Italy, at the base camp after the ascent, and 75 days after the expedition. It was shown that memory performance decreased both at base camp and, to a lesser degree, at sea level 75 days after the climb. However, tests of fluency and ideomotor ability (ability to perform skilled limb movements on command) were unaffected by altitude. In a more recent study, persistent changes in memory, reaction time and concentration were reported 75 days after a single ascent over 5000 m (Cavaletti and Tredici 1993).

Cortical atrophy and brain magnetic resonance imaging (MRI) changes have been reported in 26 climbers who ascended to over 7000 m without supplementary oxygen (Garrido *et al.* 1993). No MRI studies were performed prior to the climbs; the measurements were made 26 days to 36 months after return to sea level. The controls were 21 normal subjects, and 46% of the climbers showed MRI abnormalities. A sophisticated study of brain MRI in 14 normal subjects who ascended to 6206 m was reported by Zhang *et al.* (2012). They found abnormalities of brain white matter in various regions including the bilateral corticospinal tract, corpus callosum, and reticular formation of dorsal midbrain. However, there were no significant changes in cognitive tests.

Miscio *et al.* (2009) reported a study of cortical excitability using transcranial magnetic stimulation in seven subjects after 3–5 days at the Capanna Margherita, altitude 4559 m. Comparisons were made with the same subjects at sea level. They found that the resting motor threshold was significantly higher at altitude, but the short intracortical inhibition was significantly lower. Symptoms of acute mountain sickness were significantly correlated with the increased resting motor threshold.

Not everyone has found CNS abnormalities following return after ascent to very high altitude. For example, Clark *et al.* (1983) tested 22 mountaineers before and 16–221 days after Himalayan climbs above 5100 m with a battery of psychological and neurophysiological tests but found no evidence of cerebral dysfunction. This was a well-designed study and it is not clear why these climbers showed no abnormalities. In another study, Anooshiravani *et al.* (1999) carried out brain MRI studies and performed neuropsychological testing on eight male climbers before and after ascents to over 6000 m without oxygen. Although they found increases in symptoms of acute mountain sickness, there were no alterations in brain imaging or neuropsychological tests between 5 and 10 days after returning to sea level.

Measurements from the 1985 Operation Everest II confirmed the changes in psychometric function found on the 1981 AMREE, and extended the observations in an interesting and unexpected direction. During Operation Everest II, eight normal subjects spent 40 days in a low-pressure chamber and were gradually decompressed, ultimately being exposed to the simulated altitude of the Everest summit. Impairments in motor speed and persistence, memory, and verbal expressive abilities were found after the simulated ascent just as with the 1981 Everest expedition (Hornbein *et al.* 1989).

The new finding was a significant negative correlation between hypoxic ventilatory response and neurobehavioral function measured after the expedition. In other words, those climbers with the largest hypoxic ventilatory response showed the greatest decrement in neurobehavioral function. This was unexpected; indeed, the prediction might have been that those who increased their ventilation most would protect their CNS function by preserving their alveolar and therefore arterial P_{O_2}.

A hypothesis to explain these unexpected findings was advanced by Hornbein *et al.* (1989). They argued that the subjects with the highest hypoxic ventilatory response would reduce their arterial P_{CO_2} the most and therefore develop the most cerebral vasoconstriction. This, in turn, would cause the most severe cerebral hypoxia even though their arterial P_{O_2} would actually be higher than that in the subjects with the smaller ventilatory responses to hypoxia.

Note that this hypothesis is not supported by the measurements of cerebral blood flow against arterial P_{CO_2} in anesthetized dogs shown in Fig. 17.2. Those data show that cerebral blood flow apparently levels off at values of P_{CO_2} below approximately 15 mmHg. However, the situation with acclimatization may be different because the arterial pH returns towards normal and this may improve cerebral blood flow. In addition, the scatter in the data is such that this result may not be reliable. It should also be pointed out that the relationship between cerebral blood flow and arterial P_{CO_2} is very sensitive to the systematic arterial pressure (Harper and Glass 1965). Hypotensive dogs show a much smaller change in cerebral blood flow for a given change in P_{CO_2} than normotensive animals. Whether changes in systemic blood pressure occur at extreme altitudes is not known although there are no obvious alterations at 5800 m (Pugh 1964).

The correlation between hypoxic ventilatory response and residual impairment of CNS function leads to an interesting paradox. On the one hand, a brisk hypoxic ventilatory response is advantageous for a climber to reach extreme altitudes because otherwise the alveolar P_{O_2} cannot be maintained at the required levels. However, the only way of maintaining the P_{O_2} is by extreme hyperventilation, which reduces the arterial P_{CO_2}, which in turn reduces cerebral blood flow. Thus, such a climber is likely to suffer more residual central nervous impairment. In other words, the climber who is endowed by nature to go the highest is likely to suffer the most severe nervous system damage.

17.6 EFFECT OF OXYGEN ENRICHMENT OF ROOM AIR ON NEUROPSYCHOLOGICAL FUNCTION AT HIGH ALTITUDE

Increasing numbers of people are commuting to high altitude for commercial purposes such as mining, and scientific purposes such as astronomy (see Chapter 28). In order to reduce the neuropsychological impairment that occurs at high altitudes, oxygen enrichment of room air is now used extensively. This is remarkably effective because every 1% increase in oxygen concentration (for example, from 21 to 22%) reduces the equivalent altitude by about 300 m. Gerard et al. (2000) evaluated the effectiveness of enriching room air oxygen by 6% at simulated 5000 m altitude. A randomized double-blind study was carried out on 24 subjects who underwent neuropsychological testing in a specially designed facility at 3800 m that could simulate both an ambient 5000 m atmosphere and an atmosphere of 6% oxygen enrichment at 5000 m. The 2-hour test battery of 16 tasks assessed various aspects of motor and cognitive performance. Compared with simulated breathing air at 5000 m, oxygen enrichment resulted in higher arterial oxygen saturations, quicker reaction times, improved hand–eye coordination, and a more positive sense of well-being, each significant at the $p < 0.05$ level.

It is interesting that other aspects of neuropsychological function were not significantly improved by 6% additional oxygen. One reason may be that short-term concentration may temporarily overcome real underlying deficits. The problem was succinctly stated by Barcroft et al. (1923) reporting on the 1921–22 International High Altitude Expedition to Cerro de Pasco, Peru, altitude 4330 m. He wrote:

Judged by the ordinary standards of efficiency in laboratory work, we were in an obviously lower category at Cerro than at the sea-level. By a curious paradox this was most apparent when it was being least tested, for perhaps what we suffered from chiefly was the difficulty of maintaining concentration. When we knew we were undergoing a test, our concentration could by an effort be maintained over the length of time taken for the test, but under ordinary circumstances it would lapse. It is, perhaps, characteristic that, whilst each individual mental test was done as rapidly at Cerro as at the sea-level, the performance of the series took nearly twice as long for its accomplishment. Time was wasted there in trivialities and 'bungling,' which would not take place at sea-level.

(Barcroft *et al.* 1923)

A study of oxygen enrichment at 3800 m altitude showed that sleep quality, especially deep sleep stages, total sleep time, and efficient sleep index were all improved with oxygen enrichment (Luks *et al.* 1998). This and other studies of oxygen enrichment on sleep are discussed in Chapter 14.

In view of the above, it would be very interesting to develop neuropsychological tests which were embedded in the normal daily activities of the subject. In other words, it would be valuable to be able to measure the mental efficiency of the subjects when they were unaware of being tested. A formal study along these lines has not yet been carried out at high altitude.

The addition of extra oxygen to any environment also may carry some hazards, such as increased fire risk. This has been carefully analyzed and guidelines for safe levels of oxygen enrichment have been described (West 2001). The intervention of supplemental oxygen may be beneficial not only in professional settings where mental acuity is essential but also in areas of recreation where altitude illness can be a limiting factor to enjoyment of the sojourn (West 2002).

18

High altitude populations

SUMMARY

Differences between different highland populations and between highlanders and lowlanders are likely to be due to either the effect of being born and brought up at altitude or to genetic differences which have been selected for over many generations as having survival advantage for life at high altitude. There have been great advances in this latter area and these are considered in Chapter 4, which is new to this edition. This chapter deals with differences in physiology between highlanders and lowlanders and between different groups of highlanders. Also it considers diseases peculiar to residence at high altitude.

Many people live permanently at high altitude which has a significant effect on their physiology (see Chapter 3 for numbers and world distribution). Studies of such populations are hampered by the problem of appropriate comparison groups. Often a group of high altitude residents is compared with a group of lowlanders from a different ethnic, socioeconomic and genetic background so that it is difficult to know to what factors any differences may be attributed. Also it is becoming clear that not all high altitude residents are the same. Recent studies have found interesting differences between South American, central Asian and Ethiopian high altitude residents.

Altitude residence does not seem to have important demographic effects; economic factors are of greater importance. Fertility, which is reduced in newcomers to altitude, seems to be normal in peoples resident for generations, especially on the Tibetan plateau. Fetal growth in the last stages of pregnancy is retarded, and birth weight falls with increasing altitude of residence. Growth in childhood has been claimed to be retarded but continues for longer, though again this could be due, in part at least, to economic or nutritional factors rather than altitude per se.

The physiology of high altitude residents differs from that of lowlanders at altitude in some respects. The former have lower total ventilation at rest and exercise and blunted hypoxic ventilatory response (though in Tibetans this is less so than in South American highlanders). Despite lower ventilation their oxygen saturation and P_{O_2} are similar to those of lowlanders at altitude at rest and on exercise their P_{O_2} is less reduced. They have slightly larger lungs which contributes to higher lung diffusing capacities than lowlanders. This is an important advantage at altitude, where diffusion limitation results in lowered Sa_{O_2} and hence reduced work rate. Animals adapted to high altitude have very little pulmonary artery pressor response to hypoxia. Tibetans show a degree of this adaptation, but not South American high altitude residents. There are also differences in hemoglobin concentration and oxygen saturation between these populations, all suggesting that the Tibetans, with their longer lineage at altitude, have undergone a greater degree of altitude adaptation.

Certain diseases are found commonly among altitude residents. Again, some are the result of socioeconomic factors and are common in poor populations at sea level. Cold and cold injury are more common at altitude but, of course, not confined to it. The most common disease due to altitude hypoxia is chronic mountain sickness and high altitude pulmonary edema. This is covered in Chapter 22. Others include chemodectoma, a benign tumor of the carotid body, and a high incidence of patent ductus arteriosus in infants. Goiter, though not strictly confined to high altitude, is much more prevalent there since iodine-deficient soils are more common at high elevations and possibly the demands for iodine are greater at altitude. However, with iodine supplementation goiter is less common than in the past. Finally, sickle cell disease, though not caused by altitude, is more serious there.

18.1 INTRODUCTION

This chapter considers the characteristics of people born and raised at high altitude and whose ancestors have resided at high altitude for many generations. In Chapter 3 the locations of these populations are discussed. In general, the altitude considered is above 3000 m. The duration of residence of the population is impossible to determine; it ranges from perhaps 50 000 to 100 000 years in Tibet and perhaps 15 000 years in the Andes to a few generations in the high mining towns of Colorado, USA. The enormous developments in the field of human genetics have enabled scientists to carry out many studies of the genetics of high altitude populations since the previous edition of this book. Therefore, we have included an entire new chapter (Chapter 4) on the genetics of high altitude. The present chapter will explore differences in physiology, including pre- and post-natal development, between highlanders and lowlanders and between different groups of highlanders. Also it considers diseases peculiar to residence at high altitude.

Our knowledge of the effect of lifelong residence at altitude has come from studies of particular peoples. A major problem in interpreting results is to decide whether the characteristics found to differ from lowland populations are really due to the high altitude environment (hypoxia or cold) or due to racial, nutritional or economic factors.

Some studies have sought to eliminate racial factors by using low altitude residents of the same ethnic background as controls. It is difficult to control for nutritional factors since high altitude residents may well be economically disadvantaged when compared with their low altitude controls. This seems to be the case in the Andes. The effects of poor nutrition and chronic hypoxia are similar on factors such as growth and development, thus confounding the interpretation of results. The economic advantage may be reversed, as in Ethiopia, where the highland regions are free from malaria and the residents more wealthy and better fed. The result is that studies from this part of the world do not show the differences between high and low altitude residents that are reported from the Andes. There are fewer studies from the Himalayas and Tibet than from the Andes, though this has been redressed in recent years with an increasing number of studies from Lhasa.

However, if these reservations are kept in mind, some conclusions can be drawn from the many surveys about the effects of lifelong residence at high altitude, especially on birth weight and childhood development. Recent studies have addressed the question of differences between South American and Tibetan high altitude residents and the related one of whether there has been natural selection for giving a biological advantage to either of these populations. Moore reviewed some of these areas of interest (Moore 2001).

18.2 DEMOGRAPHIC ASPECTS

18.2.1 Population age and sex distribution

A few high altitude groups have been analyzed in some detail and the population of the Nunoa district (4000 m) of Peru showed some differences compared with the total Peruvian population (Baker and Dutt 1972). The high altitude population was somewhat younger, and the ratio of females to males was larger during infancy and childhood, but in addition there appeared to be more elderly people among the high altitude than the general population.

The explanation seems to be that, in the high altitude population, there was a high birth rate and high adult emigration rate. Male mortality was higher than female in infancy, childhood and early adolescence. The larger number of older individuals may have been due to the prestige associated with telling observers that they were of a great age. Claims to longevity are hard to substantiate because birth certificates and baptismal registers are seldom kept, and some individuals lie outrageously about their age. Areas noted for longevity, the Villcambamba region of Ecuador, the state of Georgia in Russia and the Hunzas of Northern Pakistan all claimed inordinant longevity, but many of these claims are unsubstantiated. For instance, in north Bhutan the oldest individuals were over 80 but not above 90 years old as claimed (Jackson *et al.* 1966, p. 99), and some Tibetan lamas claim to have lived to a great age. There seems to be little concrete evidence for unusual longevity at high altitude.

In the Khumbu region of north-eastern Nepal, male infant mortality was higher than female. There was little permanent emigration but a higher percentage of males were involved in accidents. In north-west Nepal, the number of males born relative to females was higher but mortality in male infants was increased (Baker 1978).

18.2.2 Fertility

Adaptation to the environment must include the ability of the species to reproduce. The Spanish who occupied the high altitude regions of South America in the sixteenth and seventeenth centuries found that neither their animals nor their womenfolk had live offspring. This was in contrast to the indigenous animals and peoples. Clegg (1978) quotes two well-observed Spanish accounts of La Calancha (1639) and Cobo (1653). The former recounts the early history of the city of Potosí (4060 m) in present day Bolivia with a population of 20 000 Spaniards and 100 000 Indians. Children born to Spanish couples died either at birth or within 2 weeks. Pregnant Spanish women developed the habit of returning to low altitude for their pregnancy and delivery and keeping their babies there until a year old. Han Chinese women living in Tibet follow a similar pattern. The cause of failure to thrive in these infants may well have been high altitude pulmonary hypertension (Chapter 22). The Amerindians, of course, had no such problems nor do the indigenous Tibetans. It was not until 53 years after its foundation that the first Spanish child was born and reared in the city. Cobo says that Jauja (3500 m), the early capital of Peru, was considered 'a sterile place' where horses, pigs or fowl could not be raised, whereas 100 years later it was a principal area producing pigs and poultry and supplying Lima with these products. Cobo also pointed out that infant survival depended upon the proportion of Indian blood in the child, with pure-blooded Spanish children mostly dying, children of mixed blood faring rather better, and pure-blooded Indian children having the lowest mortality, despite much poorer living conditions.

What is the cause of this lack of fertility in lowlanders at altitude? Sperm counts in lowland men fall temporarily on going to altitude but then recover. Testosterone levels also fall and then recover after a week or two (Chapter 16, section 16.10.3). In the female, on going to altitude, there may be temporary disturbances in menstruation (Sobrevilla *et al.* 1967). Conception rates are virtually impossible to measure, especially since chronic hypoxia may increase the frequency of early abortions. The reduced fertility may be due to a number of factors, possibly reduced conception, probably increased numbers of early abortions, stillbirths and neonatal deaths.

In altitude residents fertility was thought to be reduced. Hoff and Abelson (1976), using aggregate data from Peru, found that fertility, measured as the number of children under the age of 5 divided by the number of women aged 15–49 years, fell linearly with altitude ($p < 0.01$) but they were cautious when interpreting the data on which this was based. They also found that high altitude women who migrate to low altitude increase their fertility. However, both Carrillo (1996) and Gonzales *et al.* (1996) found global fecundity rates higher than at sea level.

Determining the factors which affect fertility in populations with many socioeconomic variables has been extremely difficult. Vitzthum *et al.* (2000) studied progesterone levels in Andean women to determine menstrual and thus ovarian function and concluded that hypoxia per se did not alter ovarian function compared to low altitude patterns. This group also found that bias in the data may arise from the low rate of conception in non-lactating women. Kapoor *et al.* (2003) studied Himalayan populations and found that since the high altitude populations are in such socioeconomic flux, there were few variables which were solely responsible for an apparent decrease in fertility in these groups. Coital frequency, late age of menarche, prolonged lactation and thus slower restoration of post-partum fecundity, rural versus urban habitation are all factors which play a role in fertility, and most investigators do not find specific variables which result from hypoxia, per se, which impair conception (Vitzhum 2001; Crognier *et al.* 2002; Vitzhum and Wiley 2003).

18.3 FETAL AND CHILDHOOD DEVELOPMENT

18.3.1 Pregnancy

ABORTION

Abortion rates are notoriously difficult to measure, but Clegg (1978) quotes a number of Andean studies giving incredibly low rates ranging from 0 to 1% (compared with worldwide rates of about 15%). He suggested this might be due to a high rate of very early abortions (before 2 weeks) which would be unrecognized and would

help to account for the low fertility. In Ethiopian women, Harrison *et al.* (1969) reported a rather higher rate (9.1%) at 3000 m compared with less than 1% in an ethnically similar population at low altitude; however, both rates are low compared with rates in many populations. Beall *et al.* (2004) studied Tibetan women with hemoglobin with high and low affinity for oxygen and found a lower offspring mortality in women with alleles for high affinity characteristics and suggested that hemoglobin affinity may be an agent for natural selection in this population. Non-B haplogroups, as compared to B groups, had higher adverse outcomes (fetal demise and neonatal deaths), but the molecular basis for these events is not known (Myres *et al.* 2000).

PLACENTAL GROWTH

Placentas are not significantly heavier at high altitude but since birth weights are low the placental/birth weight ratio is significantly increased (McClung 1969; Mayhew 1986), clearly an adaptation which would benefit fetal oxygenation. Villous vascularization is increased in the placentas from high altitude women; this increases the surface area for diffusion (Clegg 1978), although Mayhew (1986) found a smaller surface area of villi but a thinner diffusion barrier, thus resulting in an increase in the membrane diffusing capacity (Zamudio 2003). Placental infarcts are more common in altitude placentas and more frequent in women with a European admixture of genes (McClung 1969).

There is a decrease in the primary nutrient transporter GLUT1 in the placenta of women at altitude (3100 m) (Zamudio 2006). In this study while there was an increase in erythropoietin and other growth factors and thus vascularization, a decrease in glucose and other nutrient transporters, along with hypoxia, could contribute to intra-uterine growth retardation (IUGR).

FETAL GROWTH

The evidence suggests that, after the hazards of the first few weeks of pregnancy, growth is probably normal until the last trimester, when it slows to produce a lighter baby at term. The cause of this growth retardation is not clear, since the evidence reviewed by Clegg (1978) suggests that the fetus at this altitude is not hypoxic compared with lowland fetuses.

There does appear to be different adaptation strategies in high altitude populations in the Andes versus the Himalayas. Moore *et al.* (2001) studied Tibetan and Han Chinese women at 3658 m and found that Tibetan women had a higher percentage of common iliac blood flow contributing to the uterine artery. They felt that the higher birth weight of the Tibetan babies may be attributable to a compensation for a lower hemoglobin level by a higher oxygen delivery from a greater blood flow. On the other hand, in the Andes, Tissot van Patot *et al.* (2003) found a marked increase in vascular remodeling in placentas of women at 3100 versus 1600 m; but since these infants are of lower birth weight than low altitude ones, the investigators felt that this degree of angiogenesis was not adequate to restore the normal degree of oxygen delivery.

Another factor in the regulation of blood flow and thus oxygen delivery is the vasomotor regulators of flow. Moore *et al.* (2004) compared the hypoxia-inducing factor (HIF)-1 targeted vasoconstrictor, endothelin-1 (ET-1) in European and Andean women. Andean women were found to have a lower level of ET-1 suggesting less vasoconstriction and thus increased blood flow in the high altitude-adapted women. The mechanism of this phenomenon is thought to be related to a single nucleotide polymorphism in the ET-1 gene and may be a model for identifying women at any altitude prone to vascular problems such as pre-eclampsia.

In a recent study from La Paz (3600 m), Wilson *et al.* (2007) found that after adjustments for maternal height, gestational age and parity, Andean mothers had heavier babies than European mothers (209 g greater). They also found that the Andean mothers had higher uterine artery diameter and flow (60% greater) in the later stages of pregnancy. Thus oxygen delivery to the placenta was greater in the Andean than European mothers. In a companion paper (Vargas *et al.* 2007), they showed that in the same group of women, the determinants of oxygenation during pregnancy (Ca_{O_2}) was maintained near non-pregnant levels in both groups.

In a larger and more recent study (Julian *et al.* 2009), these findings were confirmed. This study looked at groups of women of Andean and European ancestry at both high (3600 m) and low (400 m) altitude in Bolivia. At high altitude, babies of Andean mothers were, after adjustment, 253 g heavier and uterine blood flow, at 20 weeks' pregnancy, was twice as great in Andean as European mothers. At low altitude there were no ancestry-related differences in pregnancy-related rise in uterine blood flow or birth weight. They also found, at altitude, that in mothers with mixed ancestry, the degree of admixture correlated with the rise in uterine blood flow.

18.3.2 Birth weight and infant mortality

Results from a number of studies in the Andes and Tibet showed lower birth weight at altitude (Haas 1976; Li 1985). The mean weight declined from about 3.5 kg in Lima to 2.8 kg at Cerro de Pasco (4300 m) and, although there is the possibility that the nutritional status of mothers may be a factor, it is unlikely to account for more than a proportion of this difference. Andean infants at 4340 m also had a marked delay in equilibration of Sa_{O_2} and lower Apgar scores compared to babies in Lima at 150 m (Gonzales and Salirrosas 2005). In Bolivia, where infant mortality and stillbirth rates are high, there is also a high prevalence of IUGR, pre-eclampsia and miscarriage (Keyes *et al.* 2003). This lower birth weight at altitude has been confirmed in a more recent study by Hartinger *et al.* (2006) who compared birth weights of babies born in Lima (150 m) with Huancayo (3280 m), Cuzco (3400 m) and Juliaca (3800 m). They found that there was no difference between low and high altitude babies born between 28 and 35 weeks but for those born between 36 and 42 weeks, those born at all three high altitude sites had significantly lower birth weights. Between the three altitude cities, the duration of residence of the population was of more importance than the actual altitude. Populations with the longest altitude residence have higher birth weight babies. This suggests that it is in the last trimester that the important effect of altitude impinges on the growing fetus, presumably because it outruns its oxygen supply from the placenta.

A similar effect of altitude has been reported from the USA (Lichty *et al.* 1957; Grahn and Kratchman 1963; Unger *et al.* 1988). Women native to high altitude who descend to low altitude have heavier babies at low altitude (Hoff and Abelson 1976). These studies include women from both indigenous high altitude populations and low altitude stock, and indicate that it is the high altitude environment rather than genetics which results in low birth weights. A study from Colorado also concludes that altitude is an independent factor in causing low birth weights. The authors obtained data from 3836 birth certificates and found that none of the characteristics associated with low birth weight – gestational age, maternal weight gain, parity, smoking, hypertension, etc. – interacted with the effect of altitude; the decline in birth weight averaged 102 g per 1000 m (Jensen and Moore 1997). However, genetic factors may play a role.

In a study in Lhasa (3658 m), Niermeyer *et al.* (1995) reported that Han Chinese infants had lower birth weights than Tibetan babies born at the same altitude. They also had lower Sa,O_2 and higher hemoglobin levels. Possibly the genetic factors work through giving better oxygenation to Tibetan mothers (see section 18.5.2). Not all investigators have found that Tibetan fetuses are spared IUGR (Tripathy and Gupta 2005), and others have documented significant malnutrition (Dang *et al.* 2004). Of interest is the finding that maternal anemia is inversely proportional to birth weight at altitudes from 2220 to 4850 m (Nahum and Stanislaw 2004). The authors attributed this finding to the decreased oxygen delivery with increasing viscosity known to occur at high altitude, but it is not clear that the degree of polycythemia was high enough to decrease blood flow.

Infant mortality depends heavily on living standards and medical facilities, and the very high infant mortality rates reported probably reflect these factors more than the effect of altitude per se. In Ethiopia, Harrison *et al.* (1969) reported a rate of 200 per 1000 live births at high altitude and 176 per 1000 at low altitude, whereas in the Andes a rate of 180 per 1000 was found in the rural area of Nunoa (4000 m) but only 73 per 1000 in urban La Paz (Baker 1978). In Himalayan Sherpas, Lang and Lang (1971) gave a figure of 51 per 1000 at 4300 m, and in North Bhutan the rate was 189 per 1000 (Jackson *et al.* 1966, p. 99). In experimental animals under controlled conditions, hypoxia increases neonatal mortality, so probably the high rates found in mountain peoples are at least partly due to the altitude. Apart from the direct effect of hypoxia an important indirect effect may be through the reduced amount of liver glycogen present at birth, an important energy store until suckling becomes established (Clegg 1978).

18.3.3 Growth through childhood

The high altitude baby starts life smaller than the average low altitude baby does, and its early growth is slower. Milestones such as sitting and walking are slightly later, but the differences between high and low altitude residents of the same race are less than those between different races or between urban and rural populations (Clegg 1978).

In Quechua Indians in Peru, throughout childhood the high altitude child lags behind his low altitude counterpart in height by about 2 years. The adolescent growth spurt is less pronounced in high altitude youths but their growth continues for about 2 years longer and their adult stature is not reached until 22 years of age (Frisancho 1978). In Ethiopia, there were no such differences. Indeed, high altitude males were taller and heavier for their age than lowlanders. In the Himalayas, a comparison of high altitude Sherpa children (3075–5050 m) with Tibetan children resident at 1400 m was made by Pawson (1977) who found no difference in the height of children in these populations. Both groups lag behind those from other high altitude populations, though other indices of maturation (skeletal and dental development and menarche) show the Sherpa children to lag behind the low altitude Tibetans. A study from Ecuador found very little difference in rates of body weight increase in children at high altitude compared with children from low altitude. There were some minor differences in rates of height increase but the authors conclude that hypoxia plays a relatively small role in shaping growth in the first 5 years after birth (Leonard *et al.* 1995).

On the other hand, investigations among the children of Kirghiz tribes of the Tien Shan mountains showed delayed growth in the high altitude children, equivalent to a lag of about 1 year. The altitude of residence was 2300–2800 m, but in the summer months they go up to 3500 m to graze their cattle (Frisancho 1978).

Menarche is a milestone well documented in studies from various high altitude regions; and, in girls living in the Andes, Himalayas and Tien Shan, it is 1–2 years later than in low altitude girls (Jackson *et al.* 1966, pp. 40–4; Frisancho 1978). The Ethiopian highlanders again are the exception as no difference was found (Harrison *et al.* 1969). Adrenarche, the increase in serum androgens, also occurs 1–2 years later in children at altitude compared with sea level in Peru (Goñez *et al.* 1993).

18.4 PHYSIOLOGY

18.4.1 Stature, lung development and function

Compared with Europeans and North Americans, most high altitude residents have a smaller stature and are lighter in weight, but when compared with people of similar race and living standards most of this difference disappears. The delayed growth (see above) is almost counteracted by the prolongation of active growth to beyond 20 years. The Han Chinese who have more recently migrated to high altitude regions do show some retardation of growth and stature, but respiratory adaptations which are similar to high altitude populations (Weitz and Garruto 2004). It is important to note, however, that Tibetans who were second-generation lowlanders adapted more quickly to high altitude than lowland Caucasians (Marconi *et al.* 2004) which suggests an inherent characteristic to adaptation.

One of the most quoted aspects of lifelong adaptation to high altitude is the deep-chested development of the thorax in high altitude residents (Barcroft 1925). This has been documented by measurement of chest circumference and vital capacity in South American Indians living above 4500 m but is quite a small difference even in this population. Vital capacity was about 300 mL higher than predicted when corrected for body size (Velasquez 1976). However, at 3500 m these measurements were smaller and less than the values published in the USA. High altitude residents in the Himalayas do not have larger circumference chests or bigger vital capacities than lowlanders (Frisancho 1978) nor do younger white residents of Leadville (3100 m), but those over 50 years of age did have significantly larger vital capacities, by 440 mL, than predicted (DeGraff *et al.* 1970). Sun *et al.* (1990) compared Tibetans and Han Chinese residents of Lhasa. Their mean ages, heights and weights were similar, but, whereas the Tibetans were lifelong residents, the Han have been resident for a mean time of 8 years. The Tibetans had vital capacities significantly greater than the Han did, 5080 mL compared with 4280 mL. High peak flows (>139%) were measured in both Tibetans and Ladakhis at 3300 m (Wood *et al.* 2003).

In Andean residents at 4540 m, the total lung capacity is about 500 mL greater than at sea level, most of the increase being due to increased residual volume (Velasquez 1976). Infants born at high altitude have greater thoracic compliance than infants of the same ethnic background born at low altitude (Mortola *et al.* 1990). In adults, the thoracic blood volume is increased and the residual volume/total lung capacity ratio increases from 21 to 28% in high altitude compared with low altitude residents. There may be some benefit from this since it would have the effect of reducing the breath-by-breath oscillations of $P\text{CO}_2$ and, hence, pH. At altitude these oscillations would otherwise be increased due to the reduction in plasma bicarbonate as part of the acclimatization process (Chapter 6, section 6.13.2). However, these changes in lung volumes, even when found, are quite small and probably have little effect on performance. Vital capacity decreases with age at sea level but this reduction is much greater at altitude, at least in Andean residents (Monge *et al.* 1990), which may account in part for the increasing incidence of chronic mountain sickness with age (Chapter 22).

The increased lung capacity may allow for an increased area for gas diffusion which, together with the increased blood volume, results in increased lung diffusing capacity. Details of studies in Andean and Caucasian residents are given in Chapter 7, section 7.5.2. This increase in gas transfer should give the altitude resident a distinct performance advantage over the newcomer to altitude. Work from Tibet by Chen *et al.* (1997) indicates that Tibetan highlanders also have higher lung diffusing capacities when compared with Han Chinese. The increase in pulmonary gas exchange can be induced after as little as 2 years in dogs brought up during maturation at 3800 m (McDonough *et al.* 2006). These findings suggest plasticity in this response if individuals are exposed to a hypoxic environment during important growth phases. Samaja *et al.* (1997), who studied Sherpas and Caucasian lowlanders at 3400 and 6450 m, found that the Sherpas were less alkalotic at the higher altitude due to a higher P_{CO_2}, although the P_{O_2} and $Sa_{,O_2}$ were the same as those of Caucasians. This indicates that their oxygen transport was more efficient.

18.4.2 Ventilatory control at rest and exercise

Newcomers to high altitude find, often to their surprise, that they have to hyperventilate on the slightest exertion. They may notice that high altitude residents seem to be relatively unaffected in this way. Reviews (Lahiri 2000; Moore 2000; Donnelly and Carroll 2005; Wilson 2005; Leon-Velarde and Richalet 2006) provide rich sources for the biochemical, genetic, cellular and physiologic responses that are known to exist in high altitude populations.

Measurements of resting and exercise ventilation in high altitude residents confirmed that high altitude natives in the Andes do, in fact, hypoventilate compared to sojourners. Chiodi (1957) showed that resting ventilation was higher in newcomers to altitude than in residents. At 3990 m the values were 5.3 and 4.5 L min^{-1} m^{-2}, and at 4515 m, 5.6 and 4.9 L min^{-1} m^{-2} for newcomers and residents, respectively. The $Pa_{,CO_2}$ values were in accordance with these differences. Santolaya *et al.* (1989) studied workers at the Aucanquilcha mine (5950 m) in Chile. Their

mean $Pa_{,CO_2}$ was 27.5 mmHg whereas lowlanders at that altitude had a value about 5 mmHg lower, indicating ventilation 22% higher. They also showed no respiratory alkalosis (pH 7.4), which lowlanders would have at that altitude.

On exercise, Buskirk (1978) found a similar distinction in Andean high altitude residents as did Lahiri *et al.* (1967) in Sherpa subjects compared with lowlanders at altitude. It is likely that this lower ventilation in high altitude residents is due to their low hypoxic ventilatory response (HVR), especially the ventilatory response to prolonged hypoxia as opposed to acute hypoxia (Gamboa *et al.* 2003 and Chapter 6). HVR correlates with exercise hyperventilation (Schoene *et al.* 1984) and thus would be associated with both the objective and subjective response to exercise ventilation at high altitude. As discussed in Chapter 6 this blunting of the HVR appears to take place over decades at altitude. Children resident at high altitude have normal HVR, and this blunting is seen in white subjects resident in Leadville (3100 m) in Colorado, so it does not seem to be genetically determined (Weil *et al.* 1971; Lahiri *et al.* 1976). There does, however, appear to be some differences in the ventilatory response to hypoxia between genders with women breathing more than men (Joseph *et al.* 2000).

Work by Zhuang *et al.* (1993) showed some interesting differences between lowland born Han Chinese and highland born Tibetans studied in Lhasa (3658 m). The Han had migrated to altitude in childhood, adolescence or adulthood. They showed the decline in HVR with length of residence at altitude as seen in Colorado altitude residents, but the Tibetans, who had a higher HVR than the Han, showed very little decline with age. However, Tibetans showed a paradoxical increase in ventilation on breathing 70% oxygen, a response not seen in Han subjects. Tibetan lifelong residents at 4400 m when studied at 3658 m and compared with Tibetans living there had blunted HVRs though their resting ventilation was similar (Curran *et al.* 1995). Recently, the same team has looked at a group of men of mixed Han–Tibetan parentage. They found that HVR was decreased with time of residence at altitude, but that resting ventilation did not decrease, as is the case with Han subjects. They exhibited the same paradoxical response to oxygen breathing as did Tibetan subjects (Curran *et al.* 1997).

Beall and colleagues have compared Tibetan and South American Aymara highlanders. They found resting ventilation was roughly 1.5 times higher in the Tibetans and HVR about double that of the Aymara. They also found that the contribution of genetic differences to the variance in ventilation was 35% in the Tibetan population and nil in the Aymara. The figures for HVR were 31 and 21%, respectively (Beall *et al.* 1997a; see also section 18.5.2).

18.4.3 Hemoglobin concentration

The increase in hemoglobin concentration at altitude is one of the best-known adaptations to altitude hypoxia. It is found in both acclimatized lowlanders and lifelong residents at altitude. This is discussed in detail in Chapter 9.

In the Andes, some workers have found very high hemoglobin concentration in residents (Talbott and Dill 1936; Dill *et al.* 1937; Merino 1950) and suggested that this is part of their long-term adaptation to altitude. However, subjects may have been included in these study populations who would now be considered to have chronic mountain sickness or Monge's disease (Chapter 22). Other studies have not found such high levels or a significant difference between residents and acclimatized lowlanders (Peñaloza *et al.* 1971). Frisancho (1988) reviewed the published data and showed that hemoglobin concentration values from mining areas in the Andes were higher than from non-mining areas, and that if studies from non-mining areas were compared with those from the Himalayas there was no significant difference. In mining areas, cobalt sometimes leaches into the drinking water, and having been ingested has the effect of stimulating erythropoiesis thus increasing the hemoglobin levels (Reeves and Weil 2001; Jeffereson *et al.* 2002 and Chapter 22.2.5).

However, Beall *et al.* (1998) found Aymara Andean high altitude natives to have hemoglobin concentrations significantly higher than Tibetans at a similar altitude, by 3–4 g dL^{-1}. Normal values were established by Vasquez and Villena (2001) in natives to 4000 m in Potosi, Peru, and found

to be 52.7 and 48.3% hematocrit and 18.3 and 15.8 g dL^{-1} hemoglobin for men and women, respectively. Villafuerte *et al.* (2004) modeled optimal values in the Andean (hemoglobin 14.7 g dL^{-1}) population and concluded that other factors have influenced the mean values which are higher and thus may not be optimal for oxygen delivery. Leon-Velarde *et al.* (2000) showed a gradual increase in erythrocytosis in both men and women with age, which was felt to be excessive and thus not beneficially adaptive.

Much of the polycythemia persists in populations, both children and adults, who have low iron stores. This phenomenon has been studied in Bolivia (Cook *et al.* 2005), and nutritional intervention with weekly iron supplementation has been found to be beneficial (Berger *et al.* 1997), but intervention on a public health scale has not been universally undertaken.

In the Himalayas and on the Tibetan plateau, residents tend to have rather lower hemoglobin concentration than acclimatized lowlanders (Wu *et al.* 2005). As discussed in Chapter 9, it is thought that although a modest rise in hemoglobin concentration (to perhaps 18.0 g dL^{-1}) is advantageous, values much above this level are probably detrimental. Thus the Tibetans' lower hemoglobin concentration values are considered to be evidence of better altitude adaptation.

18.4.4 The carotid body and chemodectoma

Chronic hypoxia causes an increase in the size and weight of the carotid body. This was first reported in high altitude Andean natives by Arias-Stella (1969). He found the weight of the two carotid bodies in residents of Lima to be just over 20 mg, whereas in altitude residents they totalled over 60 mg. Heath and co-workers found a similar increased weight of carotid bodies in patients with chronic hypoxic lung disease. They found a good correlation between carotid body and right ventricular weight, suggesting that a common correlation with hypoxia was the cause of the hyperplasia (Heath 1986).

The principal cell involved in this hyperplasia is the sustentacular (type II) cell with compression and obliteration of clusters of chief (type I) cells. This type of hyperplasia is similar to that seen in systemic hypertension (Heath 1986).

Chemodectoma, a tumor of the carotid body, is rare at sea level, but appears to be relatively common at high altitude. Saldana *et al.* (1973) reported its occurrence in a higher proportion of Peruvian adults born and living at 4350 m than in those living at 3000 m. All were benign and the incidence was higher in women. An association between chemodectoma and thyroid carcinoma has been noted in two patients at 2380 m (Saldana *et al.* 1973). No cases of chemodectoma have yet been reported from the Tibetan plateau or the high Himalayan valleys.

18.4.5 Cardiovascular adaptations

PULMONARY CIRCULATION

Andean high altitude residents share with newcomers the raised pulmonary artery and right ventricular pressure due to the hypoxic pulmonary pressor response (Chapter 8), resulting in right ventricular hypertrophy (Recavarren and Arias-Stella 1964). Indeed, in Andean children at high altitude, the usual involution of the muscular coat of the pulmonary artery after birth does not take place, or does so only partially, so that the pulmonary arteries, both large and small, show far greater muscularization than is normal in sea level residents (Saldana and Arias-Stella 1963a; Saldana and Arias-Stella 1963b; Saldana and Arias-Stella 1963c; Huicho and Niermeyer 2006).

This finding of right ventricular hypertrophy, continued muscularization of the pulmonary arteries and raised pulmonary artery pressure in residents at high altitude should be regarded as a response to high altitude rather than an adaptation, since there is no evidence that it has any physiological benefit. Indeed, it merely throws more strain on the right heart.

The purpose of the hypoxic pressor response in humans at sea level, apart from its vital role in prenatal life, is presumably to redistribute blood away from areas of the lung that are hypoxic because of, for instance, atelectasis, and thus improve matching of ventilation and blood flow in various clinical situations. It would probably be beneficial to lose this response at altitude, and the altitude-adapted yak would seem to have done this (Chapter 8, section 8.5).

Studies in Tibetan highlanders suggest that they have achieved a similar adaptation to the yak and do not have raised pulmonary artery pressures at altitude and little rise on exercise (Groves *et al.* 1993) though the numbers studied were small. Neither do they develop the structural changes in their pulmonary arterial tree that are found in Andean highlanders (Gupta *et al.* 1992). The incidence of right ventricular hypertrophic signs in the electrocardiograph (ECG) was found to be only 17% in Tibetans and 29% in Han Chinese at the same altitude (Halperin *et al.* 1998). Lifelong residents also have an increase in the number of branches to the main trunks of their coronary arteries (Arias-Stella and Topilsky 1971) and presumed adaptation by angiogenesis to optimize perfusion to tissues that are chronically more hypoxic.

In the last few years the importance of nitric oxide (NO) and its metabolites in vascular response has become apparent and despite the technical difficulties, many studies have sought to document the effect of altitude on this system and some studies have compared high altitude residents with lowlanders. Beall *et al.* (2012) have reviewed these studies and conclude that Tibetans had NO levels in the lung, plasma and red blood cells that were at least double and in some cases orders of magnitude greater than other populations. Red blood cell-associated nitrogen oxides were more than 200 times higher. Other highland populations had higher levels than lowlanders but not as high as Tibetans. Presumably these findings are at least part of the explanation of the lack of pulmonary hypertension in Tibetans at altitude.

HEART RATE

Another adaptation of high altitude residents is that, on exercise at altitude, their maximum heart rate does not seem to be limited, as is the case for acclimatized lowlanders. They maintained their heart rate variability both at low altitude and upon re-ascent to high altitude, also found in rats acclimatized to high altitude (Melin *et al.* 2003).

This is discussed more fully in Chapter 8 and in relation to the adrenergic system in Chapter 16. A study by Passino *et al.* (1996) looked at the spectral analysis of ECGs of high altitude residents compared with lowlanders at altitude. The high altitude residents did not show the reduced vagal tone seen in lowlanders, which may indicate the mechanism which allows this higher maximum heart rate in highlanders. These high altitude natives maintained higher heart rate responses while running a marathon at 4220 m (Cornolo *et al.* 2005) as well as after they had descended to low altitude (Gamboa *et al.* 2001), suggesting a maintained sympathetic tone after the hypoxic stress had been removed. Some genetic advantage must be conveyed to high altitude natives of uninterrupted lineage, as those high altitude inhabitants with Spanish admixture demonstrated a greater decrease in $V_{O_{2,max}}$ when exercised at 4228 m than did pure natives to these altitudes (Brutsaert *et al.* 2003).

WORK ECONOMY

One further curious finding is that Tibetans demonstrate improved work economy (Marconi *et al.* 2005). In other words, they have been shown to carry out workloads at a lower energy expenditure than low altitude controls (Ge 1994; Curran *et al.* 1998; Marconi *et al.* 2005; Marconi *et al.* 2006). The reasons for such improvement are not fully understood but provide a fertile area for further investigation as understanding such adaptation may provide insight into more optimal functioning of patients with a variety of diseases with impairment of oxygen delivery.

18.5 ADAPTATION TO HYPOXIA OVER GENERATIONS

Most of the adaptations to hypoxia that have been shown in humans appear to develop during a lifetime of exposure. Even the blunting of the hypoxic ventilatory response has been shown to develop in people of lowland origin over a period of decades (Weil *et al.* 1971). The lower hemoglobin concentration in Sherpa and Tibetan subjects has been suggested as an example of adaptation over many generations in Tibetan stock. Recent work on the genetics of high altitude populations are discussed in Chapter 4.

18.5.1 The hypoxic pulmonary pressor response

Hypoxic pulmonary vasoconstriction to varying degrees is a response universal to most mammals which has sparked the curiosity of many physiologists (Moudgil 2005; Reeves and Grover 2005; Rhodes 2005). A better understanding of the cellular, biochemical and genetic aspects of this response has been unraveled over the last decade.

In animals, Harris (1986) has shown elegantly that in cattle the pulmonary pressor response, or lack of it, is genetically determined. The yak has little or no response, whereas the cow has a brisk response. The crossbred dzo has the blunted response of its yak parent, but the second cross of dzo and bull produces 50% brisk and 50% low response offspring. That is, the gene responsible for a low response is dominant and the characteristic is inherited in a Mendelian way. This vasomotor reactivity is mediated, in part, by the production of NO in Tibetan highlanders (Hoit *et al.* 2005), Tibetan sheep (Koizumi 2004), as well as in other animals, including the yak (Ishizaki 2005). Presumably, a low response is an advantage at altitude such that lower pulmonary vascular resistance results in better cardiac output and exercise capacity. A brisk response is a risk factor for brisket disease (named after the brisket, the loose skin at the animal's throat). Thus, we have a true adaptation achieved presumably by environmental pressure selecting for the low response gene. Similar adaptation has been found in the llama.

There is evidence that in populations of Tibetan origin a similar adaptation may have taken place. Jackson (1968) found little ECG evidence of pulmonary hypertension in Bhutanese and Sherpa subjects at altitude, in that their mean frontal QRS axis differed by only 10 from healthy Edinburgh adults, in contrast to both lowlanders and Andean residents at altitude, who have marked right axis deviation due to pulmonary hypertension (Chapter 8). Groves *et al.* (1993) found pulmonary artery pressures and resistance in five Tibetan subjects in Lhasa (3658 m) to be within normal sea level values at rest and exercise. This suggests that the Tibetan population demonstrates genuine altitude adaptation, presumably by natural selection over very many generations.

18.5.2 Arterial oxygen saturation

In 1994, Beall and her colleagues reported that the level of SaO_2 was influenced by a single gene in a population of Tibetan women they had studied at 4850–5450 m (Beall *et al.* 1994). They later studied another Tibetan population in the Lhasa region (3800–4065 m) and calculated that this gene accounted for 21% of the variance in SaO_2 (Beall *et al.* 1997b). More recently, the same group compared Tibetan with South American Aymara women. They found that the Tibetans had SaO_2 on average 2.6% higher than the Aymara, and also that whereas much of the variance of SaO_2 in the Tibetan women could be attributed to genetic factors, no significant proportion of the variance could be so attributed in the South American population (Beall *et al.* 1999). Therefore there is the potential for natural selection towards higher SaO_2 in the Tibetan but not in the Aymara population.

Beall *et al.* (2002) reported an unusual adaptation of Ethiopian highlanders at 3530 m who had a modest polycythemic response (15.9 and 15.0 g dL^{-1} in men and women, respectively) with surprisingly high SaO_2, approximately 95.3%. This is the first description of this form of adaptation in a population which, because of sociopolitical circumstances in the past, is just beginning to be studied. Understanding of this observation is yet to be unraveled.

18.6 CLINICAL CONDITIONS ASSOCIATED WITH ALTITUDE RESIDENCE

In this section we consider those conditions which are either unique to high altitude residence, such as chronic mountain sickness, or which occur at low altitude as well but are more common in high altitude populations at their altitude of residence, such as pre-eclampsia. Also mentioned are some conditions which seem to be less common in high altitude populations, such as atherosclerosis.

18.6.1 Birth defects

Apart from congenital heart disease, considered in the next section, a high frequency of other birth defects has been noted by Castilla *et al.* (1999). In a collaborative study from three hospitals situated between 2600 and 3600 m in Bogota (Colombia), La Paz (Bolivia) and Quito (Ecuador) they found a high frequency of craniofacial defects, cleft lip, microtia, pre-auricular tag, brachial arch complex, constriction band complex and anal atresia; there was a low frequency of neural tube defects, anencephaly and spina bifida. The incidence of patent ductus arteriosus was not addressed.

18.6.2 Cardiovascular disease

CONGENITAL HEART DISEASE

Congenital cardiovascular malformations are common at altitude, with patent ductus arteriosus being 15 times more common at Cerro de Pasco (4200 m) than at sea level in Lima (Peñaloza *et al.* 1964). Marticorena *et al.* (1959) reported an incidence of 0.72% of patent ductus arteriosus in children born around 4300 m, compared with an incidence of 0.8% for all congenital heart disease at sea level.

In Xizang (Tibet), among the resident Tibetan population the incidence of congenital heart disease has been shown to range from 0.51 to 2.25%, with patent ductus arteriosus being the most frequently encountered abnormality (Sun 1985). The greater the altitude the higher the prevalence; the highest documented incidence (2.5%) occurred in Chinese emigrants (Zhang 1985). Presumably the cause of these high rates is the lack of a sudden increase in oxygen levels in the few hours after birth, which normally triggers the reduction in pulmonary vascular resistance and the closure of the ductus.

ATHEROSCLEROSIS

Studies of populations in the Andes suggest that both coronary artery disease and myocardial infarction are uncommon among high altitude residents. No cases were found in one series of 300 necropsies carried out at 4300 m, and epidemiological studies in South America have shown that both angina of effort and ECG evidence of myocardial ischemia are less at altitude than at sea level (Ramos et al. 1967). In the Tibetan ethnic population of North Bhutan no autopsy studies were available but angina seemed uncommon, and, as judged by ECG recordings, evidence of coronary artery disease was minimal. Studies from the Tien Shan and Pamir also suggest that degenerative cardiovascular disease is rare in these regions (Mirrakhimov 1978).

In autopsy studies of 385 Tibetan adults living in the Lhasa area, arteriosclerosis of the aorta and its main branches occurred in 81.8% and of the coronary artery in 65.5%. In Qinghai, coronary artery disease was common and autopsies on Tibetans showed the same incidence as in lowlanders, but the incidence of coronary infarction was low (Sun 1985). Serum cholesterol levels were low in Andean natives and in the Bhutanese high altitude group studied; in the latter there was no progressive increase with age (Jackson et al. 1966, p. 96).

Faeh et al. (2009) studied mortality from coronary artery disease and stroke in Switzerland. They found a lower mortality rate in those born at high altitude (up to 1900 m). This was true even if subjects moved to lower altitude later in life.

Moderate altitude and presumably a more active lifestyle of physical activity conveys some protection against obesity. A modernization of lifestyle in some high altitude populations migrating to low altitude with decreased activity is associated with a higher prevalence of hypertension, obesity and cardiovascular disease (Smith 1999; Cabrera de Leon et al. 2004). Serum leptin levels, a marker as a risk for cardiovascular disease, is usually lower in the active, non-obese high altitude populations (Lindegarde et al. 2004). Even in the presence of relative obesity (BMI >30), an active lifestyle in Aymara natives of Chile was associated with a low prevalence of type 2 diabetes mellitus (Santos et al. 2001). Obesity per se is also associated with pulmonary hypertension and respiratory disturbances during sleep (Valencia-Flores et al. 2004).

HYPERTENSION

Hypertension is uncommon in high altitude populations in South America. In a study of 300 high altitude natives in Peru no significant rise in either systolic or diastolic pressure occurred with age. Of individuals aged between 60 and 80 years in the same area, few had a systolic pressure above 165 mmHg or a diastolic pressure above 95 mmHg (Baker 1978). By contrast, Sun reports (Sun 1985; Sun 1986) a relatively high incidence of hypertension among indigenous Tibetans. He also found an age-associated increase in blood pressure. There was no tendency for hypertension to decline at higher altitudes and the blood pressure was higher in women than in men. The incidence was greater in the urban population around Lhasa than in rural populations. Similar observations have been made in Tibetans living in high altitude areas of western Szechuan. However, Han (Chinese) immigrants to Tibet showed a lower incidence of hypertension than did the Tibetans. In Qinghai province (which contains the north-eastern part of the Tibetan plateau) the incidence of hypertension appears to be lower than in Xizang (Tibet). Zhao et al (2012) found similar high rates of hypertension in Tibetan men and women at an altitude of 4300 m in Yangbaling (Tibet). They found 56% of their subjects had blood pressure over 140/90, of which 61% had blood pressure of over 160/100.

The incidence of hypertension and lack of rise in blood pressure with age in the South American and Himalayan populations studied may be the product of diet and behavior associated with a traditional lifestyle. The cause of hypertension among Tibetans is not clear. On the plateau, obesity is uncommon and traditionally few smoke (though this is changing). However, they do have a very high intake of salt, estimated at up to 1 kg per month, much of it taken in their tea. They also add yak butter, which is often slightly rancid. In the Bhutanese and Sherpa varieties of 'Tibetan' tea neither the salt nor the butter content appears, by taste, to be as high. In all houses and nomad dwellings there is a continuous supply of this tea, which is offered to every visitor. Even when they have migrated to low levels, Tibetans still drink large quantities of it and may become very obese. The high salt and butter intake may be a factor in the high incidence of hypertension in Tibetans.

However, a 15-year survey of Tibetan native highlanders living on the Tibetan plateau showed a low incidence of systemic hypertension. A total of 7797 men and 8029 women were studied. Just over 2% of this group had hypertension compared with over 4% of Chinese immigrants to Tibet. The intake of salt varied. Tibetans in Zadou county (4068 m) had the highest intake with an average of 14.6 g day^{-1} and an incidence of hypertension of 3.48%. In Zhidou county (4179 m) the average salt intake was 2.2 g day^{-1} and hypertension was found in 2.62% (Wu 1994a). By contrast, in lowland Chinese the incidence of hypertension is 7.9% (Liu 1986).

18.6.3 Infection

Direct exposure to increased solar radiation inhibits the growth of some bacteria because of the ultraviolet component of sunlight. *Staphylococcus aureus* is greatly inhibited, but *Escherichia coli* is more resistant (Nusshag 1954). The number of bacteria in ambient air decreases with altitude, and a study on the Jungfraujoch (3400 m) in Switzerland showed that, despite a large number of tourists, few bacteria were present in the air.

High altitudes do not influence human bacterial flora per se. However, a lower incidence of many common infections of bacterial, viral and protozoal origin was observed in soldiers at altitudes up to 5538 m (Singh *et al.* 1977). Examination of nasal swabs in a high altitude population in north Bhutan showed that there was only a 4% carrier rate of coagulase-positive staphylococci; normally the incidence is between 29 and 40% in Western communities. A high frequency of β-hemolytic streptococci, highly sensitive to penicillin, was found in throat cultures, whereas in Western communities sensitivity to penicillin would be minimal (Selkon and Gould

1966), though this may well be changing in more developed areas.

In the highlanders of Peru, Colombia and Ecuador, oroya fever is found, which is caused by *Bacillus bacilliformis* becoming parasitic in the red blood cells. Various hemorrhagic fevers are described in the highlands of Bolivia. These are considered to be viral in origin, the virus belonging to the same group as that which causes Lassa fever. Hemorrhagic disorders have also been described in north-eastern Nepal.

Mosquitoes, which transmit malaria and yellow fever, are absent at high altitude, but typhus appears to be commoner than at lower levels. This may be because bathing is not usual at higher altitudes, because of the cold, and so lice are common.

Pulmonary disease also appears common at altitude and this in part may be related to the exposure of highlanders to the smoke from open fires inside their houses or tents. In Xizang (Tibet) the incidence of chronic bronchitis was 3.7% in a low altitude population and 22.9% in a population at 4500 m. This was complicated by emphysema in 5–12% of cases and by cor pulmonale in 0.98% (Sun 1985). In Qinghai province, chronic obstructive airway disease is relatively common but smoking is prevalent, particularly among immigrants to high altitude.

In Nepal and throughout the subcontinent, pulmonary tuberculosis was relatively common, whereas in Ethiopia it was rare. In Ethiopia the major communicable diseases were measles, malaria, dysentery, scabies and syphilis, and the total incidence of communicable disease was greater in the low altitude population (Harrison *et al.* 1969).

In northern Bhutan, respiratory infections appeared to be commoner in the younger age groups but were rare in adults; antibodies to a number of common viral infections were found. A high proportion of the population had been exposed to influenza, mumps, measles, herpes simplex and the common cold (Jackson *et al.* 1966, p. 96).

Leprosy occurs in Nepal and Bhutan (Ward and Jackson 1965) and was reported in Tibet in the nineteenth century and in the western Himalayas (Moorcroft and Trebeck 1841, Vol. 1, p. 180).

Chronic eye infections are seen in the populations of the Pamir, Himalayas and Tibetan plateau; the smoke of yak dung fires exacerbates them. In summary, where certain infections are common they are due to the low living standards of the people rather than to altitude per se.

18.6.4 Goiter

The frequency of goiter in mountainous areas has been recognized for centuries, but it is not confined to the mountains (Fig. 18.1). Iodine deficiency is due to low iodine content of the soil and therefore the water. Soils poor in iodine are found where the land remained longest under quaternary glaciers. When the ice thawed, the iodine-rich soil was swept away and replaced by new soil derived from iodine-poor crystalline rocks. Seaweed, which is rich in iodine, and other folk remedies have been used since ancient times for prophylaxis and treatment (Hetzel 1989).

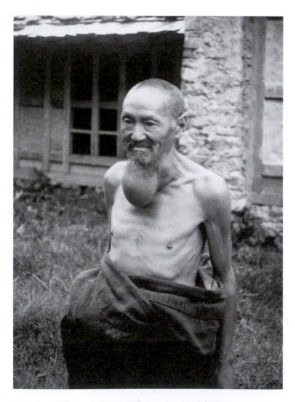

Figure 18.1 Tibetan from north Bhutan with large pendulous goiter.

Scientific proof that goiter was due to iodine deficiency was not available until Marine and Kimball (1920) published a controlled trial in high-school children in Akron, Ohio. They showed a reduction in the size of goiters and prevention of their development in children treated with iodine. Iodine deficiency causes hyperplasia and retention of colloid in the thyroid, resulting in goiter and, eventually, hypothyroidism in adults. Children born to iodine-deficient mothers have a range of neurological and skeletal defects known collectively as cretinism, an association noted for centuries. This term covers a range of clinical conditions which seem to vary in frequency and importance from locality to locality and includes dwarfism, goiter, facial dysmorphism, deafness, deaf mutism and intellectual impairment. In populations with goiter, the overall work capacity of the population may be impaired, as, in addition to cretinism, there is a marked morbidity, infant mortality is raised and mental subnormality common.

Iodine deficiency may result from insufficient intake, goitrogenic substances and deficiency in intrathyroidal enzymes; an excess of calcium or fluoride in the presence of iodine deficiency may increase the incidence of goiter. McCarrison (McCarrison 1908; McCarrison 1913) carried out a classical study of goiter and endemic cretinism in the Gilgit Agency of Kashmir (Karakoram). In 1906, McCarrison found a goiter incidence of 65%.

The incidence of goiter may vary widely within a few miles; some 100 miles (160 km) north of Gilgit where goiter was endemic, it was not observed in the semi-nomadic Kirghiz tribesmen who inhabit the Pamir plateau of southern Xinjiang. Direct questioning of the nomads revealed that they knew about goiter but they were adamant that there was no history of its occurrence among them (Ward 1983), although Marco Polo noted a large population of people with goiter in Yarkand (Shache). However, hearsay evidence is notably unreliable. Anecdotal evidence of goiter in other regions of the Himalayas, the Shimshall region of the Karakoram, and west Bhutan, suggests also that the incidence may vary considerably within a few miles (Saunders 1789; Shipton 1938).

Rockhill (1891, p. 265) also observed goiter, particularly in women in eastern Tibet, and other travelers noted the condition in northern Tibet

(Bonvalot 1891, p. 116) and in the gorge country of south-east Tibet (Bailey 1957). The incidence of goiter in Himalayan valleys is high, and in the Tibetan ethnic population of north Bhutan it was the most common clinical condition. In subjects less than 20 years old it was less marked, and younger individuals had a diffuse enlargement, whereas with age a nodular goiter was more common. No cases of cancer or thyrotoxicosis were seen, and two cretins were found in 349 individuals examined. The incidence of goiter was 60% in females and 19% in males (Jackson *et al.* 1966, pp. 40–4).

Ibbertson *et al.* (1972), in a survey of Sherpas (also of Tibetan ethnic origin) in the Sola Khumbu region of north-eastern Nepal, found that 92% had a palpable goiter, which was visibly enlarged in 63%; 75% had below normal protein-bound iodine levels in the blood and 30% were clinically hypothyroid. Classical myxedema was present in 5.9% of the population, deaf mutism in a further 4.7% and isolated deafness in a further 3.1%. Pitt (1970) describes Nepalese babies born with goiter.

In many of these areas the incidence of goiter is much lower now after various projects for giving iodine by tablets or depot injections have been carried out. However, in a survey carried out in 1980–81 in Ethiopia, the gross goiter prevalence was found to be 30% among schoolchildren and 19% in household members (Wolde-Gebriel *et al.* 1993). A recent survey in Ethiopia (Abuye *et al.* 2008) still found rates of 25–63% in various regions. As well as iodine intake, altitude and consumption of cassava were identified as risk factors. The effect of the latter was thought to be due to the intake of cyanide.

18.6.5 Sickle cell disease

Adzaku *et al.* (1993) reported on 136 patients resident at about 3000 m in Saudi Arabia and compared them with 185 patients living at sea level. Patients at both locations included those with homozygous disease (Hb SS), hemoglobin C (Hb SC) and sickle cell trait (Hb AS).

The main finding was a marked increase in 2,3-diphosphoglycerate (2,3-DPG) in patients with sickle cell disease compared with normal controls at altitude and patients at sea level. Their hemoglobin concentration was not different from sea level patients; they were anemic, with values around 8.0–9.0 g dL^{-1}. Sickle cell patients resident at low altitude have a high risk of crises on going to altitude. Adzaku *et al.* (1993) attribute the relative well-being of their patients at altitude to their high 2,3-DPG, which, at this relatively modest altitude, would help tissue oxygenation, in contrast to the situation at extreme altitude (Chapter 13).

18.6.6 Pre-eclampsia

The incidence of pre-eclampsia is increased among mothers at altitude. Keyes *et al.* (2003) reported that the incidence of pre-eclampsia in La Paz, Bolivia (3600 m) was 1.7 times that in Santa Cruz (300 m) and in primiparous women the figure was 2.2 times. In Saudi Arabia, Mahfouz *et al.* (1994) reported a significant increase in pregnancy-associated hypertension in women resident at an altitude as low as 2744 m compared with sea level subjects. Palmer *et al.* (1999) found the case incidence of pre-eclampsia was 16% at 3100 m and 3% at 1260 m in two Colorado rural communities. They also noted that the usual fall in blood pressure during pregnancy was not seen in the altitude group, even in women who remained normotensive.

Zamudio (2007) has reviewed this topic and has discussed how the findings of many studies of pregnant women at altitude of uterine blood flow etc. may support or cast doubt on four possible mechanisms that have been proposed for the development of pre-eclampsia. She concludes that there is no single mechanism and that different factors may be important in different cases. Altitude residence by increasing the degree of hypoxia in the placenta increases the risk of pre-eclampsia to a higher level and hence a greater percentage of pregnant women will develop the condition.

Acute mountain sickness

SUMMARY

Individuals who ascend too rapidly to high altitude are at risk for developing one of three forms of acute altitude illness, acute mountain sickness (AMS), high altitude cerebral edema (HACE) and high altitude pulmonary edema (HAPE). In this chapter, we consider AMS in greater detail while HACE and HAPE are considered further in Chapters 20 and 21.

The primary symptoms of AMS, which may come on as early as 6–24 hours following ascent include headache, anorexia, nausea, vomiting, lack of energy, malaise and disturbed sleep. In untreated individuals, they are often worst on the second and third days at altitude, usually disappear by the fifth day, but may reappear on ascent to a higher altitude. Scoring systems have been devised to diagnose and grade the severity of AMS but these are largely reserved for research purposes to ensure standardization across studies.

The incidence of AMS depends upon the rate of ascent and the altitude reached. It is uncommon below 2000 m but is very common among those flying directly to altitudes above 3800 m. It occurs in both sexes and at all ages. Fitness confers no protection, and so far no factors have been identified which can predict susceptibility to AMS in individuals with no prior record of travel to high altitude. The pathophysiologic mechanism underlying the development of AMS remains unclear despite many years of research into this question. The leading theory is that cerebral edema and elevated intracranial pressure play a significant role in this process, but such findings are lacking in patients with mild disease. To the extent that cerebral edema is playing a role, it is likely the result of multiple factors including altered fluid and sodium balance, changes in cerebral blood flow and cerebrovascular autoregulation and altered blood–brain barrier permeability. Blunted ventilatory responses to hypoxia and the subsequent decrease in oxygen saturation have been found in some studies of AMS and may also contribute to its development.

Although there remains considerable debate about the mechanisms of AMS, there is consensus about the best means for prevention and treatment. AMS can be prevented or ameliorated by a slow rate of ascent, which allows for normal acclimatization to occur and by drugs, of which acetazolamide is the best studied and most widely used. Dexamethasone has also been shown to be quite effective in preventing and treating AMS. Patients with mild disease may not require anything more for treatment than stopping their ascent and using acetaminophen or non-steroidal anti-inflammatory medications for relief of headache. In more severe cases, acetazolamide or dexamethasone can be added and are effective at speeding symptom resolution. Individuals in whom symptoms resolve with appropriate treatment can continue their ascent and might consider remaining on pharmacologic prophylaxis during this time. Those individuals in whom symptoms do not resolve after a few days of appropriate treatment should descend to lower elevation.

19.1 HISTORICAL PERSPECTIVE

Following the earliest descriptions of altitude illness by Acosta, described in detail in Chapter 1, section 1.3, the first modern account of acute mountain sickness (AMS) was put forth by Ravenhill (1913) who pointed out that fatigue, cold and lack of food complicated previous descriptions by explorers and mountain climbers. He was serving as a medical officer of a mining company whose mines at 4700 m in Chile were served by a railway and, as a result, had the opportunity to observe individuals suffering from the effects of altitude alone. While the local Bolivian name for AMS was *puna* and the Peruvians called it *soroche*, Ravenhill referred to the illness as *puna* of the 'normal' type. (Traditional Tibetan names for AMS include *ladrak* (poison of the pass), *damgiri*, *duqri*, *yen chang* (from the Koko Nor region), *chang-chi* (from Szechuan) and *tuteck*.) In describing AMS in greater detail, Ravenhill wrote:

> It is a curious fact that the symptoms of puna do not usually evince themselves at once. The majority of newcomers have expressed themselves as being quite well on first arrival. As a rule, towards the evening, the patient begins to feel rather slack and disinclined for exertion. He goes to bed but has a restless and troubled night and wakes up next morning with a severe frontal headache.
>
> There may be vomiting, frequently there is a sense of oppression in the chest but there is rarely any respiratory distress or alteration in

the normal rate of breathing so long as the patient is at rest. The patient may feel slightly giddy on rising from bed and any attempt at exertion increases the headache, which is nearly always confined to the frontal region.

> (Ravenhill 1913)

Ravenhill went on to describe *puna* of the nervous and cardiac types, which correspond in our present nomenclature to high altitude cerebral edema (Chapter 20) and high altitude pulmonary edema (Chapter 21), respectively. After Ravenhill, altitude illness was well recognized, but the distinction and importance of the two complicating forms seem to have been lost, at least in the English-speaking world, until Houston (1960) and Hultgren and Spickard (1960) described high altitude pulmonary edema and Fitch (1964) described high altitude cerebral edema. High altitude pulmonary edema was recognized earlier by South American physicians, however, as Lizárraga (1955) gave the first detailed description of the condition after Ravenhill. A fuller account of the history of acute altitude illness is given in West (1998).

19.2 TERMINOLOGY

Although the terms *puna* and *soroche* are used loosely in South America in reference to acute mountain sickness, the dyspnea normal to exertion at high altitude (Ravenhill 1913) as well as chronic mountain sickness, it is important to use more explicit terminology when describing these conditions. Acute altitude illness refers to the three disorders that can occur within the first several days of arrival at high altitude, acute mountain sickness (AMS), high altitude cerebral edema (HACE) and high altitude pulmonary edema (HAPE). This chapter will focus on AMS, while the latter two entities, which are both severe, potentially fatal illnesses, are discussed in greater detail in Chapters 20 and 21, respectively.

All three acute altitude illnesses are distinct entities from chronic forms of altitude illness, chronic mountain sickness and high altitude heart disease, that develop over many months to years of residence at high altitude. This latter group of entities is discussed further in Chapter 22.

19.3 CLINICAL FEATURES AND DIAGNOSIS OF AMS

19.3.1 Symptoms, signs and time course of AMS

Acute mountain sickness is a self-limiting condition affecting previously healthy individuals going rapidly to altitudes above 2300 m. The altitude at which symptoms start varies between individuals with very susceptible people developing symptoms below this elevation and others not developing symptoms until much higher elevations, if at all. Anywhere from 6 to 24 hours following ascent to a given elevation, affected individuals gradually develop a constellation of symptoms, including headache, anorexia, nausea, vomiting, fatigue, light-headedness and sleep disturbance. Even though periodic breathing is a common cause of sleep disturbances in AMS, it can be present in individuals who remain free of AMS. Importantly, individuals with AMS should have no neurologic symptoms aside from headache and dizziness. Symptoms typically peak on the second to third day in untreated individuals, disappear by the fourth or fifth day and do not recur as long as the individual remains at the same elevation. Symptoms may recur with subsequent gains in elevation, however. Individuals who remain at high elevation for many days and descend to lower elevation can often re-ascend quickly to high altitude without developing symptoms, although the likelihood of a safe ascent will be a function of how high they went on their first excursion, how long they remained there and how long they spent at the lower elevation before re-ascent. As a result, it is difficult to provide firm guidelines for how individuals should approach this situation.

There are no characteristic physical examination findings in AMS, although crackles on auscultation and peripheral edema may be present in a minority of cases (Hackett and Rennie 1979). Variable changes in body temperature have also been reported with some studies reporting a mild increase of between 0.5 and 1.2°C depending on the level of AMS severity (Maggiorini et al. 1997) and others reporting a decrease of 1.7°C with no change in metabolic rate (Loeppky et al. 2003). Various studies have also reported lower oxygen saturation values in individuals with AMS compared to those who remain healthy (Roeggla et al. 1996; Basnyat et al. 1999) but AMS can still be seen in those with relatively preserved oxygenation. Elevated diastolic blood pressure has also been shown to correlate with AMS severity (Koehle et al. 2010).

19.3.2 Making the diagnosis of AMS

Acute mountain sickness is diagnosed solely on the basis of the patient's symptoms and there are no diagnostic laboratory tests. There must be a history of recent gain in elevation and, if individuals ascend rapidly by car, plane or cable car, a period of several hours may pass before the onset of symptoms. Individuals who ascend more gradually by climbing or hiking can have symptoms immediately upon arrival as they will have already spent time above their threshold for developing symptoms. In order to say that an individual has AMS and nothing more severe, the neurologic exam and mental status must be normal. Otherwise, consideration must be given to whether the patient has HACE or another diagnosis.

Traditionally, the presence of headache has been required for diagnosis of AMS, as specified in the Lake Louise scoring system (discussed further below under section 19.3.4), but, following a large Chinese study on altitude illness in military recruits in Tibet that used a set of Chinese criteria that did not require headache (Ren et al. 2010), there has been debate as to whether headache is necessary to make the diagnosis (Roach et al. 2011; West 2011).

Diagnosis can be difficult in pre-verbal children less than 4 years of age who cannot adequately report symptoms to their parents. To address this problem, Yaron et al. (1998) created the Children's Lake Louise score which uses a fussiness score in lieu of the headache score in the standard Lake Louise criteria and a pediatric symptom score to assess appetite, vomiting, playfulness and ability to sleep. They showed that parents were capable of using this scoring system in an appropriate manner. In general, the safest course is to assume that behavior such as irritability, tearfulness and refusal of food in a child who has gained altitude in the previous hours or days indicates AMS until proved otherwise. The standard Lake Louise scoring system can be used in children aged 4–11 years, although a different diagnostic threshold may be necessary for this group, as children in this age range tend to over-report symptoms (Southard *et al.* 2007). The issue of children at altitude is described in greater detail in Chapter 27.

19.3.3 Differential diagnosis of AMS

Although AMS is the most likely cause of symptoms shortly following a large acute gain in altitude, it is important to remember that the symptoms of the disease are non-specific and, as a result, may be caused by other disorders such as exercise-associated hyponatremia (Ayus and Moritz 2008), dehydration, viral syndrome, migraines or carbon monoxide poisoning. The last entity may occur in individuals who use cooking stoves in poorly ventilated tents, although a study from Denali did not reveal any correlation between carbon monoxide levels and AMS symptoms (Roscoe *et al.* 2008). The prudent approach is to attribute all symptoms that develop following ascent to acute altitude illness but to consider alternatives when clinical features are suggestive or the patient

does not respond to appropriate therapeutic interventions.

19.3.4 AMS scoring systems

In clinical situations, the diagnosis of AMS is largely made in an informal manner based on the patient's reported symptoms. In research studies, however, there is a need for a more systematic approach and for all researchers to use the same system in order to facilitate comparison of results between studies. The most complicated scoring system is the Environmental Symptom Questionnaire (ESQ) (Sampson *et al.* 1983), which consists of 67 questions, many of which are overlapping and of uncertain relevance to AMS. An observer can administer the questions or the subject can complete a self-assessment; the two methods give similar results. A more simplified approach, referred to as the Lake Louise Scoring System, was created at the Hypoxia Symposium in 1991 and later modified at the following Hypoxia Symposium in 1993 (Table 19.1; Roach *et al.* 1993). As noted above, an important feature of the Lake Louise score (LLS), which has become the subject of debate, is that headache must

Table 19.1   Lake Louise consensus: scoring of acute mountain sickness (AMS) (from Roach *et al.* 1993) (a) AMS self-assessment. The sum of the responses is the AMS Self-report score. Headache and at least one other symptom must be present for the diagnosis of AMS. A score of 3 or more is taken as AMS. It is suggested that this part of the scoring system be always used and reported separately. The question relating to sleep will not always be relevant, e.g. in short 1-day studies or in evening assessment when twice daily scoring is used.

Symptom	Scoring
1. Headache	0 None at all
	1 Mild headache
	2 Moderate headache
	3 Severe headache, incapacitating
2. Gastrointestinal symptoms	0 Good appetite
	1 Poor appetite or nausea
	2 Moderate nausea or vomiting
	3 Severe, incapacitating nausea and vomiting
3. Fatigue and/or weakness	0 Not tired or weak
	1 Mild fatigue/weakness
	2 Moderate fatigue/weakness
	3 Severe fatigue/weakness

4. Dizziness/light-headedness	0 None
	1 Mild
	2 Moderate
	3 Severe, incapacitating
5. Difficulty sleeping	0 Slept as well as usual
	1 Did not sleep as well as usual
	2 Woke many times, poor nights sleep
	3 Could not sleep at all

(b) Clinical assessment. This portion of the scoring system contains information gained by examination. The Clinical Assessment score is the sum of scores in the following three questions.

Sign	Scoring
Change in mental status	0 No change
	1 Lethargy/lassitude
	2 Disorientated/confused
	3 Stupor/semiconscious
	4 Coma
Ataxia (heel/toe walking)	0 None
	1 Balancing maneuvers
	2 Steps off the line
	3 Falls down
	4 Unable to stand
Peripheral edema	0 None
	1 One location
	2 Two or more locations

(c) Functional score. The functional consequences of the AMS Self-reported score should be further evaluated by one optional question asked after the AMS Self-report questionnaire. Alternatively, this question may be asked by the examiner if clinical assessment is performed.

Overall, if you had any of these symptoms, how did they affect your activities?	0 Not at all
	1 Mild reduction
	2 Moderate reduction
	3 Severe reduction (e.g. bedrest)

be present for the diagnosis. Whether or not a study measuring AMS incidence uses the LLS or a system that does not require headache for diagnosis has the potential to affect the measured incidence of disease.

There have been a number of studies comparing the ESQ with the LLS. Bärtsch et al. (1993) for example, found the percentages of subjects diagnosed as having AMS in Alpine huts at four altitudes was comparable whichever system was used. Maggiorini et al. (1998) applied questionnaires to 490 climbers in Alpine huts

up to 4559 m. Using a Lake Louise score of 4 or more as the cut-off, they found a sensitivity of 78% and specificity of 93% compared with the ESQ AMS-C. Ellsworth et al. (1991) found similar results in 400 climbers on Mount Rainier. Given the comparability between the two systems, the LLS has become the preferred method because of its greater simplicity.

Another important question regarding the LLS is the appropriate scoring cut-off for making the diagnosis. The consensus report from the Hypoxia Symposium suggested a score ≥3 (with headache) was sufficient to diagnose AMS, although Maggiorini *et al.* (1998) showed that using a threshold of ≥4 had better sensitivity and specificity when compared to the ESQ. It is also not clear whether or not to include the Clinical Assessment and Functional Score sections of the LLS in the diagnostic strategy. These components are used in some, but not all studies. Clearly, if the scores from these sections are added to the scores from the self-reported symptom section, a greater cut-off value would be appropriate. In the paper by Bärtsch *et al.* (1993) a score >5 for the total Lake Louise score was suggested. Until more data are available on the other parts of the assessment, reliance should be placed mainly on the self-reported score, which has been well-validated. Finally, the LLS and ESQ are English language questionnaires. Although many studies in international settings translate the instruments into other languages, translation is not always performed and some non-English speakers may be using the English language questionnaire. This issue may be significant for comparing results between studies as Dellasanta *et al.* (2007) has shown that use of English questionnaires affected measured outcomes in some nationalities.

Given some of the issues associated with the ESQ and LLS, Wagner *et al.* (2007) proposed the use of a visual analog scale (VAS) to diagnose and grade the severity of AMS. Kayser *et al.* (2010) however, showed that the utility of this approach is limited and comparisons between studies done using either approach may be difficult. Even though the VAS and LLS scores had a reasonable correlation ($r = 0.84$), the respective scores do not scale linearly and instead show a threshold effect; with low LLS scores, the VAS scores all fell below the identity line while in the higher range of LLS scores, VAS scores fell above the line of identity.

19.4 INCIDENCE OF AMS

Documented incidence rates vary significantly between different high altitude regions and likely reflect the effect of multiple factors. Incidence rises, for example as measurements are made at steadily higher elevations. This change in incidence with altitude was demonstrated best by Maggiorini

et al. (1990) who found an incidence in climbers to European Alpine huts of 9% at 2850 m, 13% at 3050 m and 34% at 3650 m. Similarly, Honigman *et al.* (1993) documented an incidence of 25% in tourists traveling to 1900–2400 m in Colorado compared to an incidence rate of 43% among trekkers at 4343 m in Pheriche, Nepal (Hackett and Rennie 1979).

The rate or mode of ascent will also affect the reported incidence rate at a given elevation with faster ascent rates being associated with higher incidence. In their study of trekkers in Nepal, Hackett and Rennie (1979), for example found that trekkers who flew into Lukla had an incidence of 49%, compared to 31% in those trekkers who walked the entire distance. The rates in either group, however, were markedly lower than those individuals who directly flew into an airstrip at Syangboche (3800 m) in the same region (Murdoch 1995). Similarly, Basnyat *et al.* (2000) noted a very high incidence of AMS (68%) among religious pilgrims, who travelled by bus to 2000 m and then rapidly ascended on foot to the festival site at Gosainkunda Lake (4300 m). All of the pilgrims in this study normally reside below 2300 m and the majority (78%) made the ascent over only two nights. There is also an important interaction between the rate of ascent and the ultimate altitude achieved. Ranging between 75 and 77%, AMS rates on Kilimanjaro are some of the highest reported for any region (Karinen *et al.* 2008; Davies *et al.* 2009), likely reflecting the high elevations achieved on the climb as well as the notoriously fast ascent profiles on many of the routes.

Even at a given elevation reached by the same means in all subjects, incidence rates may differ for a variety of reasons. Assessment of AMS symptoms after only a few hours of exposure may lead to lower incidence than if subjects remain at the same elevation for longer periods of time. Studies from Aconcagua (6962 m) and the Capanna Margherita (4559 m) also demonstrate that the risk of AMS was lower in individuals with prior exposures to high altitude (Schneider *et al.* 2002; Pesce *et al.* 2005). The background of the study subjects may also be important, as Cabada *et al.* (2010) showed that the incidence of AMS in Cuzco, Peru (3400 m) varied between North

American and western European travellers despite similar ascent profiles to that elevation. They attribute the differences to variability in pre-travel preparation but the observed differences may have also reflected difference in pre-trip exposure to high altitude, for which they did not control. Lower incidence rates may also be documented at a given elevation over time as education and awareness about AMS increase (Gaillard *et al.* 2004; Vardy *et al.* 2005).

An under-recognized factor affecting reported incidence rates may also be proximity of a given region to the equator. West *et al.* (1983) have shown that barometric pressure at a given elevation is latitude-dependent due to differences in air mass over the equatorial and polar regions. As a result, ambient oxygen tensions and AMS risk at 4000 m near the equator, for example, may be different than those observed at the same absolute elevation at other latitudes. This issue was nicely demonstrated by Anderson *et al.* (2011) who noted an incidence rate of 52% in workers arriving at the South Pole (2835 m). This rate is significantly higher than that reported at similar elevations elsewhere and may be attributable, in part, to the fact that the barometric pressure at that elevation resulted in physiologic altitudes of about 3400 m, as well as the fact that workers were flown to that elevation.

19.5 FACTORS AFFECTING RISK FOR AMS

By far the most important reason individuals develop AMS is that they go too high, too fast. An individual, for example, who travels to and sleeps at 4500 m over only 2 days is more likely to develop symptoms than someone who spends 5 days reaching the same sleeping elevation. Beyond this important principle, however, there are many factors that may affect susceptibility to the disease.

19.5.1 Individual susceptibility

For any given altitude/time profile there is significant variation in individual susceptibility. This variability is likely driven by inherent genetic

differences but no specific genetic polymorphisms have been identified to this point. Studies have examined the role, for example, of the bradykinin receptor B2 gene (Wang *et al.* 2010) and ACE gene polymorphisms (Kalson *et al.* 2009) but no definitive links were found with AMS susceptibility. The genetics of high altitude physiology are discussed further in Chapter 4.

19.5.2 Physical fitness

A common misperception is that good physical fitness is protective against the various forms of altitude illness. This is not the case, as demonstrated by Milledge *et al.* (1991a) who found no correlation between fitness as measured by $V_{O_2,max}$ before an expedition to Mount Kenya and AMS symptom scores during the first days at altitude. Similarly, Bircher *et al.* (1994) studied 41 mountaineers who traveled over 20–22 hours to 4559 m and found no correlation between a measure of fitness (PWC_{170}) and AMS scores, while Savourey *et al.* (1995) found no correlation between $V_{O_2,max}$ and subsequent AMS on an Andean expedition. Despite the lack of a relationship between fitness and AMS risk, being in good physical shape for mountain travel is still important as it provides a margin of safety in any mountaineering situation, improves exercise tolerance at high altitude and may prevent physical exhaustion, which can mimic AMS.

19.5.3 Gender, age and body habitus

Inconsistent data have been reported regarding the effect of gender and age on AMS risk. Regarding gender, for example, Kayser (1991) found women to have a higher rate of sickness than men (69 versus 57%) among trekkers going over the Thorong pass in Nepal (5400 m), while Honigman (1993) found no difference in this regard. In terms of the effect of age, data from Hackett *et al.* (1976) and Roach *et al.* (1995) suggested that older individuals were at lower risk than younger travelers but Yaron *et al.* (1998) found a similar incidence of AMS in young children and adults. Graham and Potyk (2005) suggest that the reason for observed age-related differences in some studies may be due to the fact that non-specific symptoms of AMS may be attributed to comorbid conditions that increase in prevalence with age, thereby leading to under-reporting of AMS.

Data regarding the effects of body habitus are more consistent as multiple studies suggest that obese individuals are at greater risk for AMS than the non-obese (Hirata *et al.* 1989; Kayser 1991; Honigman 1993; Ri-Li *et al.* 2003). The reasons for this observation are unclear but may relate to lower average minute ventilation in these individuals relative to the non-obese.

19.5.4 Smoking and diet

There has been an impression among mountaineers that smokers have less AMS than non-smokers, perhaps because, being habituated to a modest level of carboxyhemoglobin they have, in effect, some pre-acclimatization. Aside from a study by Yoneda and Watanabe (1997), in which smokers had fewer subjective symptoms compared to non-smokers but no differences in time for useful consciousness following acute onset of severe hypoxia equivalent to 7260 m, there have been no systematic studies demonstrating support for this impression.

While a high carbohydrate diet may have some physiological benefit at altitude (Chapter 15, section 15.8.1) and is preferred by many mountaineers, there is no clear evidence it reduces AMS. In a chamber study of 19 subjects given either a high (68%) or normal (45%) carbohydrate diet for 4 days prior to 8 hours of exposure to 10% normobaric oxygen, Swenson *et al.* (1997) found that there was no difference in the AMS scores between individuals taking the two diets.

19.5.5 Hypoxic ventilatory responsiveness

From a theoretical perspective, it would make sense that impaired hypoxic ventilatory responses (HVR) would predispose to AMS. Individuals with a blunted response would have lower alveolar and arterial P_{O_2} values at any given altitude and might, therefore, become more symptomatic than those with stronger responses and higher oxygen tensions. Several experiments in the laboratory setting have provided support for this concept (Lakshminarayan and Pierson 1975; Hu *et al.* 1982; Matsuzawa *et al.* 1989). Similarly, Richalet *et al.* (1988) studied a large group of climbers before they went on various expeditions to the great ranges and found that a low ventilatory and cardiac response to hypoxia during exercise were risk factors for AMS. This finding has since been confirmed in a subsequent study by the same group (Richalet *et al.* 2011).

However, a number of other field studies have failed to find a relationship between HVR measured prior to high altitude travel and subsequent development of AMS (Milledge *et al.* 1988; Milledge *et al.* 1991b; Savourey *et al.* 1995). Hackett *et al.* (1987), for example, studied 106 climbers on Denali and found that, while a low Sa_{O_2} predicted the likely development of AMS, there was no good correlation between HVR and Sa_{O_2} on arrival at altitude. Hohenhaus *et al.* (1995) found that compared with healthy individuals, HVR was significantly lower in subjects who developed HAPE but not in subjects with AMS. Finally, Bärtsch *et al.* (2002) found no relationship between HVR, measured at sea level, and subsequent AMS upon ascent to 4559 m but did document that failure to raise the HVR on the first day at altitude was associated with a higher incidence of AMS.

19.5.6 Hypoxic pulmonary vasoconstriction

In the pulmonary circulation, alveolar hypoxia triggers hypoxic pulmonary vasoconstriction which leads to a rise in pulmonary artery pressure. While this phenomenon clearly plays a role in the development of HAPE (Chapter 21), there is no apparent effect on the incidence of AMS. Hohenhaus *et al.* (1994) for example showed that nifedipine, a calcium channel blocker with pulmonary vasodilatory properties prevents the development of HAPE but not AMS.

19.5.7 Oxygen saturation

A large number of studies have attempted to determine whether an individual's oxygen saturation at high altitude affects the likelihood of developing AMS with some studies reporting a link between hypoxemia and development of AMS (Roeggla et al. 1996; Roach et al. 1998; Basnyat et al. 1999; Tannheimer et al. 2002; Burtscher et al. 2004; Karinen et al. 2010) and others reporting no relationship (Roach et al. 1995; O'Connor et al. 2004). In considering these studies, however, it is important to note that only a few of the studies use a prospective approach and ask whether the presence of hypoxemia early in the trip predicts the subsequent development of AMS later in the stay at high altitude (Roach et al. 1998; Tannheimer et al. 2002; Karinen et al. 2010). Roach et al. (1998) for example measured oxygen saturation in 102 climbers at 4200 m on Denali, questioned them about AMS symptoms on their return from their summit bids and found that the Sa,O_2 measured before climbing from base camp correlated with subsequent AMS scores. The remainder of the studies on this question measured S_pO_2 at the same time the subjects were assessed for AMS (Roeggla et al. 1996; Basnyat et al. 1999; O'Connor et al. 2004; Koehle et al. 2010) and, as a result, do little to inform the discussion about whether a low saturation upon arrival at high altitude predisposes the individual to develop AMS at a later time.

The fact that the oxygen saturation may be lower in people with AMS suggests that AMS patients may have hypoventilation or underlying gas exchange problems as a result of subclinical pulmonary edema. The issue of subclinical edema was studied by Ge et al. (1997) who measured pulmonary diffusing capacity for carbon monoxide (DLCO) in a group of 32 subjects at 2260 m and following ascent to 4700 m. In non-AMS subjects there was an increase in DLCO at the higher altitude while in AMS patients the increase was insignificant. Dehnert et al. (2010) investigated this same question and found no difference in the DLCO (adjusted for alveolar volume) between individuals with and without AMS both upon arrival and following 2 days at 4559 m.

19.5.8 Exercise and AMS

High altitude travelers are often counseled to avoid heavy exercise immediately following ascent, but it remains unclear whether exercise is, in fact, associated with the development of AMS. Roach et al. (2000) for example exposed seven subjects to approximately 4800 m altitude in a chamber for 10 hours on two separate occasions, keeping the subjects at rest for the duration of one of the exposures but exposing them to intermittent exercise during the other exposure. AMS scores were significantly higher during the exposure with exercise. These results differ, however, from earlier data from Bircher et al. (1994) who found no difference in the incidence of AMS in relation to intensity of work (as assessed by heart rate) in groups of subjects who ascended on foot to the Capanna Margherita (4559 m).

19.5.9 Prior history of AMS

Prior outcomes at high altitude are a reasonable, although not perfect, predictor of well-being on future ascents. Individuals who developed AMS in the past are likely, although not guaranteed, to develop AMS with ascent to a similar elevation while those individuals who remained well on prior trips to high altitude are likely to do well on future trips provided they ascend to the same elevation at the same or slower rate.

Richalet et al. (2011) recently provided systematic evidence for this long-standing clinical observation. In a large, prospective study of 1326 individuals traveling to altitudes over 4000 m, they found that a prior history of severe high altitude illness (severe AMS, HACE or HAPE) was, along with several other variables associated with an increased likelihood of severe altitude illness on future ascents.

It is important to note, however, that prior altitude illness does not, in and of itself, cause altitude illness on future occasions. What it does, instead, is simply provide evidence that the individual's physiologic responses to high altitude are such that they are predisposed to problems in the future. With proper ascent rates and, perhaps pharmacologic prophylaxis (discussed further below in section 19.7), these individuals can still avoid AMS.

19.5.10 Predicting who will develop AMS

Given the high incidence of AMS among travelers to certain elevations, identifying those susceptible to the disorder would be useful as it would assist in the development of preventive strategies for a given individual. Several prediction tools have been proposed in this regard. Conducting a systematic review of the literature on oxygen saturation following arrival at high altitude, Burtscher *et al.* (2008) concluded that an arterial saturation determined 20–30 minutes following exposure to a simulated altitude of 2300–4200 m accurately predicted susceptibility in 80% of cases. Tannheimer *et al.* (2009) proposed that the time necessary to complete a running task at high altitude and nadir oxygen saturation during this task were predictive of an individual's risk of developing altitude illness with further ascent. Finally, in the study mentioned above, which is clearly the most comprehensive one to date on this issue, Richalet *et al.* (2011) proposed a multivariate predictive model to identify individuals susceptible to severe high altitude illness (severe AMS, HACE or HAPE) with the key factors being a prior history of severe altitude illness, a history of migraine headaches, decreased ventilatory responses during hypoxic exercise and desaturation >22% during hypoxic exercise. The study did not, however, address susceptibility to less severe forms of AMS.

A problem with many of these proposed decision tools, however, is that they involve testing strategies, such as a hypobaric chamber or a cardiopulmonary exercise system that might not be available to all providers trying to assess risk for a given individual. Whether the expense and time necessary to complete these tests is warranted in light of the self-limited and mild nature of the symptoms that many individuals will develop at high altitude and the ease of using simple, less costly preventive strategies (discussed further below) is also an open question.

19.6 PATHOPHYSIOLOGY OF AMS

Unlike the situation with HAPE, where the mechanism underlying its development is relatively well understood (Chapter 21), the underlying pathophysiology of AMS remains unclear despite a significant amount of research devoted to this issue. Clearly, hypoxia is a crucial starting mechanism for AMS but it is not the direct cause of symptoms. Within a few minutes of exposure to high altitude, the alveolar, arterial and tissue P_{O_2} fall but AMS onset is delayed for at least 6–24 hours, suggesting that hypoxia initiates some process, which, in turn, causes the symptoms of the disorder. Hypobaria itself, rather than just hypoxia, may also be playing a role through a variety of mechanisms, such as increased fluid retention (Loeppky *et al.* 2005b). In the text that follows, we consider some of the hypotheses that have been advanced regarding the specific processes linking hypoxia and, perhaps, hypobaria to the development of AMS. Figure 19.1 outlines several possible mechanisms by which hypoxia potentially leads to AMS but the reader must recognize that these are proposed pathways and that a definitive mechanism has yet to be elucidated.

19.6.1 Cerebral edema, intracranial pressure and AMS

One of the long-standing concepts advanced regarding AMS pathophysiology is that symptom onset is related to the development of cerebral edema and increased intracranial pressure (ICP). Recent magnetic resonance imaging (MRI) studies actually suggest that all individuals experience generalized brain swelling upon exposure to acute hypoxia as a result of vasogenic edema but that this mild increase in brain volume is not generally associated with the development of AMS (Kallenberg *et al.* 2007; Schoonman *et al.* 2008; Dubowitz *et al.* 2009). Instead, it is likely the development of cytotoxic edema and further increases in brain volume beyond that seen in all individuals, which likely lead to headache and other symptoms of the disorder (Kallenberg *et al.* 2007; Schoonman *et al.* 2008). Additional evidence of increased ICP includes early case series of AMS patients demonstrating elevated ICP during AMS compared to after recovery (Singh *et al.* 1969), as well as more recent studies using surrogate measures of ICP elevation

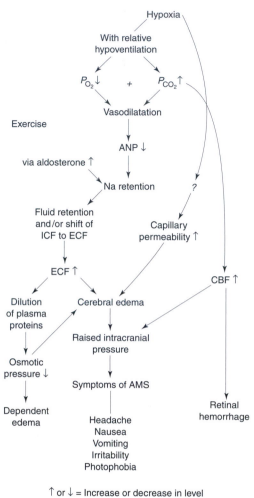

Figure 19.1 Possible mechanisms underlying acute mountain sickness (AMS). ICF, intracellular fluid; ECF, extracellular fluid; CBF, cerebral blood flow; ANP, atrial natriuretic peptide.

including ultrasound assessment of optic nerve sheath diameter (Fagenholz et al. 2009) or optic disk measurements based on fundus photography (Bosch et al. 2008) which noted a relationship between elevated ICP and AMS scores.

A relatively appealing idea that derives from these concepts is referred to as the tight-fit hypothesis. First proposed by Ross (1985), the hypothesis suggests that individuals with a higher ratio of cerebrospinal fluid to brain and blood volume have greater ability to compensate for cerebral edema or increased blood volume by displacing cerebrospinal

fluid (CSF) from the intracranial compartment and, as a result, are protected against the development of AMS compared to those individuals with a lower ratio. The hypothesis has not been tested extensively but several studies do provide some support for this concept. Wilson and Milledge (2008) analyzed previously unpublished data, including invasive ICP measurements, collected at 5030 m by Brian Cummins during a field study in 1985, and found an inverse correlation between ventricular size and headache scores. In their MRI study of individuals exposed to normobaric hypoxia equivalent to 4500 m in elevation, Kallenberg et al. (2007) also found that anatomic features consistent with a 'tight-fit' brain increased susceptibility to cytotoxic edema and the development of AMS.

A lingering problem in attempts to attribute the development of AMS to cerebral edema and elevated ICP is the fact that evidence of elevated ICP in mild disease is lacking. Several studies have measured ICP in milder cases and found no relationship between measured pressures and the symptoms of the disorder (Wright et al. 1995; Roach and Hackett 2001). Because headaches occur in early AMS at a time when edema and significant increases in ICP may not be occurring, alternative explanations such as changes in the blood–brain barrier in response to inflammation or free-radical formation, activation of the trigeminovascular system and altered cerebrovascular autoregulation have been proposed as potential contributors to AMS pathophysiology. Several of these topics are considered in further detail below.

19.6.2 Other potential contributing mechanisms for AMS

There are several other potential mechanisms that have been proposed to play a role in the development of AMS either by increasing the propensity for cerebral edema and elevated ICP or contributing to symptom development in the absence of these phenomena.

ALTERATIONS IN FLUID BALANCE

Subjects with AMS may develop a state of expanded plasma and extracellular fluid volume similar to that seen in subjects starting day-long exercise at low altitude. Examples of peripheral and periorbital edema that can be seen in AMS are shown in Fig. 19.2. Evidence of such fluid retention is provided by the clinical observation of lower urine output in soldiers with AMS than in soldiers free of symptoms (Singh *et al.* 1969) and by the finding that trekkers with AMS gained weight, while trekkers without AMS had lost weight by the time they reached 4243 m (Hackett *et al.* 1982). More recently, Loeppky *et al.* (2005a), exposed healthy men and women to hypobaric hypoxia (426 mmHg, approximately 4880 m) for 8–12 hours and noted significant fluid retention among the 16 individuals with the highest AMS scores. The 'normal' response to altitude seems to be a mild diuresis, whereas subjects destined to get AMS have an anti-diuresis.

The mechanism for the observed anti-diuresis remains unclear. In the study noted above, Loeppky *et al.* (2005a) found that anti-diuretic hormone levels fell in those who remained free of AMS but increased and continued to rise in those with AMS, and closely correlated with symptom severity and fluid retention. Other studies have implicated alterations in the renin–aldosterone axis and atrial natriuretic peptide levels, but the evidence has been inconsistent. With regard to aldosterone activity, AMS symptom scores were found to correlate with aldosterone levels and with reduced 24-hour urine sodium output on the first day at altitude in subjects who had ascended to 4300 m on foot on Mount Kenya (Milledge *et al.* 1989), while a similar result was reported from a study in the European Alps (Bärtsch *et al.* 1988). Hogan *et al.* (1973) however, found in a chamber study that subjects with AMS had lower aldosterone concentrations than did asymptomatic subjects, while Loeppky *et al.* (2005a) showed no difference in plasma renin activity or aldosterone levels in those with and without AMS. Similar variability has been seen in studies of atrial natriuretic peptide, with some studies reporting a tendency to higher levels in subjects more resistant to AMS (Milledge *et al.* 1989) but two other studies demonstrating the opposite result (Bärtsch *et al.* 1988; Cosby *et al.* 1988).

CEREBROVASCULAR BLOOD FLOW AND AUTOREGULATION

Severinghaus *et al.* (1966) demonstrated that cerebral blood flow (CBF) increased following ascent to high altitude but decreased with acclimatization, likely due to the erythropoietic response and subsequent increases in arterial oxygen content and oxygen delivery. Differences in the CBF response may account to some extent for the development of AMS. While Jensen *et al.* (1990) found no difference in CBF between subjects with and without AMS, other studies relying on Doppler ultrasound showed greater increases in middle cerebral artery velocity in subjects with AMS compared to asymptomatic controls (Baumgartner *et al.* 1994; Jansen *et al.* 1999).

The differences in cerebral blood flow between those who develop and do not develop AMS may relate, in turn, to the subjects' ventilatory responses and the subsequent changes in the arterial P_{CO_2} and P_{O_2}, two variables that have potent effects on CBF. The possibility that hypocapnia over a number of hours might be a factor in the genesis of AMS was tested by Maher *et al.* (1975). They

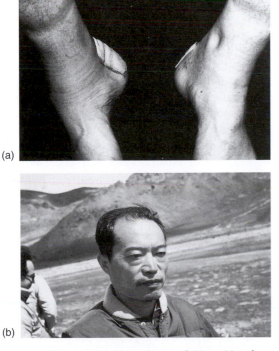

(a)

(b)

Figure 19.2 (a) Pitting edema of the ankle after hill walking at low altitude. (b) Periorbital edema at high altitude.

exposed two groups of subjects to simulated altitude in a hypobaric chamber. One group had CO_2 added to the atmosphere to maintain their P_{CO_2} at control levels; the other group breathed air and became hypocapnic. Hypoxia was similar in the two groups, although to achieve this outcome, the group with CO_2 added was taken to a lower barometric pressure. Far from alleviating symptoms of AMS the added CO_2 increased their severity. Other studies have shown that AMS symptoms correlate well with the P_{CO_2} (Forwand et al. 1968; Sutton et al. 1976; Hackett et al. 1982), suggesting that failure to decrease the P_{CO_2} as a result of blunted ventilatory responses plays a key role in AMS onset, as these individuals will have greater CBF and overall intracranial volume compared to those individuals who hyperventilate and decrease their P_{CO_2}. Individuals with blunted ventilatory responses will also have greater degrees of hypoxia compared to those who adequately raise their minute ventilation, which should also contribute to increased CBF.

In addition to the P_{CO_2} and P_{O_2}, CBF is also regulated in response to changes in mean arterial pressure. In particular, through a mechanism referred to as cerebrovascular autoregulation, constant CBF is maintained over a range of mean arterial pressures. Recent evidence suggests that impairment of this mechanism following ascent may contribute to the development of AMS. Van Osta et al. (2005) studied 35 volunteers following ascent over 20 hours to 4559 m and found that those subjects with a low cerebral autoregulation index, a marker of impaired autoregulation, had lower S_aO_2 and higher AMS scores compared to those with normal indices. They proposed that impaired autoregulation led to increased capillary perfusion, increased hydrostatic pressures and, as a result, cerebral edema. Cochand et al. (2011) have also shown that a lower autoregulatory index at sea level may predict the development of AMS following ascent, although this study did not include assessment of the autoregulatory index at altitude to determine if those individuals with altered autoregulation at sea level demonstrated similar problems in this environment. Subudhi et al. (2011) cast some doubt on this concept, however. They studied cerebral autoregulation prior to and after 9 hours of exposure to a simulated altitude of 4875 m in subjects taking dexamethasone and acetazolamide for AMS prophylaxis and found that although both drugs decreased symptoms of AMS, there were no clear relationships between these effects and changes in cerebral autoregulation.

INFLAMMATORY RESPONSES, FREE RADICALS AND REACTIVE OXYGEN SPECIES

While the changes in CBF noted above potentially affect blood–brain barrier permeability and edema formation by increasing hydrostatic pressure, it is also possible to increase permeability through other mechanisms including inflammatory pathways and reactive oxygen species.

Inflammation

Several forms of indirect evidence have implicated inflammation in the development of AMS. Richalet et al. (1991), for example, found a rise in plasma levels of most of the six eicosanoids measured in subjects taken abruptly to the Vallot observatory on Mount Blanc (4350 m), all of whom subsequently developed AMS, and noted that the time course for elevation of the levels of these vasoactive mediators paralleled the development of AMS symptoms. Roach et al. (1996) measured urinary leukotriene E_4 in subjects taken to 4300 m with a 4-day stopover at 1830 m and noted a significant increase in levels of urinary leukotriene E_4 although they were unable to demonstrate a statistically significant correlation with AMS. Other studies have not yielded consistent evidence of increases in inflammatory markers. Swenson et al. (1997), for example, measured a number of cytokines in the plasma of 19 subjects exposed to 10% oxygen for 8 hours and found no change in the concentration of the measured cytokines by the end of the exposure time. The exposure in this study was short in duration, however, and may not reflect changes that would occur over a longer time period. More recently, Julian et al. (2011) studied changes in inflammatory biomarkers in healthy individuals exposed to 10 hours of hypobaric hypoxia (425 mmHg) and found that while resistance to AMS was associated with downregulation of the inflammatory and permeability responses, the converse did not appear to be true; AMS susceptible individuals did not show evidence of an exaggerated inflammatory response.

The potential link between inflammatory pathways and AMS is weakened by the fact that multiple studies have shown that leukotriene blockade does not prevent AMS upon rapid exposure to hypoxia (Muza *et al.* 2004; Grissom *et al.* 2005; Luks *et al.* 2007). The negative results in these studies may be due to the fact that the intervention targeted just one small arm of what may be a very complicated inflammatory cascade, however. Gertsch *et al.* (2010) have shown that the less specific non-steroidal anti-inflammatory, ibuprofen, may prevent AMS but this study did not include an analysis of inflammatory mediator levels and how these might have been affected by the medication and, as a result it is difficult to use this study as proof of a link between inflammation and AMS.

Vascular endothelial growth factor

Vascular endothelial growth factor (VEGF) is another permeability factor inducible by hypoxia that may also alter blood–brain barrier integrity. Schoch *et al.* (2002) showed in mice, for example, that hypoxia induced an increase in VEGF, as well as evidence (documented by fluorescein marker) of cerebral edema that was prevented by inhibition of VEGF by a neutralizing antibody. Tissot van Patot *et al.* (2005) studied free plasma VEGF and found higher levels in subjects at 4300 m who had AMS. Walter *et al.* (2001), however, documented an increase in VEGF upon ascent to 4559 m, but found no difference between subjects with and without AMS or HAPE.

Reactive oxygen species

Recently, considerable attention has been focused on the role of reactive oxygen species (ROS) in altering vascular permeability and causing AMS. Bailey *et al.* (2001), for example, documented free radical-mediated vascular permeability in male volunteers ascending to high altitude, especially in the muscle vascular bed, which they contended may be related to the cerebral leak in AMS. In a subsequent study, rapid ascent to 4559 m induced an increase in cytokines, markers of muscle damage, neuronal damage, and ROS, which suggested tissue damage, but no correlation with

AMS could be substantiated (Bailey *et al.* 2003). In another study (Bailey *et al.* 2005), ROS were induced in humans by hypoxia (F_IO_2 of 0.12 for 18 hours) and lumbar punctures, brain MRI, AMS scores and ROS measurements were performed. Although 50% of the subjects developed AMS, there was no correlation between mild evidence of cerebral edema, clinical symptoms of AMS, or increase in intracranial pressures.

While these latter studies seem to cast doubt on the role of ROS in the pathophysiology of AMS, it may be that they are exerting a cerebral effect independent of changes in blood–brain barrier permeability. Bailey *et al.* (2009b) for example, showed that individuals with AMS following 6 hours of exposure to hypoxia (F_IO_2 of 0.12) were more hypoxemic and had greater increases in free radical-mediated lipid peroxidation than AMS-negative individuals without any evidence of blood–brain barrier disruption or neuronal-parenchymal injury. In another study, Bailey *et al.* (2009c) noted net positive cerebral output of lipid-derived free radicals and lipid hydroperoxides during 9 hours of exposure to an F_IO_2 of 0.13, that correlated with AMS scores but did not find evidence for altered blood–brain barrier function. How the free radicals and ROS lead to AMS without disruption of the blood–brain barrier and edema formation remains unclear, but Bailey *et al.* (2009a) have proposed that it may be related to their interaction with the trigeminovascular system.

As the discussion above has likely made clear, there remain many potential mechanisms for the development of AMS. While each proposed mechanism is plausible in its own right, there is conflicting evidence with regard to most of these ideas and we still lack a coherent explanation for the development of the disorder. Further work will be necessary until we have a level of understanding similar to that which exists at present for HAPE.

19.7 PROPHYLAXIS OF AMS

While various treatment strategies are available for those who develop AMS, the best approach is to prevent its development in the first place. In the majority of cases, AMS can be prevented through non-pharmacologic measures, while in other cases, drug prophylaxis is warranted and can be of great use. In considering these measures, it is important to remember that physiologic responses to high altitude and susceptibility to altitude illness vary significantly between individuals. As a result, a strategy that works for one individual may not be suitable for another.

19.7.1 Non-pharmacologic measures

Providing time for the body to acclimatize to high altitude is the single best way to prevent AMS, a principle made clear by the fact that AMS only occurs during the first few days at a given altitude. There are limits to acclimatization, however, which vary between individuals. Even after acclimatization to lower altitudes has been achieved, individuals may be at risk for AMS, HACE or HAPE with ascent to higher elevations.

RATE OF ASCENT

Slowing the rate of ascent provides adequate time for acclimatization and is perhaps the best means of preventing AMS. Rather than focusing on the speed at which someone walks or climbs, the key issue is the rate at which they increase their sleeping elevation. Recently published consensus guidelines from the Wilderness Medical Society, for example, recommend that once an individual travels above 3000 m, they should not increase the sleeping elevation by more than 500 m day^{-1} and should include a rest day every 3–4 days, during which they sleep at the same elevation for another night (Luks *et al.* 2010). Various resources make similar recommendations (Hackett and Roach 2001) but despite the widespread use of this approach, there is little in the way of data to support it. The recommendations likely originated following an epidemiological study of trekkers on the route to Everest Base Camp (Hackett *et al.* 1976) in which trekkers who walked from Jiri rather than flying to Lukla or who spent an extra night in Pheriche had a lower rate of AMS than trekkers who followed faster ascent profiles. While subsequent survey

data (Basnyat *et al.* 1999) have provided further evidence in support of this approach, there has been only one attempt to systematically study the effect of ascent rate on AMS incidence. Bloch *et al.* (2009) randomized climbers on Muztagh Ata (7546 m) to one of two ascent profiles and found that those individuals randomized to a slower ascent had lower symptom severity, incidence of AMS and greater chance of summit success than those randomized to the faster profile.

Slower ascents are clearly important at preventing AMS but the wide inter-individual variability in susceptibility makes it very difficult to be dogmatic about the precise ascent rates that individuals should follow. This principle was demonstrated nicely in a study by Murdoch (1999) in which he surveyed 283 trekkers in the Everest region of Nepal asking about AMS symptoms and speed of ascent. Half the trekkers ascending at the very low mean rate of 100–200 m day^{-1} became sick while almost half the trekkers ascending at 500–600 m day^{-1} remained free of AMS. Obviously there was a process of self-selection, with those feeling fine going fast and those feeling less well going slowly. His conclusion was that while the recommended ascent rates are likely slower than necessary for many trekkers, they should continue to be the guideline, in the interest of a substantial minority. With repeated travel to high altitude, individuals will learn their personal tolerances over time and can adapt the rules of thumb as necessary, being careful to choose slower rates when accompanied by individuals making their first trip to this environment.

FLUID INTAKE

Trekkers and climbers are often urged to drink plenty of fluids in order to prevent AMS but there is little sound evidence to support this recommendation. Basnyat *et al.* (1999) surveyed trekkers at Pheriche (4243 m) and found that individuals with higher fluid intake (up to 5 L day^{-1} in some cases) had a lower incidence of AMS (odds ratio 1.54). This study is limited, however by the retrospective nature of the data collection, the high likelihood of recall bias and difficulty establishing causality, as only those individuals who were feeling well may have been able to keep up with the higher fluid intake. Other, more systematic studies have not found any support for a relationship between hydration status and AMS incidence or severity. Aoki and Robinson (1971), for example, found no differences in AMS scores during 2 days of exposure to a simulated altitude of 4270 m between individuals made hypovolemic with furosemide diuresis and those receiving placebo or vasopressin to maintain euvolemia. More recently, Castellani et al. (2010) showed that although hypohydration degraded aerobic performance at simulated high altitude, there was no effect on the development of AMS. Richardson et al. (2009) did show that dehydration was associated with an increase in AMS scores with exposure to hypobaric hypoxia but also noted increased symptoms in the setting of hyperhydration.

The question remains as to why this recommendation persists despite the lack of supporting evidence. What likely accounts for the perception of benefit is the fact that individuals maintaining adequate volumes of fluid intake are preventing dehydration, a problem for which individuals are at higher risk at high altitude due to the lower humidity and whose symptoms often mimic those of AMS. While preventing dehydration is an important end in and of itself, too much fluid intake may also be problematic. Not only may overhydration create symptoms mimicking those of AMS (Richardson 2009), but also excessive free water consumption in the absence of adequate salt intake could lead to symptomatic hyponatremia during sustained exercise (Ayus and Moritz 2008).

PRE-ACCLIMATIZATION

Recent work suggests that hypoxic exposures prior to the planned ascent may decrease the risk of illness during that ascent, provided those exposures occur within a certain time frame relative to the planned ascent. Beidleman et al. (2004) for example, showed that 4 hours of daily exposure to the equivalent of 4300 m significantly decreased the incidence of AMS upon subsequent rapid ascent to 4300 m in a hypobaric chamber, and demonstrated in a later study (Beidleman et al. 2009) that 6 days of staging at 2200 m

decreased the incidence and severity of AMS during rapid ascent to terrestrial 4300 m. Similarly, Wu et al. (2009) showed that workers on the Tibet Railway who spent 7 months working at approximately 4500 m interspersed with 5 months living near sea level had a lower incidence of AMS with subsequent ascents when compared to people traveling to altitude for the first time. Despite the data in this regard, implementation of a pre-acclimatization program is challenging, as the precise timing and regimen of exposures necessary to produce a benefit remains unclear. Some exposure is good and more is likely better but how high and how often one should be exposed beforehand is not known. The question also remains as to whether most travelers have the time to invest in such programs.

OTHER MEASURES

Other strategies, such as avoiding alcohol or caffeine or choosing diets rich in carbohydrates, are often recommended but lack supporting evidence. In the case of caffeine, abrupt cessation of intake may even provoke withdrawal symptoms that resemble AMS (Hackett 2010). Another common-sense recommendation with good physiologic rationale but little supporting evidence is to avoid opiate pain medications, particularly at night, as the respiratory depressant effects could worsen oxygenation and possibly provoke AMS. Johnson et al. (2010) showed that use of non-invasive positive pressure ventilation during sleep improves nocturnal oxygen saturation and decreases AMS symptoms, but this strategy is logistically infeasible for the majority of high altitude travelers.

19.7.2 Pharmacologic prophylaxis

For the majority of individuals, an adequately slow rate of ascent is enough to prevent AMS. In other cases, however, pharmacologic measures may be necessary to further decrease the risk, with the decision to use pharmacologic prophylaxis being based on the individual's prior history at high altitude and the risk associated with the planned ascent (Luks et al. 2010).

ACETAZOLAMIDE (DIAMOX®)

Acetazolamide remains the mainstay of pharmacologic prophylaxis against AMS. After Cain and Dunn (1965) first showed that the medication increases ventilation and Pa,O_2, and decreases Pa,CO_2, multiple double-blind, placebo-controlled field studies have shown it to reduce the incidence and severity of AMS (Forwand et al. 1968; Birmingham Medical Research Group 1981; Larsen et al. 1982). Doses as high as 250 mg every 8 hours or 250 mg every 12 hours were used in the early studies but recent studies suggest that 125 mg every 12 hours may be as effective with fewer side effects (Basnyat et al. 2006; van Patot et al. 2008). Based on the results of these studies, the Wilderness Medical Society guidelines now recommend the lower dose although the proper dosing regimen remains a subject of debate (Dumont et al. 2000; Kayser et al. 2012). The pediatric dose is 2.5 mg kg^{-1} dose^{-1} every 12 hours up to a maximum of 125 mg dose^{-1}.

Regardless of which dose is used, the medication is best started the day before ascent to high altitude, but can be started following arrival as well. The duration of treatment depends upon the circumstance and situation. For subjects climbing steadily to a high point, such as the summit of a mountain, and then descending, the last dose is taken on the morning of summit day. In situations where subjects go to a given altitude and remain there for many days, the risk of AMS is limited to the first 4 or 5 days and treatment can be stopped after that time. Although it is of no use for preventing AMS after that point, Bradwell et al. (1986) showed that taking acetazolamide for 3 weeks at 4846 m decreased loss of body weight and muscle bulk and maintained better exercise performance compared to those on placebo. Despite the results of the study, use of the medication for preventing deterioration during long stays at high altitude has not become standard practice.

The primary side effects include parasthesias in the hands and feet, which tend to diminish with continued use of the drug and cease when the drug is withdrawn, as well as altered taste of carbonated beverages. The latter side effect is due to inhibition of carbonic anhydrase in the tongue, which blocks conversion of CO_2 to carbonic acid as the drink passes over the tongue, thereby preventing stimulation of acid-sensing buds. These side effects are generally mild and well tolerated, although in rare cases they can be more extensive and distressing for the individual. For this reason, individuals who have never used acetazolamide before may consider a trial of the medication for 48 hours in their home environment before embarking on their high altitude sojourn to ensure they tolerate it well.

The safety of acetazolamide is assured by its widespread use in glaucoma where it is used for years at doses similar to that recommended for AMS prophylaxis. There is a small chance of cross-reactivity in individuals with a history of sulfa allergy and caution should be used when prescribing the medication to these individuals, particularly with planned travel into remote areas (Luks and Swenson 2008; Kelly and Hackett 2010).

Acetazolamide is a mild diuretic and will increase the frequency and volume of urination at high altitude. The diuretic action itself plays little role in AMS prevention, however, and drinking fluids to replete losses caused by acetazolamide will not counteract its benefits in this regard. The primary mechanism by which acetazolamide protects against AMS is inhibition of carbonic anhydrase and the subsequent effects on acid–base balance and central respiratory control. Acetazolamide acts as a respiratory stimulant by promoting the excretion of bicarbonate in the kidneys, causing a metabolic acidosis that counteracts the respiratory alkalosis that results from the hypoxic ventilatory response and slows the rise in minute ventilation. The importance of this renal effect is shown in several studies demonstrating that benzolamide, a selective inhibitor of renal carbonic anhydrase with no cerebral action, decreases the incidence of periodic breathing (Swenson et al. 1991) and prevents AMS (Collier et al. 1996).

In addition to its renal effects, acetazolamide has several important effects on central respiratory control that further raise minute ventilation. By blocking brain vascular endothelial carbonic anhydrase and preventing conversion of carbon dioxide to bicarbonate, acetazolamide causes small rises in tissue PCO_2 near the central and peripheral chemoreceptors that stimulate increases in minute ventilation. (Swenson and Teppema 2007). Central carbonic anhydrase inhibition also leads to increased hydrogen ion concentration in the central chemoreceptors, which counteracts the inhibitory effect of the respiratory alkalosis. A more thorough discussion of the multiple means by which acetazolamide increases minute ventilation and prevents AMS is provided in several excellent reviews on the topic (Swenson 1998; Leaf and Goldfarb 2007; Swenson and Teppema 2007).

DEXAMETHASONE

For those individuals with an allergy or intolerance to acetazolamide, dexamethasone provides a valid alternative for AMS prophylaxis, as several prospective, randomized field and chamber studies have demonstrated a benefit in this regard (Johnson *et al.* 1984; Ellsworth *et al.* 1987; Ellsworth *et al.* 1991). A chamber study by Rock *et al.* (1989) suggested that 4 mg every 12 hours was the minimum effective dose, although another regimen providing an equal total daily dose (2 mg every 6 hours) is mentioned by several other sources (Hackett and Roach 2001; Luks *et al.* 2010). For those highly susceptible individuals, the combination of acetazolamide and dexamethasone may be more effective than acetazolamide alone (Bernhard *et al.* 1998), although for the majority of individuals single agent prophylaxis should be sufficient. Dexamethasone should be avoided for prophylaxis in children.

Unlike acetazolamide, dexamethasone does not affect ventilation or facilitate acclimatization. As a result, individuals must be careful to monitor for symptom onset if the drug is abruptly discontinued. It can be an important adjunctive therapy for individuals ascending rapidly to altitudes higher than 3000 m for a rescue, but should never be taken as a means to mask symptoms of moderate or severe AMS or HACE while the climber continues to ascend. Individuals should not use dexamethasone for prophylaxis for greater than 7–10 days. If longer use is necessary for some reason, the drug must be tapered off, rather than abruptly stopped, to avoid problems with adrenal suppression, as demonstrated in a recent case report of a climber who developed Addisonian crisis in Everest Base Camp following abrupt cessation of the drug (Subedi *et al.* 2010).

OTHER DRUGS

The prophylactic effects of multiple other drugs have been examined but none of these agents have become part of standard prevention protocols. Conflicting data have been presented regarding spironolactone (Jain *et al.* 1986; Basnyat *et al.* 2011) while several studies have shown that theophylline, a respiratory stimulant, prevents AMS and decreases periodic breathing (Kuepper *et al.* 1999; Kupper *et al.* 2008). Use of the latter agent might be challenging at high altitude, however, due to the medication's narrow therapeutic window and risk of toxicity. Sumatriptan may be effective against AMS (Jafarian *et al.* 2007) while antioxidants have not proven effective (Baillie *et al.* 2009) despite the work discussed earlier regarding the role of free radicals in the underlying pathophysiology of the disease.

Burtscher *et al.* (1998) demonstrated that aspirin was an effective prophylactic agent, but in a subsequent study lacking a placebo arm (Burtscher *et al.* 1999) it was effective at preventing headache only when used in conjunction with dexamethasone. A related medication, the acetylsalicylic acid analog, calcium carbasalate, was shown to have no benefit (Kayser *et al.* 2008). Gertsch *et al.* (2010) showed in a randomized, placebo-controlled trial that ibuprofen was as effective as acetazolamide at preventing high altitude headache and AMS but it is hard to determine how much of the effect on AMS in this study was driven by the effect of headache, a key component of the AMS score. More recently, Lipman *et al.* (2012) compared ibuprofen (600 mg every 8 hours starting 6 hours prior to ascent) to placebo in healthy individuals rapidly ascending from 1240 m to 3810 m and noted a decreased incidence of AMS in the ibuprofen group (odds ratio 0.3, 95% confidence interval 0.1–0.8) although there were no statistically significant changes in severity of AMS symptoms between the two groups or headache score measured by use of a visual analog scale.

Despite the suggestion of benefit from ibuprofen, clinical experience with prophylactic use of the medication remains limited and, as noted above, it has not been adopted as part of consensus guidelines for management of altitude illness. In addition, given concerns for potential for gastrointestinal bleeding in this environment (Chapter 25, section 25.6.1) use of non-steroidal anti-inflammatory agents for long durations at high altitude should likely be avoided until further data are available on this issue.

Several studies have demonstrated that the herbal extract *Ginkgo biloba* is effective at preventing AMS (Roncin *et al.* 1996; Moraga *et al.* 2007), but multiple negative studies have also been published (Gertsch *et al.* 2004; Chow *et al.* 2005) that raise questions about its utility. The discrepant results in these trials likely result from important differences in the source and composition of the *Ginkgo* products used in the studies. Because individuals purchasing the herbal remedy from a local health food store cannot have any confidence in the true composition of the *Ginkgo* product they obtain, it should not be used for AMS prophylaxis.

Despite its widespread use for prophylaxis in South America, there is no evidence that coca, in the form of either chewed coca leaves or coca tea is effective at preventing AMS.

19.8 TREATMENT OF AMS

19.8.1 Non-pharmacologic measures

Descent to lower elevation remains the single best treatment for all forms of acute altitude illness but is generally not necessary unless an individual shows evidence of HACE or HAPE, or has AMS and is not responding to appropriate treatment. In many cases, rest alone relieves the symptoms of AMS (Bärtsch *et al.* 1993), a fact that must be borne in mind when considering the results of trials of therapy in AMS. Affected individuals should try to rehydrate themselves to eliminate any element of dehydration that can mimic AMS and efforts should be made to exclude other AMS mimics such as hyponatremia. By simulating descent, supplemental oxygen will improve symptoms but besides being impractical in most cases, its use may actually impede acclimatization. Voluntary hyperventilation or pursed lip breathing are of more theoretical than practical benefit as they are difficult for ill individuals to sustain for adequate periods of time. Portable hyperbaric chambers, discussed further in Chapter 20, are rarely necessary for AMS and are typically reserved for more severe disease.

19.8.2 Pharmacologic measures

Individuals with AMS can use acetaminophen, non-steroidal anti-inflammatory drugs (NSAIDs) and anti-emetics to relieve the symptoms of AMS. No controlled trials have assessed the utility of acetaminophen or NSAIDs in treating the full spectrum of symptoms in AMS but several studies have shown that these agents are effective at treating high altitude headache (Broom *et al.* 1994; Harris *et al.* 2003).

Individuals not responding to these conservative measures or with more severe AMS can consider adding either acetazolamide (250 mg every 12 hours) or dexamethasone (4 mg every 6 hours). The utility of the former in this regard has been demonstrated in a single randomized trial (Grissom *et al.* 1992) while the benefits of the latter have been demonstrated in multiple studies (Ferrazzini *et al.* 1987; Hackett *et al.* 1988; Levine *et al.* 1989). Both agents can be used to treat AMS in children (Pollard *et al.* 2001). Research studies have not compared which agent is more effective at AMS treatment but clinical experience suggests that dexamethasone is a faster, more reliably effective treatment for any degree of AMS (Luks *et al.* 2010). As noted earlier, however, unlike acetazolamide, it will not have any effect on acclimatization, which may be important upon further ascent.

19.8.3 Subsequent action

Affected individuals should never ascend further in the face of ongoing symptoms of AMS, as symptoms will only worsen and the individual risks progression to HACE and/or HAPE. Those individuals whose symptoms resolve with appropriate treatment can continue their ascent to higher elevation and should consider prophylactic acetazolamide or dexamethasone during this time. If individuals fail to improve after several days of appropriate therapy or worsen at any time, they should descend until symptoms resolve. Re-ascent can be considered after symptom resolution and 1–2 days of rest and acclimatization.

19.9 FUTURE TRIPS TO HIGH ALTITUDE

Individuals respond reasonably consistently with repeated trips to high altitude, so that performance on one occasion is a guide to future performance. Those individuals who have been sick with ascent to a given elevation in the past are likely, but not guaranteed, to become sick with future ascents to the same elevation, while those individuals who remained well on prior ascents are likely, but also not guaranteed, to remain well with future ascents to similar elevations.

This clinical impression has been confirmed in a study by Forster (1984) who studied workers at Mauna Kea observatory in Hawaii (4200 m). These workers alternated 5 days at the observatory with 5 days at sea level, which allowed Forster to score the symptoms of AMS in 18 men on two altitude shifts. He showed that the rank order of scores correlated significantly on the two occasions and also demonstrated a tendency to acclimatize better on each subsequent trip to altitude.

While prior performance is a reasonably good predictor of future performance, there are numerous exceptions to this rule. For instance, someone who has had little trouble on the first two trips may develop AMS on a third, perhaps because they ascended at a slightly faster rate. They might also develop dehydration or a viral infection that could be mistaken for AMS (Bailey *et al.* 2003). Predictability of incurring altitude illness is greater in the case of individuals who have had HAPE than it is AMS.

Knowing that prior performance is a reasonable predictor of future performance, individuals who make repeated trips to high altitude can learn about their personal tolerances of the environment and may deviate from the ascent rates recommended for preventing altitude illness. For example, individuals who have repeatedly been sick on prior trips should opt to ascend at a slower rate than recommended, while those who have tolerated the environment without difficulty on earlier excursions may, within reason, choose to move at a faster rate. The latter strategy should always be undertaken with caution, however, particularly when moving to altitudes higher than they have ever attained before, and the individual should always be prepared to descend and/or slow the rate of ascent if problems develop.

Individuals who have developed AMS on repeated trips in the past may consider consultation with their primary care physician, travel clinic provider or a physician familiar with high altitude issues in order to consider appropriate means to mitigate the risk of ascent on future trips so they can continue to enjoy the opportunities available in mountain environments.

20

High altitude cerebral edema

SUMMARY

High altitude cerebral edema (HACE) is a severe form of acute mountain sickness (AMS) characterized by the same symptoms, headache, malaise and fatigue which can progress to ataxia, altered consciousness, hallucinations, coma and death. Signs include papilledema, extensor plantar responses and other neurological signs. There may be mild fever, cyanosis (which may be secondary to concomitant high altitude pulmonary edema (HAPE)), increased pulse and respiratory rates. Computed tomography (CT) and post-mortem appearance indicate cerebral edema, and magnetic resonance imaging (MRI) scans show lesions in the splenium and corpus callosum. In untreated cases remaining at altitude, death can occur in a few hours or days.

The incidence of HACE is less than for HAPE, usually occurs at a higher altitude, but many patients have a mixed picture with signs and symptoms of both conditions.

Prevention of HACE is the same as for AMS; that is, to make a slow ascent to altitude and to descend if symptoms do not improve. The diagnosis is made on the history and clinical examination. In a patient with symptoms of AMS, if any neurological signs appear or if there is any clouding of consciousness or hallucinations, then HACE is the likely diagnosis. Often, the earliest sign is ataxia, which is easily missed in a patient lying in a tent with a headache, especially as he may be irritable, and insist that he is all right.

The most important action in treatment, as in HAPE, is to get the patient down. If this is impossible or while awaiting evacuation, oxygen, if available, will help. Dexamethasone 4–8 mg initially, followed by 4 mg every 6 h often relieves the neurological symptoms and signs, and treatment in a portable compression bag (Gamow or Certec) is also beneficial, at least for a few hours. Recovery is often rapid on descent, but a number of cases have been described in which recovery was delayed by days or weeks, and, of course, some victims die regardless of descent or medication, and some cases with residual neurologic have been reported.

The mechanism of development of cerebral edema is not understood. It is probably the same as in AMS at first, but instead of being self-limited, it progresses to an advanced stage giving rise to the signs and symptoms described and eventually to death. Recent opinion about the mechanism of the edema is that it is both vasogenic and cytotoxic in origin with an increase in the permeability of the blood–brain barrier (BBB).

20.1 INTRODUCTION

The symptoms of AMS are probably due to mild cerebral edema, which, though unpleasant, are not serious. In a small minority of cases, usually at altitudes higher than 3500 m, the condition progresses to more severe symptoms. Unmistakable signs of cerebral edema and increased intracranial pressure become manifest and can progress to coma. Death can occur if the patient is not treated and has been reported even if descent or other interventions have been initiated. This severe form of AMS is called HACE.

Ravenhill (1913) called the condition 'puna of a nervous type.' He describes three cases who recovered on being sent down to low altitude. As with acute pulmonary edema of high altitude, his work was forgotten, and it was only during the 1960s that description of this serious form of acute cerebral edema of high altitude emerged (Fitch, 1964; Singh et al. 1969).

20.2 CLINICAL PRESENTATION

20.2.1 Epidemiology

Symptoms of AMS usually precede HACE (Chapter 19). HACE can occur in unacclimatized individuals usually at 3000 m or higher. Because of difficulty in knowing the number of people exposed, its incidence has never been accurately determined, but HACE certainly is much less common than AMS or HAPE. A 1% incidence in trekkers in Nepal between 4200 and 5500 m was reported by Hackett et al. (1976). An extraordinarily high incidence of 31% was reported by Basnyat et al. (2000) in a group of pilgrims who ascended rapidly in Nepal. Often HACE and HAPE may coexist (Yarnell et al. 2000). Symptoms of stupor and coma were described in 13% of 52 patients with HAPE (Gabry et al. 2003) which is similar to the findings of Hultgren et al. (1996) in the Canadian Rockies. Sometimes in HAPE, the severity of hypoxemia is so great that it is difficult to know whether the symptoms are secondary to cerebral edema or the effects of hypoxemia.

The age and sex distribution, like that for AMS, shows no group to be immune. Possibly the younger male is rather more at risk, perhaps because he is more likely to push on to higher altitude with symptoms, a feature of many histories

in fatal cases. People native to high altitude can become victims of HACE. The impression is that the incidence in them is lower, but there are no good published data.

20.2.2 Symptoms and signs

Symptoms of AMS usually precede those of HACE by 24–36 h, but the presence of milder cerebral edema before the progression to HACE has not been confirmed (Fischer et al. 2004). Headache, loss of appetite, nausea, vomiting and photophobia are common. Climbing performance decreases dramatically, and in fact, patients may just stop any activity and become irritable and withdrawn and wish only to be left alone. Behavior may become bizarre and irrational, and survival instincts cease. The clinical transition from AMS to HACE is often difficult to ascertain, but the appearance of ataxia, irrationality, hallucinations or clouding of consciousness should alert one to the likelihood that the patient now has HACE. The patient may report blurring of vision which may be due to retinal hemorrhages or to papilledema. Deep-tendon reflexes may be brisk, and later the plantar reflexes may become extensor. There may be ocular muscle paralysis with diplopia. The pulse is often rapid, and cyanosis usual.

As the condition progresses, all symptoms and signs become more evident. The headache becomes worse, and ataxia intensifies so that the patient can no longer sit up (truncal ataxia) or walk in a coordinated manner. If coma ensues, breathing becomes irregular. Death may come in a few hours or in a day or two in untreated cases. Residual and permanent neurologic impairment, including dementia (Usui et al. 2004), have been reported.

Although with a recent ascent to high altitudes greater than 3000 m and the symptoms described above, good clinical evaluation must be made, as many of the symptoms are non-specific and may be secondary to many other conditions, including structural (tumors), psychiatric (psychosis), metabolic (hypoglycemia, ketoacidosis, hyponatremia), toxic (ingestions), epileptic (Firth and Bolay 2004; Daleau et al. 2006) or cerebrovascular (stroke, hemorrhage, migraine) abnormalities.

20.2.3 Case histories

CASE 1

As reported by Houston and Dickinson (1975), a 39-year-old Japanese female flew from 1500 to 2750 m, and during the next 2 days, climbed to 3500 m, where she developed a severe headache. On day 4, at 3800 m, she began to vomit. On day 5, at 3960 m, she became breathless and weak, was vomiting and needed assistance to walk. On day 6, she lost consciousness and was carried down to 3350 m where she was found to be deeply unconscious and cyanosed, with a temperature of 40.6°C and a pulse of 140 beats min^{-1}. Crackles filled the chest. Reflexes were brisk and plantars flexor. Slight papilledema was present. She was treated with oxygen, furosemide and penicillin. On day 8, she was flown to a hospital at 1500 m where she was found to be in the same condition but with extensor plantar reflexes. Lumbar puncture showed a pressure of 270 mm H$_2$O, but examination of the cerebrospinal fluid (CSF) was normal. She slowly improved over 2 weeks and eventually recovered completely.

Comment. The symptoms of HACE are dominant in this case but the patient also had signs of HAPE.

CASE 2

As reported by Dickinson *et al.* (1983), a 46-year-old man trekked from 1500 to 3650 m in 2 days. On the way, he began to feel unwell, was tired, anorexic and later began to vomit. At 3650 m, he became unconscious and was evacuated to a hospital at 1500 m. On examination, he was deeply unconscious, responding only to pain. He was cyanosed and hyperventilating. There were crackles and wheezes in the lungs; papilledema and retinal hemorrhage were present. Respirations were 40 breaths min^{-1}, the pulse was 120 beats min^{-1}, and the temperature 40°C. He remained unconscious and died after 4 days in the hospital.

Comment. This is a typical case of HACE, which seemed to have reached an irreversible stage before descent.

CASE 3

As reported by Houston and Dickinson (1975), a 42-year-old fit man reached 3600 m from sea level in a few days. He spent 2 days at this altitude and on day 3 climbed to 4940 m, returning to sleep at 3960 m. On day 4, after carrying about 25 kg to 4940 m, he complained of severe headache, and went to sleep on arrival at the camp. Next morning, he was confused and unable to talk coherently. He could not coordinate hand and foot movements and was disorientated in time and space. He was carried down to 3600 m where he became coherent and was able to walk without assistance. He was given an intramuscular steroid and by late afternoon seemed normal. The next day he was taken down to 2130 m where he was completely normal.

Comment. A typical case of HACE where prompt action in bringing the patient down saved his life.

CASE 4

In an abridged study from Howarth (1999), a 42-year-old member of a scientific expedition had trekked to Kangchenjunga Base Camp (5100 m) and spent a week at this altitude including climbing twice to about 5400 m on day outings without illness or incident. With three companions, he set out to climb a 6200 m peak on the return trek. On the first day from Base Camp, their porters took the wrong route to their intended camp at 5500 m necessitating some climbing over very rough ground. During the early part of the day, the patient had been going strongly, but later he was slow and reached camp at 2.45 p.m., cold and exhausted. He complained of a bad headache but took some hot soup and painkillers. AMS was diagnosed, and it was hoped he would improve with rest. However, over the next 2 h he deteriorated and became ataxic. He was given acetazolamide and dexamethasone, but vomited most of the tablets. Evacuation was started, but it required a man on each side to support him and over the boulder-strewn ground, going was very slow. He continued to deteriorate, and they had to stop for rest every 20 yards or so. The party was benighted, but fortunately was able to radio other members of the expedition for help. The rescue party met them with oxygen and injectable dexamethasone after which the patient improved though descent over now steepening scree was still very slow. A temporary camp at about 4900 m was reached at 11.30 p.m. By next morning, the patient was much better, and during the day was able to walk slowly back to Base Camp.

Comment. This case illustrates the unpredictability of AMS in that typical HACE developed in a climber who would seem to have acclimatized well. In some subjects who have no problems up to a certain point, there seems to be a critical altitude above which they quite abruptly start having symptoms. It also emphasizes the importance of making an early diagnosis and getting the patient down as soon as possible. Of course, this is easier with hindsight.

20.2.4 Investigations

Unless the case of presumed HACE is, in fact, another condition, such as mentioned in section 20.2.2, blood counts and biochemistries are usually normal, but white counts may be high. Chest radiographs may show evidence of concomitant pulmonary edema. Although normally not necessary to perform except to rule out a central nervous system (CNS) infection or hemorrhage, lumbar punctures show raised pressures, 44–220 mmH$_2$O (Singh *et al.* 1969; Houston and Dickinson 1975), but normal CSF chemistries and

cell counts. Computed tomographic scanning of the brain in 12 patients with HAPE and HACE (Koyama *et al.* 1984) showed evidence of cerebral edema with diffuse low density of the entire cerebrum and compression of the ventricles. Recovery to normal CT findings occurred within a week in three cases, but abnormal findings persisted for 1–2 weeks in two cases; one case took over a month to clear.

Hackett *et al.* (1998) reported MRI in nine patients with HACE compared with three with HAPE and three who had been to altitude with no illness. They found intense T2 signals in white matter, especially in the splenium and corpus callosum in the subjects with HACE. There were no lesions in the grey matter (Fig. 20.1). With this one study, there was no correlation between the severity of edema on imaging and the subsequent clinical course.

Microhemorrhages were found in the brains of subjects with non-fatal HACE (Kallenberg *et al.* 2008). MRIs were performed in victims of both HACE and severe AMS 2–31 months after the clinical event. Multiple hemosiderin deposits primarily in the corpus callosum were found in the HACE victims but not those who suffered severe AMS with comparable altitude exposure. These findings suggest vascular permeability, especially in the corpus callosum where the blood vessels are small perforating arteries unprotected by adrenergic tone and this may be more vulnerable to stress failure.

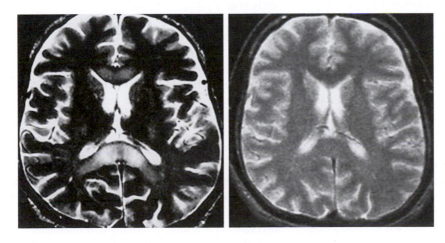

Figure 20.1 Left, Axial T2-weighted magnetic resonance image of patient showing markedly increased signal in corpus callosum including both the genu and the splenium, as well as increased signal of periventricular and subcortical white matter. Right, same patient 11 months later showing complete resolution.

20.2.5 Treatment

The treatment for HACE is very similar to that for HAPE. Victims should go to lower altitude as soon as possible, especially before their condition renders them unable to care for themselves and thus impose greater risk to their fellow climbers. Recognizing the symptoms early while the victim is still ambulatory may mean the difference between a successful descent, with recovery, and death on the mountain. While awaiting evacuation, oxygen therapy is advised but often is only of marginal benefit. Dexamethasone has been shown to be of benefit in a double-blind, randomized, placebo-controlled trial in AMS (Ferrazzini et al. 1987). It is particularly the cerebral symptoms which seem to be helped by this drug, so it is a critical drug to have available and use in this situation. The dose utilized in the trial was 8 mg initially, followed by 4 mg every 6 h. Enthusiasm for dexamethasone should be tempered by the finding that, although symptoms are relieved, the physiological abnormalities (fluid shifts, oxygenation, sleep apnea, urinary catecholamine levels, chest radiograph, perfusion scans and the results of psychomotor tests) are not improved (Levine et al. 1989). The drug is no substitute for descent.

Some authors have recommended diuretics, but the delicate balance between cerebral perfusion and pre-existing hypovolemia in the mountains accentuated by diuresis is a risk not worth taking in the field setting. Once in the hospital setting where monitoring is possible, the usual measures taken to decrease intracerebral edema (mannitol, hypertonic saline, etc.) are reasonable.

Portable hyperbaric bags (Gamow bags) are now available, and their use in HAPE is discussed in Chapter 21. In HACE, their use is less well documented (Freeman et al. 2004); but, if available and if descent is necessarily delayed, a hyperbaric bag should be tried. Its use may have therapeutic benefit and make it possible for a patient to descend unaided, instead of having to be carried. Recovery after descent may not be as rapid as is usually the recovery from HAPE (Dickinson (1979) and cases 1 and 2). Some reports detail recoveries from 2 to 14 days or even longer (6 weeks; Hackett et al. (1998)) with some reports

of persistent neurologic impairment. Better education about altitude maladies (Vardy et al. 2005) and the increasing availability of helicopter rescue in remote areas of the Himalayas (Graham and Basnyat 2001) are improving the outcomes of HACE and other altitude illnesses.

20.2.6 Post-mortem appearance

There have been a few reports of post-mortems in HACE (Singh et al. 1969; Houston and Dickinson 1975; Dickinson et al. 1983). The usual findings in the brain are of cerebral edema with swollen, flattened gyri, and compression of the sulci. There may be herniation of the cerebellar tonsils and unci. Spongiosis, especially in the white matter, may be marked. In many cases, there are widespread petechial hemorrhages; in some, there are ante-mortem thrombi in the venous sinuses or there may be subarachnoid hemorrhages. There seems to be considerable variation in the findings. It must always be remembered that the few cases that reach autopsy are highly selected and may be unrepresentative of the condition as seen clinically in the field.

20.3 MECHANISMS OF HACE

20.3.1 Cytotoxic versus vasogenic edema

The mechanism for the development of cerebral edema at altitude is reviewed in Chapter 19, and there may be many responses of edema formation which AMS and HACE have in common. There is agreement that hypoxia induces an increase in extracellular fluid. It may also cause increased microvascular permeability. The images on MRI suggest that the leak is vasogenic in origin, i.e. an increase in permeability of the vascular endothelium, but these findings do not differentiate between a leak caused by increased pressures or factors such as inflammation that increase the vulnerability of the endothelial lining.

Cytotoxic edema results from hypoxic-induced failure of cellular ion pumps with a rise in intracellular sodium and osmolarity and consequent cellular swelling from an influx of water (Fishman 1975). Bailey *et al.* (2009) have put forth a detailed review of evolving theories of brain edema at high altitude. As mentioned above, there is strong evidence that acute exposure to hypoxia results in some vasogenic edema and subsequent intracranial hypertension with displacement of the unmyelinated pain-sensitive fibers in the trigeminovascular system, leading to headache. The authors cite studies (Bailey *et al.* 2006; Kallenberg *et al.* 2007; Schooman *et al.* 2008) which confirmed formation of mild vasogenic edema in the susceptible areas (corpus callosum) after hypoxic exposure, but also evidence of intracellular edema in those with symptoms of more severe AMS. Attempts to study HACE victims were difficult since their clinical illness had been at least 6 days before. The authors invoke a role for inflammation, especially from reactive oxygen species (ROS), whose free radicals cause a disruption of the Na^+/K^+-ATPase pump and astrocyte swelling. HACE may then reflect a more extreme variety of osmotic-oxidative stress leading to blood–brain barrier dysfunction, cerebral microvascular stress failure, as well as brain cell swelling.

Zhou *et al.* (2011) took rats to 5000 m for 9 days and measured markers of inflammation, such as TNF-alpha, superoxide dismutase, endothelin, glutathione, and others in brain tissue, as well as brain morphology by electron microscopy, and brain water. There was a significant increase in all of these markers by 9 days, as well as evidence of disruption of the blood–brain barrier. The increase of brain water correlated with the increase in inflammatory markers.

20.3.2 Cerebral blood flow

An inordinate increase in cerebral blood flow would seem a likely culprit, leading to cerebrovascular damage and subsequent leak of fluid from the intra- to extravascular space. Hypoxia increases cerebral blood flow (Severinghaus *et al.* 1966; Borgstrom *et al.* 1975), particularly when there is no marked reduction in P_{CO_2}. The usual increase in alveolar ventilation upon ascent to altitude and the resulting hypocapnia lead to cerebral vasoconstriction. The body's response upon rapid ascent, though, is to optimize blood

flow and oxygen delivery such that the increase in cerebral blood flow from hypoxia overrides the vasoconstriction from the hypocapnia.

Attempts to find a correlation between AMS and HACE and cerebral blood flow have not given consistent results. While Baumgartner *et al.* (1994) found a correlation between cerebral blood flow (CBF) and AMS, Jensen *et al.* (1990) found none. Furthermore, a doubling of CBF by hypercapnia in sheep did not cause brain edema (Yang *et al.* 1994). These same factors may become more pronounced to cause the symptoms of HACE, but that theory is mere speculation.

In an attempt to find a relationship between autoregulation of CBF with hypoxia and systemic blood pressure, Jansen *et al.* (2000) studied subjects at low altitude and Sherpas who had not experienced HACE and sojourners at high altitude and found an inconsistent decrease or maintenance of autoregulation of CBF in response to hypoxia and an increase in systolic blood pressure (SBP) raised by phenylephrine in all groups. Thus, it does not seem likely that one could base an etiology for the mechanism of HACE on normal autoregulation of CBF. On the other hand, a subsequent study in subjects rapidly ascending to 4559 m showed a correlation between CBF, Sa_{O_2}, and AMS scores (Van Osta *et al.* 2005).

Imray *et al.* (2005) found intriguing results when they measured cerebral perfusion and oxygenation in unacclimatized subjects at 150 and 5260 m during progressive exercise. Whereas cerebral oxygenation was maintained throughout exercise at low altitude, at high altitude it increased up to 30% of maximal exercise and then fell progressively as the exercise intensity increased (Fig. 20.2). The authors speculate that this phenomenon may contribute not only to performance at high altitude but also to the brain's vulnerability to edema.

CBF autoregulation is largely successful in optimizing oxygen delivery to the brain, but recently has been shown to be impaired even after acclimatization (Iwasaki *et al.* 2011). Eleven healthy subjects were studied at low altitude, acute hypoxia (10.5%), and after a month at 5260 m altitude. A number of signals of CBF velocity were measured and although predictably increased with both acute and chronic hypoxic

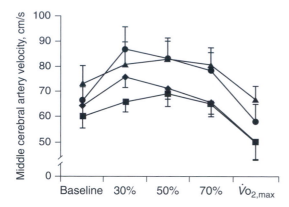

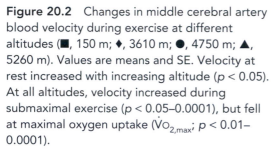

Figure 20.2 Changes in middle cerebral artery blood velocity during exercise at different altitudes (■, 150 m; ♦, 3610 m; ●, 4750 m; ▲, 5260 m). Values are means and SE. Velocity at rest increased with increasing altitude ($p < 0.05$). At all altitudes, velocity increased during submaximal exercise ($p < 0.05$–0.0001), but fell at maximal oxygen uptake ($\dot{V}O_{2,max}$; $p < 0.01$–0.0001).

exposure, a number of signals of impaired dynamic autoregulation were found in both hypoxic conditions. It is not clear from this small study whether inter-individual variability can account for AMS or HACE susceptibility.

20.3.3 Cranial vault capacity

The question of why certain individuals are susceptible while others are not is as puzzling in HACE as in other forms of AMS. One possible factor might be the relative sizes of the brain and cranial cavity. In a recent review of etiology, Hackett (1999) discusses this 'tight fit' hypothesis. Those with a tight fit brain in the box of their cranial cavity will have a greater rise in pressure for a given increase in fluid volume in the brain. Those with looser brains are less susceptible. As we get older, our brains shrink which may be why older people are less susceptible to AMS and HACE. More data are necessary to make this hypothesis stronger. Furthermore, the percentage increase in brain volume from the edema of HACE, whether it be vasogenic and/or cytotoxic, is not thought by many to be adequate to result in

impingement of the cranial vault, except perhaps in the most extreme and terminal cases of HACE (Kallenberg *et al.* 2007; Schoonman *et al.* 2008).

20.3.4 Increased central venous pressures

Venous thrombosis has been found on CT scan in one patient (Asaji *et al.* 1984) and in some post-mortem studies of HACE. It may develop late in the condition as a consequence of intracranial hypertension. It will certainly exacerbate the condition.

Others have hypothesized that the symptoms of altitude headaches and HACE could be accounted for by elevation of central venous pressures (Wilson *et al.* 2011). In this expansive theoretical paper, these authors review a number of physiologic and clinical situations where functional increases of effluent blood flow result in a rise in intracerebral vascular pressures and can result in headaches not necessarily associated with microvascular leak. Their hypothesis encompasses mechanisms that could explain HACE.

20.3.5 Vascular endothelial growth factor

Severinghaus (1995) suggested that vascular permeability, operating in situations of angiogenesis and induced by vascular endothelial growth factor (VEGF), may be involved in HACE. Hypoxia stimulates the release of transforming growth factor which attracts macrophages. These, in turn, release VEGF and other factors which eventually give rise to growth of new capillaries. The more immediate effect is to increase capillary permeability as capillary basement membranes are broken down. He suggests that even earlier than these events, hypoxia may case osmotic brain swelling. Dexamethasone is very effective in preventing angiogenesis, and it may be this action which explains its effectiveness in HACE. This theory received support from the finding of VEGF mRNA in rat brains after only 3 h of hypoxia (Fig. 20.3). The level reached a

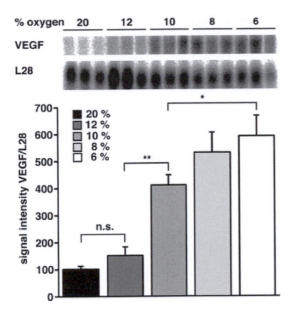

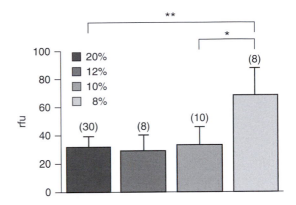

Figure 20.4   Two-fold increase in vascular permeability after exposure to 8% oxygen. Sodium fluorescein injected intravenously in controls or hypoxic mice was quantified following homogenization of brain hemispheres. Results are expressed as relative fluorescence units (rfu). Values are mean and standard deviation. **$p < 0.0001$; *$p < 0.001$; $n = 8$–30 as indicated.

Figure 20.3   Increased expression of **VEGF mRNA in mouse brain after hypoxic stimulation. Total RNA was extracted from brains of normal mice and mice exposed to 6–12% oxygen for 24h. (Upper panel) Northern blots of total RNA sequentially hybridized with a 32P-labelled probe for murine VEGF and the ribosomal protein L28. (Lower panel) Mean and standard deviation (n 5 3) of vascular endothelial growth factor (VEGF) mRNA pixel densities as quantified with a Phosphoimager and corrected for L28. Normoxic control was set to 100%. **$p < 0.001$; *$p < 0.05$; n.s., not significant.

peak of three times control at 12–24 h (Xu and Severinghaus 1998). This could explain the increased permeability of the blood–brain barrier and the vasogenic edema.

Two studies lend credence to this theory. Schoch *et al.* (2002) found increased VEGF expression and increased vascular permeability, as measured with a fluorescein marker in mice brains, which correlated with the degree of hypoxic exposure which was prevented by inhibition of VEGF activity (Fig. 20.4). By measuring free VEGF upon acute ascent to 4300 m, investigators found a correlation between free VEGF and AMS symptoms (Tissot van Patot *et al.* 2005). These studies are strongly suggestive of induction of

vascular permeability by VEGF in its response and attempt to initiate angiogenesis secondary to a hypoxic stimulus.

20.3.6 Nitric oxide and cerebral edema

Clark (1999) suggested that the mechanism of cerebral edema in HACE may be via the induction of inducible nitric oxide synthase (iNOS) in the brain by hypoxia. This gives rise to increased levels of nitric oxide (NO) which by increasing vascular permeability causes edema. In most cases, this is quite mild and self-limiting, giving rise to the symptoms of benign AMS. However, if there are even low levels of cytokines as well, due to a mild infection for instance, there will be a synergistic effect on iNOS induction and permeability. This results in HACE.

20.3.7 Conclusion

HACE is a potentially fatal form of altitude illness usually occurring at higher altitudes than AMS or HAPE and is thought to be a more severe form of AMS with more profound clinical signs and symptoms. It has largely been thought to be caused by vasogenic edema with microvascular leak. Recent evidence suggests that in addition to initial vasogenic edema, there is violation of the BBB with an evidence of inflammation contributing to both the vascular leak, as well as astrocytic swelling of a cytotoxic nature.

21

High altitude pulmonary edema

SUMMARY

High altitude pulmonary edema (HAPE) is a potentially lethal form of mountain sickness which, like acute mountain sickness (AMS), affects previously healthy people who go rapidly to high altitude. A few hours after arrival, patients most commonly suffer the usual symptoms of AMS, but then become more breathless than their companions. Over the next few hours, the breathlessness increases, a cough develops which is first dry but later productive of frothy white sputum. The sputum may become blood-tinged. The signs of obvious pulmonary edema are found, and cyanosis may be detected. Some patients literally drown in their own secretions and become comatose and can die if no action is taken. Patients have tachycardia and tachypnea with mild pyrexia and leukocytosis and a characteristic x-ray appearance. The pathology, in fatal cases, is of patchy edema of the lungs.

The most important management is to get the patient down; if there is unavoidable delay, oxygen, if available, and drugs which vasodilate the pulmonary vasculature are helpful. If descent is not feasible, hyperbaric treatment in a Gamow® (or Certec®) bag gives temporary relief and may be useful in enabling a patient to improve and walk down rather than having to be carried.

The mechanism of the edema formation is not left ventricular failure since wedge pressures on cardiac catheterization are normal. However, there is severe pulmonary hypertension. There are a number of hypotheses about how this results in edema. The most favored mechanism is that the hypoxic vasoconstriction is uneven. Vessels which are not downstream from the constricted vessels are exposed to higher pressures which suffer stress failure of these vessels allowing proteins and later blood cells to leak out into the interstitial space and then alveolar spaces. Later, there is evidence of inflammation, as cytokines and arachidonic acid metabolites are found in the edema fluid, and these contribute to the vascular leakage. Exercise seems to be a risk factor presumably by raising the pulmonary artery pressure.

Many patients who suffer HAPE show susceptibility to the condition on subsequent altitude exposure. These subjects are found to have a brisk hypoxic pressor response in their pulmonary circulation and it is thought that this susceptibility may have a genetic origin. The role of the balance between endogenous pulmonary vasoconstrictors and vasodilators and the alveolar fluid clearance, as well as genetic factors, has emerged in the unravelling of the mechanism of HAPE.

21.1 INTRODUCTION

There are a number of accounts in the early climbing literature of climbers dying of 'pneumonia.' In retrospect many, if not most, of these fatalities were probably due to HAPE. One of the best known was the death of Dr Jacottet on Mont Blanc in 1891. He died in the Vallot hut (4300 m) after taking part in a rescue on the mountain. Refusing to go down, he spent a further two nights in the hut with obvious symptoms of AMS. He died during the second night. The post-mortem showed 'acute edema of the lung' (*oedème considerable*) (Mosso 1898).

In 1913, Ravenhill described what he called *puna* of the cardiac type as a lethal form or development of AMS. Though he was wrong in attributing the condition to cardiac failure, his description of three cases fits well with HAPE. However, his work was forgotten.

For the first half of the twentieth century, the condition would not be at all common in the European Alps, because few unacclimatized people spent nights above 2500 m or in the Himalayas where approach marches to the mountains were long enough for acclimatization to take place. However, in South America, as Ravenhill's experience showed, railways and later roads had been built to altitudes up to 3000 or 4000 m, thus putting large numbers of people at risk. However, even in these countries, the condition was not recognized for many years after Ravenhill. West (1998) has unearthed a description of a case reported by Alberto Hurtado in 1937 in an obscure booklet. However, the case is atypical in a number of ways and Hurtado says (in translation from the Spanish),

> this is undoubtedly a type of Soroche (mountain sickness) which is quite rare and infrequent and is characterized by intense congestion and edema of the lung. Possibly there is in these cases a prior cardiac condition. …

This case also had further long-term problems suggestive of a cardiac condition. Although this could be considered as the first case report of HAPE after Ravenhill, there was mention of some cases of soroche who had cough with pink frothy sputum and who made a rapid recovery on descent to low altitude. This was in an article by Harold Crane, the chief surgeon of a hospital at the mining town of Oroya (3750 m) in Peru. The article was published in the *Annals of the Faculty of Medicine*, Lima in 1927. The first series of cases (seven) to be published was by Leoncio Lizárraga Morla in 1955 in the same journal. He mentioned that the condition was recognized by Carlos Monge M as early as 1927. The cases described were typical of HAPE and included chest x-rays and electrocardiograms (ECG) typical of HAPE. This paper was followed by others, including Bardáles, from Peru in the later 1950s. The first reference in English to the condition we now call HAPE was in a letter to the *Journal of the American Medical Association* by Bardáles in 1956. In it he describes the condition briefly in high altitude residents returning to altitude, saying it is particularly common in young people. For a fuller description of these papers and the full references, see West (1998).

An interesting side light showing the situation in the English-speaking world in the mid 1950s is given by a letter to Dr Griffith Pugh which he published with a comment in *The Practitioner* (Pugh 1955). Dr Pugh was the leading authority on altitude medicine and physiology in UK at the time. The letter gave an excellent account of a fatal case of HAPE and asked whether acute pulmonary edema is a common symptom of high altitude sickness. Pugh, in his response, indicates that he knew of no such case from his experience or from the literature. The original letter and response together with a commentary are to be found in West (1999).

Herbert Hultgren visited Peru in 1959 and saw cases of HAPE. He and his companion Spickard wrote up their experiences in the *Stanford Medical Bulletin* published in May 1960 under the title, 'Medical experiences in Peru'. In it they mention 41 cases of acute pulmonary edema in residents returning to altitude after a stay of 5–21 days at low altitude. They correctly suggested that the mechanism was not left ventricular failure, but related to pulmonary hypertension. Not surprisingly, this important observation was not recognized at the time, and so the condition was brought to the notice of the English-speaking medical world by Houston (1960) who published his landmark paper on 'acute pulmonary edema of high altitude' later in the same year in the *New England Journal of Medicine*. Houston said 'this single case is presented in the hope of stimulating further reports' and 'pulmonary edema of high altitude deserves further study.' Both hope and declaration have been amply fulfilled in the succeeding years by the description of hundreds of cases from all the major mountainous areas, and hundreds of studies aimed at elucidating the mechanism of the condition have been conducted, some of which will be reviewed in this chapter.

21.2 CLINICAL PRESENTATION

HAPE, like AMS, affects previously healthy individuals on ascent to altitude and often presents in the absence of AMS. There is a wide range of altitude of presentation from 2000 to 7000 m (Lobenhoffer *et al.* 1982). A typical history is that the subject ascends rapidly to altitude and is very active getting there or on arrival. Within 12–36 hours of arrival, the subject suffers the symptoms of AMS, though not necessarily very severely, and then becomes more short of breath and lethargic. The patient may experience chest pain. Physical signs are of tachycardia, tachypnea and crackles at the lung bases. A dry cough develops which later progresses to one productive of frothy white and eventually blood-tinged sputum. Over a few hours, the condition progresses with increasing respiratory distress, orthopnea, cyanosis, and bubbling respirations and may proceed to coma and death.

21.2.1 Case histories

Case histories 1–3 are taken from Houston (1960).

CASE 1

A male patient left sea level, reaching 5090 m by car and on foot 5 days later. He had no symptoms until 1 day later when he noted dyspnea progressing to severe orthopnea. Within a few hours, his breathing became progressively more congested and labored. He sounded as though he was literally drowning in his own fluid with an almost continuous loud bubbling sound as if breathing through liquid. A white froth resembling cotton candy had appeared to well up out of his mouth, even though he was sitting up with his head tilted back. The patient died within 8 hours of the onset of symptoms.

CASE 2

A Sherpa on a large expedition had carried a load from 6400 to 7000 m and returned. The following morning, he complained of severe headache and malaise. He was anorexic and remained in his sleeping bag. On examination at mid-morning, he was found to be cyanotic and breathless on the slightest exertion, and he had a dry cough. His pulse and respiratory rate were increased. Fine crackles were heard at the lung bases. At noon he started down for a lower camp at 5800 m accompanied by two expedition members. It was at once apparent that he could not carry even a light load. Every 100–200 m, he had to stop even though the route was over an easy downhill glacier. He began coughing frothy white sputum, which later became blood-tinged. At about 100 m above the camp, he was given oxygen and was able to complete the journey without stopping. After breathing oxygen for about 3 h at the camp, he declared himself well and refused any more oxygen. He descended unaided to a lower camp next day, carrying a load.

CASE 3

A 20-year-old college student from Chicago flew in the morning to Denver, Colorado, and drove that afternoon from the airport to the Keystone ski resort in Summit County (3000 m) where he was going to spend the week skiing. By mid-afternoon, he was skiing at 3700 m. That night he developed a headache which progressed to malaise, dyspnea and a dry cough which by morning had progressed to one with frothy sputum. He could not sleep and went to the resort clinic where he was found by pulse oximeter to have an oxygen saturation of 70%. His examination revealed crackles, a tachycardia, cyanosis and tachypnea. His chest radiograph showed patchy opacities in both lung fields. Application of 3 L min^{-1} flow of oxygen by nasal prongs resulted in a rise in his oxygen saturation to 91%. He was sent to his hotel room with oxygen therapy with his family. Emergency medical help was available 24 h each day. He was seen daily in the clinic and had improved by the fourth day such that he was able to ski the last 3 days of his vacation.

21.2.2 Incidence

Because of the problem of knowing the number of people at risk, it is difficult to obtain data on the incidence of HAPE. As with AMS, its incidence will depend upon the rate of ascent and the height reached. Hackett and Rennie (1976) saw seven cases in 278 trekkers who passed through Pheriche (4243 m) on their way to Everest Base Camp, giving an incidence of 2.5%. The incidence of AMS in the same group was 53%. Menon (1965) found an incidence of 0.57% in Indian troops flown to the modest altitude of Leh (3500 m). Hultgren and Marticorena (1978) gave an incidence of 0.6% in adults going to La Oroya, 3750 m. In these series, a diagnosis was only made in clear, overt cases. If the chests of all newcomers to altitude are auscultated, crackles will be heard in many who would not be otherwise diagnosed as HAPE, and radiographic signs are also found on chest x-ray in many subjects after intense exercise (Anholm *et al.* 1999; Cremona *et al.* 2002). There is controversy as to whether subclinical pulmonary edema exists in many climbers. This topic was keenly debated in a point–counterpoint piece (Cogo and Miserocchi 2011; Swenson 2011a; Swenson 2011b) which had been preceded by a strong argument for the presence of pulmonary edema in heavily exercising athletes even at low altitude (Hopkins 2010a). These observations were explained by stress failure of the fragile pulmonary capillaries from high cardiac outputs in aerobic athletes (Hopkins 2010b). The concept of pulmonary capillary stress failure will be discussed later. Thus, a degree of subclinical edema may be present in active subjects with and without simple AMS which contributes to the reduced Sa,O_2 (section 19.4.8). However, in simple AMS or in subjects without any symptoms of altitude illness,

the edema is self-limiting, whereas in HAPE it is progressive.

The incidence will be affected by health education of people going to altitude. It is the impression of health workers at the aid post at Pheriche (4243 m) in Nepal, as well as on Denali (4300 m), that the incidence is less following some years of publicity about the dangers of HAPE among trekkers and climbers.

21.2.3 Symptoms of HAPE

Table 21.1 shows the symptoms from the largest series managed by a single physician (Menon 1965) who reported 101 cases. The frequency of chest pain, second only to breathlessness is unusually high. Only 21% of patients complained of chest pain in a German series (Lobenhoffer *et al.* 1982). Hallucinations are not uncommon and, with confusion and irrational behavior, may make management difficult. Nocturnal dyspnea and the symptoms of AMS – headache, nausea and insomnia – are all common, and almost all patients have marked limitation in their exercise capabilities.

21.2.4 Signs

These depend upon the stage of the condition. Probably the earliest signs are crackles at the lung bases and tachycardia, although the former is not always reliable. Crackles may be heard in subjects

Table 21.1 High altitude pulmonary edema: symptoms in 101 cases (Menon 1965)

Symptom	No. of cases
Breathlessness	84
Chest pain	66
Headache	63
Nocturnal dyspnea	59
Dry cough	51
Hemoptysis	39
Nausea	26
Insomnia	23
Dizziness	18

who have no other signs of HAPE and who do not progress to the full blown condition (Maggiorini 2006). The presence of early edema may be the cause of dry cough on exertion and of the shift to the left of the pressure/volume curve of the lung (Mansell *et al.* 1980; Gautier *et al.* 1982), the reduction in forced vital capacity (Welsh *et al.* 1993; Fischer *et al.* 2005), and the increase in closing volumes (Cremona *et al.* 2002). The pulse rate increases early and was over 120 in 70 of 101 patients in Menon's (1965) series. The respiratory rate was over 30 in 69 cases; cyanosis was detected in 52 subjects.

The pulmonary artery pressure is high in this condition (section 21.2.7) giving the signs of right ventricular heave and accentuated pulmonary second sound in about half the patients. Signs of right ventricular failure are not prominent, but 15 of Menon's patients had raised jugular venous pressure, and dependent edema is found in a number of cases. The temperature is normal in at least 25% of cases but was found to be elevated (37–39°C) in 70% of Menon's cases. In only two cases was it above 39°C. Maggiorini *et al.* (1997) found temperature to be elevated by a mean of 0.8°C compared with climbers without HAPE. The systemic blood pressure is either normal or

mildly elevated (systolic 130–140 mmHg) as is found in some subjects on ascent to altitude who do not have HAPE. These findings suggested stress failure of the fragile pulmonary capillary bed with leak of proteinaceous fluid from the intra- to extravascular space.

Some subjects (15 in Menon's series) have mental confusion and amnesia following recovery. This may be due to hypoxia or cerebral edema (Chapter 20).

21.2.5 Radiology

A number of studies have reported patchy infiltrates (Hultgrem and Spickard 1960; Menon 1965; Vock *et al.* 1989; Vock *et al.* 1991; Koizumi *et al.* 1994).

Figure 21.1 shows a chest radiograph of a patient with HAPE and a second radiograph 4 days later after treatment. The typical features are of cotton wool blotches irregularly positioned in both lung fields, best seen by computed tomography (Fig. 21.2). They are frequently asymmetrical; possibly being denser on the side which has been dependent. Very often, the right side is more densely shadowed (Menon

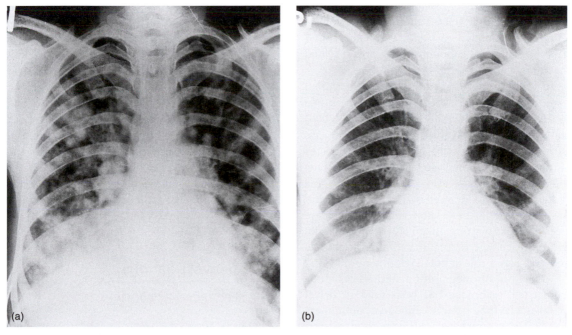

(a)   (b)

Figure 21.1   Radiograph of a patient with high altitude pulmonary edema: (a) on admission and (b) 4 days later. (Reproduced with permission of Dr T Norboo of Leh, Jammu and Kashmir, India.)

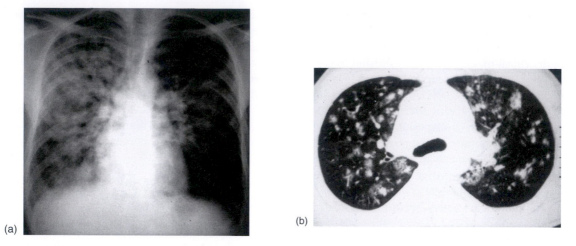

(a)

(b)

Figure 21.2   (a) Radiograph of a 37-year-old male mountaineer with high altitude pulmonary edema (HAPE) which shows a patchy to confluent distribution of edema, predominantly on the right side. (b) Computed tomography scan of 27-year-old mountaineer with recurrent HAPE showing patchy distribution of edema (from Bartsch *et al.* 2005).

1965). Quite frequently, the lower zones, especially the costophrenic angles, are spared as well as the apices. The pulmonary vessels may be seen to be engorged (Marticorena *et al.* 1964). The radiographic appearance in early cases shows more pathology than would be expected from clinical examination (Menon 1965). In patients with a second attack of HAPE, there is no consistent pattern in the areas of lung involved. In treated cases, the radiographic lesions clear rapidly (see Fig. 21.1), often within 2 days (Houston 1960), though usually lagging behind the improvement in symptoms.

In an attempt to clarify further unusual hemodynamics of those who are susceptible to HAPE (HAPE-S), Sherrer and Seiler (2006) studied 16 HAPE-S and 19 HAPE-R subjects with echocardiography at low and high (4559 m) altitude to determine the relationship between arterial oxygen saturation, HAPE-S, and the presence of patent foramen ovales (PFO). PFO was present in the HAPE-S subjects four times more frequently, suggesting that PFO hemodynamics and gas exchange is accentuated at high altitude and may play a role in the development of HAPE.

In chest ultrasonography, a method called the 'comet-tail' technique has been used to detect extravascular lung water in cardiogenic pulmonary edema. Two groups have used this method to detect pulmonary edema in subjects at high altitude in Nepal. Fagenholz *et al.* (2007a) studied subjects

with and without HAPE at Pheriche (4240 m) and found higher comet-tail scores (CTS) in the HAPE subjects than the healthy individuals with a negative correlation with oxygen saturations. With clinical improvement, scores returned to normal values. On the other hand, Pratali *et al.* (2010) documented CTS in 18 subjects ascending to high altitude. Findings were negative at low altitude (1350 m), but CTS were positive in 15 of 18 subjects at 3440 m and in 18 of 18 at 4790 m. Scores continued to increase as oxygen saturations decreased upon further ascent to 5130 m in the absence of clinical HAPE. Echocardiography documented normal right and left ventricular function in site of modest elevations in calculated pulmonary artery pressures. These authors felt that there is increased interstitial lung water in spite of no clinical evidence of HAPE and that the ultrasonography technique utilizing CTS was a valid way to document lung water, but there was no other technique to validate the data.

21.2.6 Investigations

THE ELECTROCARDIOGRAPH

The ECG shows tachycardia. The *P* waves are often peaked (*P* pulmonale), and there is right axis deviation of the QRS (mean, 1123°). Some patients show elevation of the S–T segment (Marticorena *et al.* 1964). T-waves may be inverted in the precordial leads but this may be seen in asymptomatic subjects at altitude (Milledge 1963). The ECG appearances can be attributed to the very high pulmonary artery pressure and the consequent increase in right ventricular work.

HEMATOLOGY

Menon (1965) found that hemoglobin concentration was 14.0–16.0 g dL^{-1} and the sedimentation rate was normal. The white cell count, predominantly neutrophils, was raised in 75 of 95 cases.

BLOOD GASES

P_{O_2} and arterial oxygen saturation are low compared with normal values for altitude. P_{CO_2} is very variable and is not significantly different from controls (Antezana *et al.* 1982; Schoene *et al.* 1985).

URINE

Proteinuria was present in four of 101 cases (Menon 1965), but using more sensitive tests, he found an increase in urine protein in all subjects during the first few days at altitude with the degree of proteinuria correlating with the severity of AMS (Pines 1978; Chapter 16).

21.2.7 Cardiac catheter studies

There have been a number of catheter studies carried out on patients with HAPE before treatment (Penaloza and Sime 1969; Antezana *et al.* 1982) or soon after starting treatment (Fred *et al.* 1962; Hultgren *et al.* 1964; Roy *et al.* 1969). In all these studies, there was found to be a high pulmonary artery pressure compared with healthy subjects at the same altitude (Table 21.2). The wedge pressures were normal. The pulmonary artery pressure ranged up to 144 mmHg systolic at the high end (Hultgren *et al.* 1964), but were still quite high at the mean at 60–80 mmHg systolic (Table 21.2). The normal wedge pressure implies normal pulmonary venous and left atrial pressures; in one subject, direct measurement of left atrial pressure was made via a patent foramen ovale and was normal (Fred *et al.* 1962). The cardiac output was within the normal range so the calculated pulmonary resistance was markedly raised. There was no evidence of left ventricular failure. Breathing 100% oxygen resulted in a fall of pulmonary artery pressure to normal values within 3 min in two of five subjects. However, in the other three, pressures fell, but plateaued out at 40–50 mmHg pulmonary artery pressure, well above the upper limit of normal at that altitude (Antezana *et al.* 1982).

Non-invasive echocardiography has afforded investigators the opportunity to evaluate patients during and after their bouts of HAPE (Kawashima *et al.* 1989; Yagi *et al.* 1990; Hackett *et al.* 1992; Vachiery *et al.* 1995; Busch *et al.* 2001; Berger *et al.* 2005). Similar responses were found during hypoxic exercise (Fig. 21.3). These findings have confirmed the earlier catheterization studies (Table 21.2).

21.2.8 Population at risk

The etiology of HAPE is similar to that of AMS (section 19.4), all ages and both sexes being susceptible. There is an impression that children

Table 21.2 Cardiac catheter studies in high altitude pulmonary edema (HAPE) at 3700 m (data from Antezana *et al.* 1982)

Group	Pulmonary artery pressure (mmHg)		Wedge pressure (mmHg)	Cardiac output (L min^{-1})
	Systolic	Diastolic		
HAPE (*n* = 5)	81	49	5	5.8
Controls (*n* = 50)	29	13	9	6.4

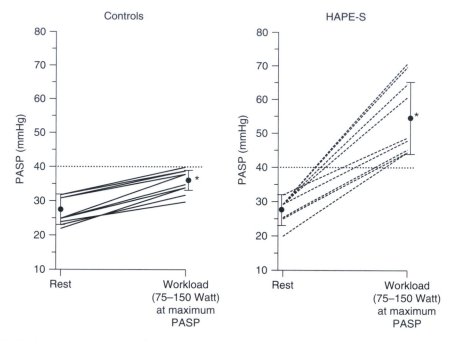

Figure 21.3 Pulmonary artery systolic pressure (PASP) response to exercise. Discrimination between controls and HAPE-S subjects by their PASP response to exercise estimated by Doppler echocardiography. HAPE-S, subjects susceptible to high altitude pulmonary edema (n = 9); controls, control subjects (n = 11). No significant differences at rest between both groups (p = 0.28). *Mean maximal PASP in controls (36 ± 3 mmHg) vs. HAPE-S (55 ± 11 mmHg) subjects, p < 0.002.

and young adults are more prone to HAPE than older people. Individual susceptibility for HAPE is more clear cut than for AMS in that subjects (HAPE-S) who have suffered HAPE on one occasion are very likely to have problems on subsequent altitude trips. HAPE has been described in both South (Hultgren and Spickard 1960) and North America (Scoggin *et al.* 1977) in permanent high altitude residents, mostly children, who have made brief forays to low altitude (1–14 days) and upon return to high altitude have subsequently developed HAPE. The role of smooth muscle remodeling and vasoconstrictive reactivity has been speculated as an etiology of this sporadic and unpredictable clinical presentation. Peñaloza *et al.* (2008) reviewed the literature pertaining to pulmonary hemodynamics in children and found that pulmonary artery pressures are elevated in children at 4000 m or higher, but regress as the child ages. There also is a higher prevalence of patent ductus arteriosus and more sustained moderate and severe pulmonary hypertension

that leads to right heart failure. Finally, individuals with congenital absence of a pulmonary artery are predisposed to developing HAPE (Hackett *et al.* 1980).

21.2.9 Physiologic characteristics

LUNG VOLUMES

One possibility is that HAPE-susceptible individuals have a restricted lung vasculature or just smaller lungs. Surface area of the pulmonary vascular bed may influence vascular resistance encountered when hypoxic pulmonary vasoconstrictive responses (HPVR) and augmented blood flow merge to stress the microvasculature. A study by Steinacker *et al.* (1998) tested this idea by comparing eight such subjects with controls at rest and on exercise in normoxia and hypoxia. The HAPE-prone group had 35% smaller functional residual capacities,

7–10% smaller vital and total lung capacities and less of an increase in their diffusing capacities on exercise under hypoxia. This lends support to the hypothesis of smaller lungs in HAPE-susceptible individuals. A similar conclusion had been reached by Podolsky *et al.* (1996) who studied the pulmonary response to exercise in HAPE-susceptible subjects at sea level and 3810 m. They found greater vascular reactivity in HAPE subjects. The reactivity was not affected by altitude or oxygenation so was due to either flow-dependent pulmonary vasoconstriction or a reduced vascular cross-sectional area.

There has been a debate for some time that many mountaineers ascending to high altitude have some element of interstitial pulmonary edema perhaps early HAPE. A recent study by Dehnert *et al.* (2010) reported extensive pulmonary function tests in a group of 34 individuals ascending to 4559 m. There were no changes noted between healthy individuals and those with AMS and minor decreases in forced vital capacity, diffusing capacity, lung compliance and closing volume in subjects with radiographically supported diagnosis of mild HAPE. Within the limits of these techniques, the findings supported the contention that extravascular lung water does not routinely accumulate in healthy people ascending to altitude, but in HAPE the findings are consistent with what physiologic changes would occur with some pulmonary edema. The study was not intended to test the hypothesis that HAPE-S individuals have smaller lung volumes.

VENTILATION

Susceptible subjects have characteristics which appear to accentuate the effects of hypoxia on acute ascent to high altitude. For instance, the primary defense against hypoxemia is the hypoxic ventilatory response (HVR). Several studies have demonstrated that HAPE-S subjects have relatively blunted HVR responses (Hyers *et al.* 1979; Hackett *et al.* 1988; Matsuzawa *et al.* 1989; Selland *et al.* 1993; Schirlo *et al.* 2002). A more blunted HVR results in greater alveolar hypoxia, the effect of which can be especially strong in individuals with brisk HPVR. One case study of a man with Holmes-Adie syndrome and HAPE

exists. The syndrome is a neurologic disorder, characterized by a markedly blunted ventilatory response to hypoxia. This patient developed profound hypoxemia with modest exercise at 2100 m and the development of HAPE, suggesting that defense of arterial oxygenation is an important factor in minimizing the development of HAPE (Richalet *et al.* 2011).

PULMONARY HEMODYNAMICS

As mentioned previously (section 21.2.7), susceptible subjects have a greater HPVR than control subjects who had been to altitude previously without problems (Hultgren *et al.* 1971; Vachiery *et al.* 1995; Eldridge *et al.* 1996; Scherrer *et al.* 1996). Hohenhaus *et al.* (1995) studied both the pulmonary pressor and hypoxic ventilatory responses in HAPE-susceptible subjects and concluded that they had lower HPVR than controls, but not significantly different from subjects who had simple AMS. The latter had a wide range of HPVR. Some HAPE-susceptible subjects had very brisk pressor responses, but not all subjects could be separated from controls by this test. Mounier *et al.* (2011) studied estimated systolic pulmonary artery systolic pressure (PASP) with echocardiography in eight HAPE-resistant (R) and eight HAPE-susceptible (S) subjects during mild exercise and hypoxia. They found that there was no overlap in systolic PASP in the HAPE-R (range 6.7–18.5 mmHg) and HAPE-S subjects (range 19.2–30.4 mmHg) which provides further strongly suggestive evidence that HAPE-S individuals have an inherent or acquired characteristic of accentuated pulmonary vascular response to hypoxia.

PULMONARY VASOACTIVE MEDIATORS

An imbalance of vasoactive mediators may be responsible for an accentuated HPVR (Dehnert *et al.* 2007), and there may be genetic predisposition to such disarray. An increased concentration of thromboxane B_2 was found in bronchoalveolar lavage fluid of HAPE victims compared to controls (Schoene *et al.* 1986; Schoene *et al.* 1988), but more recently attention has shifted to the opposing influences of nitrous oxide (NO), an endothelial-derived molecule that is a potent pulmonary vasodilator, and endothelin-1 (ET-1), a potent pulmonary vasoconstrictor. During the development of edema in HAPE-S at 4559 m, exhaled NO was 30% lower than in control subjects which also showed an inverse relationship with pulmonary artery pressure (PAP) (Fig. 21.4a) (Duplain *et al.* 2000). It was hypothesized that a defect in NO synthesis predisposed HAPE-S individuals to accentuated PAP and thus HAPE. A subsequent study (Fig. 20.4b) (Busch *et al.* 2001) noted that when HAPE-S subjects were exposed to 2 hours of acute hypoxia, exhalation of NO decreased, whereas control subjects had no change in NO exhalation. These findings also correlated with an increase in PAP as NO fell. Hypoxia per se may induce systemic endothelial dysfunction in HAPE-S subjects compared to controls (Berger *et al.* 2005). This response is not isolated to the pulmonary vasculature and results in decreased NO production which correlated with an increase in PAP in this study. HAPE-S subjects have also been found to have impaired release of NO when exposed to hypoxia (Berger *et al.* 2005).

Bailey *et al.* (2010) studied the transpulmonary concentrations of free radicals as markers upon ascent, as well as bioactive metabolites of NO in 26 mountaineers before and after ascending to 4559 m. Subjects were also evaluated for clinical HAPE and AMS. All subjects had an increase in free radicals and decrease in NO metabolites, but this difference was much more pronounced in the three subjects with HAPE. The findings suggest that part of the decrease in the vasodilatation of the pulmonary vasculature caused by NO is attenuated by the presence of free radicals which is more pronounced in HAPE.

Endothelin-1 is a potent vasoconstrictor, and plasma levels were found to be 33% higher in HAPE-S subjects compared to controls at 4559 m (Sartori *et al.* 1999b). PAP values were higher in HAPE-S subjects, and these levels correlated with the increase in ET-1. It is not clear though whether these higher values are secondary to increased ET-1 production or decreased clearance. Berger *et al.* (2008) studied transpulmonary ET-1 levels and calculated echocardiographic determinations of PASP in 34 subjects ascending to 4559 m. An increase in ET-1 and decrease in nitrites across the pulmonary vasculature correlated with a rise in PASP. The findings suggest opposing influences of NO and ET-1 on pulmonary vascular tone, but do not clarify the mechanism responsible for this balance.

Inherent sympathetic activity may play an important role in HAPE-susceptibility. Duplain

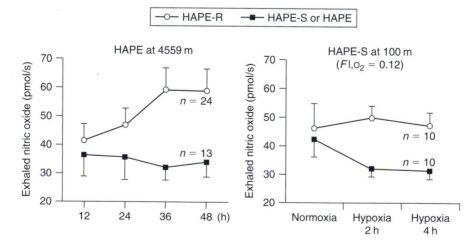

Figure 21.4   *Left*: exhaled nitric oxide (NO) after 40 h at 4559 m in individuals developing high altitude pulmonary edema (HAPE) and in individuals not developing HAPE (HAPE-R) despite identical exposure to high altitude (Duplain *et al.* 2000). *Right*: exhaled NO in HAPE-susceptible subjects (HAPE-S) and HAPE-R individuals after 4 h of exposure to hypoxia ($Fl,o_2 = 0.12$) at low altitude (elevation 100 m) (Busch *et al.* 2001). *n*, No. of subjects.

et al. (1999a) measured sympathetic activity directly from postganglionic nerve discharge in HAPE-susceptible subjects in response to a short hypoxic test. They found at both high and low altitude that the test subjects had two to three times the response compared with controls suggesting that sympathetic over-activation may be a part of the susceptibility. Berger *et al.* (2011) measured transpulmonary catecholamines in 34 mountaineers after 20 hours at 4559 m and looked at the rise in PASP. Both exercise and high altitude increased PASP, but there was no difference in the transpulmonary concentrations in catecholamines nor was there any correlation between those levels and PASP. Thus, the direct role of catecholamines in the pulmonary vascular response remains unlikely.

ALVEOLAR FLUID CLEARANCE

Most of the early studies of HAPE focused on leak from the microvasculature, but fluid flux in the lung also involves clearance of fluid from the alveolar and interstitial spaces to the lymphatic drainage. This process of active water and sodium transport across the alveolar epithelial cells is mediated by a Na^+–K^+-ATPase pump which is inhibited by hypoxia (Fig. 21.5) (Planes *et al.* 1997; Pham *et al.* 2002). It was hypothesized that individuals with impaired alveolar fluid clearance (AFC) would be HAPE-susceptible.

Similar sodium and water transport mechanisms exist in the nasal epithelium and are thought to be reflective of the alveolar epithelium (Mairbaurl *et al.* 2003; Sartori *et al.* 2004). Scherrer and colleagues (1996) have reinforced the proposition that pulmonary hypertension by itself does not cause pulmonary edema (section 20.7.3 and Sartori *et al.* 1999b). However, in transgenic mice with disruption of the gene for the α subunit of the amiloride-sensitive epithelial sodium channel, hypoxia did induce pulmonary edema. The same group has found a similar defect in epithelial ion transport in HAPE-susceptible human subjects (Lepori *et al.* 1999).

Taking advantage of the fact that one of the effects of beta-2 receptor agonists is to facilitate AFC, Sartori *et al.* (2002) used high doses of inhaled salmeterol in 37 HAPE-susceptible climbers

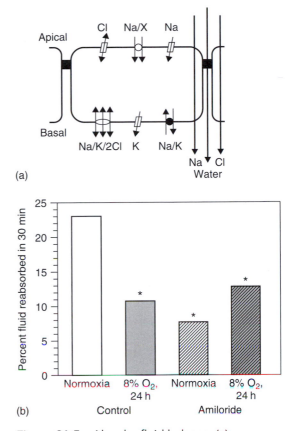

(a)

(b)

Figure 21.5   Alveolar fluid balance. (a) Removal of alveolar fluid is driven by the active reabsorption of Na^+ that enters the cell via Na channels and Na-coupled transport (Na/X) and is extruded by Na^+–K^+-ATPases. Thus, active Na reabsorption generates the osmotic gradient for the reabsorption of water. (b) Hypoxia inhibits the reabsorption of fluid instilled into lungs of hypoxia-exposed rats, which is fully explained by inhibition of amiloride-sensitive pathways (mostly Na channels). *$p < 0.05$ vs. control values in normoxia. Modified from Vivona *et al.* (2001).

taken to 4559 m and reduced the incidence of HAPE by 50%. Compared to controls, the HAPE-S subjects also had trans-nasal epithelial sodium transport that was 30% lower than non-HAPE controls. Beta-agonists lower PAP and decrease inflammation so that beneficial effect in decreasing HAPE may not be totally attributable to the facilitation of AFC. Mason *et al.* (2003) tracked the association of AFC by use of nasal transmembrane potentials and lung volumes (vital capacity) before, during and after an ascent to 3800 m. The findings suggested that an altered respiratory epithelial transport may play a role in the accumulation of extravascular water.

ET-1 may play more than just a vasoconstrictive role in the pulmonary vasculature. Berger et al. (2009) used isolated, ventilated, constant pressure perfused rat lung to assess the role of ET-1 in AFC and fluid balance. AFC was measured in lungs instilled with 5% albumin solution with and without ET-1. Hemodynamic and fluid flux was measured. In the fluid-instilled lungs with ET-1, AFC was reduced by 65% resulting in a net accumulation of 20% of fluid with increased pulmonary capillary pressures and greater lung water weight. This effect was blocked by use of an ET-1 B-receptor antagonist. These results suggest that in humans experiencing a greater increase in ET-1 upon ascent to high altitude, i.e. HAPE-S individuals, there is an accentuated effect on lung edema formation by a decrease in AFC.

GENETIC MARKERS

With an increasing array of genetic markers at the disposal of investigators, HAPE has come within the sights of researchers who are studying genes and disease states. A number of candidate genes have been investigated with some preliminary findings that are promising. Hanoka et al. (1998) found an association of certain HLA complexes (HLA-DR6 and HLA-DQ4) in patients with a history of HAPE. Hypothetically, there could be an association of angiotensin converting enzyme (ACE) insertion/deletion (I/D) gene polymorphism and vasoconstriction and fluid retention and thus potentially related to HAPE susceptibility. Morrell et al. (1999) reported that Kyrghyz highlanders with pulmonary hypertension had a high incidence of the D allele of the ACE gene compared with subjects suspected but found not to have pulmonary hypertension, but two more recent studies in a large number of subjects at altitudes from 3000 to 4559 m (Dehnert et al. 2002; Kumar et al. 2004) demonstrated no relationship between ACE I/D gene polymorphisms and HAPE. In 49 HAPE-susceptible and 55 healthy climbers, Hotta et al.

(2004) also found no relationship between ACE-I/D genes and HAPE susceptibility, but in a subset of HAPE subjects the D allele of the ACE-I/D polymorphism was associated with pulmonary vascular hyper-responsiveness in patients who were catheterized and challenged with hypoxia. A meta-analysis of 305 HAPE cases and 662 controls found no difference in ACE D and I alleles between the two groups and thus concluded that the ACE D or I gene was not associated with HAPE-susceptibility (Qi et al. 2011). In a study of 140 HAPE patients compared with 144 controls from workers on the construction of the Qinghai–Tibet railroad, the ACE gene and its polymorphisms were studied with other candidate genes. The conclusions suggested that this gene may play a synergistic role in predisposition to HAPE.

As mentioned earlier, an impairment of NO synthesis can lead to less pulmonary vasodilatation with hypoxic stress which may be a permissive factor in the development of HAPE. Gene polymorphisms for endothelial-derived NO synthase (e-NOS) were studied in HAPE-susceptible subjects, and two variants of the e-NOS gene were present in 25.6 and 23.2% versus 9.8 and 6.9% in HAPE-S versus controls. These results suggest a genetic etiology to e-NOS-related pulmonary vascular reactivity and HAPE susceptibility. Lorenzo et al. (2009) studied three generations in a family who had developed HAPE. They did entire gene arrays and did in fact not find that this family had similarities in the e-NOS gene, but did find consistency in the HIF-2A haplotype in those who developed HAPE in this family. The story may be much more complex than just looking at the e-NOS gene. Complex interactions of the gene polymorphisms may be responsible as suggested by the work of Sun et al. (2010) where they found just two haplotypes to have strong association in their population of HAPE-susceptible subjects.

In another line of genetic investigation, Saxena et al. (2005) studied polymorphisms of the pulmonary surfactant protein A1 and A2 genes (SP-A1 and SP-A2). SP-A is a potent anti-oxidant which protects against inflammatory reactions and oxidative damage and thus lung injury. The polymorphisms have been associated with respiratory distress syndrome, chronic obstructive pulmonary disease, and pulmonary infection. In this study, HAPE subjects homozygous for SP-A1 and SP-A2 had a higher degree of oxidative damage. HAPE subjects heterozygous for the polymorphisms had a lower degree of oxidative damage, while control subjects without a history of HAPE and no gene polymorphisms had little to no oxidative damage. Further investigation along these lines was carried out by Ahmad *et al.* (2011). They found upregulation of apolipoprotein A-1 and haptoglobin which quickly suppress inflammation. These markers were thought to come to play early in the development of HAPE before other anti-inflammatory mechanisms can evolve. The discussion of the role of inflammation in HAPE is discussed more completely in section 21.6.9. Other gene polymorphisms of the Hsp70 family which help to mediate perfusion and reperfusion injury in vascular beds have also been studied in HAPE patients (Qi *et al.* 2009). There was a high correlation of one of these genes especially which suggest that allowance of reperfusion injury may play a role in HAPE-susceptible individuals. Vascular endothelial growth factor (VEGF) has long been touted as playing a role in the vascular permeability of HAPE, but earlier investigations have been inconclusive. Hanaoka *et al.* (2008) looked at gene polymorphisms of VEGF in HAPE-susceptible subjects compared to controls and found no difference in frequency of variants of the VEGF gene.

These studies are just the beginning of what will become a plethora of genetic studies in the future which will further unravel the fascinating and clearly complex mechanism of HAPE.

21.2.10 Summary of HAPE susceptibility

A number of physiologic, cellular and genetic markers have provided investigators with important insight into the underlying mechanisms of HAPE:

- Smaller lung volumes and presumed vascular bed
- Blunted ventilatory responses to hypoxia
- Accentuated hypoxic pulmonary vasoconstriction
- Imbalance of vasoactive mediators that enhance (endothelin-1) and relax hypoxic pulmonary vascular tone
- Impaired transalveolar epithelial sodium and water clearance
- Gene polymorphisms which mediate *e-NOS*, *ACE* and surfactant.

21.3 PREVENTION AND TREATMENT

21.3.1 Field reports

Anecdotes and case reports convey a strong impression that HAPE victims are over-treated with every known proven and hypothetical remedy available. It is not uncommon to hear that HAPE patients in the field with reasonable access to descent get oxygen, if available, the Gamow bag, nifedipine, sildenafil, acetazolamide, lasix, and dexamethasone, all at the same time. Because of the relatively low incidence of HAPE, it has been difficult to do a comparative treatment study, but some guidelines are available that give rational approaches to situation-specific cases such that patients are well treated and not over-treated at the risk of dangerous side effects (Luks *et al.* 2008; Luks *et al.* 2010).

21.3.2 Slow ascent

It is thought that HAPE occurs in individuals who have not yet acclimatized with special disposition in those who have characteristics which make them susceptible. It can occur in individuals with AMS; therefore, if a sufficiently slow ascent is undertaken both AMS and HAPE may be avoided (section 19.6.1). However, because of the rush of modern-day life, people often ascend at a rate that puts them at risk of AMS and HAPE.

21.3.3 Exercise

Many case histories from Houston (1960) onwards emphasize the point that patients have been very energetic while getting to high altitude or on arrival there. Ravenhill (1913) was of the opinion that physical exertion rendered a man more susceptible to AMS in general. The Indian Army, with great experience of HAPE since the war with China in the Himalayas in 1962, advises all inductees to altitude to take no unnecessary exertion for the first 72 h. Exercise, by increasing cardiac output, raises the pulmonary artery pressure, especially in subjects susceptible to HAPE, and it is believed that the higher the pulmonary artery pressure, the greater the risk of HAPE. In healthy subjects at altitude, Eldridge et al. (1998) have shown that strenuous exercise results in the appearance of red blood cells (RBC), white blood cells (WBC) and gamma/delta T cells in the lavage fluid. The latter cells indicate damage to the endothelium and play a role in inflammation. Anholm et al. (1999) found radiographic evidence of pulmonary edema in a group of cyclists at the end of a run at modest altitude. However, HAPE can occur in the absence of hard physical exertion; 66 of Menon's 101 cases had taken no exercise more strenuous than office work, traveling as passengers in a truck or walking about on level ground (Menon 1965). Nevertheless, the anecdotal evidence is strong enough to advise people who have to make a rapid ascent to altitude to avoid hard physical exertion for 2 days or more.

21.3.4 Drugs

Some of the emerging suggestions for therapy to prevent HAPE have evolved from important physiologic observations which, as mentioned previously, are associated with susceptibility to HAPE. This section will address a number of pharmacologic interventions which are potentially effective for both prevention and treatment.

ACETAZOLAMIDE

Acetazolamide (section 19.6.2), by preventing or at least reducing AMS, probably also reduces the risk of HAPE, but no studies have directly addressed this issue. On the other hand, acetazolamide, not by carbonic anhydrase inhibition or NO release, has been shown to reduce HPVR (Höhne et al. 2004; Höhne et al. 2006; Swenson 2006) and may

by its effect on calcium channels reduce HPVR and subsequent susceptibility to HAPE.

CALCIUM CHANNEL BLOCKERS

Oelz et al. (1989) showed that nifedipine was of value in the treatment of HAPE. Six subjects with clinical physiological and radiographic evidence of HAPE were treated with 10 mg of nifedipine sublingually and 20 mg slow release orally every 6 h thereafter. Despite continued exercise at 4559 m, this treatment without oxygen resulted in clinical improvement, better oxygenation, reduced $(A-a)P_{O_2}$ gradient and pulmonary artery pressure, and clearing of alveolar edema. The sublingual preparation is very rapidly absorbed and occasionally results in systemic hypotension. Therefore most physicians now do not use it.

Bartsch et al. (1991) took advantage of the strong relationship between an accentuated HPVR and HAPE, used a calcium-channel blocker, nifedipine, in a group of HAPE-susceptible individuals in a controlled trial upon ascent to the Margherita hut at 4559 m and essentially prevented HAPE while also mitigating the expected rise in PAP in these subjects.

NITRIC OXIDE

NO produced by endothelial cells is a naturally occurring potent vasodilator. It was first used in the treatment of HAPE by Scherrer et al. (1996) who took 18 HAPE-susceptible subjects to 4559 m. Their pulmonary artery pressures were higher and $Pa_{,O_2}$ lower than control, non-susceptible subjects. NO lowered their PAP and raised their $Pa_{,O_2}$ whereas in control subjects $Pa_{,O_2}$ fell. The latter was thought to be due to increasing V/Q mismatching. In HAPE subjects, NO goes preferentially to ventilated, non-edematous areas dilating the vessels there. This shifts blood flow from edematous to non-edematous areas with improvement in V/Q matching. The beneficial effects of NO were confirmed by Anand et al. (1998) in 14 patients with established HAPE. They compared NO treatment with 50% O_2 and NO plus O_2 50%. Both NO and O_2 were effective in reducing PAP and improving $Pa_{,O_2}$ but the combination had an additive effect. Omura et al. (2000) exposed rats to normobaric hypoxia ($FI,O_2 = 0.10$) with one group on 83 ppm NO and the other controls. Mortality was reduced from 39.5 to 6.2% on NO with heavier lung weight in the controls, suggesting that NO was beneficial in minimizing pulmonary edema in this rat model of HAPE. These studies are of great interest in understanding the mechanisms of HAPE, but NO is not suitable for use in the field, and if the patient reaches a hospital, the descent, calcium channel blockers and oxygen are almost always effective in relieving the condition.

PHOSPHODIESTERASE-5 INHIBITION

Other interventions may affect e-NOS which result in pulmonary vasodilatation. There has been recent interest in phosphodiesterase-5 (PDE-5) inhibitors (sildenafil, tadalafil) which inhibit cGMP in the lungs, lower PAP and increase exercise performance at high altitude (Ghofrani et al. 2004; Richalet et al. 2005a) and prevent HAPE (Maggiorini 2006). Of note though was the comparative study by Fischler et al. (2009) of tadalafil and dexamethasone and placebo (see below). Although tadalafil did increase $VO_{2,max}$ and decrease echocardiographic calculations of pulmonary artery pressure, it was not as effective as the steroid. Bates et al. (2011) used placebo and sildenafil over 5 days at 5200 m altitude in Bolivia and found no difference in pulmonary artery pressures by echocardiographic calculation but did show higher scores of AMS with sildenafil. Whether this latter finding was merely a side effect of the drug itself rather than AMS is not clear. The utility of PDE-5 inhibitors in altitude illness and performance remains unclear.

GLUCOCORTICOIDS

Maggiorini et al. (2006) also noted that high-dose dexamethasone prevented the increase in PAP as much as tadalafil which initially seemed surprising. Dexamethasone may promote e-NOS synthase by inhibiting hypoxia-induced endothelial dysfunction (Murata et al. 2004), which would have some of the same salutary effects as other vasodilators in preventing HAPE. Other effects of glucocorticoids, however, make dissecting this beneficial mechanism difficult. For instance, dexamethasone increases the $Na^+–K^+–$ATPase pump at the epithelial layer (Noda et al. 2003), and pulmonary vascular permeability was reduced in rats treated with hypoxia (Stelzner et al. 1988).

Although the mechanism behind their findings is not clear, Fischler et al. (2009) compared dexamethasone with placebo and tadalafil in subjects after ascent to 4559 m. Maximum oxygen uptake was highest, VE/VCO_2 the lowest, and echocardiographic estimates of pulmonary artery pressure the lowest in the subjects on dexamethasone at 8 mg twice a day. In a subsequent study at the same site, 24 HAPE-susceptible subjects were exercised first at low altitude and then at 4559 m. Subjects were divided into placebo and dexamethasone groups (Siebenmann et al. 2011). The HAPE-susceptible subjects had a higher $VO_{2,max}$ and a higher oxygen pulse (VO_2/heart rate, an indirect measure of cardiac stroke volume). Of note was that the SpO_2 at maximum exercise was not different between the groups, but the resting SpO_2 was higher in the dexamethasone group.

OTHER VASODILATORS

Hackett et al. (1992) have shown that several vasodilators are beneficial in HAPE as indicated by a reduction in pulmonary artery pressure, pulmonary vascular resistance and improved gas exchange (Fig. 21.6). Nifedipine and hydralazine were of equal benefit but rather less effective than oxygen. Phentolamine, an alpha-blocker, was more effective than oxygen and, when combined with oxygen, was even more effective.

Of interest is the finding that ET-1 blockers do not have the beneficial effect that would be expected (Modesti et al. 2006; Faoro et al. 2009; Scheult et al. 2009) based on the hypothesis that ET-1 plays a role in increasing PASP in HAPE-susceptible subjects. Thus, blocking ET-1 receptors should result in lowering pulmonary vascular resistance (PVR) and the propensity of individuals to have microvascular leak. Perhaps some fluid-retaining characteristics of some of the ET-1 blockers may mitigate the vasoactive effect.

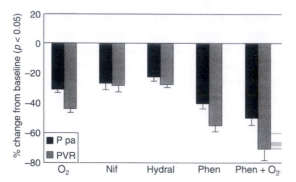

Figure 21.6 Percentage change in mean pulmonary artery pressure (Ppa) and pulmonary vascular resistance (PVR) with five different interventions in subjects with high altitude pulmonary edema (HAPE). Nif, nifedipine; hydral, hydralazine; phen, phentolamine (reproduced with permission from Hackett *et al.* 1992).

21.3.5 Field treatment

In mild to moderate cases of HAPE in an environment where medical help is available, e.g. a ski resort, and when Sa,O_2 can be improved to greater than 90% on low-flow oxygen, patients can be treated with oxygen and close observation without going down unless the clinical situation worsens (Zafren *et al.* 1996). In other situations when the patient is more severely ill and where medical care is not available, the single most important maneuver in treating HAPE is to get the patient down as fast and as far as possible. Even a descent of as little as 300 m may improve a patient's condition dramatically (report of case 2, in section 20.2). However, there are often unavoidable delays while awaiting evacuation and there are a number of therapeutic possibilities.

OXYGEN

Breathing air enriched with oxygen, if available, is an obvious and invaluable treatment. It relieves hypoxia and reduces pulmonary artery pressure (section 20.2.6), but, while most patients benefit, in some, the relief is only partial, and in a few, deterioration may continue. The dosage of oxygen is usually dictated by its supply. If there is sufficient availability, a flow of 6–10 L min⁻¹ is indicated for the first few hours, reducing to 2–4 L min⁻¹ when there is improvement.

DIURETICS

Since the patient has edema, diuretics have been used in the treatment of HAPE (Singh *et al.* 1965); however, since subjects at high altitude are often volume depleted to begin with, any presumed benefit of diuretics is outweighed by the risk of further volume depletion and the dangers in the field setting thereof.

ANTIBIOTICS

Many cases of HAPE have mild fever and leukocytosis suggesting that infection may play a part; however, there has never been any evidence that pneumonia initiates or perpetuates HAPE. Menon (1965) discontinued the use of antibiotics in his last 44 cases of HAPE with no apparent disadvantage to the outcome. Unless there is evidence of a concurrent infection, antibiotics should not be used in HAPE.

OTHER DRUGS

Digoxin has been used in cases of HAPE in its early clinical history. Menon (1965) observed the effect of an intravenous dose of 0.5–1.5 mg in 66 patients and claimed that the response was uniformly good within a few hours, even in patients given only 1 L min⁻¹ of added oxygen. However, there was no evidence of myocardial failure nor was there atrial fibrillation, the current indications for digoxin therapy, and its use is no longer advised.

Morphine (15–30 mg i.v.) has been used, again with the clinical impression that this resulted in a reduction in pulmonary edema. As it does in acute left ventricular failure, it also makes the patient more comfortable, possibly by causing peripheral vasodilatation and a decrease in preload on the right ventricle and thus a shift of blood from central to peripheral circulations. However, its respiratory depressant effects should make for caution in its use, especially in the field setting.

EXPIRATORY POSITIVE AIRWAYS PRESSURE

Feldman and Herndon (1977) suggested that expiratory positive airways pressure might be beneficial in HAPE by analogy with its use in other forms of pulmonary edema. They proposed a simple device in which the subject exhaled through an underwater tube to achieve the desired positive pressure, while inspiration was direct from atmosphere.

Schoene *et al.* (1985) used a commercial expiratory positive pressure mask on four patients with HAPE on Mount McKinley. They showed that, using the mask, arterial saturation was increased with increasing positive pressure (up to 10 cm water). There was a concomitant rise in P_{CO_2}, but not of heart rate. The intrathoracic pressure would be negative during inspiration so the cardiac output would probably not be reduced.

PORTABLE HYPERBARIC CHAMBER: THE GAMOW OR CERTEC BAGS

A lightweight rubberized canvas bag has been developed into which a patient can be placed and sealed in the bag which can be pressurized using a foot pump. There is a pressure relief valve set to 2 psi. This pressure gives the equivalent altitude reduction of almost 2000 m from a typical base camp altitude of 4000–5000 m. There are currently two commercially available bags: the Gamow from the United States and Certec from France. There have been numerous accounts of their use in HAPE and HACE, with good results (Robertson and Shlim 1991). One report draws attention to the considerable placebo effect of the procedure. Roach and Hackett (1992) have reviewed the efficacy of hyperbaric treatment. They conclude that both oxygen and hyperbaria are effective. There may be a rebound effect some hours after treatment (typically 1–2 h duration). A recent controlled trial in benign AMS has shown that 1 h in the bag at pressure (193 mbar) was significantly more effective in reducing symptoms than control (1 h at the trivial pressure of 20 mbar) (Bärtsch *et al.* 1993). The effort of maintaining the necessary pumping for even 1 h is considerable, especially at altitude where the number of rescuers might be limited. Duff (1999b), reporting a case, makes the useful point that some patients with severe HAPE or HACE may be orthopneic when made to lie flat in a compression bag and in their confused state may become belligerent. Their condition may be confused with claustrophobia. The solution is to position the bag at a 30° head-up angle.

21.3.6 Summary of prevention and treatment

Prevention of HAPE should be undertaken in individuals with a previous history of HAPE, especially if they are undergoing an unavoidably rapid ascent. These measures are:

- Encourage slow ascent, if at all possible, to allow for acclimatization.
- Use of nifedipine or other pulmonary vasodilators (PDE-5 inhibitors, maybe acetazolamide or dexamethasone) if rapid ascent is unavoidable, especially in HAPE-S subjects.
- Use of drugs which increase alveolar fluid clearance (inhaled beta-agonists, dexamethasone) upon ascent.

The treatment of HAPE should consist of:

- Mild to moderate HAPE patients where medical help is available can be treated with oxygen and observation unless the clinical situation deteriorates.
- With more severe HAPE or in areas where medical help is not available, getting the patient down in altitude as fast and as low as possible is the most prudent approach.
- While awaiting evacuation, or if evacuation is not possible, give oxygen or hyperbaria. Nifedipine 20 mg slow release should be given and a broad-spectrum antibiotic should be considered. Sildenafil or tadalafil may also be beneficial.
- The use of expiratory positive airway pressure, with a respiratory valve device, or failing that, by pursed lips breathing, will give some temporary improvement.

21.4 OUTCOME

In fully established cases, where evacuation to lower altitude is impossible and no intervention is undertaken, death within a few hours is usual. If cases are recognized early and taken down, patients usually recover completely in 1 or 2 days, but occasionally they continue to deteriorate and die even after being brought down to lower altitude, especially if there are symptoms of cerebral edema (Dickinson *et al.* 1983). Only one case has been reported as progressing to adult respiratory distress syndrome (Zimmerman and Crapo 1980). The remarkable characteristic of HAPE is the usual rapid resolution of the condition upon descent which distinguishes its underlying pathophysiology from other types of pulmonary edema. In other words, the stress failure of the endothelial lining is quickly reversed with removal of the hypoxic stress. Usually, the pulmonary hypertension decreases rapidly on going to low altitude and the inverted T waves on the ECG return to normal (Fig. 3 in Singh *et al.* 1965). However, Menon (1965) mentions two soldiers (out of 101 cases) who, having recovered from HAPE, had to be evacuated later because of breathlessness, precordial pain and inverted T waves in their EGC, and Fiorenzano *et al.* (1997) reported one case with prolonged T-wave inversion in the precordial leads suggesting prolonged pulmonary hypertension. Even patients who have apparently fully recovered have been shown to have significant hypoxemia and widened $(A-a)P_{O_2}$ gradients for up to 12 weeks (Guleria *et al.* 1969). However, after recovery at lower altitudes, many climbers have returned within a few days to climb their peaks without further trouble (Schoene *et al.* 1986; Schoene *et al.* 1988).

21.5 PATHOLOGY

21.5.1 Post-mortem examination

There have been a number of post-mortem studies which have shown a similar pathology in the heart and lungs (Hultgren *et al.* 1962; Arias-Stella and Kruger 1963; Marticorena *et al.* 1964; Nayak *et al.* 1964; Singh *et al.* 1965; Dickinson *et al.* 1983; Hultgren *et al.* 1997). The lungs are heavy and feel solid. The cut surface weeps edema fluid, usually blood stained, but a striking feature is the non-uniform nature of the edema. Areas of hemorrhagic edema alternate with clear edema and with areas which are virtually normal (or over-inflated). Pulmonary arterial thrombi are commonly found.

On microscopy, alveoli are filled with fluid containing red blood cells, polymorphs and macrophages, though not in great numbers. Hyaline membranes are found in the alveoli, identical with those seen in respiratory distress syndrome of the newborn. The pulmonary capillaries are congested with small arteries and veins containing thrombi and fibrin clot. Perivascular edema and hemorrhage are found. In post-mortem studies of high altitude natives from South America, the pulmonary arteries are very muscular and the right ventricle is hypertrophied. In lowlanders, the pulmonary vessels have normal musculature (Dickinson *et al.* 1983).

21.5.2 The edema fluid

The hyaline membranes are probably formed by coalescence of proteins, suggesting a high protein edema. It has been shown in life that the edema fluid is rich in protein. Hackett *et al.* (1986) sampled pure edema fluid by bronchoscopy in one case and showed it to have a plasma/fluid ratio of 0.8:1.1 for total protein. Schoene *et al.* (1986) took bronchoalveolar lavage fluid from three cases of HAPE and compared it with lavage fluid from three controls at the same altitude (4400 m). The fluid from patients was rich in high molecular weight protein, red blood cells and macrophages. These findings suggest a 'large pore' leak type of edema. In further studies, the same group (Schoene *et al.* 1988) also found that the fluid was rich in alveolar macrophages and a high concentration of high molecular weight proteins. There was evidence of activation of complement (C5a) and release of thromboxane B_2 and leukotriene B_4. Tsukimoto *et al.* (1994) also showed under tightly controlled laboratory conditions in the rat, that elevation of the capillary pressure alone resulted in the appearance of leukotriene B_4 in the bronchoalveolar lavage (BAL) fluid. A Japanese group (Kubo *et al.* 1998) carried out BAL in seven patients with early HAPE and found increased cell counts of macrophages, lymphocytes and neutrophils plus markedly elevated concentrations of proteins, lactate dehydrogenase, IL-1β, IL-6, IL-8, and TNFα. IL-6 and TNFα were shown to correlate with the Pa,O_2 and pulmonary artery driving pressure ($P_{PA} - P_{wedge}$). Swenson *et al.* (2002) carried out BAL in HAPE-S subjects as soon as they arrived at the Margherita hut and developed signs of HAPE. The BAL fluid showed a high protein concentration but no signs of inflammation. This important study determined that an inflammatory response does not play a role in the initiation of HAPE.

21.6 PATHOGENESIS OF HAPE

There is evidence suggesting that a degree of subclinical pulmonary edema is common during the second and third days at altitude. There is a reduction in vital capacity, a shift of the pressure/volume curve of the lung (Mansell *et al.* 1980; Gautier *et al.* 1982), and an increase in alveolar arterial oxygen difference (Sutton *et al.* 1976). This might simply be part of a generalized increase in extracellular fluid volume which shows itself as subcutaneous edema in the face on rising in the morning and in the ankles later in the day. In the skull, the same edema raises the intracellular pressure and may give rise to the symptoms of AMS, but the progression from this mild edema to clinical pulmonary edema requires a further mechanism or mechanisms.

21.6.1 Facts that require explanation

Any hypothesis that seeks to explain the mechanism of HAPE must take into account the following facts:

- The edema is of the high protein type
- The patchy distribution of the edema seen on post-mortem and radiology (Fig. 21.1)

- The very high pulmonary artery pressure and normal wedge (and left atrial) pressures (Table 21.2); the improvement which follows treatment with different drugs which reduce the pulmonary artery pressure indicates the importance of this factor in the mechanism of HAPE
- The presence of vascular thrombi and fibrin clots in pulmonary vessels (section 21.4.1)
- The individual susceptibility which is associated with an increased hypoxic pulmonary pressor response (Hultgren *et al.* 1971) and response to exercise (Kawashima *et al.* 1989)
- The increased risk of HAPE with exercise on arrival at altitude.

21.6.2 Left ventricular failure

Although HAPE resembles left ventricular failure (LVF) clinically, which is why Ravenhill (1913) called it *puna* of the cardiac type, it is not now thought to be due to left ventricular failure per se. Most catheter studies have shown normal wedge pressures and the edema fluid is of the high protein permeability type. On the other hand, Maggiorini *et al.* (2001) found elevated pulmonary capillary wedge pressures, consistent with pulmonary venoconstriction, but the chest radiograph and pathology are not typical of LVF.

21.6.3 Pulmonary hypertension

The extraordinarily high pulmonary artery pressure found in HAPE must play a role in the mechanism of the condition (Dehnert *et al.* 2007). High pulmonary artery pressure by itself does not cause edema, as for instance in primary pulmonary hypertension, or in a group of men studied by Sartori and colleagues (1999b). These individuals had suffered a period of hypoxia in the neonatal period and as a result had exaggerated pulmonary hypoxic pressor responses. When taken up to high altitude, they had high PAP, but did not develop HAPE. This is perhaps not surprising since the resistance vessels, the arterioles, are upstream of capillaries and therefore capillary pressure should be normal. One must therefore postulate some further mechanism as well as, but related to, the pulmonary hypertension. The following have been proposed.

21.6.4 Uneven pulmonary vasoconstriction and perfusion

Hultgren (1969) suggested that the edema is caused by a very powerful, but uneven, vasoconstriction so that there is reduced blood flow in some parts of the lung and torrential blood flow in others. He showed (Hultgren et al. 1966) that if one progressively ties off more and more of the pulmonary arterial tree in a dog, thus forcing the total cardiac output through only a portion of the lung, pulmonary edema results in that part of the lung that remains perfused.

A case report by Dombret et al. (1987) provides confirmation in humans of Hultgren's experimental findings. The reported patient had a massive pulmonary embolus resulting in perfusion being reduced to only the left upper and middle lobes. She developed symptoms and signs of pulmonary edema, which on radiograph were shown to be confined to those same perfused lobes.

Evidence in favor of this mechanism as being the cause of HAPE is provided by Viswanathan et al. (1979) who, at sea level, studied 12 subjects who had recovered from HAPE. They showed that, on being given 10% oxygen to breathe, they had a greater pulmonary pressor response than controls and on lung scanning their perfusion was more uneven.

This hypothesis accounts well for the patchy distribution of the condition. High flow through less severely constricted areas might well produce edema by capillary stress failure (section 21.6.5). Added support for this hypothesis came from a paper by Hackett et al. (1980), who collected four cases of HAPE occurring at very modest altitudes (2000–3000 m) in subjects who had a congenital absence of the right pulmonary artery. The edema developed in the left lung, which received the total cardiac output. That four cases of HAPE developed in such an uncommon condition (only 50 cases have been described in the world literature) strongly suggests a causative

rather than a coincidental association. Pulmonary blood flow was redistributed in rats when exposed to severe hypoxia (Kuwahira et al. 2001), while Hanaoka et al. (2000) demonstrated a more marked cephalad distribution of blood flow in HAPE-susceptible subjects when exposed to hypoxia. Using magnetic resonance imaging in HAPE-susceptible subjects and controls, Hopkins et al. (2005) found marked heterogeneity of blood flow in the HAPE-susceptible subjects when exposed to hypoxia.

21.6.5 Stress failure of pulmonary capillaries

It has been proposed that HAPE is caused by damage to the walls of pulmonary capillaries as a result of high wall stresses associated with increased capillary transmural pressure (West et al. 1991; West and Mathieu-Costello 1992a). These high capillary pressures are the result of uneven hypoxic pulmonary vasoconstriction as originally proposed by Hultgren (1969). Extensive laboratory studies have now shown that raising capillary transmural pressure causes ultrastructural damage to the capillary walls, including disruption of the capillary endothelial layer, alveolar epithelial layer, and sometimes, all layers of the wall (Tsukimoto et al. 1991; West et al. 1991; Costello et al. 1992; Elliott et al. 1992; Fu et al. 1992). The result is a high permeability form of pulmonary edema (Tsukimoto et al. 1994). Figure 21.7 is an electron micrograph showing rupture of a pulmonary capillary wall in a rat exposed to a barometric pressure of 294 mmHg for 4 h. Note the red blood cell in the process of moving from the capillary lumen to the alveolar space (West et al. 1995).

The work on stress failure began because of two key observations about HAPE. The first is that, as described above, there is a very strong relationship between the occurrence of HAPE and the height of the pulmonary arterial pressure. This suggests that HAPE is caused in some way by high vascular pressures in the pulmonary circulation. The second observation was that samples of alveolar fluid obtained by bronchoalveolar lavage in patients with HAPE show that the fluid is of the high permeability

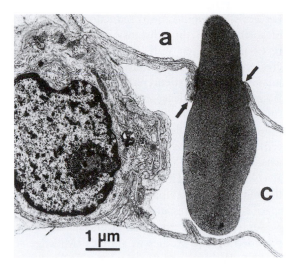

Figure 21.7 Electron micrograph of a pulmonary capillary in a rat exposed to a barometric pressure of 294 mmHg for 4 h. Note rupture of the capillary wall with a red cell moving out of the capillary lumen (c) into an alveolus (a) (from West *et al.* 1995).

type with a large concentration of high molecular weight proteins and many cells. This observation strongly suggests that HAPE is associated with damage to the walls of the pulmonary capillaries by some mechanism. The problem, therefore, was to reconcile a hydrostatic pressure basis for the disease with the development of abnormalities in the capillary walls. As a result, extensive studies of the effects of raising pulmonary capillary pressure on the ultrastructure of pulmonary capillaries were carried out. These showed that stress failure is common in rabbit lung when the capillary transmural pressure rises to 40 mmHg and that when it occurs it causes a high permeability type of pulmonary edema.

It is not at all surprising that pulmonary capillaries break under these conditions because the calculated wall stress of the capillary is extremely high (West *et al.* 1991; West and Mathieu-Costello 1992b). The surprising thing is not that the capillaries fail, but that they do not fail more often. Stress failure is now believed to play a role in a number of lung diseases (West and Mathieu-Costello 1992c) and is also the cause of bleeding into the lungs of racehorses who have very high pulmonary artery pressures with exercise, which is extremely common (West *et al.* 1993).

Bronchoalveolar lavage studies in patients with HAPE show the presence of inflammatory markers including leukotriene B_4, other lipoxygenase products of arachidonic acid metabolism, and C5a complement in the lavage fluid (Schoene *et al.* 1988). These lavage studies were not done in early stages of HAPE as was the study of Swenson *et al.* (2002), where no inflammatory markers were found. At first sight, these findings might seem to argue against stress failure of pulmonary capillaries as a mechanism. However, an important feature of the ultrastructural changes in stress failure is that the basement membranes of capillary endothelial cells are frequently exposed (Tsukimoto *et al.* 1991). The exposed basement membrane is electrically charged and highly reactive, and can be expected to activate leukocytes and platelets. In bronchoalveolar studies of the rabbit preparation, leukotriene B_4 is seen in the lavage fluid (Tsukimoto *et al.* 1994). Platelet activation will result in the formation of fibrin thrombi, which are a feature of the pathology of HAPE (Arias-Stella and Kruger 1963). As mentioned above, the study of Swenson *et al.* (2002) put to rest the role of inflammation in the initiation of HAPE as they found no evidence of inflammation in BAL fluid in HAPE-S subjects in the early stages of the development of HAPE.

A striking feature of stress failure of pulmonary capillaries is that some of the breaks are rapidly reversible when the pressure is reduced. In one study carried out in rabbit lung, it was found that about 70% of both the epithelial and endothelial breaks closed within a few minutes of the pressure being reduced (Elliott *et al.* 1992). This rapid reversibility of most of the disruptions may explain why patients with HAPE often rapidly improve when they descend to a lower altitude.

Stress failure of pulmonary capillaries had not previously been suggested as the mechanism of HAPE. However, Mooi and co-workers (1978) studied the ultrastructural changes that occurred in rat lungs when the animals were exposed to acute decompression in a hyperbaric chamber. The appearances that they described are consistent with the findings seen in stress failure.

The mechanism of stress failure has clear implications for therapy. The main objective should be to reduce the pulmonary artery pressure.

The pressure is high because of hypoxic pulmonary vasoconstriction, and the best way to reduce it is by rapid descent to a lower altitude, which reduces the alveolar P_{O_2}. In addition, oxygen should be given if this is available. Calcium channel blockers, such as nifedipine, are also effective because they reduce pulmonary artery pressure (Oelz *et al.* 1989).

A recent case report by Grissom *et al.* (2000) indicates that alveolar hemorrhage occurs early in HAPE. They report a case of HAPE in a climber who made a rapid ascent of Denali, Alaska and on whom they carried out BAL. The fluid yielded an abundance of hemosiderin-laden macrophages. These have been reported at necropsy and indicate bleeding into the alveoli. They appear from 48 h after bleeding. Bronchoscopy was performed in this case less than 48 h after symptoms started, so the timing of this result indicates bleeding occurred well before the onset of symptoms. This finding is consistent with capillary stress failure early in the course of the condition due to high pulmonary artery pressure.

21.6.6 Venular constriction

Since patients with HAPE have such a powerful arteriolar constriction in response to hypoxia, perhaps they have some degree of venular constriction as well. There is some pathological evidence for this from Wagenvoort and Wagenvoort (1976). This would not give high wedge pressures because, when the catheter is wedged, the blood in that segment runs off even through constricted venules and the wedge pressure reflects only the large vein and left atrial pressures, not the pressure in capillaries when the blood is flowing. To explain the patchy nature of the condition, one must further postulate that the venular constriction is uneven.

21.6.7 Arterial leakage

Severinghaus (1977), impressed with the extraordinarily high pulmonary artery pressure in these patients, suggested that perhaps the fluid leak was upstream of the resistance vessels (i.e. in the arteries). He pointed out that when there was generalized arterial vasoconstriction,

Laplace's law would mean reduction in diameter of small vessels, but distension of large vessels (even though their wall tension was as great or greater). Radiography frequently shows distended hilar vessels (Marticorena *et al.* 1964). These larger vessels, not designed for such high pressure, suffer minor ruptures or fenestrations, which then leak high protein fluid and eventually red blood cells. The leakage is into the perivascular spaces which, when full, 'back up' to eventually cause alveolar flooding. This sequence occurs wherever the initial leak takes place since the perivascular space is the low pressure region of the lung.

Some evidence for such a mechanism was provided by two studies in animals (Milledge *et al.* 1968; Whayne and Severinghaus 1968) and in excised dog lungs (Iliff 1971). This evidence was reviewed by Severinghaus (1977), who quoted Hultgren's report on two horses which died suddenly after running at altitude. Both were found to have a ruptured pulmonary artery. Both this and the preceding hypothesis would account for exercise being a risk factor since it increases both flow and pressure in the pulmonary artery.

21.6.8 Multiple pulmonary emboli

Multiple scattered pulmonary emboli, even of inert substances, such as glass beads, cause a rapid profuse pulmonary edema in animals (Saldeen 1976) and this has been shown to be of the protein-rich increased permeability type (Ohkuda *et al.* 1978). The finding in post-mortem studies of frequent vascular thrombi and fibrin clots has led to the microembolization hypothesis for HAPE on the premise that there is a derangement of the clotting system. The effect of hypoxia on coagulation has been studied by a number of workers (section 19.5.4). It seems that most clotting factors are unaffected by hypoxia; they are not disturbed in AMS. Some evidence of *in vivo* fibrin formation was found by Bärtsch *et al.* (1987) in patients with HAPE, but this was considered to be an epiphenomenon and not causative. If it does occur it will cause further deterioration in the patient. It is possible that changes in the red blood cells with hypoxia might alter their rheological properties and be a factor in AMS and HAPE. However, Reinhart *et al.* (1991) found no difference between subjects with and without AMS with respect to a number of rheological parameters. Platelets are clearly activated at high altitude and show signs of clumping as the day progresses (Lehmann *et al.* 2006), but there is no difference in the groups in terms of developing HAPE.

It has even been suggested that rapid ascent may cause bubble formation by decompression and thus air microembolization (Gray 1983). If this were the case, HAPE should be much more common in chamber studies than in the mountains, but this is not so.

21.6.9 Hypoxia, vascular permeability and inflammation

Hypoxia may increase vascular permeability, either directly, or more likely, via the release of chemical mediators. Against this suggestion is evidence that, in dogs, hypoxia does not alter the threshold for edema formation at a given microvascular pressure (Homik *et al.* 1988). However, it may require some other agent acting with hypoxia to produce the effect, as suggested by the work of Larsen *et al.* (1985). They showed in rabbits that neither hypoxia alone nor activation of the complement system (by infusion of cobra venom) alone caused pulmonary edema, but the two insults together did. Such a mechanism may well produce secondary intravascular coagulation, which would result in further pulmonary edema. On the other hand, Duplain *et al.* (1999b) found in a group of HAPE-susceptible individuals, some of whom developed HAPE at altitude, that there was no tendency for the exhaled nitric oxide to increase with HAPE. Exhaled NO is a marker for inflammation, so this is evidence against inflammation being a factor in the genesis of HAPE. As discussed earlier, in a well-designed study, after baseline studies at low altitude, Swenson and colleagues (2002) took HAPE-susceptible subjects to 4559 m. At the first sign of HAPE, subjects underwent bronchoscopy and BAL. The fluid was high in protein, but there were no markers of inflammation in the BAL fluid of their HAPE subjects. This study complemented the earlier

field studies (Schoene *et al.* 1986; Schoene *et al.* 1988). In those studies, the investigators could not control the stage of the illness in which the subjects were studied. These studies were the first to use BAL which demonstrated high proteins and inflammatory mediators in severe cases of HAPE. Thus, the speculation that inflammation played a role in the permeability leak was put to rest with Swenson's research which supports the mechanism of the leak being primarily secondary to high pressures.

Reactive oxygen species (ROS) have been suggested as culprits leading to vascular permeability. Irwin *et al.* (2009) studied human pulmonary artery endothelial cell monolayers and exposed them to 24 hours of severe hypoxia (3%) to investigate the effect of anti-oxidation on vascular permeability and the ROS-HIF-1a-VEGF pathway. They also studied mice at 5500 m. Treatment with an anti-oxidant mixture (ascorbate, glutathione, and a-tocopherol) resulted in a substantial decrease in marker of permeability (albumin, H_2O_2 production, HIF-1-a, VEGF) that had been produced by hypoxic exposure. Cobalt has also been shown to decrease vascular leak from reperfusion. Shukla *et al.* (2011) preconditioned rats for 7 days with cobalt Cl (12.5 mg kg^{-1}) and then exposed them to extreme altitude (9142 m for 5 hours). Markers of vascular leak (fluoroscein dye, lung water, albumin and cytokines) were all lower in the cobalt-treated animals.

21.6.10 Hypoventilation

Grover (1980) has pointed out that hypoventilation has two disadvantages for a subject in relation to HAPE. It will mean that the subject is more hypoxic at a given altitude than a subject with the normal altitude hyperventilation and also has a higher P_{CO_2}. The higher P_{CO_2} means that there is no peripheral vasoconstriction and reduction in plasma volume on going to altitude; hence the plasma osmotic pressure is not raised. The subject is, therefore, more susceptible to pulmonary edema. A number of studies have found subjects with a history of HAPE to have low hypoxic ventilatory responses (Hackett *et al.*

1988; Matsuzawa *et al.* 1989). This might lead to relative hypoventilation at altitude, although Hackett *et al.* concluded that the low HVR played a permissive rather than a causative role in the pathogenesis of HAPE, allowing hypoxia to cause depression of ventilation. They found oxygen breathing increased ventilation in some of their subjects at altitude.

21.6.11 Neurogenic pulmonary edema

In some cases of head injury, a form of acute pulmonary edema is found which can be mimicked in experimental animals by creating lesions in the fourth ventricle. High levels of catecholamines are found, and the edema can be prevented by pretreatment with α-adrenergic blocking drugs; therefore, it is assumed that the edema is caused by a surge of sympathetic activity. During the first few days at altitude, there is increased sympathetic activity and possibly a similar mechanism is at work. The effectiveness of the alpha-blocker, phentolamine, in HAPE (Hackett *et al.* 1992) suggests that this may be the case, findings also supported by the study of Duplain *et al.* (1999a). Fagenholz *et al* (2007b) used optic nerve sheath diameter (ONSD) as a surrogate measure of intracranial pressure in five HAPE victims at 4240 m in Nepal and compared their data with 32 healthy controls. ONSD was significantly higher in the HAPE subjects and decreased with clinical resolution of HAPE. Irwin *et al.* (2008) used an experimental canine model of cerebral hypoxia by infusing hypoxic venous blood for 2 hours versus controls dogs with normoxic blood infusion. The hypoxic dogs had higher norepinephrine levels, and the lungs of the hypoxic dogs were markedly abnormal with necropsy evidence of alveolar edema and hemorrhage, neutrophils and macrophages. The mechanism of the leak from hypoxia alone remains controversial and evasive.

21.6.12 Infection

Before 1960, many cases of HAPE were attributed to pneumonia. While in some cases, infection plays no part in HAPE, in others it may be a factor, especially in those where individuals who are not normally susceptible to AMS but develop a secondary infection and succumb. Carpenter *et al.* (1998) showed that rats given a mild respiratory infection and allowed to recover had greater lung edema and higher cell counts and protein concentration in BAL fluid when exposed to 10% O_2 a week later than control rats. This gives support to the clinical impression that a concomitant or even previous respiratory infection is an important risk factor for HAPE.

21.6.13 Mechanisms: conclusions

It is now agreed that the genesis of HAPE is from high pressures in the fragile pulmonary microvasculature. The mechanism of abnormally powerful pulmonary hypoxic vasoconstriction, which is uneven and leads on to capillary stress failure, seems to have the most evidence in its favor. Other inherent characteristics, above and beyond the brisk hypoxic pulmonary vasoconstriction, include slower alveolar fluid clearance, and blunted hypoxic ventilatory response, and others, all play additive roles in the clinical spectrum of the disease. A HAPE database is functional such that a larger collection of patients may allow more highly powered studies to unravel the complex mechanisms of HAPE (iharc.partners.org).

Chronic mountain sickness and high altitude pulmonary hypertension

SUMMARY

Chronic mountain sickness (CMS) was first recognized by Carlos Monge M in Peru and is also known as Monge's disease. It is found in all populations who remain at altitude for a number of years. The incidence is increased with altitude and with age; it is higher in males than females and is more prevalent in South America than in Asia or Africa. In Tibet, it is more common in immigrant Han Chinese than in native Tibetans. It is characterized by excessive erythrocytosis with hematocrit values greater than 75%, hypoxemia and pulmonary hypertension. The condition improves after descent to low altitude.

In cases without overt lung disease various factors which cause relative hypoventilation, such as a reduced hypoxic ventilatory drive or disturbed breathing patterns during sleep, may be involved in the mechanism. Patients with underlying conditions, such as chronic obstructive lung disease (chronic bronchitis, emphysema), kyphoscoliosis and other lung diseases, may also have excessive erythrocytosis and in the past were sometimes diagnosed as 'CMS (or Monge's disease) with lung disease,' but are now generally excluded from the diagnosis of CMS (León-Velarde *et al.* 2005).

The symptoms that result from this excessive erythrocytosis are rather vague and include headache, dizziness, physical and mental fatigue, anorexia and breathlessness. There may be symptoms of burning hands or feet. Signs are few and include cyanosis and a ruddy complexion.

Prevention, apart from remaining at low altitude, can only be directed at secondary risk factors, such as smoking and occupational dust air pollution. Relocation to low altitude cures the condition, but many patients, because of occupation or family, are not able to take this option. The removal of 1–3 units of blood is beneficial, but needs to be repeated as the hemoglobin concentration rises again. Respiratory stimulants have been used with reported success, including, recently, acetazolamide.

High altitude pulmonary hypertension (HAPH), previously termed sub-acute mountain sickness or high altitude heart disease, is a condition affecting either infants born or brought up to altitude within their first year, or adults resident or coming and remaining at altitude for months or years. In Tibet, the infants are usually the children of lowland

Han Chinese; the highland Tibetan infants are less susceptible. As the condition develops, the infants become breathless, irritable and edematous. The pathology is of pulmonary hypertension and right heart failure. In adults, it has been reported in Han Chinese and, much less often, in the Tibetan population, in Kyrgyz highlanders and in Indian soldiers stationed at about 6000 m for long periods. When symptoms and signs develop, they are those of right heart failure. Descent results in reversal of signs and symptoms. Short-term trials of drugs such as nifedipine and sildenafil have shown them to be effective in lowering pulmonary artery pressure while remaining at altitude, but there have been no long-term trials to observe the effects on disease progression.

22.1 INTRODUCTION

There are two chronic conditions which affect people resident at high altitudes for months or years or infants born at altitude. There are numerous terms used in the literature for these conditions. Two consensus statements have been published on this topic which include an attempt to clarify these terms (León-Velarde 1998; León-Velarde 2005). Table 22.1 sets out a schema of terms and synonyms abstracted from the latest statement (2005).

Following the consensus statement, the terms 'chronic mountain sickness,' for the condition of excessive erythrocytosis, and 'high altitude pulmonary hypertension,' for the condition where pulmonary hypertension predominates, will be used. There is considerable overlap in the two conditions. Most patients with CMS are also found to have pulmonary hypertension and may go on to develop right heart failure, while some patients with HAPH have a degree of excessive erythrocytosis. However, in most patients one or other response to chronic altitude hypoxia dominates, so the consensus group decided to keep the two diagnoses though recognizing that some patients had both conditions. The situation is, perhaps, analogous to that of high altitude pulmonary edema (HAPE) and high altitude cerebral edema (HACE). It is interesting that excessive erythrocytosis (CMS) is the common pathology in the Andes, while HAPH is more common in the high altitude areas of Asia.

Table 22.1   Nomenclature for chronic high altitude diseases and previous terms or synonyms and essential features

Suggested name	Synonyms	Features
Chronic mountain sickness	Monge's disease	Excessive erythrocytosis
	High altitude excessive polycythemia	Hypoxemia
	Excessive erythrocytosis	Pulmonary hypertension in some cases. Right heart failure
	High altitude pathologic erythrocytosis	Headache, dizziness, fatigue. Recovery on descent to low altitude
High altitude pulmonary hypertension	CMS of the vascular type	Pulmonary hypertension
	High altitude heart disease	Right ventricle hypertrophy
	Hypoxic cor pulmonale	Right heart failure
	Infant subacute mountain sickness	Moderate hypoxemia
	Pediatric high altitude heart disease. Adult subacute mountain sickness	No excessive erythrocytosis

Abstracted from the ISMM Consensus statement (León-Velarde et al. 2005).

Chronic mountain sickness has been well known for many years. The other condition, HAPH, has only been recognized as a chronic condition in adults in the Andes since 1971 (Peñalosa *et al.* 1971) and in China reported in the Chinese literature by Chen *et al.* (1982). A more acute condition was reported by Anand in Indian soldiers stationed at between 5800 m and 6700 m for several months (mean 1.8 years). The condition was recognized rather earlier in children born or brought up to altitude at an early age (Khoury and Hawes 1963).

22.2 CHRONIC MOUNTAIN SICKNESS

22.2.1 Historical

In 1925, Carlos Monge M reported a case of polycythemia in a patient from Cerro de Pasco (4300 m) in Peru to the Peruvian Academy of Medicine (Monge 1925). In 1928, he reported a series of such patients with red cell counts significantly higher than normally found at altitude (Monge and Whittembury 1976). (*Note*. Carlos Monge M is the father and Carlos Monge C the son: the M and C are the initial letters of the mothers' names, as is Spanish custom.) This condition has come to be known also as Monge's disease. The 1935 international expedition, led by Bruce Dill, reported one case of CMS in the English literature (Talbott and Dill 1936). In 1942, Hurtado published detailed observations of eight cases, outlining the symptomatology and hematological changes at altitude and the effect of descent to sea level and return to altitude (Hurtado 1942).

Outside South America, CMS was observed in Leadville (3100 m), a mining town in Colorado, USA, by Monge M in the late 1940s (Winslow and Monge 1987, p 15) and from the 1960s the condition has been studied there by Weil and colleagues (1971) from Denver (section 22.2.3). Reports of CMS from the Himalayas indicate the condition to be prevalent in immigrant Han Chinese in Lhasa (3658 m), but less common in the indigenous Tibetan population (Pei *et al.* 1989; Xing *et al.* 2008).

22.2.2 Clinical aspects of CMS

DEFINITION OF CHRONIC MOUNTAIN SICKNESS

The latest consensus statement defines CMS as:

> A clinical syndrome that occurs in natives or long-life residents above 2500 m. It is characterized by excessive erythrocytosis ([Hb] ≥ 19 dL^{-1} for females and ≥ 21 dL^{-1} for males), severe hypoxemia and in some cases moderate or severe pulmonary hypertension, which may evolve into cor pulmonale, leading to congestive heart failure. The clinical picture of CMS gradually disappears after descending to low altitude and reappears after returning to high altitude.
>
> León-Velarde *et al.* (2005)

The consensus statement also excludes from the definition of CMS patients with any chronic pulmonary disease or any other chronic condition which worsens the hypoxemia of altitude, though it does allow a diagnosis of secondary CMS in such cases.

SYMPTOMS

Patients typically have rather vague neuropsychological complaints including headache, dizziness, paresthesia, somnolence, fatigue, difficulty in concentration and loss of mental acuity. There may also be irritability, depression and even hallucinations. Dyspnea on exertion is not commonly complained of, but poor exercise tolerance is common and patients may gain weight. Poor sleep quality has also been described and is associated with decreased cognitive function in soldiers with polycythemia on the Tibetan plateau with a wide range of CMS scores (Kong *et al.* 2011). The characteristic feature of the disease is that the symptoms disappear on going down to sea level, only to reappear on return to altitude.

A symptom more recently reported in CMS is that of burning feet or hands. This was first described by León-Velarde and Arregui in 1994 (quoted by Thomas *et al.* 2000). In a study by Thomas *et al.* (2000), this symptom was present in all 10 unselected CMS patients, but also four out of five control subjects, resident at the same altitude, and free of CMS. They complained of intermittent burning usually confined to the feet. The symptoms subsided in patients who went down to low altitudes and reappeared on return to high altitude.

SIGNS

Although normal people are mildly cyanotic at an altitude of 4000 m, patients with CMS stand out since, with a high hemoglobin concentration and lower oxygen saturation, they have a far higher concentration of reduced hemoglobin. In Andean natives, the population with the greatest number of patients, the signs may be florid:

> The combination of virtually black lips and wine red mucosal surfaces against the olive green pigmentation of the Indian skin gives the patient with Monge's disease a striking appearance.
>
> Heath and Williams (1995, p 193)

The conjunctivae are congested and the fingers may be clubbed. In Caucasians and at lower altitudes such as Leadville (3100 m), the appearances are rather less striking, resembling patients with polycythemia secondary to hypoxic lung disease at sea level. Some patients show very little in the way of signs.

INVESTIGATIONS

The red cell count, hemoglobin concentration and packed cell volume are raised; values as high as 28 g dL^{-1} hemoglobin and a hematocrits of over 80% (Hurtado 1942) and even 91% (Jefferson *et al.* 2002b) have been recorded. Like secondary polycythemia at sea level and unlike polycythemia rubra vera, there is no increase in white cell numbers. Blood gases, compared with healthy controls at the same altitude, show a higher Pa,CO_2 and lower Pa,O_2 and oxygen saturation (Peñaloza and Sime 1971; Kryger *et al.* 1978a). The lower Pa,O_2 is partly due to hypoventilation as shown by

the increased Pa,CO_2 and partly (in many cases) by an increased alveolar–arterial oxygen pressure, (($A–a)O_2$ gradient).

Manier *et al.* (1988) found a mean ($A–a)O_2$ of 10.5 mmHg in CMS patients at La Paz (3600 m) compared with the normal ($A–a)O_2$ of 2.9 mmHg at this altitude. Using the multiple inert gas technique, they attributed most of this to increased blood flow to poorly ventilated areas of lung rather than to true shunting. Tewari *et al.* (1991) found a reduced diffusing capacity (DLCO) in lowland soldiers with excessive polycythemia on return to low altitude. The DLCO improved with time at low altitude and return to a normal hematocrit. The DLCO was lower in smokers than non-smokers, although both were well below predicted values. In some cases of CMS, standard pulmonary function tests show abnormalities indicating obstructive and/or restrictive defects, suggesting that patients have coexisting chronic lung disease. Using chest ultrasound, Pratali *et al.* (2011) exercised 15 patients with CMS and 20 control subjects at 3600 m altitude and found accumulation of lung water in those with CMS which may give insight to impaired gas exchange as well.

Using flow-mediated dilation, Rimoldi *et al.* (2011) demonstrated arterial stiffness in the systemic circulation of patients with CMS, as opposed to hypoxemic controls, who showed normal vascular reactivity. They felt that these findings may be an important reflection of global vascular pathology in CMS which may give insight into the predisposition of these patients to cardiovascular disease.

Thomas *et al.* (2000) investigated the pathology underlying the burning feet and hands symptom by taking peripheral nerve biopsies (sural nerve) in 10 CMS patients who all had this symptom. They found a neuropathy consisting of a thinning of the basal laminal layer of endoneural microvessels. This is the opposite of that seen in diabetic neuropathy but has been reported in severe chronic hypoxia due to chronic obstructive pulmonary disease (COPD) (Malik *et al.* 1990).

HEMODYNAMICS AND PATHOLOGY

There has been growing interest in cardiac hemodynamics and CMS (Hainsworth and

Drinkhill 2007; Peñaloza and Arias-Stella 2007; Maignan 2009; Richalet *et al.* 2009; León-Velarde 2010; Naeije 2010; Stuber *et al.* 2010). Peñaloza and Arias-Stella (2007) published an excellent review of heart disease and CMS in South America and pointed out the profound public health problem of heart disease that exists at high altitude with CMS. The very high hematocrit increases the viscosity of the blood. The systemic blood pressure may be moderately elevated and the pulmonary artery pressure is significantly higher than that of healthy high altitude residents. Peñaloza *et al.* (1971) found a mean pulmonary artery pressure of 64/33 mmHg in 10 cases of CMS compared with 34/23 mmHg in controls. Cardiac output was not significantly different, so that calculated resistance was just over twice that of controls. As well as the effect of increased viscosity, there would also be pulmonary vasoconstriction due to hypoxia. In present terminology, we would say patients who have high pulmonary artery pressure have both CMS and HAPH.

In spite of higher pulmonary artery pressures and right ventricular hypertrophy in patients with CMS as compared to both low altitude and high altitude controls, Maignan *et al.* (2009) did not find any evidence for overt right-heart failure in their study population. Stuber *et al.* (2010) also used echocardiography in 30 patients with CMS and 32 controls at 3600 m to study the pulmonary vascular response to modest exercise. Although at rest, there was a modest increase in right-sided pressures in the CMS patients, modest exercise (50 watts on a cycle ergometer) demonstrated a three-fold greater difference in the pressures in the CMS subjects which suggests a low pulmonary vascular compliance. Their findings suggest that resting measurements may underestimate the hemodynamic differences between normal and CMS groups.

In an attempt to gain insight into the underlying mechanism of the hemodynamic response in CMS, Ge *et al.* (2011) looked at mediators which have an effect on vasoreactivity and fluid balance. They looked at B-type naturetic peptide (BNP), vascular endothelial growth factor (VEGF), endothelin-1 (ET-1) and endothelial nitric oxide synthase (eNOS) in 24 CMS patients living at 4300 m and compared their results with 50 controls. Both BNP and ET-1 correlated positively with echocardiographic PAP and negatively with SaO_2. VEGF was inversely correlated with SaO_2. eNOS correlated negatively with PAP and positively with SaO_2. These findings suggest that vasoactive mediators play an important role in the pathophysiology of CMS and may afford opportunities for future prevention and treatment.

PREVENTION

Descent to low altitude without return is a sure preventative measure, but not an option for many altitude residents whose family or financial livelihood depends upon their living at altitude. Attention to any secondary risk factors such as smoking is obvious. Since many patients are miners, efforts can also be made to avoid occupational health risks, such as dust and air pollution, but these are frequently difficult to eliminate. In this respect, pollution of drinking water by cobalt may be important in some cases (see section 22.2.5). Prevention could also come from being able to predict the susceptibility to CMS. Genetic markers are being investigated (see section 22.2.5). Moore *et al.* (2007) have looked to see if clinical conditions at birth (hypoxemia, small for gestational age, preterm or pre-eclampsia) were present in patients who went on to get CMS. Impaired fetal growth was associated with adult CMS. Such information could lead to counseling for children who may have alternatives as they become adults to living at lower altitudes.

TREATMENT

A number of options are available to treat CMS (Rivera *et al.* 2007). As already mentioned, symptoms and signs classically clear up on going down to sea level. However, many patients want to remain at altitude for family or economic reasons. In these cases, venesection is beneficial. Venesection not only lowers the raised hematocrit but also improves many of the neuropsychological symptoms. It also improves pulmonary gas exchange (Cruz *et al.* 1979) and exercise performance in some subjects (Winslow and Monge 1987, p 212). In Leadville, Colorado, with about 60 patients being regularly bled for therapeutic purposes, the blood bank has no need of any other donors (Kryger *et al.* 1978a)!

An alternative to venesection for residents at high altitude is the long-term use of respiratory stimulants. Kryger *et al.* (1978b) have reported success with medroxyprogesterone acetate. They showed a fall in hemoglobin concentration after 10 weeks' treatment in 17 patients. The drug stimulated ventilation, raised Po_2 and reduced Pco_2 by a modest amount. Although the changes in blood gases were small, they suggest that the main benefit may have been in oxygenation at night since hypoxemia may be much greater then. The only side effect reported was of loss of libido in four patients. In all but one, this could be overcome by lowering the dose to a level that still kept the hemoglobin concentration down. In one patient, the dose had to be reduced to a point which did not hold down the hemoglobin concentration.

In previous editions of this text, it was reported that there had been no trials of acetazolamide in CMS. There has now been a double-blind controlled trial of acetazolamide in CMS (Richalet *et al.* 2005b). Three groups of patients ($n = 10$ in each group) were treated with either acetazolamide 250 or 500 mg daily or placebo for 3 weeks. There was significant decrease in hematocrit, serum erythropoietin, and soluble transferrin and an increase in nocturnal Sa_2O_2 of 5%. The results for the 250-mg group were as good as for the 500 mg. In a six-month follow-up study, ongoing benefits were noted with acetazolamide as well as decrease in pulmonary artery pressures (Richalet *et al.* 2008). The beneficial mechanism of this drug is thought to be as a respiratory stimulant, noted at doses of both 250 and 500 mg/day (Rivera *et al.* 2008). This simple low cost therapy would seem to offer benefit to the large number of patients with this condition.

22.2.3 Epidemiology of CMS

There has been growing interest in the regional differences and distribution of CMS around the world (Beall 2006; Beall 2007; Xing *et al.* 2008). Different degrees of severity and presentation from Africa, Asia, and North and South America provide a rich supply of information for fascinating speculation about human migration and evolution. CMS is curiously positioned to look at human adaptation over many generations to a constant physiologic stressor, hypoxia.

ANDES

CMS is found most commonly in the Andes, where it was first described mainly affecting the local Amerindians, especially the Quechuan population living on the altiplano at altitudes about 3300–4500 m. Men are affected far more commonly than women. The average age is 40 years with a range from 22 to 51 years in one reported series (Peñaloza *et al.* 1971). Occasional cases are seen in expatriate mining company staff. It used to be thought that CMS was virtually confined to the Andes but this is not the case, as is discussed below.

HIMALAYAS AND TIBET

Until recently, there have been few reported cases of CMS in the Himalayas. Winslow noted one Sherpa on the American Medical Research Expedition to Everest to have a hematocrit of 72% (Winslow and Monge 1987, p 17). Pei *et al.* (1989) describe their experience of CMS in Lhasa (3658 m). The condition is not uncommon among male cigarette-smoking Han Chinese. These subjects had immigrated some years before becoming polycythemic and then displayed the usual signs and symptoms of CMS. In a 12-month period, there were 24 patients admitted to their hospital with CMS. All were male, 23 were Han and only one Tibetan. Six were non-smokers, the rest, including the one Tibetan, were smokers. The mean duration of altitude exposure in the lowlanders was 26 years (range 9–43 years). However, though the incidence in Tibetans may be less than in Han immigrants, CMS is now being reported in this population. Wu *et al.* (1992) reported a series of 26 cases in native-born Tibetans living at between 3680 and 4179 m with typical symptoms of CMS and hemoglobin concentration of 22.2 g dL^{-1} mean compared with 16.6 g dL^{-1} in healthy controls at the same altitude.

One of the adaptations of the Tibetan high altitude dweller may be an upregulation of NO production which has been found in Tibetans

(Erzurum *et al.* 2007). They studied forearm blood flow and circulating concentrations of NO production in 88 Tibetans compared with 50 low-altitude controls. Tibetans had double the forearm blood flow and 10 times the concentration of circulating NO products. These findings suggest greater oxygen delivery to the tissues and a presumed mechanism for lower PAP which has been documented in Tibetans.

In Himalayan residents, hemoglobin concentration tends to be lower than the values from the Peruvian Andes, although much of this difference disappears if results from mining towns are excluded (Frisancho 1988). It is speculated that this may be because the geography allows residents to move to lower altitudes more easily than from the altiplano of the Andes, and the way of life of the Sherpas, with seasonal migration, contributes to this movement in altitude. Like the inhabitants of the Andes, Tibetans live on a high altitude plain and cannot easily move up and down.

Although more evidence is needed, it would seem that people of Tibetan stock are less at risk of CMS than Andean highlanders, and certainly than lowland Han subjects long resident at altitude. This may be due to genuine genetic adaptation to altitude over very many generations.

A review comparing incidence of CMS in the Andes with that in Tibet seems to bear out this earlier speculation (Moore *et al.* 1998b). This review also presents more evidence on incidence at various altitudes, men versus women, and Tibetan versus Han Chinese. In an attempt to understand who in the immigrant Han population was more susceptible to acquiring CMS, Li *et al.* (2012) found that workers living in an urban environment doing construction work had a higher prevalence of CMS than rural inhabitants, those living in oxygen-generating systems, and non-physical jobs. Such information may be helpful in the future for populations living at high altitude to institute public health measures to minimize the development of CMS.

ETHIOPIA

The political climate for many decades in Ethiopia has resulted in a delayed investigative effort. The Ethiopian highlands are not quite as high as Tibet or the Andes, and there is greater genetic heterogeneity in the various peoples who inhabit Ethiopia. What is known though is that there is no documented CMS in the Ethiopian highlanders. However, intriguing data are beginning to emerge from this area. Xing *et al.* (2008) explored hypoxia-related genes in Ethiopians, Tibetans, and Himalayan high altitude residents. Markers of the response of the cerebral circulation and hypoxic ventilatory response were low in the Himalayas and Ethiopia, and another gene that was expressed in CMS (*PDP2*) was not present in the Ethiopians. Clearly, more physiologic and genetic work will be forthcoming from the highlands of Ethiopia.

NORTH AMERICA

CMS is well recognized in Leadville, Colorado (3100 m). Kryger *et al.* (1978a) described 20 cases, all male, and mentioned that, of about 60 cases known to physicians there, only two were female. One case of apparently classical CMS in a 67-year-old woman has been reported from as low as 2000 m in California (Gronbeck 1984). Of note is the finding that CMS in North America has less pulmonary vascular involvement than in the Andes.

22.2.4 Scoring of chronic mountain sickness

A symptom/sign scoring system for CMS was proposed at the 6th World Congress of Mountain Medicine in Qinghai in August 2004 and included in the consensus statement (León-Velarde *et al.* 2005). The purpose was to provide a means of comparing cases from one study to another. Symptoms/signs are scored as 0 to 3 indicating: 0, no symptom; 1, mild; 2, moderate; and 3, severe symptom/sign. The list of symptoms/signs is as follows: breathlessness/palpitations, sleep disturbance, cyanosis, dilatation of veins, paresthesia, headache, tinnitus. Hemoglobin level: males >18 but <21 dL^{-1} = 0; >21 dL^{-1} = 3; females >16 but <19 dL^{-1} = 0, >19 dL^{-1} = 3. A summation of the scores reflects the severity of the disease (absent 0–5; mild 6–10; moderate 11–14; severe >15).

22.2.5 Mechanisms of CMS

CMS WITH NORMAL LUNGS

Patients with CMS have lower Pa,O_2 and Sa,O_2 and higher Pa,CO_2 values than healthy subjects at the same altitude. The greater hypoxemia results in higher erthropoietin levels and thus greater erthrocytosis. So what is the cause of this more severe hypoxia? The raised Pa,CO_2 points to a degree of hypoventilation, but there may also be some gas transfer defect as well. As mentioned above, a widened $P(A–a)O_2$ gradient has been shown in CMS patients (Manier et al. 1988). As mentioned before, Pratali et al. (2011) documented increased lung water after exercise in subjects with CMS which certainly can result in impaired gas exchange.

Severinghaus et al. (1966a) found that CMS patients had an extremely blunted hypoxic ventilator response (HVR) compared with healthy resident controls of the same age. Perhaps people at the low end of the spectrum for HVR in the population are destined to get CMS if they remain for years at altitude. The HVR decreases with age (Kronenberg and Drage 1973) and with duration of stay at altitude (Wiel et al. 1971); perhaps patients with CMS are those in whom the process is faster than average.

Kryger et al. (1978a), however, found no difference in HVR between patients and age-matched controls in Leadville, Colorado. They did find that their patients had a greater dead-space/tidal volume ratio and that their ventilation increased on breathing 100% oxygen; they therefore appeared to have hypoxic ventilatory depression. They concluded that blunted chemical drive to breathing is not the cause of CMS.

SLEEP

During sleep, even in normal subjects, the ventilation is depressed. If there are frequent periods of apnea, either central or obstructive, Sa,O_2 will be further reduced and could contribute to the etiology. A study by Sun et al. (1996) found that CMS patients had more disordered breathing and lower mean Sa,O_2 values when asleep than a group free of CMS. In periods of disordered breathing non-CMS controls increased their cerebral blood flow; whereas, the CMS group did not. Therefore, the latter had a reduction in their calculated brain oxygen delivery. Recently, Spicuzza et al. (2004) in a study of CMS patients and controls at 4300 m confirmed the greater hypoxemia in CMS patients when awake and showed that they were also more hypoxemic when asleep. In particular the total time spent with Sa,O_2, 80% was significantly greater in the CMS patients. This level of desaturation would be expected to trigger a greater erythropoietin release. Reeves and Weil (2001) in their review of over 900 patients with CMS studied over the years emphasize the profound hypoxia in these patients, when asleep. Kong et al. (2011) found poor sleep quality in patients with CMS to be associated with cognitive impairment.

GENDER

Women (at least before the menopause) seem to be protected from CMS as from the hypoventilation syndrome (the Pickwickian syndrome) at sea level, possibly by the stimulating effect of progesterone on ventilation. León-Velarde et al. (1997) compared pre- and postmenopausal women at Cerro de Pasco (4300 m) in Peru and found significantly higher hematocrit and lower Sa,O_2, and peak expiratory flows in the postmenopausal group, supporting the protective role of female sex hormones.

AGE

Age has effects on lung function, as well as its effect on HVR. The Pa,O_2 declines with age and, although this has little effect on oxygen saturation at sea level, it has much more effect at altitude because subjects are already on the steep part of the oxygen dissociation curve. A study by León-Velarde et al. (1993) at 4300 m in Peru found an increasing incidence of CMS with age. Taking a hemoglobin concentration of above 21.3 g dL^{-1} as 'excessive erythrocytosis,' the incidence at 20–29 years was 6.8% which increased to 33.7% at age 60–69 years. This study also found a decreasing vital capacity with age at altitude, in both those with and without CMS, but the reduction was significantly more marked in the CMS group. Sea level subjects showed no reduction in vital capacity between 20–29 years and 60–69 years.

COBALT

Cobalt is a known stimulant of erythropoiesis. In a review of their experience over many years, Reeves and Weil (2001) collected details of more than 750 men and 200 women with CMS. They noted that one of the contributing factors to the variation in the erythropoietic response to altitude was ingested toxins and minerals such as cobalt. Jefferson *et al.* (2002) in a study from Cerro de Pasco (4300 m) found that 11 of their 21 subjects with CMS had detectable cobalt levels in their serum compared with none in their controls. However, Bernardi *et al.* (2003) in their study also in Cerro de Pasco found normal cobalt levels in CMS patients. Cerro de Pasco is a mining town and cobalt is one of the many minerals in the rocks. It was not found in samples of drinking water tested by Jefferson *et al.*, but perhaps leaches in at times. It may, therefore, act as a risk factor in some cases of CMS in some localities.

CEREBRAL BLOOD FLOW IN CMS

Polycythemia (rubra vera) results in reduced cerebral blood flow (CBF) (Thomas *et al.* 1977) due to increased viscosity. However, the few studies of CBF (measuring blood velocity by Doppler ultrasound) in CMS have either shown no significant differences between subjects with and without CMS when awake breathing air (Sun *et al.* 1996), or the expected reduced flow in CMS patients compared with controls (Claydon *et al.* 2005).

GENETICS AND CMS

There seems to be a difference in response to long-term, chronic hypoxia in different populations and only a proportion of any population is susceptible to CMS. These considerations lead to the question of whether there is a genetic component to susceptibility. Mejia *et al.* (2005) in a case–control study looked at a variety of candidate genes including: erythropoietin, erythropoietin-receptor, HIF-1α (von Hippel-Lindau and others). They found no association between the polymorphisms linked to the candidate genes and severe polycythemia. In some preliminary work, León-Velarde and Mejia (2007) found insufficient information to make any consistent conclusions of hypoxia-related genes in their high altitude populations. Huicho *et al.* (2008) studied children of parents with CMS and looked at oxygen-responsive genes and those involved in glycolytic and mitochondrial pathways to see if there was a genetic signature that may predict future development of CMS. Markers of impaired adaptation to hypoxia were noted in defective coupling between glycolysis and the mitochondrial TCA cycle which may predispose these children to the eventual development of CMS. Richalet *et al.* (2011) studied 1000 patients with CMS and 1000 control subjects in Cerro de Pasco, Peru, and found that the two groups had differential gene markers for VEGF. This and other preliminary work (Buroker *et al.* 2010; Liu *et al.* 2012) could lead to the discovery of specific markers which could be predictors of those susceptible to CMS.

EXCESSIVE ERYTHROCYTOSIS WITH LUNG DISEASE

In cases of excessive erythrocytosis with definite lung disease, it is easy to understand that the combination of altitude with fairly mild lung disease precipitates polycythemia and cor pulmonale. Removal of altitude hypoxia by descent to sea level is sufficient to reverse the process. At altitude, these patients are more hypoxemic than normal people because of their lung disease, hence their stimulus to erythrocytosis via erythropoietin secretion is greater and they become abnormally polycythemic. The importance of lower respiratory tract disease is emphasized in a study by León-Velarde *et al.* (1994) which shows that subjects with chronic lower respiratory disease had higher hemoglobin concentrations, lower $Sa_{,O_2}$ and higher CMS symptom scores than healthy controls or subjects with chronic upper respiratory disease.

CONCLUSION

Altitude hypoxia and hypoventilation will result in a low Pa,O_2. This hypoventilatory response may be due to a low HVR, to hypoxic depression of ventilation or some unknown cause. If lung function is also reduced by lung or chest wall disease, this will reduce Pa,O_2 still further. Aging results in both reduced lung function and reduced HVR, especially in a life spent at high altitude, thus further lowering the Pa,O_2. The low Pa,O_2 results in a low Sa,O_2. It also stimulates secretion of erythropoietin and hence an increase in hematocrit. However, it should be noted that a study of erythropoietin levels in subjects at Cerro de Pasco (4300 m), although showing the expected higher mean values at altitude than at sea level, did not demonstrate any difference between subjects with and without CMS (León-Velarde et al. 1991). The rise in hematocrit causes a rise in blood viscosity and probably, a fall in cerebral blood flow, which, with a low Sa,O_2, results in chronic severe cerebral hypoxia and symptoms of CMS.

22.3 HIGH ALTITUDE PULMONARY HYPERTENSION

22.3.1 Introduction and history

It has been known for 60 years that exposure to hypoxia results in pulmonary hypertension. This was first demonstrated by von Euler and Liljestrand (1946) in cats and shortly afterwards by Motley et al. (1947) in man. This hypoxic pressor response is important in the fetus since blood must be diverted away from the non-functioning lung through the ductus arteriosis to the rest of the body. Its effect in life after birth may be to improve ventilation/perfusion ratios in the lung when parts of the lung are unventilated, for instance by bronchiolar occlusion in asthma or lobar consolidation in pneumonia. In these situations, the areas underventilated become hypoxic and it is clearly beneficial for vasoconstriction in these areas to reduce the blood flow and divert it to other, ventilated parts of the lung. However, at altitude, with global hypoxia there is vasoconstriction throughout the lung and the pulmonary artery pressure rises with no benefit to gas transfer apart from possibly some slight improvement in the upright lung due to rather more even perfusion. It is of note that animals adapted to high altitude, such as the yak (Harris 1986) or pika (Ge et al. 1998) do not have this pressor response, and Tibetans have a greatly diminished response (Groves et al. 1993).

As early as 1956, Rotta et al. (Rotta et al. 1956) found pulmonary hypertension in acclimatized lowlanders and residents at altitude. In 1962, Peñaloza et al. (Peñaloza et al. 1962) and Arias-Stella et al. (Arias-Stella et al. 1962) presented their data on pulmonary hypertension and pulmonary artery pathology, respectively, showing hypertension and muscularization of the pulmonary arterioles in healthy people resident at altitude in the Andes. This remodeling results in sustained hypertension even when hypoxia is relieved by oxygen breathing (see section 7.5.1) or descent to low altitude, although after some months or years at low altitude hypertension does remit.

Patients with CMS often also had pulmonary hypertension (section 22.2.2) and sometimes developed right heart failure, but the severe erythrocytosis had been described earlier and, since blood counts were so much easier to carry out than cardiac catheterization, the hypertension tended to be dismissed and attributed mainly to the increased viscosity due to high hematocrit rather than to hypoxic vasoconstriction followed by remodeling. This early work in Peru has been thoughtfully reviewed by Reeves and Grover (2005).

In 1988, Sui et al. published their experience with infants born at low altitude and taken to high altitude in Tibet. They called the condition subacute infantile mountain sickness. Shortly afterwards, Anand et al. (1990) reported a similar condition in adult soldiers stationed for some months or more at extreme altitude and called it 'adult subacute mountain sickness.' Both conditions were essentially right heart failure due to chronic pulmonary hypertension and would be called HAPH in the nomenclature suggested by the consensus statement (Table 22.1). Since then, there have been numerous reports of this condition from high altitude regions of Asia (Ge and Helun 2001; Aldeshev et al. 2002; Wu 2005), as well as an outpouring of interest worldwide (Peñaloza 2007; Xu and Jing 2009; Pasha and Gassman 2010; Lopes *et al.* 2010; Zhai *et al.* 2010; León-Velarde and Villafuerte 2011).

22.3.2 High altitude pulmonary hypertension in infants

The Spaniards who first colonized the Andes became well aware that their infants did not thrive if born at high altitude. They made it their practice to arrange delivery at low altitude and not to bring their babies to high altitude before 1 year of age.

The lowland Han Chinese colonists of Tibet face the same environmental problem. Wu and Liu (1995) described a Chinese infant of 11 months born in Lhasa (3658 m) who presented with dyspnea, cyanosis and congestive heart failure. At post-mortem, marked right ventricular hypertrophy and muscular thickening of the peripheral pulmonary artery tree were found. There was no other pathology such as congenital heart disease and the authors called the condition 'high altitude heart disease.' Sui *et al.* (1988) had reported the post-mortem findings of 15 infants who died in Lhasa of a syndrome they called 'infantile subacute mountain sickness.' The presenting symptoms were commonly dyspnea and cough, with often sleeplessness, irritability and signs of cyanosis, edema of the face, oliguria, tachycardia, liver enlargement, rales in the lungs and fever. The majority of infants had been born at low altitude but two were born at high altitude, one of Han and one of Tibetan parents. The condition was usually fatal in a matter of weeks or months. The post-mortem findings were of extreme medial hypertrophy of muscular pulmonary arteries and muscularization of pulmonary arterioles. There was massive hypertrophy and dilatation of the right ventricle and of the pulmonary trunk.

22.3.3 High altitude pulmonary hypertension in adults

Anand *et al.* (1990) described a condition in 21 soldiers who, after a full acclimatization period, had been posted to between 5800 and 6700 m for several months (mean 1.8 years). They called the condition 'adult subacute mountain sickness.' The patients presented with dyspnea, cough and effort angina. The signs were of dependent edema. They were treated at high altitude with diuretics with improvement. When they were evacuated to low altitude by aircraft, they were found to have cardiomegaly with right ventricular enlargement and, in most cases, pericardial effusion. The pulmonary artery pressure was elevated (26 mmHg) and rose significantly on mild exercise to 40 mmHg. Recovery was rapid after descent from high altitude. Investigations showed a generalized increase in the volume of the fluid compartments of the body and total body sodium, even in subjects without overt disease at these altitudes for this length of time (Anand *et al.* 1993). The increase in central blood volume is the probable cause of the decrease in forced vital capacity, and the radiographically engorged pulmonary vessels found in the subjects of Operation Everest II (Welsh *et al.* 1993). A similar condition was described by Wu (2005) in his review of CMS on the Qinghai–Tibetan plateau. It would seem that this HAPH with right heart failure is the human form of a similar condition affecting cattle taken to high altitude, and known as 'brisket disease' (Hecht *et al.* 1959). The brisket is the loose skin area of the cow's neck, which is dependent and becomes swollen with edema fluid in this condition.

Pei *et al.* (1989) reviewed their experience of CMS in Lhasa based on 17 cases. Sixteen were Han Chinese men, while the 17th was a Tibetan woman. The men had all moved from lowland China to Tibet to an altitude of 3600 m, an average of 15 years before admission to hospital. Their symptoms and signs were cough, dyspnea, dependent edema, liver enlargement and raised jugular venous pressure. The mean hematocrit was 70% and in the five patients who were catheterized the mean values of the pulmonary artery pressure was 57/28. Reviewing the natural history of the disease, they suggested that the earlier stage of the disease was dominated by polycythemia while cardiopulmonary involvement increases with the duration of the disease.

CLINICAL FEATURES

Mild or moderate pulmonary hypertension does not give rise to symptoms. There may be signs, an accentuated second heart sound and electrocardiogram (ECG) and echocardiographic evidence of hypertension, but symptoms only develop when the right heart begins to fail. The symptoms are headache, dyspnea, cough, irritability, sleeplessness and sometimes angina on exertion. Clinical signs include cyanosis, tachycardia, tachypnea, edema of face, liver enlargement and crackles in the chest (Ge and Helun 2001). Upon descending, all these symptoms and signs typically disappear in a few days or weeks, although occasionally the hypertension may be detectable for a year or more.

EPIDEMIOLOGY AND PREVALENCE

Some populations are more susceptible than others. In Qinghai and Tibet, the Han Chinese immigrants are more susceptible than Tibetans (by a factor of 3–4). Children are more susceptible than adults (by a factor of about 3). These data are shown in Table 22.2.

Men are more susceptible than women. Aldeshev and colleagues have reported on their studies of HAPH in the high altitude population in Kyrgyzstan (Aldeshev *et al.* 2002). A health survey, including ECG, was carried out in three villages between 2800 and 3100 m. ECG recordings on 741 subjects (347 males, 394 females) were analyzed. Fourteen percent had one or more criteria for cor pulmonale, 23% of males and only 6% of females, a highly significant difference.

NATURAL HISTORY OF HAPH

Aldashev *et al.* (2002) carried out right heart catheterization in Bishkek (760 m) on a group of 136 male highlanders resident between 2800 and 3600 m. Three groups were identified: (1) a group with normal pulmonary artery pressures; (2) those with normal pressures, but who had a greater than two-fold increase in pressure on breathing a hypoxic gas mixture; and (3) a group with frank pulmonary hypertension. The percentages for these groups were: 59, 21 and 20%. They were able to follow up 25 subjects 10 years later. Of the normotensive group, there was no increase in pressure. All 10 of the subjects followed up in the hyper-responsiveness group showed increase in pressures as did the seven subjects followed up in the hypertension group.

GENETIC CONTRIBUTION TO HAPH

It has been well established that brisket disease in cattle affects only certain breeds and that the pulmonary hypertensive trait in susceptible breeds is genetically determined (Cruz *et al.* 1980). HAPH is the human equivalent of this condition. Fagan and Weil (2001) have reviewed the evidence of the genetic contribution to the control of pulmonary artery pressure at altitude. They conclude that the differences among diverse altitude populations (such as indicated above)

Table 22.2 Prevalence (percentage of population) of high altitude heart disease (HAPH) at various altitudes of residence in Han and Tibetan children and adults

Altitude (m)	Han		Tibetan	
	Children	Adults	Children	Adults
<3000	0.47	0.07	0.2	0
3000–4000	1.47	0.71	0.37	0.24
4000–5000	3.64	1.72	1.04	0.46

Children are more susceptible than adults and Han Chinese than Tibetans. The prevalence increases with altitude. Data of Wu and Ge, quoted in Ge and Helun 2001.

suggest an evolutionary, genetic influence on the response of the pulmonary circulation to the hypoxia of altitude. Tucker and Rhodes (2001) reviewed the role of pulmonary vascular smooth muscle in the development of HAPH in various animals and humans. There was good evidence for the hypothesis that the amount of smooth muscle predicted the degree of response. Cattle and pigs are high responders and have thick muscle layers; sheep, dogs and a variety of animals native to high altitude are low responders and have thin muscle walls to their pulmonary arteries. Humans, rats and mice are intermediate. That these differences are genetically determined is supported by studies in cross-breeds between yak and cattle (Anand *et al.* 1986).

Aldashev *et al.* (2002) reported their results of ACE genotyping in 78 male highlanders who had undergone cardiac catheterization. There was a three-fold higher frequency of the I/I

allele in highlanders with HAPH, compared with normal highlanders and the mean pulmonary artery pressure was significantly higher in subjects with I/I than with I/D or D/D. A comparison of the frequency of these alleles between lowlanders resident in Bishkek and high altitude residents showed a significantly lower frequency of I/I and higher D/D in the highlanders, suggesting possibly evolutionary selection of D/D alleles in the high altitude population.

TREATMENT OF HAPH

The whole process of pulmonary arterial vasoconstriction and remodeling is reversed by descent to low altitude and the relief of hypoxia. However, the option of emigration from their high altitude homes and relocating to low altitude is not open to many patients with HAPH. For these patients, the possibility of drug treatment may be considered. However, such trials as have been reported are all short term, so we do not know the long-term result of drug treatment on disease progression.

Antezana *et al.* (1998) showed that nifedipine reduced the pulmonary artery pressure (*P*pa) in patients with HAPH by 20% in two-thirds of patients. The effect was greatest in those with the highest pressures and was not correlated with [Hb]. The phosphodiesterase inhibitor, sildenafil, has been shown to be effective in lowering *P*pa (and improving gas exchange) in healthy subjects taken to altitude for 6 days (Richalet *et al.* 2005a). Aldashev *et al.* (2005) studied 22 patients with HAPH in a controlled trial of two doses of sildenafil (25 and 100 mg, every 8 h) or placebo, for 3 months. The two doses were equally effective in lowering *P*pa and in increasing the length of the 6 min walking test. Sildenafil was said to be well tolerated. There do not seem to have been any trials of acetazolamide in HAPH. An interesting study on the effect of iron repletion to improve HAPH was published by Smith *et al.* (2009). The mechanism of action is not known, but may act through hypoxia-inducible factor. More work should be forthcoming.

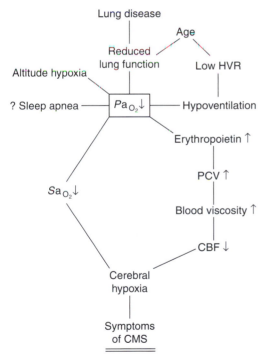

Figure 22.1 Possible mechanisms in the development of chronic mountain sickness (CMS). HVR, hypoxic ventilatory response; CBF, cerebral blood flow; PCV, packed cell volume.

CONCLUSION

HAPH, along with pulmonary hypertension in general, has become an increasingly recognized entity with many fertile areas of clinical and basic science research to understand the natural progression, underlying mechanisms, demographic variability, public health risks, and ultimately treatment with improved outcomes in millions of patients. Many of these people, especially at high altitude, go unrecognized because of lack of awareness, scant resources to diagnose, and limitations to treat and follow these patients. Questions that arise: Which patients have significant HAPH that will progress to cor pulmonale and early death? What is the natural history of the disease, and are there specific markers to identify those patients at risk for progression? What public health measures in high altitude populations might minimize the development of clinically significant HAPH?

This area of clinical disease at high altitude has emerged as one of the most exciting areas in many years, asking for research to address a public health problem. The high altitude research community should be poised to move forward.

23

Other altitude-related conditions

SUMMARY

When travelers become ill at high altitude, concern is always raised about the possibility of acute altitude illness. While disorders such as acute mountain sickness (AMS), high altitude pulmonary edema (HAPE) and high altitude cerebral edema (HACE) should always remain on the differential diagnosis, a range of other medical problems has been documented at high altitude and often merit consideration.

Thromboembolic disease: A variety of arterial and venous thromboembolic events involving the central nervous system and extra-cerebral vascular beds have been documented at high altitude raising concern that hypobaric hypoxia leads to a hypercoagulable state. The available evidence does not support such a conclusion and prophylactic measures against these events are not necessary beyond maintaining good hydration and adequate mobility. Any neurologic symptoms with rapid onset or focal neurologic deficits should prompt consideration of diagnoses other than acute altitude illness and evacuation to lower elevation.

Neurologic conditions: Aside from cerebrovascular accidents, there is a series of other documented neurologic conditions at high altitude that fall outside the realm of acute altitude illness, including migraine headaches, subarachnoid hemorrhage, transient global amnesia and focal cranial nerve palsies. Distinguishing these entities from acute altitude illness may be difficult and providers will need to rely on careful history and physical examination and should have a low threshold for moving an individual to a lower elevation for further evaluation.

Eye problems: Several important ophthalmologic problems can also occur at high altitude including the highly common but usually asymptomatic high altitude retinopathy, ultraviolet keratitis and dry eye syndrome. The cornea may also thicken in response to hypoxia at high altitude. This may potentially cause vision problems for climbers traveling at very high elevations following certain forms of refractive surgery, but is not usually associated with problems in normal individuals or those who have not had refractive surgery for near- or far-sightedness.

High altitude cough: Despite being a highly common problem associated with adverse consequences, including sleep disturbances and even rib fractures, high altitude cough has received little scientific attention until recently. Hyperventilation of cold, dry air plays an important role in its development, but other factors related to hypoxia itself likely also play a role given that increased cough frequency has also been noted in chamber experiments with careful control of environmental conditions. Management of this problem remains challenging, as many remedies have been proposed but have little scientific evidence demonstrating benefit.

Anesthesia at high altitude: Most severe medical conditions at high altitude, including problems requiring surgical intervention, will be managed with descent to lower elevation. Occasionally, however, surgical intervention including anesthesia will be necessary at high altitude and, possibly in a remote, resource-limited setting. Individuals undergoing anesthesia will be at greater risk for hypoxia due to the respiratory depressant effects of general anesthetics in the setting of low barometric pressure, a risk that persists into the postoperative period when even small concentrations of anesthetic gases can depress the hypoxic ventilatory response. Providers must also be aware of important issues that arise with monitoring devices and other anesthetic delivery equipment at high altitude and will need to consider how the altitude and temperature will affect the potency of the different anesthetic agents.

23.1 THROMBOEMBOLIC DISEASE

Over more than a century, a variety of cases of arterial or venous thromboembolic events have been reported at high altitude raising suspicion that high altitude hypoxia may provoke a hypercoagulable state that predisposes individuals to these adverse events.

23.1.1 Cerebrovascular events

Cerebrovascular accidents will typically be distinguished from acute altitude illnesses by virtue of their rapid onset and the fact that focal neurologic deficits are very uncommon in AMS or HACE. There is a long history of strokes reported at high altitude dating back as far as Robrovsky's description of his own hemiparesis and aphasia while exploring Tibet's Amne Machin range (Robrovsky 1896) and descriptions of hemiplegia in a Ghurkha soldier and Sherpa

porter on Everest expeditions in 1924 and 1936 (Norton 1925; Tilman 1948). Most recently, Jha et al. (2002) reported a series of Indian soldiers who developed strokes while stationed at high altitude and Wilson et al. (2010) described the use of transcranial Doppler ultrasound to detect evidence of middle cerebral artery occlusion that was responsible for a patient's neurologic symptoms. In addition to these events, there have been many documented cases of transient ischemic attacks (TIAs). Wohns (1986), for example, reported a series of TIAs that occurred during high altitude climbs in three separate individuals, including hemiplegia, hemiparesis, aphasia and scotomas. Similarly, Murdoch (1996) reported cases with various focal neurologic defects at altitude that also demonstrated rapid recovery. Without the aid of diagnostic studies, however, it is difficult to conclude that these cases were due to thromboembolic processes rather than ischemia due to volume depletion in the setting of hypoxemia, for example.

While events described above generally involved the arterial circulation, there have also been reports of cerebral venous infarcts at high altitude. Boulos et al. (1999), for example, reported the case of a climber in the French Alps who developed right-sided hemiparesis, dysphasia and seizures and was found to have a superior sagittal sinus thrombosis, while Torgovicky et al. (2005) reported a patient who developed sagittal and transverse sinus thrombosis following routine high altitude chamber training. Most recently, Cheng et al. (2009) reported the case of a trekker in Nepal who developed dizziness, nausea and vomiting at 4000 m and progressive obtundation following descent of over 2000 m that were subsequently determined to be due to thrombosis of the great vein of Galen and the straight sinus, while Shrestha et al. (2012) reported the case of a 47-year-old woman who presented with headache, speech deficits and visual changes, and was found to have a cerebral venous sinus thrombosis. These cases demonstrate the need to consider alternative diagnoses to acute altitude illness when neurologic or other symptoms do not improve or worsen with descent. Dickenson et al. (1983) have also noted cerebral venous thrombosis in autopsies of patients evacuated to

Kathmandu after death at altitude, while Song *et al.* (1986) made a similar finding in patients who had been at altitudes above 5000 m for more than 3 weeks.

23.1.2 Thromboembolic events outside the central nervous system

Venous and arterial thromboembolic events have also been described in sites outside the central nervous system. In addition to the noteworthy case of Art Gilkey who developed deep venous thrombosis of the lower extremities during the 1954 American expedition to K2 (Houston and Bates 1979), there have been multiple reports of pulmonary embolism (Nakagawa *et al.* 1993; Shlim and Papenfus 1995; Heffner and Sahn 1981; Ashraf *et al.* 2006). In two of those cases (Nakagawa *et al.*, 1993; Shlim and Papenfus 1995), the patients presented with high altitude pulmonary edema and were later determined to have pulmonary emboli.

Fagenholz *et al.* (2007) described the case of a previously healthy man who presented to the Himalayan Rescue Association clinic in Pheriche (4240 m) with a pale, cold right lower extremity due to thrombosis of the right superficial femoral artery at its transition to the popliteal artery and later required a below-knee amputation. Anand *et al.* (2005) have described 26 cases of portal venous thrombosis in Indian soldiers stationed above 3000 m.

23.1.3 Risk for thromboembolic disease at high altitude

As noted earlier, the large number of reported cases of thromboembolic disease has raised suspicion that hypobaric hypoxia may predispose to the development of a hypercoagulable state. To date, however, there has been insufficient evidence to support such a claim or purported etiologies, such as dehydration and/or prolonged periods of immobility in a tent.

Several large, retrospective series have attempted to establish that the risk of thromboembolic events is increased at high altitude. For example, Anand *et al.* (2001) retrospectively reviewed the records of over 20 000 hospital admissions in India over a 3-year period and found a higher incidence of venous and arterial thrombosis among high altitude dwellers compared to those from low altitude regions, while Jha *et al.* (2002) used a similar retrospective approach and reported a higher incidence of stroke in soldiers stationed at high altitude compared to those at lower elevation. The conclusions of these studies, however, are limited at best due to methodological concerns such as the narrow patient populations examined (e.g. military soldiers), limited diagnostic evaluations and the retrospective nature of the analyses. They also provide no information regarding risks associated with short-term stays at high altitude, as each of these studies concerned longer-term exposures. Zafren *et al.* (2011) sought to address the issue of risks associated with more short-term exposures in a study of climbers on Mt Everest. They attempted to characterize the incidence of deep venous thrombosis in asymptomatic individuals by performing D-dimer testing in all individuals followed by lower extremity compression ultrasound in those individuals with a positive test. Zero out of the 76 climbers had a positive test and no ultrasounds were necessary, suggesting that the incidence of asymptomatic deep venous is low.

In the absence of systematic studies demonstrating increased risk of thromboembolic events at high altitude, many studies have examined changes in various coagulation parameters as surrogate measures for thromboembolic risk. This approach also fails to provide convincing evidence of a hypercoagulable state at high altitude. Although there is consistent evidence that the activated partial thromboplastin time is shorter during acute hypoxic exposures (Maher *et al.* 1976; O'Brodovich *et al.* 1984; Bärtsch *et al.* 1988), the literature contains conflicting results about the effects of acute hypoxic exposure on platelet function (Gray *et al.* 1975; Maher *et al.* 1976; Sharma 1980; Chatterji *et al.* 1982; Lehmann *et al.* 2006), bleeding times (Bärtsch *et al.* 1989; Doughty and Beardmore 1994) and other biochemical markers of coagulation activity, such as markers of fibrinolytic activity (Bärtsch *et al.* 1988; Mannucci *et al.* 2002) and thrombin formation (Bendz *et al.* 2000; Bärtsch *et al.* 2001).

The studies noted above were generally done in healthy individuals with no evidence of underlying coagulopathy. A more recent study by Schreijer et al. (2006) suggests that the presence of underlying coagulopathy may, in fact, be the key factor that predisposes to thromboembolic events. In a study of 71 healthy volunteers, they found increased levels of thrombin–anti-thrombin complexes following 8 hours of air travel at cabin pressures equivalent to 1800–2100 m compared to following the non-hypoxic exposures. Of note, the greatest changes were noted in those volunteers with the Factor V Leiden mutation who used oral contraceptives, which suggested that the presence of a pre-existing coagulopathy may be the key factor associated with increased risk for thromboembolism at high altitude.

This result is particularly intriguing because in many of the cases of thromboembolic disease at high altitude, the affected individual was found to have some underlying predisposition to coagulopathy, such as oral contraceptive use (Shlim and Papenfus 1995), protein C deficiency (Boulos et al. 1999), hyperhomocysteinemia (Ashraf et al. 2006) or S-C hemoglobinopathy (Heffner and Sahn 1981). This finding is not universal, however, as the patients in other cases (Fagenholz et al. 2007) had no evidence of underlying coagulopathy.

Other factors not accounted for in these studies may play a role in some thromboembolic events including a combination of polycythemia and dehydration due to increased insensible losses and urinary losses (Ward 1975), and prolonged periods of immobility while tent-bound during inclement weather. Interestingly, even though polycythemia vera is known to increase the risk of thrombotic events, patients with secondary polycythemia at sea level due to, for example, chronic hypoxia do not have similar risk for such problems (Schwarcz et al. 1993). This would suggest that the polycythemia that develops with prolonged stays at high altitude may not be a predisposing factor in and of itself, unless there is some additional factor, such as dehydration and prolonged immobility. In the end, however, there is no systematic evidence that hypobaric hypoxia predisposes to a coagulopathic state or that travel to high altitude is associated with an increased risk of thromboembolic events.

One important issue with all of these studies is that they tend to assess particular facets of the coagulation system, such as thrombin–antithrombin complexes, in isolation rather than looking at the function of this complex system as a whole. To address this issue, Martin et al. (2012) performed thromboelastography (TEG), a functional test that examines the kinetics of clot formation and is reflective of all aspects of the clotting system on healthy volunteers at sea level, 4250 m and 5300 m, and actually found evidence of slowed coagulation at high altitude compared to sea level.

In the end, the evidence regarding coagulation system function at high altitude remains inconsistent and no firm conclusions can be drawn regarding an increased risk of coagulopathy.

23.1.4 Prevention and management of thromboembolic events

In the absence of evidence of increased risk of thromboembolic events at high altitude, there is no indication for any forms of pharmacologic prophylaxis, such as aspirin or subcutaneous heparin when traveling in this environment, but all individuals should remain vigilant about maintaining adequate hydration and mobility. Individuals already on anticoagulation for prior diagnoses should continue their anticoagulation at high altitude. Those taking warfarin should arrange for follow up of their pro-time or international normalized ratio (INR) in the event of prolonged stay or upon return following a short stay at altitude, as a retrospective analysis has shown that a change in altitude may lead to deviations in the INR from the therapeutic range (Van Patot et al. 2006).

Patients who develop clinical evidence of thromboembolic disease should be evacuated to lower elevation as soon as feasible. While awaiting evacuation, supplemental oxygen should be administered to help improve tissue oxygen delivery, while anticoagulation with aspirin or low molecular weight heparin, agents that do not require any monitoring of therapeutic levels, can be considered when available. However, given that central nervous system findings may be due to hemorrhage rather than thrombosis, a distinction that is often difficult to make in the field, it would be prudent to hold anticoagulation in such cases until a more definitive evaluation is completed. Whether people who have had thromboembolic events at high altitude can safely return in the future is not known. The most conservative approach is to avoid any further high altitude travel.

23.2 OTHER NEUROLOGIC CONDITIONS

In addition to the cerebral arterial or venous thromboembolic events described above, a variety of other neurologic disorders have been described at high altitude that fall outside the definition of AMS. These disorders have been reviewed by Basnyat et al. (2004) and are considered further below.

23.2.1 Migraine

While it is tempting to attribute all headaches at high altitude to AMS, it is important to consider other potential causes in the differential diagnosis. Migraine headaches are common at sea level and, as a result, they can be expected to occur at altitude as well. Although anecdotal reports suggest high altitude may be a trigger for attacks (Hackett 2001), there is no systematic evidence of such a relationship and this remains a subject of debate (Bolay and Rapoport 2011). Several reports suggest the severity of attacks may be worse at altitude and may be attended by various transient, focal neurological defects (Jenzer and Bärtsch 1993; Murdoch 1995). Jenzer and Bärtsch (1993), for example, described a healthy 25-year-old mountaineer with known migraines at low altitude who experienced very severe headache together with some aphasia and sensory impairment of his tongue and right hand following a climb above 8000 m. Four years later, he had another episode, similar in many ways to the first. Both episodes lasted a number of hours and subsequent neurological tests, including computed tomography (CT) scans, were all

negative. Distinguishing a migraine headache from AMS at altitude may be challenging particularly in those with no prior history of migraines, but the presence of aura, similarity of symptoms to those of migraine headaches experienced at sea level and the presence of focal neurologic deficits should place this diagnosis high on the differential diagnosis.

23.2.2 Subarachnoid hemorrhage

Subarachnoid hemorrhage (SAH) is another potential cause of headache that could be confused with AMS in certain circumstances. Litch et al. (1997) reported the case of an individual who developed spontaneous SAH while descending from a trek to 4700 m in Nepal. Hackett (2001), for example, has described three patients at altitude with neurological defects, two of whom were subsequently shown to have cerebral arteriovenous malformations and the third, an aneurysm. Rupture of either of these vascular abnormalities should be easy to distinguish from AMS, as the presentation – rapid onset of a maximal severity of headache often with associated nausea, meningismus or mental status changes – is very distinct from the typical headache in AMS. Similarly, the rapid onset of mental status changes seen in SAH is very different to the more gradual onset of such changes in HACE. However, pressure from a large aneurysm or a small leak from a sentinel hemorrhage may cause more subtle symptoms that are harder to differentiate from AMS. It is unclear whether ascent to altitude is a risk factor for subarachnoid hemorrhage in those with aneurysms or arteriovenous malformations. Jehle et al. (1994) have shown evidence of an association between the incidence of subarachnoid hemorrhage and changes in barometric pressure associated with changes in weather, but no studies have established a relationship with the larger barometric pressure changes seen with ascent to high altitude. From a theoretical standpoint, increased cerebral blood flow or a rise in systemic blood pressure could serve as a trigger for vascular rupture, but there is no systematic evidence of this phenomenon.

23.2.3 Seizures

Seizures have been described in men and women over a wide age range ascending to a broad range of altitudes from 2500 to 7600 m, with generalized tonic–clonic seizures being more common than partial seizures (Maa 2011). They are not typically seen as part of AMS or HACE and, as a result, their occurrence should raise suspicion for a primary seizure process or another precipitating event (e.g. head trauma, meningitis) rather than acute altitude illness. Whether altitude hypoxia triggers seizures in patients with known seizure disorders or first time seizures in previously healthy individuals is not known. Potential mechanisms by which high altitude might trigger such events include direct effects of hypobaric hypoxia, sleep deprivation, hyperventilation and cerebral edema, although systematic evidence establishing these links is lacking at this time. The majority of seizures are self-limited and field management should focus on protecting the patient by clearing the area of hard objects, protecting the head from striking hard objects and keeping the mouth clear of any material. Seizures that do not cease spontaneously should be managed as they would at sea level with benzodiazepines being the first line of treatment if such medications are available. Upon cessation of the seizure, the affected individual should be started on supplemental oxygen and acetazolamide while efforts are made to evacuate to a lower elevation and/or medical facility. Further diagnostic work up is warranted following descent or arrival back at home (Maa 2011).

23.2.4 Space-occupying lesions

Shlim et al. (1991) reported three patients who were asymptomatic at low altitude, developed neurologic symptoms at altitude and were later found to have brain tumors, while Hackett (2000) reported a case of a man who suffered diplopia and ataxia on two occasions when he ascended from sea level to 4000 m and was later diagnosed with a left frontal subarachnoid cyst. The reason for symptom onset at high altitude may relate to subclinical brain edema at high altitude (Hackett 1999), although several magnetic resonance

imaging (MRI) studies suggest that increases in brain volume may not actually be responsible (Morocz et al. 2001; Fischer et al. 2004). Rather than diffuse cerebral edema, it may be hypoxia-induced perilesional edema that is responsible for increasing symptoms (Baumgartner et al. 2007), but the frequency of this phenomenon is too small to draw any firm conclusions.

23.2.5 Transient global amnesia

Transient global amnesia is a self-limited syndrome of severe forgetful confusion marked by retrograde amnesia and disorientation except for self-identity (Hodges and Warlow 1990). Litch and Bishop (1999) described two cases of this phenomenon in mountain climbers at altitudes of 3760 and 4400 m, which resolved with descents of 750 and 450 m, respectively, while Bucuk et al. (2008) have described an individual with recurrent episodes of this phenomenon while skiing in the Alps. The etiology of this phenomenon is not clear. None of the affected individuals had other features of altitude illness suggesting that cerebral edema was likely not responsible for the observed symptoms. Given earlier reports that certain aspects of cognitive function, including recall function, are affected by moderate hypoxia (Kennedy et al. 1989), Litch and Bishop have hypothesized that the problem may have related to hypoxia of the limbic cortex and temporal hippocampus, two important structures for memory, following hypocapnia-induced cerebral vasoconstriction (Litch and Bishop 1999; Litch and Bishop 2000).

23.2.6 Cranial nerve palsies

Isolated cranial nerve palsies, including the sixth cranial nerve, the facial nerve and the hypoglossal nerve, have all been documented at high altitude, with the lateral rectus palsy being the most widely reported abnormality (Virmani and Swamy 1993; Murdoch 1994; Shlim et al. 1995; Basnyat 2001). These findings are typically not associated with AMS and are only rarely seen in patients with HACE. Given the lack of diagnostic and therapeutic capabilities in many high altitude locations, onset of cranial nerve palsies should prompt evacuation to lower elevation. Resolution with descent suggests the palsy is due to high altitude hypoxia, but further evaluation is likely warranted to rule out an alternative etiology.

23.2.7 Cortical blindness and transient visual defects

Transient blindness has been reported in otherwise healthy individuals at terrestrial (Hackett et al. 1987c) and simulated (Houston 1987) high altitude. Hackett et al. (1987c) reported six cases of this phenomenon, including four climbers on Denali in Alaska and two trekkers at the Himalayan Rescue Association clinic in Pheriche, Nepal. None of the affected individuals had retinal hemorrhage or evidence of acute altitude illness. The blindness lasted from 20 min to 24 h, with intermittent periods of normal vision. Oxygen breathing led to symptom resolution and all individuals experienced a complete recovery. It was thought to be due to hypoxia or ischemia of the visual cortex.

23.3 EYE PROBLEMS AT HIGH ALTITUDE

In addition to the transient blindness described above that likely stems from problems in the cerebral cortex, there are several other ophthalmologic issues at high altitude that are more directly related to the eye itself.

23.3.1 High altitude retinopathy

CLINICAL FEATURES AND INCIDENCE

High altitude retinopathy (HAR) refers to a broad spectrum of retinal disorders, including dilated retinal veins and arteries, diffuse or punctate preretinal hemorrhages, vitreous hemorrhage, papillary hemorrhage, prepapillary hyperemia and papilledema that occur following ascent to high altitude. Graded on a scale from 1 (mild) to 4 (severe) based on the degree of retinal vein dilation and the number and location of retinal hemorrhages (Wiedman and Tabin 1999), HAR and, in particular retinal hemorrhages, have been documented extensively in the literature (Frayser et al. 1970; Rennie and Morrissey 1975; Clarke and Duff 1976; Wiedman and Tabin 1999; Barthelmes et al. 2011; Ho et al. 2011). The reported incidence varies from zero out of 10 climbers on an expedition to Mount Kongur (7719 m) in Xinjiang, China (Clark CRA, personal communication) to 94% of climbers on an expedition to Peak Communism (7495 m) in Russia (Nakashima 1983). In two larger, more recent studies, Wiedman and Tabin (1999) reported an incidence of HAR 74% in climbers ascending to between 4950 and 7600 m and 90% in those traveling above 7600 m, while Barthelmes et al. (2011) reported a retinal hemorrhage incidence of 78% among 28 climbers during an expedition to Muztagh Ata (7546 m). Hemorrhages may be observed during all stages of travel at high altitude. In fact, in the study by Barthelmes et al. (2011), during which retinal examinations were conducted at multiple points during the expedition, the majority of hemorrhages were detected following descent to base camp at the end of the expedition. The incidence was highest among those individuals who spent the greatest duration at altitude and ascended to the highest elevation. Data from Wiedman and Tabin (1999) suggested that high altitude retinopathy may correlate with development of HACE, but other studies have not found a significant relationship between retinopathy and the development of altitude illness (Rennie and Morrissey 1975; Barthelmes et al. 2011).

Most climbers who experience high altitude retinal hemorrhages are asymptomatic because the hemorrhages typically occur away from the macula. In fact, the only reason they are identified is that systematic attempts were made to examine the retinas of climbers in each of these studies. The hemorrhages are usually multiple, often flame shaped and adjacent to a vessel (Fig. 23.1). Although lack of symptoms is the norm with these hemorrhages, vision loss can, in fact, occur, if hemorrhages involve the macular region (Wiedman and Tabin 1999; Ho et al. 2011).

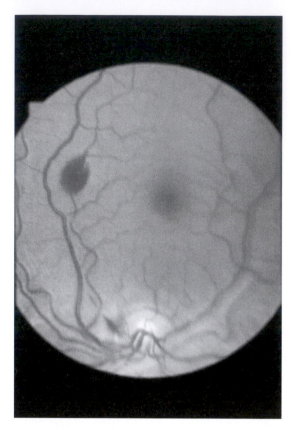

Figure 23.1 Retinal hemorrhage at altitude.

MECHANISM OF RETINAL HEMORRHAGE

The precise etiology of retinal hemorrhages is not clear. Increased cerebral blood flow (Severinghaus *et al.* 1966a) and, in particular, increased blood flow through the retinal vessels may play an important role. Frayser *et al.* (1970), for example, have shown that blood flow through the retinal vessels is increased by 105%, while Renney and Morrisey (1975) found increases in arterial and venous diameter of 24% and 19%, respectively. In the setting of increased flow and vascular dilation, any sudden increase in vascular pressure due to coughing or straining, for example, may cause microvascular rupture. However, Sakaguchi and Yurugi (1983) have produced retinal hemorrhage in animals in a chamber study when cough was presumably absent. In their study on Muztagh Ata, Barthelmes *et al.* (2011) found that increases in hematocrit correlated positively with the number of hemorrhages leading them to suggest that increased blood viscosity might increase shear stress in dilated vessels with altered endothelial integrity, thereby leading to hemorrhage.

MANAGEMENT

Individuals who develop vision loss at high altitude should descend as soon as feasible. Symptomatic hemorrhages typically resolve spontaneously over a matter of weeks at sea level, although several cases of permanent vision loss have been described (Shults and Swan 1975; McFadden *et al.* 1981). Climbers with symptomatic retinopathy have returned to summit 8000 m peaks (Mader and Tobin 2003). Whether this is safe remains a matter of debate, however, and some have argued that macular hemorrhages or any retinopathy associated with vision changes should be viewed as a contraindication to further ascent (Mader and Tobin 2003).

23.3.2 Corneal issues

CORNEAL THICKNESS

The cornea receives the bulk of its oxygen supply by diffusion directly from the environment with only a small proportion coming as a result of diffusion from the aqueous humor of the anterior chamber (Klyce 1981). As a result, when ambient oxygen tensions decrease upon ascent to high altitude, corneal oxygen supply decreases leading, in turn, to increased corneal thickness. Bosch *et al.* (2010), for example, studied climbers on Muztagh Ata (7546 m) and found that central corneal thickness increased by 13% upon ascent, but decreased rapidly following descent. Similarly, Morris *et al.* (2007) reported an increase in central corneal thickness from 543 µm at sea level to 561 µm on the first day at 5200 m, noting that this parameter continued to increase with time at the same elevation, as well as was significant inter-individual variability in the observed responses.

The precise mechanism for this observed change is not clear, but may relate to an increase in anaerobic metabolism in the cornea in response to hypoxia which leads to increased lactate concentrations in the corneal stroma and an influx of water due to altered osmotic forces. Coupled with reduced activity of the endothelial pumps, this leads to water accumulation and the subsequent thickening of the cornea. In their study on Muztagh Ata, Bosch *et al.* (2010) did find that those individuals who undertook a slower ascent profile and had higher oxygen saturations had less thickening of the cornea, leading them to suggest that systemic delivery of oxygen to the anterior chamber and diffusion of that oxygen to the cornea may provide some protective effect against the processes described above at high altitude.

The observed increases in corneal thickness do not appear to have any effect on visual acuity in normal individuals or those with myopia (Bosch *et al.*, 2010) but, as discussed further below, may have adverse effects on individuals who have undergone refractive surgery.

23.3.3 Intraocular pressure

The effect of high altitude exposure on intraocular pressure (IOP) remains unclear as various studies have reported an increase, decrease or no change in this parameter (Brinchmann-Hansen and Myhre 1989; Bayer *et al.* 2004; Ersanli *et al.* 2006). The discrepant results may be due to a variety of factors, such as failure of most studies to correct for changes in corneal thickness, differences in measurement techniques, altitudes attained and confounding effects of exercise and cold exposure. Somner *et al.* (2007) corrected for many of these issues in their study of 76 individuals as part of a non-exertional ascent to 5200 m in Bolivia and documented a statistically significant, but clinically insignificant increase in IOP from 11.4 ± 3 at sea level to 12.4 ± 3.2 mmHg at 5200 m. IOP declined over subsequent days at the same elevation, eventually falling below sea level values by day 7. The observed changes bore no relationship to the development of AMS or high altitude retinopathy.

There is no evidence that high altitude exposure worsens open angle glaucoma or provokes episodes of acute narrow angle glaucoma, although the hypoxia at high altitude could increase optic nerve damage in patients with elevated IOP at the time of their sojourn. If taken for acute altitude illness prophylaxis, acetazolamide will have the added benefit of decreasing intraocular fluid production and thereby helping limit any rises in IOP (Mader and Tabin 2003).

23.3.4 Dry eye syndrome

Dry eye syndrome is a common condition resulting from decreased tear production. Because it can be exacerbated by environmental conditions commonly seen at high altitude, including dry air, wind and glare, it is expected that many climbers and trekkers may experience this problem. Symptoms vary according to how dry the eyes become and include minor irritation, burning, foreign body sensation, light sensitivity and blurred vision (Mader and Tabin 2003). In all but the most severe cases, topical tear substitute eye drops and lubricating ointments are sufficient to treat dry eye symptoms, although high altitude travelers must pay attention to their choice of preparation. Because artificial tear preparations contain preservatives they can be reused after opening, although the preservatives themselves can cause irritation. Preservative-free preparations may avoid this problem but are prone to bacterial contamination and can only be used for 24 hours after opening. Additional protection against this problem can be attained by using wrap-around goggles that protect the eye from wind, dust and ultraviolet light and may also increase the humidity around the cornea (Mader and Tabin 2003).

23.3.5 Ultraviolet keratitis

Just as it can cause sunburn, excessive sun exposure can cause damage to the epithelial layer of the inadequately protected eye. At high altitude, the risk of such damage is significantly increased and the time-frame over which it can occur is significantly shortened as a result of the significant increase in ultraviolet light exposure as one moves higher in elevation, particularly when traveling in snow-covered terrain. Symptoms of ultraviolet keratitis, commonly referred to as 'snow blindness,' vary according to the severity of injury and include irritation, burning, foreign body sensation, increased tearing, photophobia and blurry vision. Sunglasses that protect against both UVA and UVB light are the single best way to prevent this problem, with the highest level of protection being provided by those glasses that either wrap around the lateral aspects of the orbits or include side shields. Affected individuals should use eyeglasses to protect against further injury and apply topical antibiotics to prevent bacterial superinfection. Topical scopolamine can be used for pain control in addition to systemically delivered analgesics. In severe cases, patching of one or both eyes may be necessary on a short-term basis. Symptoms typically resolve in 24–48 hours as the epithelium regenerates (Butler 2007).

23.3.6 Refractive errors, eyeglasses and contact lenses

Unless an individual has had corrective surgery and is traveling at moderate to extreme altitudes, the hypoxia at high altitude will not affect visual acuity or pre-existing refractive errors. Those individuals with refractive errors who rely on glasses or contact lenses need to consider the effect of the wilderness environment on their ability to maintain ocular hygiene and prevent significant ultraviolet exposure. The problems with glasses are obvious and most mountaineers will have found their own solutions, including prescription glacier glasses or contact lenses. A full discussion of the risks and benefits of different types of contact lenses is beyond the scope of this chapter and is provided in the review by Mader and Tabin (2003). Contact lens users must be aware of the increased risk of bacterial keratitis and the consequences of such a problem in a remote environment and, as a result, should travel with topical antibiotic drops and know how to recognize this problem.

23.3.7 Surgery for refractory errors: radial keratotomy, LASIK and photorefractive keratectomy

Three surgical procedures have been used to correct refractive errors and obviate the need for glasses and contact lenses. In radial keratotomy (RK), four to eight radial incisions are made at 90% depth in the periphery of the cornea, leading

to a change in the refractive error of the lens. In photorefractive keratectomy (PRK), a laser is used to reduce corneal curvature and create refractive changes directly on the corneal surface while in laser-assisted in situ keratomeliusis (LASIK), a thin flap is created in the cornea and lifted in order that an excimer laser can then reshape corneal stroma (Mader and Tabin 2003). Because each procedure alters the normal structure of the cornea and, as noted above, hypoxia induces corneal changes at high altitude, concern has been raised about whether travel to high altitude predisposes to visual complications in individuals who have had these procedures.

Several studies have shown that RK corneas are susceptible to problems at high altitude. Mader and White (1995), for example, compared four normal corneas with four that had undergone RK at 3658 and 5182 m. They found that the refractive error changed to 20.59 diopter and 21.75 diopters at 3658 and 5182 m, respectively, in the RK corneas, but saw no changes in the normal corneas. Mader et al. (1996) subsequently studied six subjects with RK, six with PRK and nine with myopia over a 3-day period at 4300 m and noted no change in refraction in the subjects with myopia or PRK, but significant changes in refraction in those who underwent RK. These changes occur because the peripheral corneal incisions in RK weaken the cornea in such a way that hypoxia causes preferential expansion in the periphery of the cornea that, in turn, causes flattening of the central cornea and subsequent hyperopic (far-sighted) shift (Winkle et al. 1998; Mader and Tabin 2003). Of note, the changes generally occur 24 hours or more following high altitude exposure and may be worsened during sleep when the eyelids are closed and the cornea is under increased hypoxic stress. This may result in a false sense of security for a climber with RK corneas who arrives at high altitude and initially has intact vision.

LASIK corneas are also at risk for vision changes at high altitude. Dimmig and Tabin (2003), for example, examined 12 LASIK-treated eyes in six climbers ascending Mt Everest, all of whom had 20/20 or better vision at sea level. Vision was maintained at 5365 m. One of the six climbers noted blurred vision above base camp that improved with descent, while two climbers noted problems at 8200 and 8600 m, respectively, that also improved with descent. Similarly, Boes *et al.* (2001) have documented decreased visual acuity in two climbers on Aconcagua (6963 m) that worsened with increasing altitude and declining oxygen saturation, but resolved with descent, although in one of the climbers full resolution required several weeks.

Of the three procedures, only PRK is thought to be without problems at high altitude as hypoxia causes uniform thickening of the PRK corneas, which preserves the shape of the corneal surface and, as a result, does not lead to myopic shifts (Mader *et al.* 1996; Mader and Tabin 2003).

There is an element of unpredictability to the vision changes seen following RK and LASIK at altitude and other factors including cold, drying of the cornea, duration and extent of high altitude exposure, the degree of refractive error remaining after surgery and time since surgery will affect the likelihood of any problems. For this reason, all climbers who have undergone these procedures should be prepared for problems at high altitude and should travel with back-up pairs of eyeglasses with plus lenses. Because it is hard to predict how much lens power will be needed ahead of time, it may be necessary to travel with multiple pairs of glasses (Mader and Tabin 2003).

23.4 HIGH ALTITUDE COUGH

It has been common knowledge among mountaineers that cough is a problem at high altitude, especially with ascents to extreme altitude. This is well demonstrated in Joe Tasker's account from a winter expedition on Everest's west ridge:

> Alan (Rouse) ... was still racked by frequent coughs and periodically, as if by auto-suggestion I found that I too was succumbing to a bout. Once started, there was no escape. The cold dry air compounded the irritation in the throat and the victim's body would be shaken by the hacking cough until randomly flung free of its spell. The nights

at Base Camp as well as on the mountain were often punctuated by staccato bursts of noise disturbing the sleep of the sufferer and all those around.

Tasker (1981)

This problem is exceedingly common. In a study of 283 trekkers in the Everest region of Nepal, for example, 42% of those surveyed reported having a cough (Murdoch 1995). Despite the high prevalence and its potential to cause debilitating symptoms, including rib fractures (Steele 1971), the phenomenon of high altitude cough attracted no scientific study, until Barry *et al.* (1997a) studied the issue on the British Mount Everest Medical Expedition (BMEME) in 1994. Using voice-activated tape recorders they demonstrated an increase in nocturnal cough frequency with increasing altitude, including marked increases at extreme elevations. Two of the three climbers studied experienced over 60 coughs/night at 7000 m, nearly two times higher than the highest values recorded at 5000–6000 m.

23.4.1 Mechanism

It has been generally assumed that altitude cough results from the cooling and drying of the upper airway mucosa due to hyperventilation in cold, dry air at altitude. However, anecdotal reports from Operation Everest II and systematic studies from Operation Everest III cast doubt on this theory by demonstrating that cough increased with altitude even though the air temperature and humidity were well controlled in these chamber experiments (Mason *et al.* 1999).

Identifying the precise causal mechanism has proved difficult, however. A common measure of cough sensitivity is the citric acid cough threshold test in which a subject is given increasing concentrations of nebulized citric acid and the concentration that first provokes a cough is noted. Multiple studies have shown that this threshold is reduced at high altitude (Barry *et al.* 1997a; Mason *et al.* 2009; Thompson *et al.* 2009) and that the response can be blunted with administration of salmeterol and nedocromyl (Bakewell *et al.* 1999), although observed changes have not always been associated with a change in cough frequency (Bakewell *et al.* 1999; Mason 2009). While the threshold does appear to decrease with increasing altitude, the mechanism behind the observed changes remains unclear. Earlier studies demonstrating a relationship between ventilatory responses to carbon dioxide and changes in the citric acid cough threshold (Banner 1988; Barry *et al.* 1997b) suggested a possible role for central mechanisms, but a more recent study cast doubt on this argument after finding no relationship between the threshold and hypercapnic ventilatory responses (Thompson 2009). Neuroendocrine mechanisms have also been proposed, but Mason *et al.* (2009) found no relationship between observed changes in citric acid cough threshold and changes in plasma bradykinin concentrations.

One difficulty with identifying a causal mechanism may lie in the fact that cough is probably not a uniform phenomenon at high altitude. Some individuals may have persistent cough due to a viral syndrome that is slow to resolve at high altitude, while others may cough due to exercise-induced bronchoconstriction or subclinical pulmonary edema. In a review of cough at high altitude, Mason and Barry (2007) proposed two distinct forms of cough based on the altitude at which the individual is traveling: a cough at lower altitudes that is related to exercise, persists with descent and is likely due to injury to the respiratory mucosa and a cough occurring at altitudes greater than 5000–6000 m which improves with descent, is independent of the cold, dry air and likely stems from subclinical pulmonary edema or altered central control mechanisms.

23.4.2 Treatment

Perhaps the most difficult aspect of cough for those experiencing it at altitude is the lack of proven therapeutic strategies. Inhaled corticosteroids and beta-agonists, antihistamines, throat lozenges, codeine and breathing through balaclavas have all been tried, but there is no systematic evidence demonstrating clinical benefit (Mason and Barry 2007). Antibiotic use should

be discouraged unless there is clear evidence of pneumonia and, provided that dangerous causes such as HAPE can be ruled out, the best treatment may be reassurance that the problem will resolve with descent. In some cases, the cough persists for several days following descent. Coughs lasting greater than 1–2 weeks following descent, however, should prompt evaluation for an alternative etiology.

23.5 ANESTHESIA AT HIGH ALTITUDE

Many serious medical issues that occur on climbing or trekking expeditions or at remote clinic sites at high altitude will be managed by evacuating the affected individual to lower elevation. In some cases, however, an acute problem will need to be managed without evacuation and may even require surgical intervention and possibly general anesthesia. This is demonstrated in a report by Grocott and Johannson (2007) of a woman who presented in postpartum hemorrhagic shock at 4240 m and required immediate management with ketamine anesthesia to control the source of her hemorrhage. Providers in such situations or individuals working as part of medical missions providing surgical services in high altitude facilities must be aware of unique issues that will arise in anesthetic management in this environment in order to avoid important complications.

23.5.1 Increased risk of hypoxia

During anesthesia with spontaneous ventilation, minute ventilation and, therefore, alveolar ventilation will be reduced to levels lower than appropriate for metabolic demand. Together with an increase in the alveolar–arterial oxygen difference equivalent to a shunt fraction of about 10%, this will contribute to the development of arterial hypoxemia in patients receiving anesthesia while breathing ambient air. The risk of hypoxemia is further increased by the fact that anesthesia will abolish the peripheral chemoreceptor response to hypoxia (Knill and Celb 1978). Because the peripheral chemoreceptors are severely depressed by as little as one-tenth of the anesthetic concentration of volatile anesthetic agents, this particular problem may persist well into the postoperative period and careful monitoring will still be necessary following the conclusion of any procedure. Finally, because the oxygen reservoir in the lungs at functional residual capacity is reduced compared to sea level, patients will be prone to rapid onset of hypoxemia with induction of anesthesia and onset of apnea during endotracheal intubation. To avoid these problems, the inspired oxygen concentration for the anesthetized patient at high altitude should be increased in accordance with the altitude at which the procedure is being performed (Table 23.1). Monitoring of oxygen saturation by pulse oximetry during and after any administration of anesthetic is absolutely essential.

23.5.2 Equipment issues

Several important issues may also arise with monitoring and other equipment used in the administration of an anesthetic. Floating ball or floating bobbin oxygen flow meters tend to underestimate the actual flow rate and, as a result, oxygen analyzers may be more appropriate for use at high altitude (Leissner and Mahmood 2009). Capnographs commonly used to monitor the adequacy of ventilation also malfunction at altitude due to the effects of decreased air density into the sampling chamber and the effects of lower barometric pressure on device calibration and the computer software (Pattinson et al. 2004). Particular anesthetic vaporizers (Datex Ohmeda Tec 6 and Tec 6-Plus) will require manual adjustments of the concentration control dial in order to maintain constant partial pressures of gaseous anesthetics, an important issue given that the potency of these agents is a function of their partial pressure (Leissner and Mahmood 2009). Finally, pressures in air-filled endotracheal tube cuffs or laryngeal mask airways may vary if patients are transported between altitudes with these devices in situ, leading to either significant air leaks or an increased risk of injury to the tracheal mucosa (Leissner and Mahmood 2009).

23.5.3 Choice of anesthetic agent

Although commonly used at sea level, nitrous oxide should be avoided at high altitude as it causes less analgesia and has lower potency in this environment due to the reduction in partial pressure resulting from the lower barometric pressure, a problem that is exacerbated when increasing inspired oxygen concentrations are used to prevent the onset of hypoxemia (James et al. 1982). The potency of volatile anesthetic vapors, such as halothane, is also a function of their partial pressure but, unlike nitrous oxide, the partial pressure of these agents does not vary with barometric pressure and is, instead, a function of temperature. As a result, with the exception of desflurane, these agents can be delivered at a constant potency as long as constant temperature is maintained, regardless of the altitude (Leissner and Mahmood 2009).

Propofol is a widely used anesthetic agent at sea level, but has not been studied in unacclimatized lowlanders undergoing a procedure at high altitude. Puri et al. (2008) studied responses to

Table 23.1 Minimal concentrations of oxygen in the inspired gas required to maintain a normal arterial PO_2 in the anesthetized patient

Altitude (m)	P_B (mmHg)	Oxygen concentration (%)	P_IO_2 (mmHg)
Sea level	760	40	285
2000	596	54	296
4000	462	72	298
6000	354	100	307

P_B, atmospheric pressure; P_IO_2, partial pressure of inspired oxygen.

the medication in native highlanders and showed that higher doses were necessary to achieve a target level of sedation (assessed by the bispectral index) when compared with native lowlanders. Diazepam and temazepam, long- and short-acting benzodiazepines, respectively, have been associated with ventilatory depression following administration in unacclimatized lowlanders (Roggla *et al.* 1994; Roggla *et al.* 2000). Ketamine is an appealing alternative for anesthesia at high altitude because at low doses (~2 mg/kg) it does not suppress the hypoxic ventilatory response or interfere with pharyngeal and laryngeal reflexes. Bishop *et al.* (2000) reported a series of 11 hemodynamically stable patients who underwent procedures with ketamine anesthesia at 3900 m in Nepal. Following premedication with atropine and midazolam, primary care physicians with no training in anesthesia administered 1 mg/kg of ketamine over 1–2 minutes. There were no adverse hemodynamic events and only three of the 11 patients, including two lowlanders,

required supplemental oxygen when their oxygen saturation fell below 80%. In the highest documented use of ketamine to date, Grocott and Johannson (2007) administered ketamine to the post-partum hemorrhagic shock patient at 4240 m described above. Unlike the patients in the series by Bishop *et al.* (2000), this patient did become apneic despite receiving an analgesic dose of only 0.5 mg/kg, which they attributed to the fact that she was hypoxemic and in hemodynamic shock at the time of her anesthesia.

The onset of apnea in this case despite the relatively low dose of ketamine serves as a useful reminder of the difficulties of administering anesthesia in a remote, high altitude environment. When possible, patients should be evacuated to lower elevation for definitive management of surgical issues. Aggressive interventions and the use of anesthetic agents should be reserved for those situations where life and limb are at stake and the benefits of anesthesia and surgical intervention outweigh the risks.

24

Physiology and medical aspects of heat and cold

SUMMARY

This chapter deals briefly with the physiology and pathology of heat and cold. Thermal balance, the difference between heat gain and heat loss, determines our body temperature. The various components of this balance are discussed and the ways that the body defends itself in hot and cold conditions. The processes of acclimatization and adaptation to either heat or cold are also considered.

The pathology of heat includes the effect on the whole body, heat lassitude and hyperthermia and locally, sunburn, snow blindness and prickly heat.

The body's response to cold is discussed and the pathology of cold affecting the whole body, hypothermia and locally, frostbite and non-freezing cold injury (trench foot); their diagnosis and management are addressed. However, for a more detailed account of this topic, the reader is referred to larger textbooks such as *Wilderness medicine* (Auerbach 2012).

24.1 HEAT: INTRODUCTION

The traveler, if from a cool climate, is at risk of medical problems when he or she goes to a hot climate. In these days of rapid transport, the change from cool to hot climate can be very abrupt with no time for heat acclimatization and this situation increases the risk for the newly arrived traveler. There is a variety of illnesses associated with heat from the relatively trivial, prickly heat and mild sunburn to the lethal, heat stroke. One might suppose that the mountaineer or visitor to high altitude would not be at risk of heat problems but apart from the fact that the approach to mountains is often through tropical or subtropical lowlands, the mountain environment can be hot. The great ranges are mainly at low latitudes with the sun high in the sky. At altitude, there is less air to filter out the solar radiation and snow reflects this back on a climber, further increasing the heat load. Finally, having started out in the cold early morning dressed in high insulating clothes and exercising quite hard, the climber is at real risk of suffering from overheating, dehydration and salt depletion.

The effects of sunlight in causing sunburn and snow blindness are obviously of importance to mountaineers and travelers to altitude.

24.2 HEAT: THERMAL BALANCE

Humans, like all warm-blooded animals, maintain a constant internal temperature unless the limits of their thermoregulatory systems are exceeded. These mechanisms are both physiological and technical. The technical include clothing, shelter and heating or cooling of our environment. The physiological mechanisms include regulation of blood flow to the skin, sweating and shivering. In considering the problem for subjects in a hot environment, we need to consider, on the one hand, the factors tending to make for a rise in temperature, the heat gain; and, on the other, the ways in which the body can reduce the temperature: the heat loss. The balance of heat gain and heat loss determines the temperature of the body.

24.2.1 Heat gain

Heat gain is from either external or internal sources. Externally, heat is gained via convection, conduction and radiation. The important factors are the ambient temperature and solar radiation. Internally, heat is gained as a byproduct of metabolism. At rest between 272 and 355 kJ h^{-1} (65 and 85 kcal h^{-1}) are gained from this source, but even moderate exercise raises this to 1.25–2.5 MJ h^{-1} (300–600 kcal h^{-1}). Solar radiation can add up to about 630 kJ h^{-1} (150 kcal h^{-1}).

24.2.2 Heat loss

In hot climates, it is important that heat is lost from the body down a heat gradient into the environment. Heat is lost to the environment by convection, conduction, radiation and evaporation of sweat. Normally about 65% (170–210 kJ h^{-1} (40–50 kcal h^{-1})) of heat loss is by radiation from the body to air. This depends upon the air temperature and, when the air

temperature reaches 37°C, no heat loss takes place by this mechanism. Evaporative heat loss is very important in hot climates. For every liter of sweat evaporated, 2.5 MJ (600 kcal) of heat are lost (though not all comes from the subject). However, the efficiency of sweating depends upon the humidity of the air, becoming less efficient as the humidity and temperature rise, until at 37°C and 100% humidity no evaporation can take place. At more normal humidity levels, air movement increases the rate of evaporation, hence the beneficial effect of fans in hot climates. Note that sweat that drips off the body rather than evaporating is wasted from the point of view of heat loss. The effect of sweating is to lose water and salt leading to dehydration and salt depletion if not replaced.

24.3 HEAT ACCLIMATIZATION

The human body can acclimatize to heat to some degree. Most of the research has been carried out in fit young subjects in whom a program of increasing exercise has been prescribed after an abrupt change from a cool to a hot climate. Under these conditions, it has been possible to demonstrate changes in a number of physiological systems which together mitigate the effects of high ambient temperature on physical performance. These changes take place over the first 2 weeks and are enhanced by exercise. The changes include:

- Increase in aldosterone levels leading to conservation of salt
- The reduction in the salt content of sweat
- Lowering of the temperature at which sweating starts
- Increase in sweat rates up to twice the unacclimatized rate
- Increase in the plasma volume and cardiac output.

This last adaptation allows a greater increase in skin blood flow, which increases heat transfer to the skin and increased heat loss (Armstrong and Maresh 1991).

These changes help to dissipate heat when the subject is under a heat load and reduce the risk of illnesses due to heat stress. The converse is that before acclimatization has occurred, during the first few days in a hot climate, travelers are rightly advised to avoid exercise, especially in the heat of the middle of the day.

24.4 HEAT ILLNESSES

Heat illness occurs when heat gain is greater than the subject is accustomed to. The onset is in the setting of high environmental temperature for some hours; often the patient has recently arrived in a hot country. High humidity, direct sunshine and especially exercise are aggravating factors.

There are three degrees or stages of heat illness:

1. Lassitude, heat cramps, syncope
2. Heat exhaustion
3. Heat stroke.

24.4.1 Lassitude, heat cramps or syncope

The subject feels lethargic and may have muscle cramps, often in the calves or thighs. Part of the mechanism is probably dehydration and/or salt depletion. The body temperature is normal. The treatment is the same as for heat exhaustion (see below).

24.4.2 Heat exhaustion

This is a further stage of heat illness. The setting is the same as above; often the patient has been exercising in the heat. He/she complains of weakness, faintness, anorexia, nausea, vomiting and muscle cramps. There may be flu-like symptoms. The skin is often pale and moist, or frankly sweaty. The body temperature is normal and there are no central nervous system (CNS) signs. In cases which have developed in a short time, hours or a day, dehydration is likely to be dominant, whereas in cases developing over a number of days, especially if water has been taken but little salt, salt depletion is likely to be more important. Often both are present and require correction.

Management consists of rest, reducing the heat gain, getting the patient out of the sun and into as cool a place as possible, then to replace salt and water as appropriate. One teaspoonful of salt to a liter of water is a reasonable domestic remedy. Both these stages of heat illness normally recover quickly and completely, though the patient may have a headache for a day or two.

24.4.3 Heat stroke, hyperthermia

Heat stroke is a true life-threatening medical emergency. In the 2003 heat wave in France, mortality in 345 patients admitted to intensive care, was 62.6% (Misset *et al.* 2006). The setting is the same as for heat exhaustion but with continued, more severe heat stress. The crucial difference from heat exhaustion is that the body temperature is elevated to 40°C or above. If the rise is to above 42°C for more than 45 minutes, there is danger of permanent brain damage or death (Bouchama and Knochel 2002). This explains the urgency of making the diagnosis and starting treatment.

The progression of the condition is due to the breakdown of the body's thermoregulation and the cessation of sweating. It is this cessation of sweating that triggers the rapid rise in temperature if the heat stress continues and is a very serious clinical sign. Mustafa *et al.* (2003) have shown that rabbit carotid artery responded to being heated above 37°C by vasoconstriction, which might lead to cerebral ischemia and may be part of the mechanism for heat stroke.

The clinical picture is of a patient in the setting of a high heat load who has stopped sweating. The skin, instead of being pale, cool and sweaty becomes red, hot and dry. The patient becomes confused, uncoordinated, and drowsy, and then loses consciousness. The body temperature will be found to be between 40 and 47°C. Seizures may occur during cooling. There is tachycardia and hyperventilation with $Paco_2$ often less than 20 mmHg. A quarter of patients have hypotension.

24.4.4 Primary treatment of heat stroke

The essential of treatment is to reduce the heat stress and institute cooling by whatever means are available as quickly as possible. Cooling is best effected by immersing the patient in cold water if available (Casa *et al.* 2007), or by wetting the skin and evaporating it by air movement. Water can be sprayed and fans played on the patient. Circumstances will dictate the method used, but speed is more important than sophistication. Ice packs, if available, can be used placed over superficial arteries, e.g. in the groin and axilla but, compared with a cold water bath or evaporative heat loss, are relatively inefficient. After initial treatment, it is important to admit the patient to hospital in order to be able to deal with possible complications.

24.4.5 Secondary care

On investigation in hospital, there will usually be found both respiratory alkalosis and lactic acidosis (Bouchama and De Vol 2001). Hypercalcemia and hyperproteinemia are common and reflect hemoconcentration. Hypophosphatemia and hypokalemia are also common, although hypoglycemia is rare. Rhabdomyolysis and hyperkalemia may be a problem after cooling (Knochel 1989). The most serious complications after initial treatment are those of multi-organ failure including encephalopathy, kidney or liver failure, myocardial infarction, intestinal ischemia and disseminated intravascular clotting (Bouchama and Knochel 2002).

24.5 LOCAL EFFECTS OF A HOT CLIMATE

24.5.1 Sunburn

Sunburn is caused by ultraviolet radiation, mainly by the shorter wave UV-B, 290–320 nm (Diffey 1991). It is an acute inflammatory reaction after excessive exposure to the sun. The reason that many patients are taken unawares by sunburn is that, by the time the skin reddens, the damage has been done and the burn will develop over the next few hours. There is great variation in susceptibility to sunburn depending upon the type of skin the individual has, mainly the degree

of pigmentation. Blond, blue-eyed subjects or redheads are many times more susceptible than well-pigmented black individuals. The former can burn after as little as 15 minutes in the tropical midday sun. Acquiring a tan provides some protection from sunburn, but it only increases tolerance by a factor of 2 or 3. More important in light-skinned people is the thickening of the stratum corneum of skin by sunlight exposure (Diffey 1991). Both tanning and thickening regress over a month or so of no exposure. Factors that influence the radiation load include:

- The height of the sun, time of day (75% of radiation arrives between 9 a.m. and 3 p.m.) (Diffey 1991).
- The latitude and time of year.
- Cloud cover or haze, although this can be deceptive since ultraviolet radiation is filtered less by cloud than is visible light so one can become sunburnt under light cloud cover.
- Type of terrain, which determines the reflected solar load. Snow and ice, for instance, reflect 80% of the radiation compared with 20% from sand.
- Altitude. Roughly, there is a 6% increase in radiation for every 1000 m gain in altitude (Diffey 1991).

CLINICAL PICTURE

In the setting of recent exposure to the sun, an erythema develops after 2–6 h and reaches a maximum at 12–24 h. There is a burning pain in the affected part, possibly fever, malaise and even nausea and vomiting in severe cases. The skin may go on to blister formation. The condition resolves in 4–7 days usually with peeling.

The possibility of photosensitizing drugs needs to be borne in mind. Drugs can cause either photoallergic dermatitis or just an increase in sensitivity to sunburn. There is a long list of drugs that have been reported as causing photosensitivity, but the ones most likely to be encountered in the mountain or wilderness settings are probably the tetracyclines, especially demeclocycline and doxycycline (travelers may be on this for malaria prophylaxis); quinine, topical non-steroidal anti-inflammatory drugs (NSAIDs), diuretics such as bendrofluazide, oral hypoglycemic agents and antidepressants. Sulfonamides can cause photosensitivity, but are rarely used now apart from acetazolamide. Photosensitivity is listed as a rare side effect of this drug.

TREATMENT

Most cases do not require any active treatment. Simple pain relief (paracetamol or NSAIDs) can be given. There has been debate about the efficacy of topical steroids in relieving the pain and inflammation of sunburn, but a recent controlled trial has shown two commonly used ointments to be effective (Duteil *et al.* 2002). It would seem reasonable, therefore, to use a topical steroid in cases of significant sunburn.

More severe cases may require rehydration and salt replacement and may indeed have heat exhaustion as well (see section 24.4.2). If blistering is extensive, the danger of secondary infection needs to be considered.

PREVENTION

Prevention is achieved by avoiding excessive solar radiation. The danger is particularly during midday. Travelers should either keep out of the sun or cover up with clothes, hats, etc., or apply adequate sunscreens to exposed skin areas. The latter should be of sufficient 'factor', e.g. 30, and applied liberally. If swimming, the screen should be waterproof.

LATE EFFECTS

The late effects of sunburn should not be ignored. They include an increased risk of developing skin cancers, including melanomas.

24.5.2 Snow blindness (photophthalmia, photokeratitis, ultraviolet keratitis)

Snow blindness is sunburn or inflammation of the cornea and conjunctiva due to ultraviolet light of wavelength 200–400 nm. At altitude, this makes up 5–6% of solar radiation, compared with 1–2% at sea level. Snow reflects 80% of light waves and the eyes are particularly vulnerable.

ACUTE

Within a few hours, the epithelial cells of the cornea die. There is loss of surface adhesion and the cells are brushed off the cornea by the mechanical act of blinking. The corneal nerve endings are then exposed. Within about 4 h, symptoms are felt that range from a feeling of 'grit in the eye' to excruciating pain and sensitivity to light. The slightest eye movement causes spasm of the eyelids, pupillary vasoconstriction, eye pain and headache. There is conjunctival inflammation, the eyelids are swollen and the secretion of tears profuse. The condition lasts 6–8 h and disappears in 48 h.

Treatment

Treatment includes cold compresses, an eye patch to exclude light, and the avoidance of light. The pupils should be dilated with atropine, or cyclopentolate eye drops and an ocular antibiotic used in case corneal ulceration occurs. Analgesics may be necessary, but anesthetic eye drops should not be used except for an eye examination because they may slow healing. Non-steroidal anti-inflammatory eye drops have been used, but strict evidence for their efficacy is lacking. Contact lenses should be removed.

CHRONIC

Chronic snow blindness occurs in those inhabitants of mountainous and snowy regions over a long period. Visual disturbances, with sensitivity to light and chronic conjunctival inflammation, are reported.

PREVENTION

Inhabitants of mountainous and Arctic regions have used primitive prevention methods for centuries. These include yak wool and hair pulled forward over the eyes, slits in wood, or cardboard strapped to the head. The Inuit of northern Canada have used goggles made from bone as shown in Fig. 24.1.

Glasses or goggles with lenses that cut out radiation of wavelength 250–400 nm are normally used for protection. The quality of the lens is important, and it can be made of plastic or glass. The main advantage of plastic is that it is lightweight and unbreakable, but it does not filter out all the ultraviolet light; glass is heavier, but filters out most of the ultraviolet light. Ideally, the external surface is mirror finished to reflect light, and the internal surface should not reflect light onto the cornea. Frames should have side and nasal shields for protection against sun, and a safety cord may be attached.

A consensus statement from the International Mountain Emergency Medicine Commision (Ellerton *et al.* 2009) recommends that snow goggles should have:

- Ultraviolet light absorption of 99–100%.
- Visible light transmittance of 5–10%.
- Lens material should be of polycarbonate or CR-39 glass.
- Grey lens color to reduce distortion of color perception.
- Frame design should be robust, have side shields or wrap-around design, lightweight and securely attached to the face.
- Carrying case should be rigid, to protect glasses when not in use.

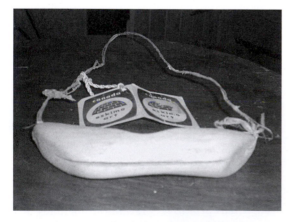

Figure 24.1 Traditional Inuit goggles made from bone used to prevent snow blindness.

A spare pair of glasses or goggles should always be carried. Goggles should have adequate ventilation to stop them steaming up (Lomax *et al.* 1991; Petetin 1991).

24.5.3 Prickly heat (miliaria rubra)

Prickly heat is a condition in which the sweat glands become blocked due to a hot humid climate. Clinically, the sufferer has an acute papulo-vesicular eruption, usually on the trunk and in the skin flexures, groin, axilla, under pendulous breasts, etc. There is a prickling sensation, hence the name, there may be itching and the patient feels the need to scratch. This may lead to secondary infection. It especially affects children, though all ages and both sexes can be susceptible.

Treatment is palliative since the condition is eventually self-limiting. Calamine lotion is traditional and gives some relief. Frequent cool showers if available are helpful, loose cotton clothes are advised.

24.6 COLD: INTRODUCTION

The situations where cold may become a serious problem are either on an adventure holiday, trekking or expedition in very cold climates or in the mountains; or when there is an emergency in the course of a normal journey that results in unexpected cold exposure, especially if there is injury or severe illness.

24.7 COLD: THERMAL BALANCE

The same underlying considerations apply as in a hot environment. The body temperature is determined by the balance of heat gain and heat loss. Heat gain is from metabolism especially during exercise. There may be some gain from solar radiation, but probably not much and none from the air. Heat loss will be by convection, conduction and radiation. The maintenance of body temperature in a cold environment depends upon reducing heat loss by technical means (clothing and footwear) and physiological mechanisms.

24.8 PHYSIOLOGICAL RESPONSE TO COLD

The body responds to cold by vasoconstriction of the skin, especially in the extremities. This conserves heat in the core of the body, the trunk and brain. The body is prepared, in effect, to sacrifice the extremities for the sake of preserving the core of the body. The other response is by shivering which increases metabolic heat production. In subjects exposed frequently to cold, cold tolerance develops to a degree, but significant cold acclimatization is difficult to achieve. Modern cold weather clothing is so efficient that the cold weather adventurer can maintain the microclimate near his skin at a comfortable temperature in almost any weather condition. However, the effect of wind is considerable. Wind chill, as is now well known, has the cooling effect on exposed skin of a much lower temperature than still air. Wind also has the effect of reducing the insulation of clothing by causing increased exchange of air within and under clothing layers.

24.9 COLD PATHOLOGY: HYPOTHERMIA

Cold can affect the body either generally to cause hypothermia or locally to cause local cold injury, frostbite or trench foot. There are broadly three settings that produce hypothermia:

1. Immersion in cold or freezing water
2. 'Exposure' on hills or wilderness in cold, wet, windy weather
3. Chronic cold due to insufficient heating especially elderly people with other illnesses.

The onset of hypothermia, in immersion cases, is in a matter of minutes, in 'exposure', in hours and in the chronic situation in days. Risk factors include lack of food and exhaustion, which in the hills, leads to stopping walking and thus losing the metabolic heat of exercise. Children are at greater risk because their smaller body to surface area ratio means they lose heat faster, as are the elderly because of their lower metabolic rate. Occult hypothyroidism is a not uncommon added factor in the elderly. Alcohol is also a risk factor. It has a vasodilator effect on the peripheral circulation, but more importantly its effect on the brain is to befuddle the victims so that they make stupid mistakes in the cold situation or just collapse, sleep in the open and drift into hypothermia.

Table 24.1 shows the stages of hypothermia and the relation of core temperature to neurological responses, signs and symptoms, but it should be appreciated that there is considerable individual variation in this relationship.

24.9.1 Clinical features: mild hypothermia

Individuals suffering from mild hypothermia complain of feeling cold and lose interest in any activity except getting warmer. They also develop a negative attitude towards the aims of the party and, as cooling continues into moderate

Table 24.1 Stages of hypothermia

Core temperature (°C)	Responses	Signs and symptoms	Classification
37–35	Normal	Cold sensation, shivering	Normal
35–32	Normal	Physical, mental impairment	Mild
32–28	Attenuated	Shivering stops, loss of consciousness	Moderate
<28	Absent	Rigid, risk of VF, appears dead	Severe

VF, ventricular fibrillation.
Note there is considerable individual variation in the relation of core temperature to signs, symptoms and neurological responses.

hypothermia, the patient becomes uncoordinated, unable to keep up and then starts to stumble. There may be attacks of violent shivering.

24.9.2 Moderate and severe hypothermia

At core temperatures below 32°C, there is altered mental function and the patient becomes careless about self-protection from the cold.

Thinking becomes slow, decision making difficult and often wrong, and memory deteriorates. There may be a strong desire for sleep and eventually the will to survive collapses with the individual becoming progressively unresponsive and lapsing into coma. Slurred speech and ataxia may suggest a stroke. Gastrointestinal mobility may slow or cease, and gastric dilatation and ileus are common (Paton 1983).

Individuals show a great range of response to cold and loss of consciousness may occur with a core temperature as high as 33°C or as low as 27°C, depending on the rate of cooling. Consciousness is usually lost at around 30°C, but patients have been reported to be conscious though confused at lower temperatures than this (Lloyd 1972; Paton 1983). As the temperature drops, heart rate slows and breathing becomes slower and shallower. These may be a physiological response to the reduced metabolic rate.

Though shivering usually stops as the temperature drops below 30°C, it has been observed at a core temperature of 24°C (Alexander 1945). Some cases have been reported to cool without shivering (Marcus 1979).

When the temperature drops to below 30°C, ventricular fibrillation may supervene. Survival depends on sufficient cardiac function to maintain output adequate for brain and heart perfusion. Cardiac function is more relevant to survival than brain temperature.

The patient with profound hypothermia may be indistinguishable from one who is dead. The skin is ice cold to touch and the muscles and joints are stiff and simulate rigor mortis. Respiration may be difficult or impossible to register; the peripheral pulses may be absent and blood pressure unmeasurable. In profound hypothermia, pupils do not react to light and other reflexes are absent.

The electrocardiogram (ECG) shows a slow rhythm with multifocal extrasystoles, broad complexes and atrial flutter (Jessen and Hagelstein 1978). There may also be J waves present (Osborne 1953).

Both hemoglobin and white cell count will be raised because of a shift of fluid from plasma to the interstitial space. Thrombocytopenia has been reported (Vella *et al.* 1988).

Even when there is evidence of a total stoppage of cardiorespiratory function, survival is possible (Siebhke *et al.* 1975). A flat electroencephalogram (EEG) is not a certain indicator of death in hypothermia. The only certain diagnostic factor is failure to recover on rewarming (Golden 1973; Lilja 1983). Before brain death can be diagnosed, the core temperature must be normal (NHS 1974); however, brain death can be the cause of hypothermia.

24.9.3 Management of hypothermia

The management of hypothermia in the field is 'the art of the possible'. Hamilton and Paton (1996) carried out a survey and concluded that most rescue groups attempting to measure temperature did so by the oral method. A low-reading thermometer was carried by a majority of teams. For reheating, commercial heating pads were used by most groups. The incidence of hypothermia was, surprisingly, the same for summer and winter. Cardiorespiratory resuscitation in the field was started in 76% of cases and the criteria for starting were the absence of a pulse, cardiac arrest and the likelihood of rapid evacuation.

MILD HYPOTHERMIA

Individuals should be stopped from walking and placed in shelter out of the wind, rain or snow. Any available warm or windproof clothing should be put on. They should be protected from further cooling and warmed by any method available.

To avoid further loss by evaporation, wet clothing should be replaced by dry, but if dry clothing is not available, wet clothing should be wrung out and put back on. If wet clothing, which has some insulating value, is left on, it should be covered with an impermeable material to prevent further heat loss. As large amounts of heat may be lost from the head, it should be covered. Warm fluids should be given, but never alcohol.

A patient with mild hypothermia can recover with these simple procedures, but recovery will be hastened if external heat is added (e.g. getting into a sleeping bag with another person). Central rewarming methods have been described (Lloyd 1973; Foray and Salon 1985) using warmed inhaled air which can be applied in the field with suitable apparatus. The added heat from these techniques is limited since gas has a low heat capacity, but the technique also prevents heat loss from expired air so that, if available, the method is worth using.

SEVERE HYPOTHERMIA

The management of severe hypothermia in the field will depend upon the local situation, possibilities for evacuation and access to specialist medical facilities. Where these are good, as in the mountains of Europe and North America, patients should be evacuated as soon as possible with the minimum of treatment in the field. However, active treatment in the field has been successful (Fischer *et al.* 1991). When bad weather delays evacuation, the patient should be rewarmed slowly and treated as gently as possible to avoid ventricular fibrillation. It is thought that ventricular fibrillation is likely to be triggered by rough handling so the greatest care should be exercised in examining and moving the patient.

If cardiac arrest occurs in a hypothermic patient, this produces a dilemma for rescuers because it may be due to some other cause and because the heart may be beating even if clinically undetectable. The mechanical irritation of chest compression may trigger ventricular fibrillation with total loss of cardiac function. However, a consensus seems to be:

- If breathing is absent, becomes obstructed or stops, then standard airway management should be started including mouth-to-mouth resuscitation.

- Chest compression should be started if no carotid pulse is detected for 60 s, if the pulse disappears, or if cardiac arrest occurred within the last 2 h.
- Resuscitation should be started only if there is a reasonable expectation that it can be continued effectively with only brief interruption until the patient can be brought to a hospital where full advanced life support is available (Lloyd 1996). Cardiac resuscitation has been continued for 6.5 h with ultimate success (Lexow 1991).
- Misguided attempts at cardiac massage may precipitate ventricular fibrillation (Mills 1983a). The mortality rate from hypothermia in the field is of the order of 50%, but with increasing expertise in management this figure should improve.
- The diagnosis of death in hypothermia should be made with caution because profound hypothermia can simulate death. Strictly, the diagnosis of death can only be made when the patient fails to revive after the core temperature has been brought to normal.

Once in hospital, it is now recognized, that along with standard intensive care, the use of extra-corporeal membrane oxygenation (ECMO) gives the best chance of success. Ruttmann *et al.* (2007) compared the results of either standard extra-corporeal circulation or ECMO and showed that the chance of a successful outcome with ECMO was six times greater than with the standard technique.

24.9.4 Prevention of hypothermia

The prevention of hypothermia in the mountains is mainly a matter of application of good mountaineering principles: good planning, adequate equipment and anticipation of possible weather conditions, accidents, etc. In addition, the risk of hypothermia in other members of the party should be appreciated and action taken in time to avert it. Modern clothing has reduced the risk of hypothermia, but it needs to be used intelligently. The concept of layering of clothing – inner thermal layers with an outer breathable, windproof and water resistant shell – needs to be understood.

Common sense and experience will inform many measures which help to prevent hypothermia. For instance, clothes should be removed before overheating, to avoid sweating and added before cooling becomes severe. When resting, get out of the wind somehow and, on a glacier, sit on a pack or rope, not directly on the ice.

24.10 COLD PATHOLOGY: FROSTBITE

Frostbite is caused by freezing of the tissues, usually skin, but in severe cases deeper tissues as well. The affected parts are usually the fingers, toes, nose and ear tips. The setting is usually in the mountains, Arctic or Antarctic wilderness and the victims are usually mountaineers, skiers or explorers. However, in northern Canada, Alaska and Siberia, victims can be ordinary residents caught out in the winter. In some cases, alcohol is an added factor in the situation. Victims of severe injury or illness in the mountains or wilderness are at particular risk (as in the case of patient A, Chapter 23 section 23.6.1).

24.10.1 Recognition and immediate management of frostbite

Frostbite often comes on insidiously. Under cold conditions, fingers and toes often become numb and this usually does not lead to frostbite. However, if there is further sufficient cooling, the tissues actually freeze and frostbite is produced without the victim realizing it. Cold fingers and toes may be pale but are soft to the touch. The frostbitten digit appears waxy white and is hard to the touch; it is in fact, frozen. The immediate management is to get the patient to a place of warmth and safety, being as gentle with the frostbitten part as possible. It is important to avoid a sequence of freeze–thaw–freeze which results in much more damage than just freeze–thaw.

Having reached a safe base the affected part should be rewarmed as rapidly as possible. This is best done in a stirred water bath at 40°C. Thereafter, clean dressings and measures to avoid infection are the key to management until the patient is admitted to hospital, if the damage is any more than superficial.

24.10.2 Secondary management of frostbite

Full management in hospital is beyond the scope of this chapter. Two points, only, will be made:

1. In severe cases where there is a question of amputation, management should be conservative. In frostbite, the early appearance of blackened skin is worse than the actuality. The underlying tissue is probably viable. This is unlike gangrene from vascular occlusion where the appearance underestimates the real extent of trouble. The difference is shown in Fig. 24.2.
2. A new grading (Table 24.2) of frostbite has been proposed by Cauchy et al. (2011). This has a strong bearing on prognosis and helps guide the timing and need for amputation. This classification is based on a series of 70 cases of severe frostbite seen and treated at the hospital in Chamonix, France. From the Technetium[99] bone scan on day 2, it is possible to make a prognosis as to the outcome and decide on the need and extent of amputation.

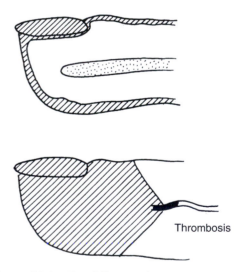

Figure 24.2 The difference between gangrene due to frostbite and due to digital artery occlusion. Top, superficial frostbite: gangrene (shaded area) is limited to the superficial 2–3 mm of tissue. Tissue damage is less than it appears. Bottom, arterial thrombosis: gangrene extends through all tissues. Tissue damage is more than it appears.

Table 24.2   Classification scheme for severity of frostbite injuries

Grade	Extent of initial lesion, day 0	Bone scan, day 2	Blisters at day 2	Prognosis at day 2
1	No lesion	Unnecessary	No blisters	No amputation
2	Lesion distal phalanx only	Reduced radiotracer uptake	Clear blister fluid	Tissue excision
3	Lesion distal, inter- and proximal phalanx	No radiotracer uptake on digit	Hemorrhagic blister fluid	Bone amputation of digit
4	Lesion in carpal/tarsal	No tracer uptake in carpal/tarsal	Hemorrhagic blisters carpal/tarsal	Bone amputation of limb

After Cauchy *et al.* 2001.
The initial assessment on arrival in hospital, day 0, is made after rapid rewarming.

3. Newer treatments are now being trialed in the hope of reducing the need for amputation. These include prostaglandins (iloprost) and thrombolysis with recombinant tissue plasminogen activator. A dramatic case report by Sheridan *et al.* (2009) highlights the use and apparent benefit of the latter therapy. A clinical trial of thrombolysis compared with aspirin plus buflomedil and aspirin plus iloprost by Cauchy et al (2011) concluded that aspirin and iloprost should be used in all cases of severe frostbite and that thrombolysis be considered on a case by case basis. Of course, to be effective, thrombolysis needs to be delivered as soon as possible after rewarming.

It must also be remembered that severe frostbite, especially in mountain rescue cases, is often accompanied by hypothermia and injuries, which will influence management. Pain is also a very real problem and, in many cases, the psychological impact of the whole experience on the patient will be severe. A recent review of frostbite is by Freer and Imray (2012).

24.11 COLD PATHOLOGY: NON-FREEZING COLD INJURY

Prolonged exposure of tissue in wet, cold conditions in temperatures below 15°C will result in non-freezing cold injury, often with lasting damage to muscles and nerves.

'Trench foot' is the most common form of this condition and is a significant cause of injury in military operations when, for combat reasons, long periods have to be spent with feet in water or in deep snow. Water both increases and accelerates the risk of injury, as does any factor that impedes circulation to the extremities, such as a cramped position, immobility, tight clothing, tight boots and tight socks. Mountaineers are at risk when powder snow gets into their boots by the ankle or is melted by foot warmth; damp socks will increase cooling.

Exactly the same sequence occurs with the hands in mittens or gloves made sodden by water or snow. However, because the hands are easier to inspect and keep dry and warm, 'trench hand' is uncommon.

Non-freezing cold injury, though initially reversible, becomes irreversible if cooling is prolonged. It often occurs in tissues immediately proximal to frostbite.

24.11.1 Clinical features

When first seen, the affected part will be pale and sensation and movement poor. The pulse may be absent, but freezing has not occurred. If these features do not improve on warming, non-freezing cold injury is present.

After a few hours the part becomes swollen, numb, blotchy pink-purple and heavy. After 24–36 h, a vigorous hyperemia develops with a bounding pulse and burning pain proximally but not distally. Edema with 'blood blisters' appears and, if the skin is poorly perfused, it will become gangrenous and slough. At night, a pain like an electric shock makes sleep difficult.

In severe cases, there is a progressive reduction in sensation. The joints become stiff and muscles cease to function. To maintain balance, the legs are kept apart and the sensation of movement has been likened to walking on cotton wool (Ungley *et al.* 1945). Hyperemia appears to be due to vasomotor paralysis with paleness on elevation and redness when the part is dependent. This phase may last from days to weeks, as may changes in sensation. Persistent anesthesia suggests neurone degeneration with the prospect of long-term symptoms (Burr 1993).

24.11.2 Prevention and treatment

With modern outdoor clothing and footwear, this condition is seen much less frequently. Nevertheless, it does still occur. In 1988, the incidence in one USA marine unit of 355 soldiers was 11%. Tobacco smoking (but not race) was associated with a higher incidence of trench foot, although the difference did not reach significance (Tek and Mackey 1993).

The patient should be removed from the cold; whole-body warming should be started (Lahti 1982) and dehydration corrected. Rapid warming of the part has been advocated. Because of pain, analgesics should be given, the patient rested and the part raised. Blisters that develop should be left unless infected, when drainage should be carried out. Gangrene may occur later, and this may be more widespread and affect deeper tissues more extensively than freezing cold injury. Conservative management should be adopted and surgical procedures kept to the minimum. A recent review of non-freezing cold injury has been published by Imray *et al.* (2011).

Pre-existing medical conditions at altitude

SUMMARY

Much of the attention regarding medical issues at high altitude focuses on the risk of developing one of several acute altitude illnesses and how to prevent and manage those problems. While this is the primary question for most high altitude travelers, it is important to remember that some of these travelers will also have underlying medical problems, such as hypertension, diabetes or asthma. In such situations, it will also be necessary to consider how high altitude will affect these problems, whether it is safe for the individual to undertake the planned sojourn and how best to manage the problem during their travels.

At present, due to lack of clinical studies addressing these issues, very little information exists to guide medical practitioners as they evaluate and advise such patients. The purpose of this chapter is to review what data are available regarding a large number of common clinical problems that adventuresome patients might have and thus provide a reasonable framework for practitioners to use when advising these individuals. Practitioners will not be able to provide complete assurance that the underlying problems will not get worse at high altitude or predispose to acute altitude illness, but through a careful weighing of the available evidence and thorough pretravel evaluation, they can increase the likelihood of a safe and successful journey by an informed patient.

25.1 INTRODUCTION

With increasing numbers of people traveling to high altitude for work, adventure holidays, expeditions, skiing and religious pilgrimages, doctors are frequently being asked to counsel patients on the risks of their planned trip. While such counseling typically focuses on recognition, prevention and treatment of acute altitude illness, providers are increasingly being asked to also evaluate whether their patients' underlying medical condition(s) will worsen at high altitude and how best to manage them during their planned sojourn. This issue is particularly common among older high altitude travelers as their increasing age increases the likelihood of their having chronic underlying medical conditions that might be affected by the environment at high altitude. The importance of such counseling is well demonstrated by the high incidence of medical problems, as well as acute altitude illness, among elderly religious pilgrims traveling to festivals and sacred sites at high elevations in Nepal, Tibet and elsewhere in the Himalayas. Many of these individuals have underlying medical conditions yet receive little pre-pilgrimage evaluation and, as a result develop severe problems during their journey (Basnyat *et al.* 2006).

Advising travelers with underlying medical conditions is challenging because there have been few clinical studies devoted to this issue. In an excellent earlier review article, Hackett (2001) has tried to synthesize the available evidence from clinical studies and case reports regarding a large number of medical conditions and, more recently, several review articles have addressed these questions for patients whose problems fall within specific disease categories including cardiac conditions (Bärtsch and Gibbs 2007; Dehnert and Bärtsch 2010; Luks *et al.* 2010), pulmonary problems (Luks and Swenson 2007; Stream *et al.* 2009), chronic kidney disease (Luks *et al.* 2008), diabetes (Leal 2005) and neurologic conditions (Baumgartner *et al.* 2007). This chapter will summarize the available evidence in these and other categories and the reader is referred to those review articles for further details.

Before considering the specific details of the various medical conditions below, it is worthwhile to review some general principles for how to approach these patients. First, while the particular concerns will vary from patient to patient depending on the patient's medical problem, there are several broad questions that can be used to guide the pretravel assessment including:

1. Will the underlying condition get worse at high altitude. For example, will a patient with hypertension experience worsening blood pressure control following ascent and need to alter their medications or will a diabetic patient experience greater difficulty controlling blood sugar.

2. Will the underlying condition predispose the patient to acute altitude illnesses including acute mountain sickness (AMS), high altitude cerebral edema (HACE), and high altitude pulmonary edema (HAPE). In general, the majority of underlying problems are not thought to increase the risk of these disorders but some diseases, such as pulmonary hypertension, may very well increase the risk of altitude illness, as described further below.

3. Is my patient at risk for developing severe, symptomatic hypoxemia at high altitude and how can this be managed in that environment. This question will be very prominent in those patients with known right-to-left shunts, such as pulmonary arteriovenous malformations, or patients with severe underlying lung disease.

4. Will the underlying condition predispose to poor exercise tolerance at high altitude. Patients with severe anemia, for example, will have decreased oxygen delivery capacity and may not be able to compensate as well for the lower arterial oxygen content, thereby limiting exercise performance.

In addition to considering these questions, the provider must consider the availability of medical resources in the area of planned travel. While many people travel to resort areas with easily accessible medical facilities, a considerable amount of high altitude travel involves venturing into remote areas away from medical care where timely evacuation might be difficult to arrange. The more severe the underlying problem, the more important it is to avoid travel into such areas and arrange plans for accessing resources if problems develop during the trip.

When traveling as part of an expedition or trek, the aphorism, 'no man is an island' applies with greater force than in normal urban life. One member's illness affects the whole team and may even imperil the safety of other members; therefore, it is ethically imperative that if a person knows he/she has some pre-existing condition which might affect performance or the ability to complete the trip, they should make that information known to the trip leader and, when available, the team's medical provider.

Providers must also stress to patients that travel should only be undertaken when the underlying disorder is under good control. For example, patients in the midst of having recently suffered from an asthma exacerbation should avoid high altitude travel particularly into remote areas, while an individual with a recent gastrointestinal bleed should defer travel until it is clear they will not experience a recurrence. In addition, individuals should be as fit as possible before they leave for a holiday at altitude. Good fitness does not protect against altitude illnesses but does add an element of safety as the fitter one is the better one can cope with long days, arduous rescues, or escapes from impending bad weather.

Finally, there is always an element of increased risk with high altitude travel, especially in individuals with pre-existing medical conditions and, given the dearth of clinical studies examining patients with various disorders at high altitude, it will be impossible to guarantee patients that they will, in fact, have a safe trip. It is only by carefully weighing the potential benefits and risks of any planned trip and doing an appropriate pretravel assessment that one can increase the likelihood of the safest possible outcome for the patient.

25.2 CARDIOVASCULAR DISORDERS

Of all the potential underlying medical problems that warrant consideration, cardiovascular disorders are perhaps one of the most important categories as the hypoxia and subsequent increase in sympathoadrenal activity seen following acute ascent have the potential to exacerbate many of the diseases that fall within this category.

25.2.1 Coronary artery disease

A key concern in patients with coronary artery disease is whether the ambient hypoxia at high altitude will provoke myocardial ischemia, particularly in the setting of any physical exertion. This question can be examined in several different clinical contexts including patients with occult coronary artery disease, those with recognized, stable disease and those who have undergone coronary revascularization.

OCCULT CORONARY ARTERY DISEASE

Resting hypoxemia does not appear to unmask previously unrecognized coronary artery disease (CAD) (Alexander 1994; Burchell et al. 1948), although ischemic changes may be seen on electrocardiography during exercise (Khanna et al. 1976). As a result, there is no indication to screen all individuals for CAD prior to ascent to high altitude, particularly if they have good exertional tolerance and no exercise-induced angina at sea level. For those individuals with strong risk factors for CAD who do not regularly engage in exercise, screening with a symptom-limited exercise test prior to the high altitude sojourn would be a prudent approach.

PREVIOUSLY DIAGNOSED CORONARY ARTERY DISEASE

Exposure to high altitude reduces the arterial Po_2 and so, other things being equal, will reduce myocardial Po_2. While hypoxia leads to coronary vasodilation and increased myocardial perfusion in normal individuals (Kaufmann et al. 2001), it may actually provoke vasoconstriction and subsequent decreases in myocardial perfusion in individuals with atherosclerotic disease and endothelial dysfunction (Gordon et al. 1989; Wyss et al. 2003; Arbab-Zadeh et al. 2009). Despite this paradoxical response, it appears that myocardial oxygen delivery might actually be adequate in most patients provided appropriate precautions are taken. Erdmann et al. (1998), for example, performed exercise studies following ascent by cable car to 2500 m in patients with coronary artery disease and documented ejection fractions <45% and noted no adverse events, arrhythmia or electrocardiographic signs of ischemia. Levine et al. (1997) also performed exercise studies in patients with stable CAD and found that the double product (the product of systolic blood pressure and heart rate) that induced 1 mm of ST segment depression, a marker of the ischemia threshold, was 5% lower with acute exposure to simulated altitude of 2500 m, but returned to sea-level values after 5 days of acclimatization at the same terrestrial altitude. More recently, de Vries *et al.* (2010) performed exercise testing and echocardiography on eight patients with a history of myocardial infarction and relatively preserved ejection fractions (54 ± 6%) at 4200 m and noted no symptoms or echocardiographic evidence of myocardial ischemia. These studies suggest that patients with known stable coronary artery disease and good exercise tolerance can ascend to moderate altitudes (~3000–3500 m) and perform physical activity, although the data from Levine *et al.* (1997) suggest it may be prudent to delay such activity for at least a few days following arrival.

Individuals with stable disease who do not engage in regular physical activity at sea level should not plan to exert themselves at altitude unless they embark on a sea-level exercise program prior to their planned trip and demonstrate good exercise tolerance. Individuals may also need to avoid excessive exertion in cold temperatures, a common environmental feature at high altitude, as data from sea level suggest low ambient temperature may be related to myocardial ischemia (Lassvik and Areskog 1980) through a possible effect on platelet function.

It should be noted, however, that these recommendations apply only to asymptomatic patients with stable disease, as the studies noted above did not include patients with unstable angina or exercise limitations at sea level. These patients should avoid high altitude travel altogether. If such travel is necessary for some reason, such as to attend an important family function, they should avoid any physical exertion or travel into remote areas and travel with a plan for accessing care or descending in the event they develop symptoms.

RECENT MYOCARDIAL INFARCTION

A recent myocardial infarction should be viewed as a contraindication to ascent to high altitude, but patients who undergo revascularization and remain asymptomatic after an adequate period of time can likely ascend without difficulty. Schmid *et al.* (2006), for example, performed exercise studies at 540 m and 3454 m in 15 patients who had undergone revascularization by either angioplasty or bypass surgery following an acute coronary syndrome and noted no adverse events or electrocardiographic evidence of ischemia at either low or high altitude. Of note, beta-blockers were held for 5 days prior to exercise testing and all of the patients had completed an ambulatory rehabilitation program and had relatively preserved ejection fractions (60 ± 8%). Additional anecdotal reports provide further evidence that individuals can travel to high altitude, even as high as 5700 m, without adverse effect (Berner *et al.* 1988). The exact duration that individuals must wait before traveling to high altitude following myocardial infarction and revascularization is not clear. Subjects in the study by Schmid *et al.* (2006) were anywhere from 6 to 18 months out from their event suggesting one-half year would be the minimum advisable duration to wait. Importantly, the patients should be asymptomatic and have regained good exercise tolerance at the time of their planned sojourn. Those patients on dual anti-platelet therapy (for example, aspirin and another anti-platelet agent, such as clopidogrel) following coronary stent placement should be careful to avoid activities that carry a risk of physical trauma, particularly in remote areas (Dehnert and Bärtsch 2010).

25.2.2 Hypertension

The available evidence suggests that when patients with mild–moderate hypertension ascend to high altitude, systolic blood pressure rises mildly (10–15 mmHg on average) and subsequently declines over days to weeks (Palatini *et al.* 1989; Savonitto *et al.* 1992; Roach *et al.* 1995; Wu *et al.* 2007b). While there is significant inter-individual variability in the observed responses, there is, unfortunately, no adequate means to predict ahead of time which individuals will experience marked rises in their pressure. There is currently no evidence that hypertension or observed rises in blood pressure following ascent are associated with increased risk of AMS or other adverse events, such as retinopathy, intracranial hemorrhage or myocardial infarction.

Given these data, individuals with well-controlled hypertension can safely ascend to high altitude without the need for medication adjustments or blood pressure monitoring following arrival. Because the studies cited above generally did not include individuals with severe hypertension, individuals with poorly controlled or labile blood pressure should plan to monitor blood pressure following arrival and adjust their medications according to a plan arranged with their physician prior to their trip (Luks 2009b). Because elevated blood pressure may improve over time at high altitude, individuals who add or change blood pressure medications in response to a pre-arranged plan should continue to monitor their blood pressure and readjust medications as needed to avoid hypotension.

25.2.3 Heart failure

There is little information about the effects of high altitude exposure on patients with heart failure. Agostoni et al. (2000) performed cardiopulmonary exercise tests on 38 heart failure patients at sea level and simulated altitudes of 1000 m, 1500 m, 2000 m and 3000 m and noted a decrease in work rate with increasing altitude with the greatest decrements seen in those patients with the greatest baseline exercise impairment. Similarly, as noted earlier, Erdman et al. (1998) noted decrements in exercise capacity in patients with ischemic cardiomyopathy similar to those seen in healthy controls following ascent to 2500 m. Neither of these studies found evidence of significant complications such as arrhythmia, myocardial ischemia or pulmonary edema.

While these studies suggest short-term exposures may be tolerated in patients with stable disease, additional issues warrant attention. AMS is often associated with fluid retention and, to the extent this occurs in a heart failure patient, it could lead to volume overload and pulmonary edema. Marked blood pressure elevations due to increased sympathoadrenal activity could increase left ventricular afterload and impair systolic function. Finally, Agostoni et al. (2006) demonstrated that carvedilol, a commonly used beta-receptor antagonist in heart failure patients, may be associated with blunted ventilatory responses in acute hypoxia, which may predispose to increased hypoxemia at high altitude. Whether these blunted ventilatory responses lead to acute altitude illness is not clear as prior studies on this question have yielded conflicting results (Milledge et al. 1988; Richalet et al. 1988; Milledge et al. 1991b; Savourney et al. 1995; Bärtsch et al. 2002; Richalet et al. 2011).

25.2.4 Pacemakers and defibrillators

Little information exists regarding pacemaker and implantable cardiac defibrillator (ICD) function at high altitude. Weilenmann et al. (2000) studied 13 patients with single chamber pacemakers and found no changes in ventricular stimulation thresholds at a simulated altitude of 4000 m, although the duration of exposure was only 30 minutes and may not accurately reflect what would happen with longer stays in hypobaric hypoxia. Kobza et al. (2008) surveyed 217 patients with ICDs who traveled to altitudes above 2000 m and found that 4% experienced an ICD shock during their sojourn. Given the retrospective nature of the study, however, it is difficult to determine if the shocks were due to alterations in the defibrillation threshold of the device or were due to the patients underlying cardiac condition.

25.2.5 Arrhythmias

Given the increased sympathoadrenal responses following acute hypoxic exposure to high altitude and reports of conduction abnormalities, such as sinus bradycardia, premature contractions, atrial flutter and incomplete right bundle branch block in healthy individuals at high altitude (Levine et al. 1997; Woods et al. 2008), one might expect an increased incidence of arrhythmias in those with pre-existing arrhythmias, but data regarding this question are limited. In one of the few studies of this question, Wu et al. (2007b) performed electrocardiograms (ECG) and 24-hour ambulatory ECG on 42 workers on the Qinghai–Tibet Railway with a variety of pre-existing arrhythmias including sinus arrhythmia, premature atrial or ventricular beats, first degree

AV-block and incomplete right bundle branch block. Assessments were made at 1 week and 3 months after exposure to 4500–5056 m and, aside from one case of asymptomatic Wolff–Parkinson–White syndrome, there were no reported exacerbations of underlying arrhythmia or other life-threatening conduction issues.

25.2.6 Adult congenital heart disease

With improvements in medical care, many patients with congenital heart disease are living into adulthood, engaging in a wider variety of activities and may, as a result, have the opportunity to travel to high altitude. Drawing conclusions about high altitude activity in this patient population is challenging given the wide variety of congenital defects and surgical repairs. From a theoretical standpoint, those patients at potential risk for problems would include those whose defects are associated with pulmonary hypertension, which, as discussed further below, may increase the risk of high altitude pulmonary edema, and those individuals with significant right-to-left shunts and baseline hypoxemia. These theoretical concerns have not been evaluated systematically, however, and overall very little information exists to help guide assessment of these patients. The limited evidence suggests that individuals with unilateral absence of a pulmonary artery (Hackett *et al.* 1980; Rios *et al.* 1985) or Down syndrome, a disorder associated with various cardiac abnormalities (Durmowicz 2001), may be associated with an increased risk of HAPE while patients who have undergone a Fontan procedure for correction of tricuspid atresia may actually tolerate submaximal exercise at 3050 m despite the lack of a functional right ventricle. Given the paucity of data in this area, individuals with complex congenital heart disease should undergo thorough evaluation prior to any planned high altitude travel, including echocardiography, to assess pulmonary artery pressures and cardiopulmonary exercise testing to assess the overall adequacy of cardiac function (Luks *et al.* 2010). Consideration can also be given to pretravel high altitude simulation testing (Dine and Kreider 2008), although this test will only give information about short-term exposures and may not reflect what will happen on a long trip.

25.3 LUNG DISEASES

Because hypoxia is one of the key challenges faced by high altitude travelers and because many of the important physiologic responses to hypobaric hypoxia involve the respiratory system, individuals with underlying lung disease are a category of patients who require careful evaluation prior to high altitude travel. This topic has been reviewed extensively elsewhere (Luks and Swenson 2007; Stream *et al.* 2009) and the risks associated with several important forms of lung disease are considered and summarized below.

25.3.1 Asthma

Given the prevalence of asthma in the general population, particularly among young otherwise healthy individuals who engage in active pursuits, it is likely that providers will be asked to evaluate the safety of high altitude travel in this patient population. This assessment may be challenging, however, due to the variety of factors that can impact asthma control at high altitude. While some factors such as the lower air density, increased sympathoadrenal activity and decreased number of dust mites may improve various biologic and clinical markers of disease activity (Spieksma *et al.* 1971; Boner *et al.* 1993; Valletta *et al.* 1995; van Velzen *et al.* 1996; Grootendorst *et al.* 2001), other factors such as hypoxia (Dagg *et al.* 1997; Denjean *et al.* 1988), hypocapnia (Newhouse *et al.* 1964; van den Elshout *et al.* 1991) and decreased air temperature (Dosman *et al.* 1991; Kaminsky *et al.* 1995) may increase airway resistance or trigger airway reactivity and potentially worsen asthma control. Predicting which of these factors may have the biggest effect in a given individual at high altitude is difficult.

The studies noted above generally try to isolate the effect of a single factor on asthma control. The reality, however, is that when a patient travels to high altitude, multiple factors will exert an effect at the same time. For this reason, clinical studies of asthma patients at high altitude may provide more useful information to guide the pretravel assessment. Golan *et al.* (2002) reported that 20% of adventure travelers with asthma, including many engaging in high altitude trekking, had their 'worst ever' asthma during the trip. This study, however, did not control for the altitudes attained during high altitude travel nor the fact that travel to such regions often requires that individuals spend time in urban centers with very poor air quality. Other field studies suggest the risks of high altitude travel may be quite manageable. Cogo *et al.* (1997) and Allegra *et al.* (1995), for example, studied mild asthmatics and reported decreased bronchial hyper-reactivity to hypoosmolar aerosol or methacholine at 4559 and 5050 m when compared to sea level. Stokes *et al.* (2008) have also documented that well-controlled mild asthmatics can ascend to 5895 m without exacerbations of their disease and with no increase in the rate of AMS compared to non-asthmatic climbers.

While these studies suggest well-controlled asthmatics will tolerate high altitude travel without problems, several studies do suggest that caution is still necessary. Louie and Pare (2004), for example, reported a decrease in peak expiratory flow of 76 ± 67 L/min during a trek to 5050 m in Nepal, although these results are difficult to interpret as some of the subjects were taking dexamethasone and acetazolamide which might have affected the degree of asthma control. Several studies have also reported an increased incidence of asthma or exercise-induced bronchoconstriction in cross-country skiers and ski mountaineers, two groups of athletes whose activity requires high minute ventilation in cold environments (Larsson *et al.* 1993; Durand *et al.* 2005; Pohjantahti *et al.* 2005). Several studies do suggest that the airway hyperreactivity in athletes at high altitude may be blocked in part by nifedipine (Henderson *et al.* 1983), acetazolamide (O'Donnell *et al.* 1992) and cromolyn sodium (Juniper *et al.* 1986), but this question has not been examined in large clinical studies.

Patients with mild-intermittent or mild-persistent asthma can safely ascend to high altitude provided their disease is under good control at the time of their trip. Patients with more severe disease or who are in an active exacerbation at the time of their trip should avoid high altitude travel, particularly into remote regions away from medical care. Individuals should remain on their pre-existing medication regimen and also carry an adequate supply of rescue inhalers and oral prednisone that can be used in the event of an exacerbation. Those individuals using metered-dose inhalers should be careful to keep the inhalers warm in cold environments and should be aware that the number of puffs delivered per inhaler may be decreased at elevations above 3000 m (Roggla and Moser 2006). Individuals can consider peak expiratory flow monitoring during their trip but should be aware that variable orifice peak flow meters may underestimate peak flows at high altitude or in cold environments (Thomas *et al.* 1990; Pollard *et al.* 1996) and may need to rely more on the trends in their measurements rather than the absolute values.

25.3.2 Chronic obstructive pulmonary disease

Chronic obstructive pulmonary disease (COPD) patients will face a variety of challenges at high altitude, including impaired oxygenation, increased ventilatory requirements and increased pulmonary vascular resistance, all of which may significantly impair performance at high altitude.

Unfortunately, the literature on this question is somewhat limited, as only a single study has examined COPD patients in the field at high altitude. Graham and Houston (1978) took eight patients with severe COPD (FEV_1 of 1.27 L) to the modest altitude of 1920 m and documented a drop in PaO_2 from 66 to 54 mmHg with no adverse clinical events. In the absence of other field studies, further information about expected changes in oxygenation can be taken from the studies examining COPD patients during commercial flight. These studies consistently demonstrate that in patients with FEV_1 1–1.5 L exposed to the equivalent of 2340 m the PaO_2 often falls below 50 mmHg, with more significant drops during mild exertion, such as walking on flat ground (Dillard *et al.* 1989; Berg *et al.* 1992; Christensen *et al.* 2000; Secombe *et al.* 2004; Akero *et al.* 2005). There are no major adverse events reported in these studies and patients only experienced mild dyspnea, fatigue and headaches.

Given the expected severe decrease in arterial oxygenation at high altitude, the question that arises is which patients will require supplemental oxygen during their journey. Prediction rules utilizing sea-level arterial blood gases (Gong *et al.* 1984), pulmonary function testing (Dillard *et al.* 1989), exercise testing (Christensen *et al.* 2000) or the high altitude simulation test (Dine and Kreider 2008) are commonly used to assess the need for supplemental oxygen during commercial flights, but it is not clear that these rules can be rigidly applied with high altitude travel. Most of these rules, for example, are based on studies involving short duration hypoxic exposures experienced on aircraft and may not reflect outcomes during longer exposures when, for example, ventilatory acclimatization and improvements in oxygenation would be expected. The lack of significant symptoms noted in those studies above also argues against strict use of oxygen in all patients in whom the PaO_2 is predicted to be low at altitude. Given these issues, a more prudent approach may be that laid out in a review on this topic by Luks (2009a) in which patients can travel with a prescription for oxygen that they can fill upon arrival at high altitude based on symptoms or pulse oximetry monitoring following arrival, rather than necessarily going through the cumbersome and costly steps of acquiring supplemental oxygen prior to their trip.

Aside from the oxygenation issue, other theoretical concerns for high altitude travel in COPD patients include whether high altitude exposure will have any adverse effect on pulmonary function or whether patients with bullous disease are at increased risk for pneumothorax. Data on the former question are mixed as multiple studies have shown either improvements, no change or worsening in various markers of pulmonary function. Regarding the latter question, despite the theoretical concerns that bullae might expand in response to low barometric pressure at high altitude, there is no evidence that risk of pneumothorax or pneumomediastinum is increased with exposure hypobaric hypoxia (Yanda and Herschensohn 1964; Tomashefski *et al.* 1966).

High altitude travel should be avoided in patients with an FEV_1 <1 L, carbon dioxide retention or pulmonary hypertension, while patients with an FEV_1 of 1–1.5 L may be able to travel with adequate pretravel evaluation, including assessment of the need for supplemental oxygen using prediction equations that take into account the patient's baseline FEV_1 (Dillard *et al.* 1989) or, where feasible, the hypoxia inhalation test (Dine and Kreider 2008). Patients in whom the PaO_2 is predicted to fall below 50 mmHg should either travel with portable supplemental oxygen or be provided with a prescription they can fill upon arrival at high altitude. Patients already on supplemental oxygen should remain on this at high altitude and will require higher flow rates. Patients should remain on their pre-existing medication regimen and carry an adequate supply of their rescue inhalers. Acetazolamide should not be used for AMS prophylaxis or treatment in patients with an FEV_1 <25% (Luks and Swenson 2008).

25.3.3 Interstitial lung disease

Only two studies have examined the effect of simulated high altitude on patients with interstitial lung diseases, with each study noting a decline in PaO_2 to around 50 mmHg with exposure to the equivalent of 2340 m (~8000 ft) at rest and more significant declines with mild exercise such as walking on flat ground for 50 m (Christensen *et al.* 2002; Seccombe *et al.* 2004). No studies have examined whether these disorders increase the risk of high altitude illness, but it should be remembered that patients with severe interstitial lung disease often develop pulmonary hypertension which, as discussed further below, may increase the risk of high altitude pulmonary edema. Furthermore, these patients have reduced lung compliance, which may increase the work of breathing in response to hypoxia at high altitude. Patients with severe restrictive physiology (total lung capacity (TLC) <50% predicted) or a pre-existing oxygen requirement should likely avoid high altitude travel altogether, while those with less severe disease can travel to high altitude with adequate pretravel assessment. The regression equation provided by Christensen *et al.* (2002) can be used to help assess the need for supplemental oxygen which the patient can either bring with them or arrange to obtain following arrival at their destination.

25.3.4 Cystic fibrosis

More and more patients with cystic fibrosis (CF) are living into adulthood and it is likely that many of these patients will seek travel opportunities that involve going to high altitude. As with the COPD and interstitial lung diseases, the available evidence suggests that exposure to moderate altitudes of 2000–3000 m is associated with a significant decrease in arterial oxygenation, with more precipitous declines being seen in individuals with severe disease or following exercise (Rose et al. 2000; Ryujin et al. 2001; Thews et al. 2004; Fischer et al. 2005). Despite the severe hypoxemia, however, the subjects in these studies had either no or minor symptoms in response to the hypoxemia. This finding must be viewed with caution as the hypoxic exposures were of only short duration and may not adequately predict what would happen with longer exposures typical of a high altitude vacation or climbing expedition. A report of two cystic fibrosis patients with baseline FEV_1 ~1 L who developed pulmonary hypertension and cor pulmonale during a high altitude trip provides some evidence that patients with severe disease can, in fact, develop severe problems at high altitude (Speechley-Dick et al. 1992).

CF patients with severe disease (FEV_1 ≤1 L or < 30% predicted) should avoid high altitude travel, but other patients can likely travel safely provided their disease is under good control at the time of their trip and they can continue their pre-existing airway clearance regimen, prophylactic antibiotics and mucolytic therapy. The hypoxia inhalation test commonly used with other lung disease patients does not perform well in cystic fibrosis patients and the decision to use supplemental oxygen should be based on pretravel spirometry, with supplemental oxygen recommended for those with FEV_1 between 30 and 50% predicted (Oades et al. 1994; Fischer et al. 2005).

25.3.5 Pulmonary vascular disease

Decreased alveolar oxygen tensions at high altitude lead to hypoxic pulmonary vasoconstriction, which, in conjunction with the rise in cardiac output (before acclimatization), leads to a rise in pulmonary artery pressure. This important physiologic response creates significant potential risk for patients with underlying pulmonary hypertension and may, in particular, predispose to high altitude pulmonary edema. The literature contains a large number of reports of patients with pulmonary hypertension due to both anatomic (Hackett et al. 1980; Rios et al. 1985; Torrington 1989) and non-anatomic causes (Nakagawa et al. 1993; Naeije et al. 1996; Durmowicz 2001) who developed HAPE following ascent to a variety of different elevations. It is not clear from these reports exactly what level of pulmonary hypertension is necessary to increase the risk of HAPE and no cases of this phenomenon have been described in patients with idiopathic pulmonary arterial hypertension, but this body of reports strongly suggests that these patients require close evaluation prior to any high altitude travel. Even if these individuals do not develop overt edema, they may still be at risk for worsening right heart function due to the rise in pulmonary artery pressure and subsequent increase in right ventricular afterload. Patients with milder disease can likely travel to high altitude, but should be placed on systemic vasodilator therapy, such as nifedipine, if not already on such therapy, while those with poorly controlled disease (e.g. NYHA class III or IV symptoms) or who require continuous intravenous vasodilator therapy should avoid high altitude altogether. If high altitude travel is necessary in those cases, strong consideration should be given to using supplemental oxygen to blunt the rise in pulmonary artery pressures.

A prior history of pulmonary thromboembolic disease presents a difficult clinical dilemma. As discussed in Chapter 23, there are case reports of thromboembolic disease at high altitude, but most of those cases occurred in patients with hypercoagulable states (Boulos et al. 1999; Folsom et al. 2002) and there is little consistent evidence that travel to high altitude predisposes people to either hypercoagulability or recurrent thromboembolism. Nevertheless, it seems reasonable to evaluate patients with pre-existing thromboembolic disease carefully. Those with no known predisposing conditions and who lack pulmonary hypertension should have no contraindications from going to high altitude for recreation. Any pre-existing anticoagulation regimen should be continued, but such medication should not be started solely for the purpose of a high altitude trip. Individuals should also remain well hydrated and avoid periods of immobility, as can happen when tent-bound in prolonged storms.

25.3.6 Diseases of ventilatory control and ventilation

Because ventilatory responses play a key role in acclimatization and adaptation to high altitude, individuals with ventilatory control disorders warrant careful consideration prior to high altitude travel. The most common clinical abnormality of respiratory control, obesity–hypoventilation syndrome is considered further below in the section 25.10, while the expected outcomes in patients with obstructive sleep apnea traveling to high altitude is considered in detail in Chapter 14. Few data exist regarding other forms of ventilatory control disorders at high altitude, but it is possible to identify several groups who might be at risk for problems. Because carotid endarterectomy can damage or obliterate the carotid body, patients who have undergone bilateral endarterectomy or ablation, an old treatment for refractory asthma, may be at risk for impaired hypoxic ventilatory responses (Honda *et al.* 1979; Roeggla *et al.* 1995) and, as a result, significant hypoxemia following ascent. Similar problems may also be seen in Parkinson's disease and myotonic dystrophy, as these disorders have been shown to be associated with impaired hypoxic ventilatory responses at sea level (Carroll *et al.* 1977; Serebrovskaya *et al.* 1998). Finally, patients with skeletal or neuromuscular disorders, such as severe kyphoscoliosis, diaphragmatic paralysis or Duchenne's muscular dystrophy, may not be able to adequately raise their minute ventilation in response to the hypoxia at high altitude, despite having adequate carotid body responses. Even if they do not have problems with ventilation while awake, bilateral diaphragmatic paralysis patients can develop arterial hypoxemia when supine (Sandham *et al.* 1977; Kumar *et al.* 2004) and as a result may experience significant desaturation during sleep at high altitude.

25.4 BLOOD DISORDERS

25.4.1 Anemia

Anemia will impair oxygen delivery and exercise performance at high altitude, but there are no data regarding the degree of anemia sufficient to provoke these problems and no data indicating that anemia increases the risk of acute altitude illness. Individuals with anemia of known cause should have their hematocrits checked prior to high altitude travel and consider pretravel transfusion if their hematocrit is below 20% or perhaps higher thresholds if physical activity is planned. Individuals with low iron stores, such as premenopausal women (Richalet *et al.* 1993) can also give consideration to iron supplementation prior to and during their trip. Those individuals in whom the cause of anemia has not been identified should complete a diagnostic work up prior to their trip to rule out ongoing bleeding or a hemolytic process.

Patients using exogenous erythropoietin (EPO) for chronic anemia may need reduced doses during prolonged stays at high altitude, as a retrospective analysis of a large number of dialysis-dependent patients in the United States found that patients living above 1800 m received 19% less EPO and had higher hematocrits than patients living at sea level (Brookhart *et al.* 2008). Any patient on EPO therapy planning a prolonged stay at high altitude will need close follow up of their hematocrit.

25.4.2 Patients on chronic anticoagulation therapy

Individuals on chronic anticoagulation with warfarin, clopidogrel or aspirin should use caution when traveling into remote areas away from medical care, as control of spontaneous or traumatic bleeding may be difficult in the absence of blood product support.

No studies have prospectively examined the effect of acute hypoxia on the anticoagulant effects of these medications, but a retrospective analysis of high altitude residents traveling to lower elevations revealed that such travel was associated with alterations in the patients' international normalized ratio (INR) (Van Patot et al. 2006). Given this, any individuals on warfarin should arrange follow-up measurement of their INR upon returning home at the end of their trip or, in the case of prolonged stays at high altitude, during the trip itself.

25.4.3 Sickle cell anemia and sickle cell trait

High altitude travel should be avoided in patients with sickle cell anemia, as hypoxia will increase sickling and provoke vaso-occlusive crises (Green et al. 1971), a problem that has even been described with pressurized airplane flights or driving over mountain passes as low as 2500 m (Mahoney and Githens 1979). Reports in the literature indicate that travel over 2000 m is associated with a 20–30% risk of vaso-occlusive crises in patients with either homozygous sickle cell disease (Hb SS) or sickle cell/hemoglobin C disease (Hb SC) (Adzaku et al. 1993). Even patients with sickle cell trait (Hb AS) may be at risk for problems, as several reports have documented splenic crises in these patients following acute altitude exposure (Franklin and Compeggie 1999; Tiernan 1999). Hb AS patients can likely still travel to high altitude, but should be vigilant about maintaining hydration and seek medical attention and/or descend with the onset of left upper quadrant pain or left-sided pleuritic pain.

25.5 DIABETES MELLITUS

The limited available evidence suggests that diabetes does not impair physiologic adaptation or exercise performance or increase the risk of acute mountain sickness at high altitude and that diabetic patients can engage in a wide range of activities in this environment (Honigman et al. 1993; Moore et al. 2001; Pavan et al. 2003; Kalson et al. 2007). In fact, a type I diabetic patient has summited Mt Everest while other studies report success rates on Mt Kilimanjaro that are similar to those of non-diabetic patients (Admetlla et al. 2001; Pavan et al. 2003; Kalson et al. 2007).

It is important to note that all of the studies above only considered type I diabetics and the literature currently lacks evidence regarding type II patients. A particular concern with the latter group of patients, particularly older individuals, is that they are more likely to have comorbid conditions, such as coronary artery disease, hypertension or obesity than a young, otherwise healthy type I patient and, as a result may need pretravel evaluation for those issues.

Besides tolerance of and performance at high altitude, an important question for diabetic patients is whether their insulin requirements and glycemic control will worsen following ascent to high altitude. The data on this question are mixed with some studies reporting increased requirements (Admetlla et al. 2001; Pavan et al. 2003; de Mol et al. 2011) and others reporting reduced requirements (Moore et al. 2001). Comparison between studies is difficult, however, due to differences in ascent profiles, duration spent at altitude, food intake and activities during the expeditions in each study. Dexamethasone will worsen glycemic control, so diabetic travelers should likely rely on acetazolamide for prophylaxis against altitude illness provided they have no contraindications to that medication.

From a practical standpoint, those individuals taking insulin should appreciate not only the considerable energy output that may be demanded over a few days, up to 25 MJ day^{-1} (6000 kcal day^{-1}) or more, but also the variation from day to day and within the day. During severe exercise, they may need less insulin than on rest days because of increased glucose uptake by muscle metabolism. During rest days, insulin requirement will be similar to that at sea level. Because of these great variations, diabetics should be encouraged to use quick acting insulin for basal and meal coverage. Long acting insulin preparations, such as glargine, should generally be avoided or used at lower doses than normal until the individual has a good idea of their insulin requirements. They must also give strong consideration to proper storage of their insulin, taking care to prevent freezing or heating of the insulin ampules throughout the expedition.

In recent years, increasing numbers of type I diabetics have been using insulin pumps rather than intermittent subcutaneous injections to regulate blood glucose levels. Whether these devices function as intended at high altitude is unclear. In the lone study on this topic, King *et al.* (2011) examined 10 insulin pumps during airplane flight with a 200 mmHg decrease in cabin pressure, as well as in a hypobaric chamber. During the chamber studies, bubbles developed in the insulin and expanded according to Boyle's Law. The authors also noted excess insulin administration during airplane flight (0.623% of the cartridge volume), likely due to bubble formation and expansion, which could, in turn, lead to hypoglycemia. Until further evidence is available, these findings suggest it would be prudent for individuals relying on pumps to either decrease their basal insulin rates or change to intermittent subcutaneous injections for the purpose of their trip.

The variability in activity and dietary intake and questions about pump function place a premium on frequent glucose monitoring in insulin-dependent travelers. Caution must be exercised in interpreting glucometer readings, however, as early studies on monitor accuracy at altitude suggested that a variety of meters using different measurement methodologies either over- or underestimate serum glucose values (Gautier *et al.* 1996; Pecchio *et al.* 2000; Moore *et al.* 2001; Fink *et al.* 2002). Two more recent studies, however, suggest that the performance of some later generation monitors may, in fact, be better. De Mol *et al.* (2010) studied glucose dehydrogenase and glucose oxidase monitors in simulated and terrestrial high altitude conditions and found no significant differences in monitor performance between the two types of monitoring systems in all of the tested glucose ranges, although all of the systems tended to overestimate glucose at high altitude. Of note, the glucose dehydrogenase systems had better within-meter variation and

accuracy when compared to reference glucose solutions than the glucose oxidase systems, perhaps because, unlike the glucose oxidase systems, the glucose dehydrogenase reaction pathway does not involve oxygen. The latter finding agrees with that of Oberg and Ostenson (2005) who found that the glucose dehydrogenase monitors performed better during testing in a hypobaric chamber. A problem in this study, however, was that both monitoring systems had accuracy issues when exposed to cold temperatures, a common environmental condition on many high altitude trips.

Given these concerns with monitor accuracy, patients should likely not maintain overly strict control for the duration of their travel as the risks associated with hypoglycemia outweigh the risks associated with short-term elevations in serum glucose values. Travelers should also maintain ready access to glucose sources that can be used in the event of hypoglycemic events. Finally, it is important for the diabetic traveler to inform their travel partners and expedition leaders of their condition so appropriate evaluation and management can be instituted in the event the individual manifests complications of their illness while at high altitude.

25.6 GASTROINTESTINAL DISORDERS

25.6.1 Gastrointestinal bleeding

Patients with prior gastrointestinal bleeding due to, for example, peptic ulcer disease or gastritis should exercise caution when traveling to high altitude as several reports indirectly suggest the risk of gastrointestinal bleeding may be increased at high altitude. Wu *et al.* (2007a), for example, studied 13 502 workers between 3500 and 4900 m on the Qinghai–Tibetan railway and found a 0.49% incidence of hematemesis, melena or hematochezia. Endoscopy was performed on all affected individuals and revealed evidence of gastric and duodenal ulcers, gastric erosions and hemorrhagic gastritis. More recently, Fruehauf *et al.* (2010) performed endoscopy on 26 asymptomatic mountaineers with normal pre-expedition endoscopy ascending to 4559 m over 22 hours and noted gastric or duodenal erosions/ulcers, hemorrhagic gastritis or duodenitis and reflux esophagitis in 28% of individuals on day 2 and 61% of individuals on day 4 at high altitude, although none of the climbers experienced active gastrointestinal bleeding. These studies do not establish a definitive link between acute hypoxia and gastrointestinal bleeding, but do suggest that patients with poorly controlled esophagitis, gastritis or peptic ulcer disease may be at risk for problems at high altitude. Individuals with these problems should be careful when using medication known to increase the risk of gastrointestinal bleeding, such as non-steroid anti-inflammatory agents or dexamathasone, to treat or prevent symptoms of altitude illness or arthralgias and should consider the possibility of occult bleeding in the event they develop unexplained weakness.

25.6.2 Inflammatory bowel disease

There are no data available regarding the effects of acute hypoxia on patients with inflammatory bowel diseases, including Crohn's disease and ulcerative colitis. Travel to high altitude should be avoided during exacerbations of these disorders. Those patients whose disease is in a quiescent phase may consider high altitude travel, but must carefully plan their diet and medications, research the availability of local healthcare resources and evacuation strategies prior to their trip and travel with medication suitable for treating exacerbations.

25.6.3 Chronic liver disease

Similarly, there are no data regarding patients with chronic liver disease at high altitude, although from a theoretical standpoint, two groups of cirrhotic patients may have difficulty in this environment. Those patients with portopulmonary hypertension may be at risk for high altitude pulmonary edema or worsening right heart function, as discussed earlier in this chapter, while those patients with hepatopulmonary syndrome may have significant hypoxemia due to worsening shunt physiology

in low ambient oxygen conditions. Regardless of whether or not they have these disorders, all chronic liver disease patients should avoid acetazolamide for prevention or treatment of AMS as the medication can provoke hyperammonemia and worsening encephalopathy in these patients (Luks and Swenson 2008).

25.6.4 Other gastrointestinal conditions

Pre-existing gastrointestinal tract conditions such as hemorrhoids, perianal hematomas, perianal and ischiorectal abscesses and anal fissures should all be dealt with prior to any prolonged expedition to high altitude as management once in the field may be challenging. Hernias should also be repaired prior to an expedition as the heavy lifting often required on such trips could lead to enlargement of the hernia and potentially increase the risk of incarceration and strangulation, problems that could have devastating consequences in a remote area away from medical care.

25.7 CHRONIC KIDNEY DISEASE

Patients with chronic kidney disease (CKD) face several potential challenges at high altitude. Because renal insufficiency impairs urinary concentration and dilution capacity, these patients may be at risk for volume depletion or volume overload, the latter of which might predispose to pulmonary edema. Mairbaurl et al. (1989b) for example, demonstrated that dialysis-dependent patients had greater weight gain between dialysis sessions at 2000 m when compared to 576 m. Due to impaired EPO production and decreased red blood cell survival, CKD patients may also have blunted erythropoietic responses to high altitude, as evidenced by several studies showing little to no change in hemoglobin concentration, EPO production and reticulocyte count over 2 weeks at altitudes between 2000 and 4600 m. While a low hematocrit might be tolerated at low elevation, the blunted hematologic response at high altitude would be expected to decrease oxygen delivery and limit exercise capacity (Mairbaurl et al. 1989a; Quick et al. 1992). Despite these blunted erythropoietic responses, as noted earlier, CKD patients on exogenous EPO therapy actually require lower doses than at sea level (Hussein *et al.* 1992; Brookhart *et al.* 2008) suggesting that individuals on EPO staying at altitude for more than several weeks will need careful follow up of their medication dosing.

Many patients with CKD have a chronic metabolic acidosis. While this could potentially raise minute ventilation and help defend the arterial P_{O_2} at high altitude, it could also theoretically increase the risk of HAPE, as data from animals (Lejeune *et al.* 1990) suggest metabolic acidosis increases hypoxic pulmonary vasoconstriction, a key pathophysiologic factor in

HAPE. CKD patients also have a 40% prevalence of mild to moderate pulmonary hypertension (Abassi *et al.* 2006), which, as noted above may be a risk factor for HAPE, particularly in individuals who cannot adequately regulate their volume status.

Finally, patients with CKD who opt for pharmacologic prophylaxis against altitude illness with acetazolamide will need to decrease the dose or choose another medication altogether based on their glomerular filtration rate (Table 25.1). Patients on diuretic therapy will also need to carefully monitor their weight and alter their diuretics according to a pre-arranged plan if they have fluid retention.

Table 25.1 Medication choices and dose adjustments for altitude illness medications in patients with chronic underlying medical conditions

Medication	Dose adjustments in renal insufficiency	Dose adjustments in hepatic insufficiency	Other issues
Acetazolamide	Avoid use in patients with GFR <10 mL/min, metabolic acidosis, hypokalemia, hypercalcemia and hyperphosphatemia or recurrent nephrolithiasis	Acetazolamide use is contraindicated	Avoid in patients on chronically high doses of aspirin Avoid in patients with ventilatory limitation (FEV_1 <25% predicted) Caution in patients with documented sulfa allergy Avoid concurrent use of topiramate and ophthalmic carbonic anhydrase inhibitors
Dexamethasone	No contraindication and no dose adjustments necessary	No contraindication and no dose adjustments necessary	Expect elevated blood glucose values when used in diabetic patients Avoid in patients at risk for peptic ulcer disease or upper gastrointestinal bleeding Caution in patients at risk for amoebiasis or strongyloidiasis
Nifedipine	No contraindication and no dose adjustments necessary	Best to avoid. If use is necessary, give at reduced dose (10 mg bid)	Caution in patients taking medications metabolized by CytP450 3A4 and 1A2 pathways Caution during concurrent use with other antihypertensive medications

Tadalafil	Dose adjustments necessary if GFR <50 mL/min; if GFR 30–50 mL/min, use 5 mg dose, maximum 10 mg in 48 h; if GFR <30 mL/min, no more than 5 mg	Child's Class A and B: maximum 10 mg daily Child's Class C: Do not use tadalafil	Increased risk of gastroesophageal reflux Caution in patients taking medications metabolized by CytP450 3A4 pathway Avoid concurrent use of nitrates or alpha-blockers
Sildenafil	Dose adjustments necessary if GFR <30 mL/min	Dose reductions recommended. Starting dose 25 mg tid Avoid use in patients with known esophageal or gastric varices	Increased risk of gastroesophageal reflux Caution in patients taking medications metabolized by CytP450 3A4 pathway Avoid concurrent use of nitrates or alpha-blockers
Salmeterol	No contraindication and no dose adjustments necessary	Insufficient data. Best to avoid the medication in these patients	Potential for adverse effects in patients with coronary artery disease prone to arrhythmia Avoid concurrent use of beta-blockers Avoid concurrent use of monoamine oxidase inhibitors or tricyclic antidepressants

25.8 ORTHOPEDIC CONDITIONS

Those with arthritis, particularly of the joints of the lower limb should carefully consider the degree and amount of exercise that has to be taken on a mountain trek. Acetaminophen and non-steroidal anti-inflammatory drugs can be very beneficial and should be started early rather than being heroic about the pain, although, given the issues discussed above regarding the risk of gastrointestinal bleeding at high altitude, individuals should exercise caution with prolonged high dose of non-steroidal anti-inflammatory agents, such as ibuprofen or naproxen. Treatment of painful joints, particularly of the hip, whether by replacement prosthesis, arthrodesis or some other method may make a short trek possible.

25.9 EAR, NOSE, THROAT AND DENTAL PROBLEMS

Nasal polyps or a deviated nasal septum that interferes with breathing should be treated prior to ascent. Patients with perennial rhinitis and sinusitis should ensure supplies of their usual medications.

Any individual planning a trip out of range of dental care, particularly long expeditions into remote areas, is well advised to have a thorough dental check-up evaluation of any suspected problems prior to their trip. Air resulting from decay in the root system or beneath old fillings could theoretically expand upon ascent to high altitude and cause increasing pain.

25.10 OBESITY

Several studies have suggested that obese individuals are at greater risk for acute mountain sickness. Ri-Li *et al.* (2003) for example, exposed obese and non-obese men to a simulated altitude of 3658 m for 24 hours and found a higher incidence of AMS and lower oxygen saturation values during sleep in the obese subjects compared to the non-obese. The results of this chamber study agree with those of Honigman *et al.* (1993) who found a higher incidence of AMS among obese individuals traveling to altitudes between 1920 and 2950 m in the Colorado Rockies as part of general tourist activities. The reason for the possible increased risk is not clear, but may relate to differences in ventilation, particularly at night, relative to the non-obese travelers. This question has not been evaluated prospectively at terrestrial high altitude and the degree of obesity necessary to increase risk remains unclear.

Morbidly obese individuals with obesity hypoventilation syndrome may be at risk for developing problems aside from AMS following ascent. These individuals often have underlying pulmonary hypertension, which as noted earlier, may increase the risk for developing high altitude pulmonary edema. In addition, the increased alveolar hypoxia at high altitude may trigger further rises in pulmonary artery pressures and induce right heart failure, a phenomenon which has been described in the setting of commercial airline flight (Toff 1993).

25.11 NEUROLOGICAL PROBLEMS

25.11.1 Headache

The presence of headaches in daily life at low altitude does not predispose to headaches upon ascent to high elevation, although the severity of high altitude headaches may be greater in such individuals (Silber *et al.* 2003). Although there is no convincing evidence that hypoxia provokes migraine headaches, migraine headache sufferers may be at greater risk for developing acute mountain sickness (Hackett 2001; Richalet *et al.* 2011) or altered character of their migraine headaches following ascent (Murdoch 1995).

25.11.2 Epilepsy

There is no systematic evidence that travel to high altitude is associated with increased frequency or severity of seizures in people taking medications for a known seizure disorder, although there are several unpublished reports of seizures in individuals who had a remote history of seizures or who were subsequently diagnosed with an underlying seizure disorder (Baumgartner *et al.* 2007). It is probably reasonable for patients with well-controlled seizures to go on a trek or other trip to high altitude but technical climbing should be avoided due to the potential adverse consequences of a seizure to the seizing individual or their climbing partners. Some anti-seizure medications may affect breathing adversely during sleep, while others in high doses may affect coordination. Patients taking topiramate for seizure prophylaxis should avoid acetazolamide as the medication has carbonic anhydrase activity and combined use of the medications can result in nephrolithiasis (Luks and Swenson 2008).

25.11.3 Sleep

Common sleep disturbances at high altitude as well as expected outcomes in patients with underlying obstructive sleep apnea are described in detail in Chapter 14. Individuals who use medications to promote sleep at sea level should exercise care at high altitude as some medications may lead to nocturnal hypoventilation and worsening hypoxemia. The available evidence suggests that temazepam, zolpidem and zaleplon are likely safe and effective at high altitude, while diazepam and opiate medications should be avoided. Eszoplicone has not been studied at high altitude but should be safe to use given that it has a similar mechanism of action as zolpidem and zaleplon. Diphenhydramine is likely also safe, but the potential for daytime drowsiness may make this a less than ideal sleep aid for those engaged in high risk or technical activities at high altitude (Luks 2008).

25.12 RHEUMATOLOGIC DISORDERS

There is no evidence that exposure to high altitude leads to exacerbation of underlying rheumatologic disorders, although the lack of information on this question may reflect the fact that people with severe rheumatologic disease may not be fit enough or feel well enough to travel to high altitude. Certain rheumatologic diseases, such as scleroderma or rheumatoid arthritis, can be associated with the development of interstitial lung disease or pulmonary hypertension. Patients with such problems should exercise caution with travel to high altitude as discussed earlier in this chapter.

Some sources (Grissom and DeLoughery 2007) warn about the possibility of increased frequency and severity of attacks of Raynaud's phenomenon at high altitude, particularly in cold conditions but there is little evidence to support this claim. Luks *et al.* (2009) tried to evaluate this issue by surveying a large number of individuals with primary Raynaud's phenomenon who travel to altitudes above 2440 m. They found that motivated individuals employing various prevention and treatment strategies were able to engage in a wide variety of activities, including winter sports, at high altitude but that there was considerable heterogeneity in perceptions of the frequency, duration and severity of attacks at high altitude compared to high elevation.

25.13 PSYCHIATRIC ILLNESS

Very little information exists regarding the effect of high altitude on patients with underlying psychiatric illnesses, such as depression, bipolar disorder or severe anxiety. Fagenholz *et al.* (2007) described six trekkers in Nepal who developed anxiety-related problems, including symptom-limited panic attacks related to nocturnal periodic breathing, excessive health-related anxiety and excessive emotionality

despite having no history of anxiety disorders or other psychiatric illnesses at low altitude. This report fits with anecdotal experiences of other medical personnel at high altitude who have interacted with individuals having difficulty coping with some of the different sensations they experience at high altitude, such as dyspnea and tachycardia. However, despite these experiences and the fact that many of the common symptoms experienced by high altitude travelers, including headaches, dyspnea, increased heart rate and awakening at night with dyspnea, are similar to those experienced in panic attacks, there is little evidence that the acute hypoxia at high altitude leads to panic attacks or increases anxiety (Roth *et al.* 2002).

Many types of high altitude travel including long duration treks in foreign countries and major mountaineering expeditions can impose stresses on the traveler that might not be experienced with less extensive trips back home. In addition, the safety of expedition members often depends not only on their own behavior and actions, but also on the well-being of others. For this reason, individuals should not embark on long duration or technical climbing trips to high altitude, particularly in remote areas, if they have any form of psychiatric illness that is not under adequate control. Any exacerbation of their illness could lead to disruption of travel plans or possibly physical harm for them or other members of the expedition.

25.14 PRE-EXISTING MEDICAL CONDITIONS AND ALTITUDE ILLNESS MEDICATIONS

Recommendations for pharmacologic prevention and treatment of acute altitude illness are largely based on studies performed in healthy individuals lacking severe chronic medical problems. For this reason, providers should exercise caution when prescribing these medications to patients with chronic medical conditions, taking care to choose the appropriate choice and dose of medication and to avoid adverse drug interactions. A full discussion of these medication issues is provided elsewhere (Luks and Swenson 2008) and a summary of these recommendations is provided in Table 25.1.

26

Women at altitude

SUMMARY

Women respond to altitude in very much the same way as men. They acclimatize in a similar way, are as likely to develop acute mountain sickness (AMS) and experience similar changes in exercise performance. Studies investigating the effect of the menstrual cycle have also failed to find significant differences in performance or susceptibility to AMS in different phases of the cycle. Women seem to have an advantage over men in that they lose less weight at altitude probably because they suffer less loss of appetite. The risk of altitude exposure in pregnancy is not known, but, based on the current state of knowledge, women known to be at increased risk for spontaneous abortion or ectopic pregnancy should avoid high altitude travel in the first trimester while in the second half of pregnancy, travel to moderate altitudes is safe provided the woman does not undertake heavy exercise or have any pregnancy-related complications, such as pregnancy-induced hypertension. Oral contraceptives are widely used for both contraception and for menstrual regulation by women at altitude and while there is a theoretical risk that altitude and increased hematocrit may lead to thrombosis, there is no direct evidence that this relationship exists at high altitude.

26.1 INTRODUCTION

While much of the early research into the effect of hypoxia on humans used fit young men as their subjects, more recent studies are now including or focusing solely on female subjects, thereby providing an opportunity to consider whether the female responses to acute hypoxia and susceptibility to altitude illness differ from those of their male counterparts. In this chapter, we consider this developing literature and examine physiologic responses, acclimatization, exercise performance and neurohumoral changes in women exposed to acute hypoxia and discuss other issues unique to the female high altitude traveler, including pregnancy and oral contraceptive use. The focus throughout will be on women exposed to acute hypoxia while the subject of women residing at high altitude is considered in Chapter 18.

26.2 CLIMBING PERFORMANCE

Since Junko Tabei, a Japanese climber, became the first woman to climb Everest in 1975, more than 75 women from varying nationalities and socioeconomic backgrounds have also made the ascent, including some without supplemental oxygen. Women have climbed other 8000 m peaks, including K2 and Kanchenjunga and, in fact, two women – Gerlinde Kaltenbrunner and Edurne Pasaban – have now climbed all 14 peaks of 8000 m. Kaltenbrunner has, in fact, accomplished this feat without the aid of supplemental oxygen. Overall, the number of women participating in high altitude climbing, particularly in the elite category, is lower than that of men, but there is no systematic evidence to suggest there are differences in climbing performance at these extreme or lower elevations.

26.3 ACCLIMATIZATION

The pattern of physiologic responses to hypoxia is similar between men and women, although there may be subtle differences in the magnitude of these responses in certain circumstances. For example, as long ago as 1911, Mabel FitzGerald (1913) documented hypoxic ventilatory responses over a range of altitudes and showed that the Pa,CO_2 is about 2 mmHg lower in women than men, thereby suggesting they may have greater levels of minute ventilation. Their PO_2, which was calculated from an assumed R, was presumably slightly higher. Multiple studies have confirmed that the PCO_2 falls more in women than in men during acclimatization (Hannon 1978; Barry et al. 1995; Loeppky et al. 2001), although Muza et al. (2001) reported no differences in end-tidal CO_2 and other measures of ventilatory acclimatization between men and women at 4300 m. The results of the latter study, however, were based on comparisons with male data from a separately conducted study and this study design issue may have accounted for the lack of agreement with the other studies noted above. The greater level of ventilation seen in these other studies is assumed to be due to the stimulatory effect of sex hormones and disappears after menopause.

Women also increase their hemoglobin (Hb) concentration, hematocrit and red cell mass in the same way as men, although the magnitude of the response may be dampened in women with low iron stores due to heavy menstrual blood losses.

In an early study on Pikes Peak (4300 m), for example, Hannon et al. (1966) demonstrated that women on iron supplementation had similar rises in Hb to men, whereas women not taking iron had a slower increase in Hb. Richalet et al. (1994) provided further evidence of this phenomenon, demonstrating suboptimal Hb responses, despite adequate erythropoietin responses in two women with documented low iron stores.

Multiple studies have reported no significant differences in the incidence of AMS between men and women (Hackett et al. 1976; Maggiorini et al. 1990; Honigman et al. 1993), which, given that development of AMS is representative of poor acclimatization, provides further evidence of the lack of significant differences in acclimatization between men and women. Furthermore, the presumed association between AMS and fluid retention (Hackett and Rennie 1979; Hackett et al. 1982) has not been documented to occur at a greater rate in women in whom some increase in fluid retention is thought to occur during the luteal phase of the menstrual cycle.

26.4 PERFORMANCE AND THE MENSTRUAL CYCLE

Studies from Mt Everest have demonstrated that men with higher hypoxic respiratory drives have greater ventilatory responses, higher arterial oxygenation and better climbing performance at extreme altitudes than those with lower hypoxic drives (Schoene 1982; Schoene et al. 1984). Given that menstruating women have higher hypoxic and hypercapnic respiratory drives and, thus greater exercise ventilation during the luteal phase of the menstrual cycle (Schoene et al. 1981), it is reasonable to consider whether exercise and high altitude performance varies depending on the particular phase of a woman's menstrual cycle. Beidleman and colleagues (1999) tested this hypothesis by studying exercise responses during $VO_{2,max}$ and submaximal exercise to exhaustion in eight menstruating women during the early follicular and mid-luteal phases at sea level and following acute exposure to the equivalent of 4300 m in a hypobaric chamber. Despite the fact that Sa,O_2 was 3% higher at altitude during the mid-luteal phase, peak and submaximal exercise ventilation, $V_{O_{2,max}}$ and time to exhaustion did not differ between menstrual phases at sea level or altitude. No studies have examined whether female climbing performance at extreme altitudes, such as those on Mt Everest, varies based on the phase of the menstrual cycle, but the results from Beidleman and colleagues suggest that timing of an ascent relative to the menstrual cycle does not play a role.

26.5 WEIGHT LOSS

Weight loss is a well-noted problem with prolonged stays at high altitude, but the available data suggest that women do not lose as much weight as men in this environment. Hannon *et al.* (1976), for example, studied men and women over a 7-day period on the summit of Pikes Peak (4300 m) and noted that women lost only 1.49% of their body weight during this period compared to a loss of 4.86% among the men. They attributed this difference to the fact that the women seemed to regain their appetites sooner than men did. Collier *et al.* (1997) studied individuals trekking to Everest Base Camp (5340 m), as well as several individuals who climbed towards the summit (8848 m) finding that among the trekkers, the women had no significant weight loss during their stay at this altitude, while the men lost an average of 0.11 kg m^{-2} day^{-1}. Among those who climbed towards the summit, seven men who reached altitudes of 7100–8848 m lost an average of 0.15 kg m^{-2} day^{-1}, while the one woman who climbed to above 8000 m lost no weight.

26.6 CATECHOLAMINES AND CARBOHYDRATE METABOLISM

In a 12-day study on Pike's Peak (4200 m), Mazzeo *et al.* (1998) found no difference in catecholamine response between men and women, nor between the follicular and luteal phases of the menstrual cycle. However, for a given noradrenaline urinary excretion, the heart rate and blood pressure response was lower in the follicular than in the luteal phase. In a subsequent study, Mazzeo *et al.* (2001) found that women have a strong sympathoadrenal response to acute hypoxia during rest and exercise, as well as strong compensatory sympathoadrenal responses (increased norepinephrine and epinephrine levels) to alpha-adrenergic blockade at both sea level and high altitude.

Consistent with results seen in men, insulin sensitivity in women appears to follow a biphasic pattern at high altitude with decreased sensitivity within the first few days of exposure and increased sensitivity after a period of acclimatization. Braun *et al.* (2001) for example, demonstrated reduced insulin sensitivity during 16 hours of exposure to hypobaric hypoxia, while Braun *et al.* (1998) found that after 9 days at altitude (4300 m), the blood glucose response to a standard meal was reduced with no changes in insulin concentrations. This result was likely due to increased stimulation of peripheral glucose uptake or suppression of hepatic glucose production. An additional finding in the latter study included the fact that the glucose response was lower in the estrogen than in the estrogen plus progesterone phase of the menstrual cycle.

Mawson *et al.* (2000) found that women's total energy requirements at 4300 m were 6% above sea-level values and that this difference could not be explained entirely by an increase in the basal metabolic rate. Unlike men, blood glucose utilization rates in young women after 10 days at 4300 m were lower at rest and no different during submaximal exercise from those observed at sea level. There was no correlation with circulating estrogens or progesterone (Braun *et al.* 2000).

26.7 PREGNANCY AND ORAL CONTRACEPTIVES

The risk to a pregnancy of going to altitude is not known with confidence and is likely to vary based on the stage of pregnancy and the health of the pregnant mother. Pregnant women known to be at risk for spontaneous abortion or ectopic pregnancy should avoid high altitude travel in the first trimester. Consideration can be given to doing an ultrasound prior to long duration high altitude travel to confirm an intrauterine location of the fetus and avoid complications of ectopic pregnancy during the sojourn (Jean and Moore 2012).

Travel to altitudes below 2500 m is likely safe for the mother and fetus in the second half of pregnancy, although increased progesterone, increased uterine bulk and raised diaphragms seen in late pregnancy may lead to a heightened sense of dyspnea. Travel during this time frame is contraindicated, however, in patients with pre-eclampsia, chronic hypertension or other factors that increase the risk of pre-eclampsia, impaired placental function, intrauterine growth retardation, or maternal heart or lung disease or anemia (Jean et al. 2005). Due to concerns about provoking fetal hypoxia or preterm labor, exercise should be delayed for 2–3 days following arrival to allow time for acclimatization and exertion levels should be maintained below those typically achieved at sea level (Jean et al. 2005). Despite its widespread use for prevention of acute altitude illness in other settings, acetazolamide is contraindicated in the first trimester due to concerns about teratogenicity while use after 36 weeks of pregnancy is also contraindicated due to a risk of provoking neonatal jaundice (Jean et al. 2005).

It is well known that oral contraceptives increase the risk of thrombosis at sea level, particularly when used in conjunction with cigarette smoking. Although cases of venous thromboembolism have been documented at high altitude, including in women using oral contraceptives (Shlim and Papenfus 1995), there have been no systematic studies assessing the risks associated with oral contraceptive use at high altitude. Miller (1999) surveyed 316 women trekking to Everest Base Camp and found that 30% were using oral contraceptives, primarily for control of menstruation. While a significant number of women reported irregularities of menstruation, particularly when pills were not taken regularly,

no episodes of venous thromboembolism or other complications were reported. The study design and relatively small numbers of patients, however, prevent any firm conclusions regarding safety of use in this environment. Given the widespread use of these medications and lack of clear evidence of complications related to their use at high altitude, women already on such therapy can remain on it during high altitude travel, but should maintain adequate hydration and avoid smoking. Women planning long high altitude expeditions, particularly in more austere environments, who would like more control over their menses or to avoid it altogether can also consider oral contraception during their sojourn, but should start the medications several months ahead of time in order to get used to the side effects.

26.8 WOMEN AND COLD

Cold injury, hypothermia, frostbite and immersion injury are seldom reported in women at altitude. The lack of reports could reflect the fact that women are not traveling to the same extent as men in environments where these injuries may occur, but could also be due to increased protective effects of the relatively thicker layer of subcutaneous fat found in women or perhaps differences in preparation for cold conditions. Women do have a higher incidence of Raynaud's phenomenon compared to men and the cold conditions at high altitude may provoke more frequent or intense episodes of this problem. The limited available evidence, however, suggests that motivated individuals using a variety of preventive and treatment strategies can engage in a wide variety of activities, including winter sports, at altitudes greater than 2440 m without experiencing severe adverse consequences (Luks et al. 2009).

27

Extremes of age at altitude: children and the elderly

SUMMARY

The physiologic responses of children to high altitude are similar to those of adults. However, infants in the first few months of life have ventilatory and hemodynamic responses that are in transition from the fetal to childhood settings, which may result in quite severe hypoxia in certain circumstances. Although the risk of acute altitude illness, including acute mountain sickness (AMS), high altitude pulmonary edema (HAPE) and high altitude cerebral edema (HACE) are similar between children and adults, preverbal children may not be able to adequately express that they are feeling unwell and, subsequently, may not be diagnosed as promptly as older individuals. As a result, any child who has recently ascended to altitude and becomes unwell must be assumed to be suffering from AMS unless there are clear signs of an alternative diagnosis. Children are more at risk of hypothermia and cold injury because of their larger surface to weight ratio, especially if they are being carried and not exercising. Infants are at risk of high altitude pulmonary hypertension (HAPH) if they remain at altitude for months. The management of all forms of acute altitude illness and hypothermia is similar to that in adults with appropriate adjustment of drug dosage. The justification for taking very young children, particularly infants, to altitude is questionable and is discussed.

Increasing numbers of elderly people are going on holidays to the mountains and, provided they are otherwise fit, age should not be viewed as a contraindication to such activities. Exercise capacity is reduced compared to younger mountaineers and goals must be adjusted accordingly. The elderly are no more likely to get AMS than young people. In fact, they seem to suffer less, perhaps because they are likely to gain altitude more slowly than younger individuals with higher exercise capacity. Travel planning in the elderly must take into account underlying medical conditions, including heart and lung disease and locomotor defects, whose incidence increases in the elderly, although the risk associated with previously unrecognized disease, specifically asymptomatic coronary artery disease, is small. Prevention and management of acute altitude illness in the elderly is the same as in younger individuals.

27.1 INTRODUCTION

Much of what is known about the effect of altitude on humans is based on studies of fit young men, and few studies have addressed the question of the effect of altitude on children or elderly individuals. The available literature on these issues is reviewed in this chapter but answers to frequently asked questions must still rely to some extent on anecdotal experience or extrapolation from young adult data. This chapter deals mainly with lowland children and elderly people going to altitude, while highland populations are considered further in Chapter 18.

27.2 CHILDREN

27.2.1 Introduction

The increased accessibility of the high altitude regions of the world to adults means that more children are now being taken on adventure holidays to these places. Infants have been carried over 6000 m peaks in Nepal (Pollard *et al.* 1998), while lowland Han Chinese children are taken to high altitude in Tibet and Qinghai and many school parties are venturing to high altitude. Are these children at risk from the effects of altitude? What advice should a doctor give to parents considering taking children to altitude? Many of these questions are addressed in a consensus statement from the International Society of Mountain Medicine, 'Children at altitude' (Pollard *et al.* 2001) and have been recently reviewed by Yaron and Niermeyer (2008).

27.2.2 Infants at altitude

There are some special considerations that apply to infants at altitude relating to the immaturity of their respiratory control mechanisms and the fact that their pulmonary arteries are undergoing involution of the thick muscular layers at this time. Following birth, the low flow, high resistance fetal circulation transitions over a variable time period to the high flow, low resistance adult circulation with closure of the ductus arteriosus serving as a key step in that process. Hypoxic exposure during this period can slow and possibly reverse this circulatory transition, making oxygenation difficult for the infant, particularly now that the placenta is no longer available for oxygenation

(Niermeyer 2007). Heath and Williams (1995) have also demonstrated that babies born at high altitude have persistence of the muscularization of pulmonary blood vessels in contrast to babies born as sea level.

Beyond the circulatory issues, there are also important considerations regarding ventilation. In the neonate, hypoxia has a depressant effect on ventilation. Normally this changes to the adult pattern of stimulation in the first few weeks of life, but a study by Parkins *et al.* (1998) found that even at 3 months infants responded to 15% oxygen breathing by frequent periods of isolated and periodic apnea. The mean saturation while breathing an F_IO_2 of 0.15 was 92% in these infants. The responses were very variable, but some infants had saturations that fell to less than 80% for up to a minute (at which time the intervention was stopped).

Niermeyer (2003) has reviewed her own and others' work on infants at high altitude. There are remarkable differences in arterial saturations in the first few months of life between infants at low and high altitudes and in different populations at high altitude. Figure 27.1 shows the Sa,O_2 during the first 4 months of life in quietly sleeping infants at various altitudes and in different populations. Infants at sea level have a saturation of 96–98% within the first few hours after birth and reach a slightly higher level with less variability over the next few months as their cardiorespiratory control goes through the transition from fetal to young infant settings. At Denver (1610 m), there is a small drop from 24 to 48 h after birth and the Sa,O_2 then remains constant. The same population at the altitude of Leadville, Colorado (3100 m) shows a profound drop 24–48 h after birth and then a rise over the next 2 months. Han Chinese infants in Lhasa (3658 m) show a similar drop, but then a continued decline over 4 months. Tibetan infants also at Lhasa have a rather higher Sa,O_2 at birth than Chinese infants but a similar drop, which then remains steady. Andean infants (not shown) have results intermediate between Tibetan and Han Chinese. The mechanisms behind these observations are complex and include changes and differences in control of breathing, maturation of the lung and control of pulmonary vascular pressures.

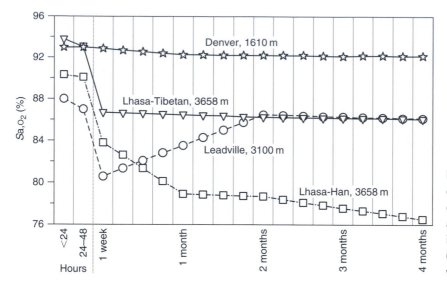

Figure 27.1 Arterial oxygen saturation in quietly sleeping infants at various altitudes and in various populations (from Niermeyer 2003, with permission).

It seems likely that hypoxia interferes with the normal transition of responses that occurs after birth (Parkins *et al.* 1998). It is the Han Chinese infants, of course, who, with their profound hypoxemia, are particularly prone to symptomatic high altitude pulmonary hypertension (previously called sub-acute mountain sickness) (Sui *et al.* 1988), described in Chapter 22.

Yaron *et al.* (2003) reported the physiological responses to altitude of children aged 3–36 months. The comparison was between Denver (1610 m) and an altitude of 3109 m. After 24 h at altitude, the children showed tachypnea, relative hypoxia, hypocarbia and a reduction in cerebral tissue oxygenation (by near-infrared spectroscopy). These changes were similar to those seen in adults. However, the reduction in cerebral oxygenation was age dependent, with lower values being seen in the younger subjects. AMS symptoms were scored, but there was no correlation between AMS scores and any physiological measurement.

27.2.3 Sudden infant death at altitude

In view of the quite severe desaturation in infants at altitude (Fig. 27.1) and the known effect of an acute respiratory infection to lower $Sa_{,O_2}$ still further, it would seem likely that altitude must be a risk factor for sudden infant death syndrome

(SIDS). However, there is very little evidence to support this assertion. One study that did address this question was by Kohlendorfer and colleagues (1998) who carried out a case–control study in Austria of SIDS deaths. They found that higher altitude districts did have higher rates of SIDS, but these districts also had higher rates for the practice of placing infants in the prone position for sleep. This effect largely accounted for the difference in rate of SIDS. The possibility that altitude is a risk factor for SIDS cannot be ruled out at present, especially at altitudes higher than in this study.

27.2.4 Older children at altitude

Little is known about the physiologic responses of children between the ages of 3 years and the early teens to altitude. Recently, Scrase *et al.* (2009) studied nine children between the ages of 6 and 13 years without previous high altitude exposure during a trek to 3500 m in Nepal and demonstrated responses similar to that seen in most adults. Over the course of the trek, the children showed a small increase in resting daytime respiratory rate, increases in resting heart rate with increasing altitude (on average 24 bpm higher at 3500 m than at sea level), an average 9% drop in daytime oxygen saturation and an average 11% decrease in nocturnal oxygen saturation and a 7 mmHg reduction in the end-tidal carbon dioxide partial pressure compared to their sea-level values. Spirometry was also performed as part of the study with both the forced expiratory volume in one second (FEV_1) and forced vital capacity (FVC) remaining within 7% of baseline values in seven of the nine children, but showing significant drops between 12 and 23% in two others. After a week of trekking and sleeping at up to 3860 m, oxygen saturation improved 3% on average, while end-tidal carbon dioxide fell by an additional 3 mmHg, changes indicative of ongoing ventilatory acclimatization.

27.2.5 Sleep at altitude in children

Sleep disturbances at high altitude are well documented in adults (see Chapter 14), but only a few studies have examined these issues in children. Yaron et al. (2004) used ankle actigraphy to continuously monitor motion in infants and young children (range, 4–33 months) during sleep at home and at just above 3100 m and found significant disturbances in sleep that were most pronounced on the first night at altitude. More recently, Kohler et al. (2008) compared sleep responses in 20 prepubertal children (ages 9–12 years) with their fathers during one night at 490 m and two nights at 3450 m and found that the children spent less time in periodic breathing on both nights at high altitude than the adults and had a lower apnea threshold, but had similar drops in their nocturnal oxygen saturations and end-tidal carbon dioxide tensions. Total sleep duration was similar between the children and adults, although the authors were unable to assess for differences in the distribution of sleep stages.

27.2.6 Diagnosis of AMS in children

In older children, the diagnosis of AMS can be made based on symptoms as in adults, although problems with both over- and underestimation of symptoms make diagnosis challenging. In their study of children trekking in Nepal, for example, Scrase et al. (2009) found that the children over- and under-reported symptoms on the Lake Louise Scoring System (LLSS) when compared to the objective physical measures or observations by parents and investigators. Similarly, Southard et al. (2007) reported that the language used in the LLSS tended to underestimate AMS symptoms in 4–11-year-old children. In younger children who cannot articulate their feelings, the diagnostic challenges are likely to be worse. In such children, AMS will manifest as lack of playfulness, fussiness, anorexia, nausea and altered sleep patterns (Yaron 2002), but such changes are non-specific and hard to distinguish from other potential causes. In the setting of a recent increase in altitude, the only safe course is to assume a young child's fractiousness is due to AMS unless there are signs clearly pointing to some other cause. Yaron et al. (1998) have proposed a 'fussiness score' in such preverbal children, analogous to the Lake Louise score for AMS (section 18.8). Fussiness is scored on a scale of 0–6 for both amount and intensity. This equates to the headache symptom in the Lake Louise system. Other symptoms are then scored 0–3 for, 'How well has your child eaten?', 'How playful is your child today?' and 'How has the child napped today?' This system may also be found as an appendix to the ISMM (International Society for Mountain Medicine) consensus statement (Pollard et al. 2001). To evaluate this scoring system, they studied 23 children aged 3–36 months who ascended over 4 days from either Denver (1609 m) or Fort Collins (1615 m) Colorado to the Keystone Summit Lodge (3488 m). There were 45 accompanying adults, 20% of whom developed AMS at Keystone. Based on the 'fussiness score,' 21% of the infants were diagnosed as having AMS. This scoring system, also referred to as the 'Children's Lake Louise score' was further evaluated in a subsequent study by this group (Yaron et al. 2002) and found to demonstrate good inter-observer agreement.

27.2.7 Incidence of acute altitude illness in children

There have been a few surveys of children at altitude. Wu (1994b) studied lowland Han Chinese adults and children at the overnight stop, Tuo-Tuo (4550 m), as they traveled the Qinghai–Tibet highway to Lhasa. A total of 5355 adults and 464 children were assessed and AMS was diagnosed based on symptoms and the response to oxygen breathing. The incidences for AMS were 38.2% in adults and 34.1% in children. In Colorado, Theis *et al.* (1993) found an incidence of AMS of 28% at an altitude of 2835 m for children aged 9–14 years, but there was no comparable figure for adults. This may seem rather high for this altitude, but a control group at sea level had a 20% incidence of similar symptoms as those seen in AMS, so some of the reported symptoms at altitude may have been due to the travel itself. More recently, Yaron *et al.* (2002) also found similar incidence of AMS in young children as in adults at 3109 m: 19 and 24%, respectively. Finally, Pradhan *et al.* (2009) reported a 47% incidence of AMS among 36 native Nepalese children between the ages of 3 and 15 years ascending from 1950 to 4380 m as part of a pilgrimage to Gosaikunda Lake.

While the incidence rates noted in these and other studies (Yaron *et al.* 1998) suggest that children and adults likely share the same susceptibility to AMS, the reproducibility of symptoms upon subsequent ascent may differ between the two groups. Rexhaj *et al.* (2011) studied 27 unacclimatized children and 29 adults during two ascents to 3450 m 9–12 months apart and found that none of the six children who developed AMS on the first ascent experienced this problem on repeat ascent compared to 14 of 18 adults who had AMS with both exposures. Four children who remained symptom free on the first ascent also developed AMS with the second exposure.

There have been no reported cases of HACE in children, while the incidence of HAPE has been only infrequently reported. In the same study noted above, Wu (1994b) diagnosed HAPE based on symptoms and chest radiography and noted an incidence of 1.51% in children compared to 1.27% in adults. Respiratory infection (Durmowicz *et al.* 1997) and underlying cardiopulmonary abnormalities, such as pulmonary hypertension (Durmowicz 2001), may predispose to HAPE in children. Like adults, children residing at high altitude have also been noted to experience a phenomenon known as re-entry pulmonary edema, whereby pulmonary edema develops following rapid re-ascent to their home elevation after a sojourn to lower elevation (Scoggin *et al.* 1977). Of note, when Hultgren and Spickard (1960) first described HAPE in Peru, several of

the cases were in children who had returned with their family to their high altitude residence after spending time at sea level.

27.2.8 Prophylaxis and treatment of altitude illness in children

Pharmacologic prophylaxis against altitude illness should generally be avoided unless overly rapid ascent is unavoidable or the child has a history of re-entry HAPE. The treatment of AMS in children is the same as in adults (section 19.7). Beyond having a high index of suspicion in the setting of a recent gain in altitude, the essential step is to get the child down to a lower altitude. In only the mildest cases is a 'wait and see' policy justified. If there is any suspicion of AMS, further ascent is out of the question. There have been no formal trials of any drugs in children in this setting, but it is assumed that the same medication can be used in children as in adults. The dosage suggested for drugs used in AMS is shown in Table 27.1. Aspirin should be avoided because of the slight risk of Reye's syndrome.

Table 27.1   Dosage for drugs used in children for acute mountain sickness, high altitude pulmonary edema and high altitude cerebral edema

Drug	Dose	Route
Paracetamol	12 mg kg^{-1} every 6 h	Oral
Dexamethasone	0.15 mg kg^{-1} every 6 h	Oral or i.v.
Acetazolamide	AMS prophylaxis: 1.25 mg kg^{-1} every 12 h; max 125 mg AMS treatment: 2.5 mg kg^{-1} every 12 h; max 250 mg	Oral
Nifedipine	0.5 mg kg^{-1} every 8 h; max 20 mg for caps, 40 mg for tabs	Oral

Source: Pollard *et al.* (2001).
AMS, acute mountain sickness.

Symptoms and signs of HAPE or HACE mandate immediate descent or transfer to a health facility with supplemental oxygen. Management of these disorders is similar to that in adults (Chapters 20 and 21). There is a report of the successful use of the Gamow bag in a 3.5-year-old child with severe AMS (Taber 1994). Given reported associations between HAPE and underlying cardiopulmonary abnormalities, such as pulmonary hypertension (Durmowicz 2001) or absent right pulmonary artery (Rios et al. 1985), children who develop exaggerated hypoxemia or other evidence of HAPE at high altitude should undergo diagnostic evaluation by their pediatrician upon return to sea level (Yaron and Niermeyer 2007).

27.2.9 Children, cold and heat

Children are not only smaller than adults but have a larger surface-to-weight ratio, so as a result, cool faster in cold and heat up more quickly in hot conditions (Kennedy and Gentle 1995). Thermal balance is less efficient in children, and during exercise they generate more metabolic heat for a unit mass than adults, have lower cardiac output and gain heat more rapidly from the environment. They also acclimatize to heat more slowly in hot conditions. In addition to their larger surface to mass ratio, they have less subcutaneous fat and may have an underdeveloped shivering mechanism. For all these reasons, they are at greater risk than adults of hypothermia in a cold environment and of overheating in hot environments.

In cold or wet conditions, a windproof and waterproof garment is essential, and particular attention should be paid to the head from which proportionally more heat is lost than in an adult. It should also be remembered that a child who is being carried is not generating heat in the way the adult carrier is and so needs more clothing. Overheating can occur when on a glacier or snowfield in sunny conditions because of direct and reflected heat. Eyes must be protected by goggles and the exposed skin by sunblock cream. Adequate fluid must be given, especially in hot conditions, to prevent dehydration (Pollard and Murdoch 1997).

27.2.10 Conclusions

Although children are at no greater risk of AMS than adults at the same altitude, the fact that young children have difficulty in articulating their symptoms means that diagnosis is more difficult and may be delayed. Children with these problems can progress from being perfectly healthy to being seriously ill at an alarming rate. The fact that, in most cases, an altitude holiday is also a holiday in a part of the world where medical help is far away and gastrointestinal infections and other diseases are common must be borne in mind. As a result of all these factors, efforts must be made to balance the risks of high altitude travel with the benefits of what may be a valuable experience in the event no one becomes ill. On balance, we would concur with Pollard et al. (1998) in a cautious approach in advising families considering high altitude trips with some minor modifications in their recommendations. They suggest that, with children under 2 years of age, parties should not sleep at over 2000 m and no higher than 3000 m for children of 2–10 years. In light of the data from Scrase et al. (2009) noted above, children over the age of 6 years, who can verbally express their symptoms, can likely sleep as high as 3500 m without problems and enjoy higher altitudes with probably little more risk than adults.

27.3 ELDERLY PEOPLE

27.3.1 Introduction

The increasing number of people going to high altitude includes a large proportion of elderly individuals. People are living longer than in the past and many retired men and women have the money, time and inclination to enjoy sightseeing or treks to the great ranges, to ski and to attend conferences. A survey of over 1900 visitors to Keystone, Colorado (2783 m), for example, revealed that 48% were aged 40–60 years and 15% were over 60 (Gillman 1993). Approximately 10% of trekkers in Nepal were 50 years of age or older (Hultgren 1992), while over 70% of Japanese trekkers were over 50 years old (Saito et al. 2002). Physicians are often asked to evaluate the risk of high altitude travel in such individuals. In considering this question, it is important to remember that older individuals often have underlying medical problems that might worsen at high altitude. The evaluation of specific conditions and their management at high altitude is considered in Chapter 25, while in this section we focus on the apparently fit elderly person at altitude.

27.3.2 Performance

All bodily functions deteriorate with age and this includes the maximum oxygen uptake both at sea level and at altitude (Pugh et al. 1964). However, the effect of age on $V_{O_2,max}$ is very variable (Dill et al. 1964). West et al. (1983c) reported the results of measurements of $V_{O_2,max}$ on two subjects. There was only a moderate deterioration in performance over a 20-year period (aged 31–51 years). Stathokostas et al. (2004) found a 14% decline in $V_{O_2,max}$ over a decade in men with a mean age of 73 years, while in a group of women, of a similar age, the decline was only 7%.

With increasing age, skeletal muscles gradually decrease in volume, mainly due to a reduced number of motor units (Porter et al. 1995). This in turn may be due to drop-out of anterior horn cells as part of the loss of neurons throughout the central nervous system (CNS). Conley and colleagues (2000) measured the reduction in cross-sectional area of the large muscles involved in cycling together with performance, measured as $V_{O_2,max}$ in a group of elderly subjects (mean age 69 years), compared with a group of younger subjects (mean age 39 years). They also measured the oxidative capacity of the quadriceps muscle. They found that the volume of the exercising muscles in the elderly was only 67% of that in the younger group. The oxidative capacity was reduced to 53% of the younger group and the $V_{O_2,max}$ was only 45% of the younger group. They conclude that the oxidative capacity decline with age resulted from a reduction in both muscle volume and capacity per unit volume and was an important determinant of the age-related reduction in $V_{O_2,max}$.

Exercise can make a big difference to the rate of decline in performance. Kasch et al. (1995) carried out a follow up of a group of men for 28 years. Twelve continued to exercise over this period and 12 dropped out of exercising. The rates of decline were 5 and 19%, respectively. Interestingly, the blood pressure in the exercising group remained unchanged at 119/75, while in the drop-out group it rose from 128/85 to 149/90. A study by Macaluso et al. (2003) showed that in healthy women aged 65–74 years, an 8-week exercise training program increases muscle strength, power and functional ability (there was no further improvement with a further 8 weeks' training).

In the end, the ability to go to altitude depends more on an individual's degree of fitness than on age. Fit men of 75 years who normally live at sea level have spent months at 5000 m without difficulty and a 76-year-old man climbed Mt Everest in 2008. The ability to carry loads may be reduced compared to younger individuals, but no one should be discouraged from going to altitude on grounds of age alone.

27.3.3 Age and acclimatization

There are very few data on the effect of age on rate and degree of acclimatization. Levine et al. (1997) studied 20 subjects with a mean age of 68 years attending a veterans' reunion at a resort at 2500 m. They found the expected decrease in Pa_{O_2}, Sa_{O_2} and $V_{O_2,max}$ and increase in pulmonary artery pressure of 43% due to the effect of hypoxic vasoconstriction and sympathetic activation. The induction of a 1 mm depression of the S–T segment occurred at a lower exercise rate at altitude, but this returned to sea level values after 5 days at altitude. They conclude that elderly men acclimatize well at this altitude and regain sea level performance after 5 days. There is no evidence that age has an effect on minute ventilation or P_{CO_2}. P_{O_2} declines with age at sea level and also at altitude due to reduced pulmonary efficiency. Burtscher et al. (2001) found that ventilatory adaptation to high altitude in the elderly (55–77-year-old men) was complete within the first 2 days at an altitude of 2000 m. The fact that the elderly are no more susceptible to AMS than the young (see below) also suggests that they acclimatize as fast and as well as young people.

27.3.4 Age and AMS

It might be assumed that older people would be more prone to AMS, but there is no evidence that this is the case. In fact, anecdotal evidence suggests that older mountaineers actually do better than the young, but this may be because they do not climb as fast as younger individuals and therefore have a lower tendency to move too high too quickly, a major risk factor for developing acute altitude illness. Despite the fact that the sensitivity of the hypoxic ventilatory response (HVR) declines with age (Kronenberg and Drage 1973; Poulin *et al.* 1993; Serebrovskaya *et al.* 2000), as well as the fact that arterial oxygen saturation is lower in older people due to both the lower HVR and the age-related decline in lung function, survey data such as those by Kayser (1991) and Stokes *et al.* (2010) find no significant age effect on the incidence of AMS or the likelihood of summiting high mountains including Mt Kilimanjaro (5895 m). Even the fact that older people have more pre-existing disease, especially heart and lung disease, does not increase the risk of AMS (Roach *et al.* 1995).

There is a hypothesis, at present unproved, that AMS is due to increases in intracranial pressure stemming from cerebral edema. According to this theory, subjects with a large brain in relation to their skull will have a greater rise in pressure for a given degree of cerebral edema compared to those with smaller brains relative to skull capacity and a similar degree of edema (Ross 1985). The elderly, who have greater age-related atrophy than younger individuals, will have more space within their skulls and, as a result, a greater ability to tolerate cerebral swelling. This could explain the apparent resistance to AMS in older subjects and provide a rare example of the advantage of growing old, but has yet to be proven in systematic studies.

27.3.5 Conclusions and advice

The available evidence indicates that age alone is no bar to a fit person going to altitude. Exercise capacity is reduced in elderly people as it is in young people, and the itinerary should be planned accordingly, but the risk of AMS is no greater. However, 'age never comes alone' and the presence of pre-existing conditions, which might reduce one's enjoyment of a holiday at best and be life-threatening at worst, should give pause for thought. Some of these conditions are considered in Chapter 25. However, anyone who can manage a full day walking on hills at low altitude without undue strain is likely to be able to enjoy a standard Himalayan trek. In a situation of having to go rapidly to altitude, for instance having to fly into an airport at high altitude, it is probably more important for elderly people than for young people to give themselves 2–3 days to acclimatize before undertaking any strenuous activity (Levine *et al.* 1997).

28

Commercial, scientific and military activities at high altitude

SUMMARY

Commercial and scientific activities at high altitude have greatly increased over the last few years. Several mines are now situated at altitudes of 4000–6000 m. Some mines, for example Collahuasi in north Chile use a commuting pattern for the workers. They live at sea level but are transported by bus up to the mine where they spend 7 days and they then return to their families at sea level for a further 7 days. The cycle is then repeated. In this mine, the ore is at about 4400 to 4600 m, but the camp where the miners sleep is at a lower area of 3800 m. In a new mine under development at Toromocho, Peru, the ore deposits are at 4700–4900 m and the camp is at about 4500 m. One plan is to offer oxygen enrichment for the workers during the night using nasal cannulas. Several telescopes have been installed at an altitude of 5000 m at Chajnantor in north Chile, including the enormous multinational radiotelescope, ALMA. Although many of the astronomers work at a lower altitude, it is necessary to have some people on the site and the rooms are oxygen-enriched to maintain an oxygen concentration of about 27%. Portable oxygen is used to service the telescope antennas in the field. A recent development is the Chinese railway between Golmud, Qinghai Province and Lhasa, Tibet. The train reaches an altitude of over 5000 m and all the passenger cars have oxygen generators that raise the oxygen concentration in the air. Construction of the railway involved as many as 100 000 people and there were numerous cases of high altitude diseases. Military operations have been conducted at altitudes up to 7000 m in the dispute between India and Pakistan with some soldiers moving rapidly to high altitudes and down again. Oxygen enrichment of room air at very high altitude improves neuropsychological function during the day and enhances sleep at night. This technique is also potentially valuable at much lower altitudes, such as ski resorts, where sleep is a problem.

28.1 INTRODUCTION

Currently, one of the most challenging and interesting topics in high altitude medicine and physiology is the increasing number of people who go to high altitude for commercial or scientific activities. Two major areas are high altitude mining and high altitude astronomy. Mining at high altitude goes back several hundred years, although the modern practice of having miners commute from much lower altitudes, even sea level, is relatively recent. Siting telescopes at high altitudes, for example over 4000 m, is also a more recent activity. Some of the most challenging problems arise in connection with placing telescopes at altitudes of 5000 m or above in north Chile. Another striking innovation is the Chinese train from Golmud, Qinghai to Lhasa, Tibet which reaches over 5000 m. The enterprising solution to the problem of hypoxia is to provide oxygen enrichment of the air in every passenger car. Finally, military operations at high altitudes involve intermittent exposure to very high altitudes.

This chapter overlaps somewhat with previous chapters. The value of oxygen enrichment of room air to improve sleep at high altitude was briefly discussed in Chapter 14. The improvement of neuropsychological function at an altitude of 5000 m as a result of oxygen enrichment of room air has been referred to in Chapter 17.

28.2 HISTORICAL

Mining activities at high altitude are very old. For example, gold has been mined in western Tibet for centuries. The open cast mines at Thok Jalung (*thok* is Tibetan for gold) were investigated in 1867 by Nain Singh, one of the early pundits, the clandestine native explorers of the Survey of India (Waller 1990). Chinese sources suggest that Tibetans worked as high as 6000 m in the Tanggula range of central Tibet mining quartz, and chromate mines are also found in central Tibet (Ward 1990). In several areas of the South American Andes, there is evidence that mining activities were carried out by the Incas before the Spanish conquest. The Spanish conquistadors founded the imperial city of Potosí (4060 m) in Bolivia, the site of an enormous silver mine, in the 1540s. According to one historian quoted by Monge (1948), there were 100 000 natives and 20 000 Spaniards in Potosí at one time. However, little information remains about the actual mining activities.

A colorful description of the mining practices in Cerro de Pasco, Peru (4340 m) was given by Barcroft *et al.* (1923) in their account of the International High Altitude Expedition to Cerro de Pasco which took place in 1921–22. Although most of the studies carried out by the physiologists were on themselves, many interesting observations were made on the native miners. One mine was 250 ft (76 m) below the surface, and the staircase which led down to it was 600 ft (183 m) in length. The porters who carried up the loads of ore from the mine varied greatly in age and stature. One boy who was said to be 10 years of age carried a load of 40 lb (18 kg) (Fig. 28.1). Another porter who was thought to be 19 years old brought up a load of about 100 lb (45 kg). The physiologists noted that the exercise was spasmodic. The climb was very slow and consisted of the ascent of a few steps, followed by a long pause during which the porter regained his breath. They noted that the

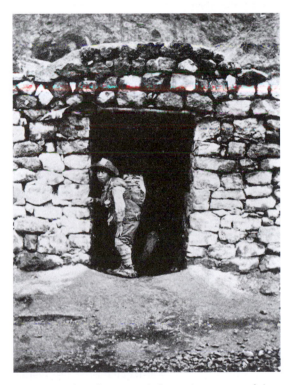

Figure 28.1   Photograph from the report of the 1921–22 International High Altitude Expedition to Cerro de Pasco, Peru, showing a young boy, said to be 10 years old, carrying a load of 18 kg, which he has just brought up from the mine 250 ft (76 m) below the surface (from Barcroft *et al.* 1923).

panting of the porters could be heard far down the staircase, before they came into view. The miners enjoyed sports, for example soccer, when they were not working. Each period of the game was 15 minutes long.

More recently, the extraordinary physical activity of miners at the Aucanquilcha mine (5950 m) in north Chile has been described (McIntyre 1987). The photograph on page 455 of that article shows the miners shattering boulders of caliche (sulfur ore) using sledgehammers. The caretakers of this mine lived indefinitely at this altitude, and they were probably the highest inhabitants in the world (West 1986a). The mine is no longer working.

28.3 MINING

Table 28.1 lists the altitudes of some of the most important commercial or scientific activities at high altitude. All of these are mines, except for two telescope sites. It can be seen that many of the mines are above 4000 m in altitude, with the highest being Aucanquilcha at 5950 m, although,

as indicated earlier, this mine is no longer operating.

The mines fall into two categories. Many of the old mines, such as those at Cerro de Pasco and Morococha, have complete communities near the mine itself. This means that the families are located there and, in particular, the children are raised at these high altitudes. Many people now question the wisdom of this because there is some evidence that children grow more slowly at high altitude (Frisancho and Baker 1970), although the issue is somewhat controversial (see Chapter 27). Certainly, the central nervous system is exquisitely sensitive to hypoxia, as discussed in Chapter 17, and, other things being equal, one would prefer to see children brought up in a more normal ambient P_{O_2}.

Another disadvantage of having whole communities at the site of the high altitude mine is that a large amount of infrastructure has to be provided. This includes schools, medical facilities and meeting halls, all of which increases the expenses of the mine. These considerations have led many modern mining operations to develop a commuting pattern where the families live at

Table 28.1   Examples of commercial and scientific activities at altitudes of 3500–6000 m

Country/state	Facility	Altitude (m)	Latitude	Product or activity
Chile	Andina	3400–4200	33°S	Copper
	Aucanquilcha[a]	5950	21°S	Sulfur
	Choquelimpie	4500	20°S	Silver
	Collahuasi	4400–4600	21°S	Copper
	El Indio	3800–4000	30°S	Copper, gold, silver
	Quebrada Blanca	4400	21°S	Copper
	Chajnantor	5000	23°S	Telescope site
Peru	Cerro de Pasco	4330	11°S	Copper, gold, lead, zinc
	Morococha	4550	12°S	Copper
	Toromocho	4700–4900	12°S	Copper, silver, molybdenum
Bolivia	Potosí	4060	20°S	Silver, tin
Hawaii	Mauna Kea	4200	20°N	Telescope site
Colorado	Climax	4350	39°N	Molybdenum
	Summitville	4050	37°N	Gold

[a]This mine is not operating at present.

or near sea level and the miners commute to the mine itself where they spend a period of 7–10 days.

As an example of a modern mine based on the commuting pattern, the mine at Collahuasi will be briefly described. This is a very large, open-cut copper mine in north Chile at a latitude of 21°S. Mining operations in this area were carried out in pre-Spanish times. It is interesting that Thomas H. Ravenhill (1881–1952), who gave the first accurate clinical descriptions of high altitude pulmonary edema (HAPE) and high altitude cerebral edema (HACE) (Ravenhill 1913), was the medical officer at this mine in 1909–11 (West 1996b). The working areas of the mine are at altitudes of 4400–4600 m, although the mining camp where the miners sleep is at the lower altitude of 3800 m. There are currently several thousand people working at the mine which makes it one of the largest copper mines in the world. Copper is a major export of Chile.

The miners' families live in Iquique on the coast in accommodation supplied by the mining company. The miners are transported to the mine by special buses which take a few hours for the trip on a new road built by the mining company. A typical schedule is that the miners spend 7 days at the mine, where they work for up to 12 h per day, and then sleep in the mining camp at an altitude of 3800 m. At the end of 7 days, they are transported by bus down to Iquique, where they spend the next 7 days with their families. This cycle is repeated indefinitely.

Richalet and colleagues (2002) have studied a group of 29 of these miners aged 25 ± 5 years over a period of 2.5 years. The subjects were extensively tested at sea level prior to their exposure to high altitude including a physical examination, ECG, hematology, maximal exercise, ventilatory and cardiac responses to an inhaled oxygen concentration of 11.4% both at rest and exercise, pulmonary vascular response to hypoxia using echocardiography, and 24 h monitoring of ECG and arterial pressure. Measurements at high altitude included a daily acute mountain sickness score, sleep characteristics, and 24 h monitoring of the ECG and arterial pressure. All the measurements were repeated after periods of about 12, 19 and 31 months.

It was found that the hematocrit increased, measured at both sea level and high altitude, after 12 and 19 months (Fig. 28.2), but interestingly it returned to values similar to the initial pre-exposure values at the end of 31 months of chronic intermittent hypoxia. In every instance, there was an increase in hematocrit on acute exposure to high altitude which continued over the 31 months and presumably can be attributed to a reduced plasma volume. Perhaps surprisingly, body weight and body composition did not change significantly over the 31 months. This may be related to the fact that although the miners were exposed to high altitude which often causes a weight loss, they had excellent food at the living facility. Mean systemic arterial pressure both during the day and night were increased at high altitude compared with sea level. The sea level pressures tended to decrease with time. Another interesting finding was that the systolic pulmonary artery pressures, measured by echocardiography, both in normoxia and after challenge with 11.4% oxygen at sea level, did not change significantly over the first 19 months, although the pressure following an acute hypoxic challenge was less after 31 months. There was a small increase in end-diastolic diameter of the right ventricle as measured by echocardiography

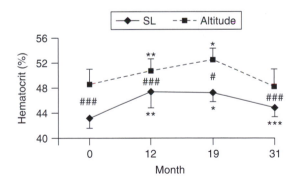

Figure 28.2 Hematocrit of miners before (0) and after 12, 19 and 31 months of exposure to chronic intermittent hypoxia. Seven days were spent at an altitude of 3800–4600 m followed by 7 days at sea level and the cycle was repeated for the whole 31 months. Mean ± SD. Time vs. 0: *, **, ***: $p < 0.05$, 0.01, 0.001, respectively. Altitude vs. sea level (SL): #, ##, ###: $p < 0.05$, 0.01, 0.001, respectively (from Richalet *et al.* 2002).

from 18.6 ± 3 mm to 22.4 ± 2.4 mm after 19 months of exposure to chronic intermittent hypoxia.

Unexpectedly, maximal exercise as measured at sea level was found to be decreased by 12.3% at the end of 31 months of chronic intermittent hypoxia. This was accompanied by a decrease in maximal heart rate of 6.8%. When the arterial oxygen saturation during exercise was measured following exposure to the hypoxic mixture, the saturation was found to be lower at the end of 12 months of chronic intermittent hypoxia than in the prehypoxia measurements, but it remained stable thereafter. On the other hand, the ventilatory response to hypoxia increased after 12 months of exposure and remained elevated. Interestingly, symptoms of acute mountain sickness were similar throughout the period of exposure to chronic intermittent hypoxia, the score always being higher on the first or second day following ascent to altitude. Consistent with this, the quality of sleep was impaired during the first two nights at high altitude (being worse on the second night) and remained unaltered during the 31 months of chronic intermittent hypoxia.

This was the first study of this pattern of chronic intermittent hypoxia and showed that some degree of acclimatization occurred during the 31 months but that, not surprisingly, the changes were less than in a group of people permanently exposed to an altitude of 4000 m. However, it was interesting that the symptoms of acute mountain sickness and the impairment of sleep at high altitude persisted during the whole of the 31 months. Incidentally, it had been hoped to extend this study for a total of 5 years, but apparently the mining company that supported the work felt that sufficient information for their purposes had been obtained after 31 months.

The 7 × 7-day schedule referred to above is not universally employed in the high altitude mines that use commuting. Periods at high altitude as long as 10–14 days have been tried. It does not make much sense from a physiological point of view to have a period at high altitude of less than 7 days because there is evidence that the ventilatory acclimatization continues for at least this period of time (Lahiri 1972; Dempsey and Forster 1982). Other features of high altitude acclimatization,

such as the development of polycythemia, take several weeks to reach a steady state. On the other hand, the physiological value of polycythemia is now less clear than it was earlier thought to be (Winslow and Monge 1987).

Another important question is the time course of deacclimatization. Ideally, the workers should not lose all the acclimatization that they have developed at high altitude during their period with their families at sea level. Relatively little information about the rate of deacclimatization is available, although some measurements suggest that the rate of change of the ventilatory response during deacclimatization is slower than during acclimatization (Lahiri 1972). Deacclimatization is discussed further in section 5.4.4.

Finally, although the physiological aspects of scheduling are important, it may be that social factors will be dominant. Experience has shown that miners are reluctant to leave their homes for more than 7–10 days, and it is probable that a schedule of 7 days of high altitude followed by 7 days at sea level, or alternatively 10 by 10 days, will be the most acceptable.

Reference was made above to the miners at Aucanquilcha (5950 m) who were breaking large pieces of sulfur ore using sledgehammers. However, the activities at a modern mine, such as Collahuasi, are quite different. The ore is dislodged using explosives, and then it is picked up by enormous diesel electric front-end loaders that can scoop up 80 tons of ore at a time. Three scoops are then placed in a gigantic diesel electric truck which can carry 240 tons (Fig. 28.3). Of course, considerable skill is necessary to operate these very large pieces of equipment, and substantial damage can be done to people or machines if the equipment is not operated correctly.

The highly skilled nature of modern mining is one reason why in mines like Collahuasi, none of the miners are people indigenous to the high altitudes. Another reason is that there is not a large indigenous high altitude population in Chile. This is in contrast to the situation in many mines in Peru where, for example at Cerro de Pasco and Morococha, there are large indigenous populations who can provide relatively cheap, unskilled labor for the mines.

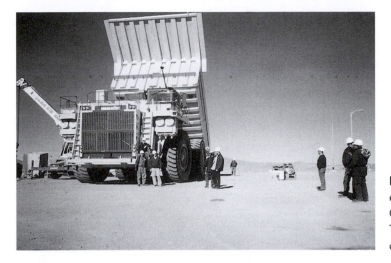

Figure 28.3 Enormous diesel electric truck at the modern Collahuasi mine in north Chile. This can transport 240 tons of copper ore.

Recently, plans for another mine have been made public and this will be described briefly because it indicates some of the striking changes in thinking about working at very high altitudes. The name of the mine is Toromocho and it is being developed by Chinalco (Aluminum Company of China). One source estimates that an investment of $16 billion will be required to bring it to production. The site is about 140 km east of Lima near the present town of Morococha where there is an old mine. Toromocho means 'a bull without horns' and refers to the shape of Mount Toromocho which is apparently a mountain composed of copper ore mixed with silver and molybdenum. A challenging problem is that part of the ore deposit is under the existing town of Morococha which will need to be moved. Houses will be provided for the present residents in the new location and they will also receive monetary compensation.

Remarkable features of the project include the high altitudes of both the mine and the accommodation for the workers. The ore deposits are at an altitude of 4700–4900 m. The camp with dormitories will be at the extraordinary altitude of about 4500 m where the proposal is to include 11 three-storey dormitories holding up to 5000 people. Lowlanders employed to run the heavy equipment, such as mechanical loaders and trucks, will find this dormitory altitude very challenging, especially for sleeping. One proposal is to provide oxygen enrichment using nasal cannulas. The alternative

of providing oxygen-enriched rooms for so many people seems prohibitively expensive. Apparently there will be no supplemental oxygen on the work site itself. The plan is to supply sufficient oxygen by cannulas to reduce the equivalent altitude to 3900 m, but even this altitude will be difficult to tolerate for many lowlanders.

Presumably the workforce will include highlanders who formerly lived in the town of Morococha, altitude about 4500 m. These people are used to the altitude of the camp and presumably will not have a problem. Therefore, one solution for the altitude of the camp would be to provide oxygen-enriched rooms only for the lowlanders, although it has been pointed out that this may be criticized as discriminatory. However, as discussed in relation to the Collahuasi mine, open-cut mining these days requires highly skilled people to operate the enormous mechanical shovels and trucks and presumably these workers will come from lower altitudes. The mine is presently under construction and it will be interesting to see how the logistics are finally worked out. However, it provides a striking example of emerging trends in commercial projects at very high altitudes.

Another challenging problem of these high altitude mines is the selection of workers. Certainly not everybody is able to work effectively at altitudes of 4400–4900 m. There is, therefore, considerable interest in possible medical tests that could predict who will be able to work well at altitude or, perhaps more importantly, who will be unable to tolerate the altitude. One possible test is the ventilatory response to hypoxia, during both rest and exercise (Rathat *et al.* 1992). As pointed out in Chapter 13, there is evidence that tolerance to extreme altitude requires a reasonable level of hypoxic ventilatory response in order to defend the alveolar P_{O_2} at a viable level. However, whether this will be a useful prognostic test for working at altitudes of 4000–5000 m is not clear. Probably the best predictor at the present time is whether a prospective worker has previously worked effectively at high altitude.

Richalet *et al.* (2012) have published a prospective study of physiological risk factors for severe high altitude illness. They used an exercise test with the subjects breathing 11.5% oxygen and found that the most important risk factors were a large fall in arterial oxygen saturation during hypoxic exercise, low response of heart rate to hypoxia during the exercise test, low hypoxic ventilatory response, young age, female gender, rapid ascent, and previous history of high altitude illness.

Even if workers have been shown to tolerate these high altitudes reasonably well, it is clear that they cannot accomplish the same amount of physical work as at sea level. The decline in maximal oxygen consumption with increasing altitude is discussed in Chapter 12, where it was pointed out that the $\dot{V}_{O_{2,max}}$ of an acclimatized subject at an altitude of 5000 m is only about 70% of the sea level value. Another way of looking at this is that the workforce would have to be increased by about 40% at this high altitude to accomplish the same amount of physical work. It is interesting that this inefficiency is not confined to human beings, but is also seen in mechanical equipment. Table 28.2 shows that, at an altitude of 4000 m, the amount of equipment to produce the same amount of work as at sea level has to be increased by 25 to 85% (Jimenez 1995).

28.4 TELESCOPES

28.4.1 Mauna Kea

As indicated previously, there were mines at altitudes over 4000 m in the South American Andes for many years prior to the Spanish

Table 28.2 Increase in mine equipment size at 3000 and 4000 m to achieve the same output as at sea level

Equipment	Output unit	Increase at altitude (%)	
		3000 m	4000 m
Diesel engines	Brake horse-power	40	55
Compressors	Airtool work	55	75
Vacuum filters	Tons solids h^{-1}	30	45
Vacuum pumps	Intake volume	30	40
Transmission lines	MVA km^{-1}	20	30
Transformers	MVA	15	25
Electrical machines	kW	15	25
Flotation	tons h^{-1}	35	50
Leach vessels	tons h^{-1}	50	85

Source: Modified from Jimenez (1995).

conquest. However, the practice of siting telescopes at high altitude is much more recent, mostly within the last 50 years. There are several advantages in placing telescopes at high altitudes. One is that the instrument is then above much of Earth's atmosphere, which otherwise absorbs some of the optical and radio waves. Another advantage is that in some areas, for example Chajnantor (see section 28.4.2), the atmosphere is extremely dry and absorption of radio waves by water vapor is therefore much less. Finally, remote mountain sites tend to have little light or radio wave pollution, although this advantage can also be achieved in other remote areas at lower altitudes.

Two telescope sites will be considered here. One is the extinct volcano at Mauna Kea in the big island of Hawaii. The summit is at an altitude of 4200 m and at least 10 instruments are located either on or near the summit. A feature of Mauna Kea is that it is less than 100 km from the city of Hilo at sea level, and it is possible to drive from one site to the other in a couple of hours. There is also an intermediate station with dormitories at 3000 m at Hale Pohaku, and some newcomers can spend a night there before going to the summit. However, the majority of the staff who operate the telescopes commute from sea level every day. The barometric pressure at the summit is about 465 mmHg, so the P_{O_2} of moist inspired gas is only 87 mmHg, as against 150 mmHg at sea level. The hypoxic stress is therefore severe (see Figure 7.4).

Forster (1986) studied the incidence of acute mountain sickness (AMS) and the arterial blood gases of some of the workers on the United Kingdom Infrared Telescope (UKIRT) on the summit of Mauna Kea. These shift workers spent 40 days working at sea level at Hilo, followed by a 5-day shift at high altitude. The first night of the shift was spent in the dormitories at 3000 m, and following that 4 days were spent on the summit of Mauna Kea, with the workers returning to 3000 m for each night. It was found that 80% of the shift workers had symptoms of AMS on their first day at the summit. Apart from breathlessness, headache was the most frequent complaint, and this affected 41% of shift workers at the start of their high altitude shift. Other common symptoms were insomnia, lethargy, poor concentration, poor memory and unsteadiness of gait. The frequency of symptoms decreased over the 5 days of the shift and, at the end, 60% of the workers were asymptomatic.

Arterial blood gases were measured in 27 UKIRT shift workers. On day 1 at 4200 m, the mean arterial P_{O_2} was 42 mmHg, rising to 44 mmHg on day 5. The arterial P_{CO_2} was 29 mmHg on the first day, falling to 27 mmHg on the fifth day. Arterial pH was 7.49 on day 1, falling to 7.48 on day 5.

It is interesting that there was no difference in the incidence of AMS between shift workers who worked at the summit after a brief sojourn at sea level (mean 4 days), compared to a protracted rest period (mean 37 days) at sea level. This suggests that in this group, the acclimatization to high altitude achieved during 5 days on Mauna Kea was lost within a few days of return to sea level. HAPE was infrequently seen at Mauna Kea, with only one case in 41 shift workers during a 2-year study period. Also only one worker on Mauna Kea had an episode of HACE.

An interesting problem related to the astronomers near the summit of Mauna Kea is their reluctance to admit that the hypoxia is affecting them, and their resistance to using oxygen enrichment of room air which is discussed in section 28.7. As Fig. 7.2 shows, the alveolar P_{O_2} for acute exposure to the barometric pressure on the summit of Mauna Kea is about 45 mmHg. This could increase to as much as about 53 mmHg if the subject becomes fully acclimatized, although this never happens on Mauna Kea because astronomers do not stay there long enough. Note that these values for alveolar P_{O_2} agree well with the arterial P_{O_2} values cited above when the arterial P_{O_2} was 42 mmHg on day 1 rising to 44 mmHg on day 5.

This is a severe degree of oxygen deprivation. As was pointed out in section 7.3, Fig. 7.2 also shows that if a patient with chronic obstructive pulmonary disease has a P_{O_2} below 55 mmHg, the patient is entitled to continuous oxygen therapy under Medicare. Clearly, the Mauna Kea astronomers are well below that level which unquestionably reduces physical and mental powers. It would be easy to alleviate some of this severe hypoxia using oxygen enrichment of room air, but for some curious reasons some of the astronomers are adamantly against this. This macho attitude is very unfortunate.

28.4.2 Chajnantor

The other telescope site that will be discussed here is Llano de Chajnantor in north Chile, southeast of San Pedro de Atacama, at a latitude of 23°S and an altitude of 5060 m. This is a remarkable site because it is fairly flat, covers a large area, and is easily accessible by road from San Pedro (altitude 2440 m). The first part of the road is an international highway leading from Chile to Bolivia and Argentina, and the final 15 km is now also paved. The drive from San Pedro to Chajnantor takes only about 1 h. There must be few places in the world where it is possible to reach an altitude of 5000 m so easily.

Several small radio telescopes have been sited at Chajnantor or nearby. The California Institute of Technology has had a radio telescope for studying the cosmic microwave background radiation since 1999. This was one of the first facilities to use oxygen enrichment of room air. The personnel have been living and working in an environment of 27% O_2 for many years. However, the main interest of Chajnantor is the recently constructed Atacama Large Millimeter/sub-millimeter Array (ALMA) which is another example of a major engineering accomplishment at a very high altitude. The project is a collaboration between the United States, Canada, Europe, Japan, Taiwan and Chile. The barometric pressure at the site, altitude 5050 m, is about 420 mmHg, with an inspired Po_2 of only 78 mmHg, so the degree of hypoxic stress is substantial.

The radiotelescope array will eventually consist of more than 50 identical 12 m reflector antennas connected by fiberoptic cables (Fig. 28.4). The configuration of the array will extend over distances of 150 m to 14 km. In addition, there will be compact arrays of 4 × 12 m and 12 × 7 m antennas. The ability to move the antenna dishes across the desert plateau over these large distances up to 14 km gives the telescope an extremely good spatial resolution and the ability to change the type of imaging required. This is similar to the zoom effect in light photography. Each of the large dishes weighs 150 tonnes. They are assembled at the Operations Support Facility at an altitude of 2900 m and moved to the 5000 m site using custom-built 28-wheel self-loading haulers each weighing 130 tonnes. A feature of these

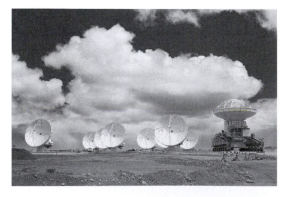

Figure 28.4 Some of the antenna dishes of the ALMA radiotelescope at an altitude of 5050 m. The huge transporter that moves the telescopes up to the site is shown on the right.

gigantic trucks is that the driver is provided with supplementary oxygen.

At the 5000 m array operations site, there is a large building with rooms for technical personnel and banks of fast computers. Optical cables transmit data down to the operations support facility at 2900 m where much of the analysis is done. The array operations site has a number of rooms that are oxygen-enriched which allows complex accurate work to be done by the personnel. The facility will be fully operational by the end of 2012, although various improvements can be expected after that date. This gigantic project is a remarkable example of very sophisticated engineering at very high altitudes.

28.5 RAILWAYS

Railways have been built at high altitude for many years. For example, the central railway of Peru was completed to Aroya in 1893 and this included crossing the Andean crest at Ticlio at an altitude of 4800 m. The cog railway up to the summit of Pikes Peak in Colorado (4300 m) was finished in 1891. However, a modern railway from Golmud in Qinghai Province, China to Lhasa, Tibet has posed enormous challenges not only for the engineers and construction workers, but indeed for the passengers. The length of the rail link is over 1100 km with more than three-quarters of the distance above 4000 m altitude. In fact, the track crosses some of the highest ranges on the Tibetan plateau, the highest altitude being just over 5000 m. Some 100 000 construction workers are reported to have been used to put in the track, and although the medical facilities were impressive, there were many cases of mountain sickness (Wu *et al.* 2007a; Wu *et al.* 2007b; Wu *et al.* 2009; Wu *et al.* 2010). Indeed, it could be argued that Chinese physicians probably have more experience of high altitude problems (including their prevention and management) than any other group in the world. One of the most challenging problems was constructing the tunnels at very high altitudes, for example the Fenghuoshan Tunnel at an altitude of 4905 m. Excavations were done with hand drills and the physical demands on the workers were enormous. To partially relieve the hypoxia, large volumes of high concentration oxygen were produced by generators located outside the tunnel, and the gas was pumped to the workface through a large pipe. It was reported that this increased the inspired P_{O_2} by as much as 15 mmHg, which would have reduced the equivalent altitude by about 1200 m. Another remarkable challenge was the Mount Kunlun Tunnel at an altitude of 4660 m which is 1686 m long and believed to be the longest permafrost tunnel in the world.

To relieve the hypoxia of the passengers who are exposed to an altitude of over 5000 m, each coach of the train is equipped with an oxygen generator. In this instance, the generator used a membrane separation technique that allowed the generator to typically produce about 40–50% oxygen. This was added to the ventilation air of each car to achieve 24–25% oxygen concentration in the car (Fig. 28.5). As indicated in the next section, each 1% of oxygen enrichment reduces the equivalent altitude by about 300 m, so that the 4% increase from 21 to 25% yielded a reduction in equivalent altitude of about 1200 m. Therefore, at the train's highest altitude of about 5000 m, the cabin altitude was reduced to about 3800 m. Of course, the passengers in the train are sedentary so they do not need as much oxygen enrichment as most workers. The train terminates at Lhasa, altitude 3658 m, which is lower than the train route.

The O_2 and CO_2 levels in the air of each car are monitored and apparently automatically modulate the oxygen-enriched airflow as the altitude changes. There is a panel on the oxygen generator in each coach that indicates both the oxygen concentration produced by the generator, and the oxygen level in the coach air (Fig. 28.5). As indicated above, each passenger car has its own generator, and parallel systems on adjacent cars can be engaged to serve as backups in case of failure. In addition, numerous oxygen outlets throughout the train allow passengers to plug in a tube connected to nasal cannulas. Each train carries a doctor and nurse who are available if necessary.

One of the potential issues is loss of oxygen when a train stops at a station and the doors are opened. However, when the author took the train a few years ago it stopped at only three stations between Golmud and Lhasa, and all the doors were opened at only one of these stations. Naturally the gangways between the carriages are gas-tight and the windows are tightly sealed. The air conditioning maintains a slight positive pressure so that any leaks are to the outside. The Golmud-Lhasa railway is a triumph of high-altitude engineering.

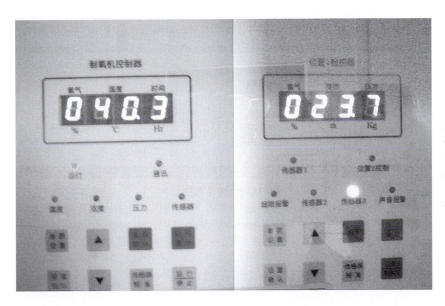

Figure 28.5 Panel on the oxygen-concentrator in one of the passenger cars of the Golmud–Lhasa railway. On the left is the O_2 concentration produced by the concentrator, and on the right is the concentration in the air of the carriage.

28.6 MILITARY OPERATIONS

To paraphrase Winston Churchill, never have so many lowlanders been transported to such high altitudes for such long periods (and it might be added, to so little avail) as in the dispute between India and Pakistan over the Jammu–Kashmir region. The unhappy result is that large numbers of soldiers have been stationed at altitudes up to 7000 m for substantial periods of time. Many of these soldiers come from altitudes near sea level, such as the plains of India. A fascinating account of some of the problems was given by Anand (2001). Indeed, this conflict was responsible for the appearance of a new medical condition initially called 'adult subacute mountain sickness' (Anand *et al.* 1990) in which young soldiers develop right heart failure with peripheral edema somewhat reminiscent of brisket disease in cattle at high altitude (see Chapter 21). Jha and colleagues (2002) reported the high incidence of stroke in these young soldiers at these great altitudes. There have been previous military operations at high altitudes, for example in the Soviet Union during the Second World War, but the altitudes near the Siachen Glacier where the India–Pakistan dispute has taken place are far above these.

28.7 OXYGEN ENRICHMENT OF ROOM AIR

An important advance in the last 20 years has been the demonstration of the feasibility and value of raising the oxygen concentration of room air at high altitude in order to relieve the hypoxia (West 1995). The possibility of doing this was originally suggested by Cudaback (1984) and plans were made to oxygen-enrich the control room of the Keck telescope at Mauna Kea, but these were never carried out at the time.

The principle of oxygen enrichment is simple. Oxygen, ideally from a concentrator or possibly from a cryogenic source, is added to the ventilation of a room, thus increasing the oxygen concentration from 21% to a higher value. The reason why oxygen enrichment is so powerful is that relatively small degrees of oxygen enrichment result in large reductions of equivalent altitude.

The term 'equivalent altitude' refers to the altitude at which the moist inspired P_{O_2}, when a subject is breathing ambient air, is the same as the inspired P_{O_2} in the oxygen-enriched environment. Figure 28.6 shows that, between altitudes of 3000 and 6000 m, each 1% of oxygen enrichment results in a reduction of equivalent altitude by about 300 m. In other words, if a room at the Chajnantor site, altitude 5000 m, is oxygen-enriched by 6% (that is, the oxygen concentration is increased from 21 to 27%), the equivalent altitude is reduced by about six times 300 m, or 1800 m. Therefore, the altitude effectively goes from one of 5000 m to one of 3200 m, which is much more easily tolerated especially as personnel usually have some acclimatization to altitude.

When this idea was originally proposed, some people argued that it would be impossible to maintain an enriched-oxygen atmosphere within a room because of inevitable leaks. However, in practice, oxygen enrichment is relatively simple and reliable. The room does not have to be gas tight. Large potential leaks, such as window surrounds, are taped, and ideally a double door is provided so that there is an air lock. However,

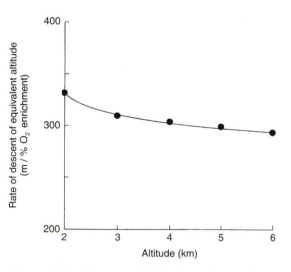

Figure 28.6 Degree of reduction of equivalent altitude (meters of descent per 1% oxygen enrichment) plotted against the altitude at which the enrichment is made. Note that at altitudes up to about 6000 m, each 1% of oxygen enrichment results in an altitude reduction of more than 300 m (from West 1995).

oxygen-enriched air is blown into the room and escapes through small leaks, and in practice it is easy to control the oxygen level within 0.25%.

Oxygen enrichment of rooms has become feasible largely because large quantities of oxygen can now be produced relatively cheaply. The simplest way to do this is to use an oxygen concentrator and thousands of these are now used in homes to provide oxygen for patients with chronic lung disease. In this case, the oxygen is delivered by nasal cannulas. The principle is that air is pumped at high pressure through a synthetic zeolite which adsorbs nitrogen from the air. The result is that the effluent gas has a high oxygen concentration, typically 90–95%. After 20–30 s, the zeolite is unable to absorb more nitrogen and the compressed air is then switched to another cylinder containing the same material. The original cylinder is then purged of nitrogen by blowing air through it at normal pressures. In this way, a continuous supply of 90–95% oxygen is available. A typical commercial unit provides 5 L min^{-1} of over 90% pure oxygen at a power consumption of 350 W. It is also possible to provide the oxygen from liquid oxygen tanks, but this is more expensive and less convenient because the tanks need to be replenished.

An important issue is what level of ventilation to use in the room. Clearly, the higher the ventilation, the larger the amount of oxygen that must be produced to maintain a given degree of oxygen enrichment. This topic has been discussed extensively elsewhere (West 1995). We use the 1975 American Society of Heating, Refrigeration and Air-Conditioning Engineers (ASHRAE) standard of 8.5 m^3 person^{-1} h^{-1}, which corresponds to 142 L min^{-1}. This is calculated to maintain the carbon dioxide concentration in the room below 0.24%, based on a carbon dioxide production rate per person of 0.3 L min^{-1}. This concentration of carbon dioxide was chosen by ASHRAE as a measure of acceptable ventilation levels. Substantially higher concentrations of carbon dioxide can be inhaled without people being aware of them. However, the carbon dioxide concentration is a useful objective marker of adequacy of ventilation, and higher levels tend to be associated with awareness of body odor.

It should be added that in 1989, ASHRAE increased the minimum standard of ventilation by three- to four-fold. This was a somewhat controversial decision, and was partially based on the possibilities that there may be smokers in the room, there are health variations among people, and some types of room furniture cause outgassing, which may be injurious. In designing a facility for use at high altitude, it can be assumed that people will not be allowed to smoke in the room, and it is also possible to choose furniture that does not result in outgassing hazards.

It is not difficult to set up a module that can be used for oxygen enrichment in the field. For example, a standard shipping container of dimensions 20 ft (6.1 m) long, 8 ft (2.44 m) wide and 8 ft high is fitted out as a living space with beds, or a laboratory or a machine shop. A larger laboratory can be housed in a standard shipping container of dimensions 40 ft (12.19 m) long by 8 ft wide by 8 ft high. Such containers are currently in use at the Chajnantor site, in connection with the California Institute of Technology radiotelescope known as the Cosmic Background Imager. The oxygen is provided from oxygen concentrators, and the concentrations of both oxygen and carbon dioxide are continually monitored inside the rooms.

The experience of the astronomers with oxygen enrichment has been very satisfactory (West and Readhead 2004). There have been few technical problems in maintaining the target oxygen concentration of 27%, and the carbon dioxide concentration is typically less than 0.25%. The CalTech project was a particularly valuable field test of oxygen enrichment because, for the first 2 weeks, the astronomers were working in ambient air conditions. They found this extremely tiring, despite the fact that they slept every night at San Pedro (altitude 2440 m). When the oxygen enrichment modules were set up, they noticed an immediate improvement in work productivity and efficiency. In fact, they soon instituted a rule that no one was allowed to control the telescope or use power tools unless using oxygen enrichment. When the astronomers were not in the oxygen-enriched modules, they used portable oxygen in order to provide oxygen enrichment. They also reported that it was feasible to sleep at the Chajnantor site in the oxygen-enriched rooms. This had not proved to be possible while breathing ambient air because of the poor quality of sleep.

Several studies have been carried out on the physiological effects of oxygen enrichment of room air at high altitude. The first studies were performed at the Barcroft facility of the White Mountain Research Station (altitude 3800 m) in California, where the oxygen concentration of the test room was raised from 21 to 24% (Luks et al. 1998). This reduced the equivalent altitude to about 2900 m. In a double-blind study, it was shown that oxygen enrichment during the night resulted in fewer apneas and less time spent in periodic breathing with apneas. Subjective assessments of sleep quality showed significant improvement. There was also a lower AMS score during the morning after oxygen-enriched sleep. An unexpected finding was that there was a larger increase in arterial oxygen saturation from evening to morning after oxygen-enriched sleep than after sleeping in ambient air. Of course, both measurements of arterial oxygen saturation were made with the subject breathing ambient air.

In another study, the mechanism of the unexpected increase in arterial oxygen saturation the following morning was investigated (McElroy et al. 2000). Because this could have been caused by a change in the control of ventilation, the ventilatory responses to hypoxia and to carbon dioxide were measured in the evening and in the morning after sleeping both in the oxygen-enriched environment and in ambient air. No effect of oxygen enrichment on the control of ventilation was found. An alternative explanation is that the increase in arterial oxygen saturation seen following sleep in the oxygen-enriched environment might have been the result of less subclinical pulmonary edema, compared with sleeping in ambient air. An additional observation that might support this explanation was that the increase in arterial oxygen saturation was transient, with the result that by midday the difference between the oxygen-enriched and ambient air treatments on oxygen saturation was abolished.

A final study was carried out on the effects of oxygen enrichment on neuropsychological function at a simulated altitude of 5000 m, as referred to briefly in Chapter 16. Again, the Barcroft facility, at an altitude of 3800 m, was used, and the concentration of oxygen in the room was manipulated to simulate ambient air at an altitude of 5000 m, and an oxygen concentration of 27% at an altitude of 5000 m. A large battery of neuropsychological tests was performed in a double-blinded manner, and it was found that there were significant improvements in reaction times, hand–eye coordination, and mood (Gerard et al. 2000). These findings are directly relevant to the project of oxygen enrichment at the Chajnantor site.

An important consideration when oxygen is added to air is whether the fire hazard is increased, compared with sea level. This has been carefully analyzed (West 1997) and it has been shown that, with the levels of oxygen enrichment considered here, the fire hazard is less than at sea level. The basic reason is that, although the P_{O_2} is increased by oxygen enrichment at high altitude, it is still far below the value at sea level. Although it is true that the reduction of the partial pressure of nitrogen at altitude also increases the fire hazard to a small extent because of the reduced extinguishing effect of this inert gas, it remains true that the fire hazard using the degrees of oxygen enrichment described here is less than at sea level. The National Fire Protection Association (NFPA) (National Fire Protection Association 1993) defines an oxygen-enriched atmosphere as having an increased fire hazard, in the sense that it will support an increased burning rate of materials, if the percentage concentration of oxygen is greater than $23.45/(P_f^{0.5})$, where P_f is the total barometric pressure expressed as a fraction of the sea level pressure. For the Chajnantor site, $P_f = 0.55$, so that if the oxygen concentration is greater than 31.6% it would exceed the NFPA threshold. The oxygen concentration of 27% is well below this value.

Up to the present time, most of the interest in oxygen enrichment of room air has been for commercial, scientific and railway activities above 4000 m. However, it is likely that the same technique could be valuable at substantially lower altitudes associated with ski or mountain resorts. Many people who visit these places have difficulties especially with sleeping during the first 2 or 3 days. Oxygen enrichment of room air can greatly improve sleep quality. Indeed, people who build houses at altitudes above 2000 m have shown great interest in oxygen enrichment of bedrooms for the same reason. A study of the appropriate oxygen concentrations at these moderate altitudes indicates that considerable alleviation of the hypoxia can be brought about without incurring a fire hazard (West 2002b).

It could be argued that oxygen enrichment of room air represents a new attitude to living and working at high altitude. Until now, most people have accepted hypoxia as something that has to be endured. However, this proactive attitude of raising oxygen concentration of the rooms to reduce the equivalent altitude could represent a major advance.

29

Athletes and altitude

SUMMARY

Recently, athletes have used high altitude training to enhance sea level performance, but many remarkable feats of endurance have been recorded in the mountains. One of the most remarkable was the first ascent of Everest without supplemental oxygen in 1978, followed by a number of phenomenally fast ascents to extreme altitude without supplemental oxygen.

In athletic competitions at altitude, faster times are recorded in sprint events because of lowered air resistance, while in endurance events, because of a lower $Vo_{2,max}$, times are slower.

The paradox is that acclimatization to altitude results in central and peripheral adaptation that enhances oxygen delivery and utilization, but hypoxia decreases the intensity of training and may even cause detraining.

As polycythemia increases, the $Vo_{2,max}$ and endurance performance decreases. This might indicate that the higher the athlete goes to train the better, but this is not the case as an increased hematocrit carries its own disadvantages, especially increased viscosity and decreased microvascular perfusion if the hematocrit is too high. There is some evidence that athletes who live at moderate altitude (2500 m) and train at low altitude (1500 m) improve their endurance performance. However, there is considerable individual variation in the results of the 'live high, train low' method. Recently, there has also been much interest in the use of intermittent exposure to hypoxic environments to see if benefits for performance can be attained this way. There has also been some work in the effect of hypoxic training on work efficiency, as well as the effect on the malleability of the level of sustainable work, i.e. the lactate threshold which affects performance.

For maximal sea level performance, it is still not clear how long or how high the athlete should live at altitude or how long they should remain at sea level before racing. These techniques have become the focus of intense debates in the governing bodies who oversee international sport. There is even a controversy on the 'legality' of athletes using exposure to hypoxic environments as an ergogenic aid and thus the use of 'unfair means.'

Unfortunately, few trials have adequate sea level controls to compare with altitude training. Until this is done, much information will remain largely anecdotal.

29.1 INTRODUCTION

In 1965, Pugh (1965) suggested that athletic performance at altitude would result in faster times in sprint events due to decreased air resistance that parallels barometric pressure; by contrast in distance events, times would be increased because the maximum oxygen uptake falls with altitude (Wehrlin and Hallen 2006).

Comparing the times of athletes in the 1965 Pan-American games held in Mexico (2250 m) with those of the Melbourne Olympics of 1956 at sea level, he showed that there was an increase in time of 2.6% in the 800 m and 14.9% in the 10 000 m events. In the 100 m and 400 m, but not the 200 m, race times at altitude were faster than at sea level.

In the Mexico City Olympics in 1968, Tommie Smith, Lee Evans and Bob Beamon set records in the 200 m, 400 m, and long jump, respectively, that stood for years, while in the longer endurance events times were slower than at sea level. This was due to the reduced $Vo_{2,max}$ which at this altitude is 84% of sea level values. However, the times were not as slow as had been predicted. In one of the most important races in those games, in an upset, Kip Keino who was born and raised at approximately 2300 m in Kenya beat the heavily favored Jim Ryun from the United States. This race was the beginning of heated debates about the value of altitude training on athletic performance. There was little note that Keino not only lived at altitude, but also had grown up running many miles back and forth to school as a child!

Marathon performance at altitude is affected mainly by a lowered $Vo_{2,max}$ which decreases by about 1.5–3.5% for every 300 m of ascent above 1500 m (Roi *et al.* 1999).

29.2 THE MOUNTAINEER AS AN ATHLETE

The first mountaineers who could be called athletes were Habeler and Messner (Messner 1979). In 1978, they made the first ascent of Everest without supplemental oxygen, and this focused attention on their birth, upbringing and training at intermediate altitude in the European Alps. A number of high altitude natives have repeated this feat on Everest, but then so have mountaineers born and bred at sea level.

Habeler and Messner's training, which included long distance running and very rapid alpine ascents up to 4875 m and later rapid ascents in the Himalayas, played a major role in their exceptional fitness and subsequent success.

With training, outstanding feats of endurance have been recorded. In 1899, a Ghurka soldier born and bred at intermediate altitude in Nepal ascended and descended an 800 m peak in Scotland and crossed 4 miles of scree and bog in 55 min. A hundred years later in 1999, this feat was repeated by a trained athlete (a fell runner) in 53 min 45 s (The Times 1999).

Other outstanding endurance feats at low and high altitude are recorded. For instance, a 49-year-old man ran 391 miles in 7 days, 1 h and 25 min over Lakeland Hills up to 850 m in the UK. This involved a total ascent of 37 000 m, an average of over 5000 m per day (Brasher 1986). In June 1988, 76 summits in the same region were reached in 24 h involving an ascent and descent of 12 000 m (Brasher 1988). At intermediate altitude, all 54 of the peaks over 4300 m in Colorado, USA were climbed in 21 days (Boyer 1978), and the ascent of Mont Blanc (4807 m) from Chamonix, with return to Chamonix (1050 m) was made in 5.5 h (Smyth 1988). At high altitude, one ascent was made from 4900 m to 8047 m with return to 4900 m in 22 h (Wielicki 1985) and from 3000 m to 6000 m in 19 h (Rowell 1982).

In 1986, an ascent and descent of Everest (8848 m) in 2 days by a new route on the North face was completed from the head of the West Rongbuck Glacier (5800 m); supplementary oxygen was not used (Everest 1987). In 1990, Marc Batard ascended from Base Camp to the summit of Everest in 22.5 h also without the use of supplementary oxygen (Gillman 1993). An astounding ascent by Sherpa Pemba Dorji from Base Camp to the summit was reported to be 8 h 10 min (www.mounteverest.net/news)!

29.3 PRESUMED MECHANISM OF HYPOXIC EXPOSURE

As is well described in more detail in earlier chapters, exposure to high altitude stimulates a number of return to low altitude at least 2 to 3 days before an important race. On the other hand, Schuler *et al.* (2007) studied the adaptation of $Vo_{2,max}$ and time to exhaustion in eight elite cyclists to 2340 m altitude where competitions are likely to take place. After an initial decline in those variables (12.8 and 25.8%, respectively), these variables improved over time such that by 21 days, the decline was only 0.7 and 1.4%, respectively. Thus, it was recommended that athletes competing at that altitude should spend 3 weeks at this modest altitude in order to return to their pre-competition fitness without losing such fitness as they would do at higher altitudes.

29.4 HYPOXIC TRAINING

29.4.1 Effect of hypoxic training

To achieve optimum physical performance in middle and long distance events at altitude, it is clear that adequate acclimatization to hypoxia, or better still being born and bred at altitude, is essential. Most evidence suggests that after a period of training at altitude, performance improves upon returning to sea level, but the timing, i.e. altitude and duration at altitude for maximum sea level performance after altitude training is not clear. However, altitude training or exposure to simulated hypoxic environments at low altitude is frequently used by competition athletes to improve their sea level performance. On the one hand, acclimatization to high altitude results in central and peripheral adaptations that improve oxygen delivery and utilization. Hypoxic exercise may increase the stimulus of training thus magnifying the effect of endurance training. On the other hand, the hypoxia of altitude limits the intensity of training and may result in detraining.

Some of the best endurance runners have been born and bred in East Africa, living at an altitude of 1500–2000 m, implying that this upbringing will contribute to their continued success. However, Weston *et al.* (1999) compared elite African 10 km runners and their Caucasian counterparts, both of whom lived at sea level. The African runners had a greater resistance to fatigue,

and higher oxidative enzyme activity, combined with a lower accumulation of lactate. With the difference between winning and losing an event being often so small, the psychological effects of altitude training should not be discounted.

Numerous anecdotal reports suggest that endurance athletes benefit from altitude training; however, when appropriate controls have been included in studies, the results are less impressive. Additionally, there have been several altitudes used such that it is difficult to know if there is a minimal altitude, above which a benefit is gained. Using controls, Roskamm *et al.* (1969) found subjects who trained at 2250 m improved their $Vo_{2,max}$ by comparison with sea level subjects and those at 3450 m, but Hanson *et al.* (1967) also with sea level controls and starting with unfit subjects ($Vo_{2,max}$, 40 mL min^{-1} kg^{-1}) found no advantage in training at an altitude of 4300 m. In well-trained subjects too, the picture is not clear. A well-controlled study by Adams *et al.* (1975) using a crossover design in experienced trained athletes ($Vo_{2,max}$ 73 mL min^{-1} kg^{-1}) showed no significant differences in low altitude performance between those who trained at altitude (2300 m) and sea level. Similar findings were reported by Debevec *et al.* (2010) where they trained two groups of subjects for 20 sessions, one at sea level and one with an FiO_2 of 0.12. They measured peak power output and time to exhaustion and found mixed but inconclusive results about the benefit of hypoxic training.

Because so many hypoxic training studies have been completed without normoxic controls, it is difficult to determine whether the physiological changes noted are due to hypoxia alone or a training effect. In one series with controls, 10 elite middle- to long-distance runners trained for 10 weeks at the same exercise rate at sea level and at a simulated altitude of 4000 m. There was no improvement in $Vo_{2,max}$, yet personal best times over 10 km improved by about 6% in the altitude-trained athletes, (Asano *et al.* 1986). Is it possible that this was due to a psychological effect or an improvement in exercise efficiency? Anaerobic performance may also improve after returning to sea level, following a stay at altitude; however, many studies have shown no improvement (Martin and Pyne 1998).

29.4.2 Dose of hypoxic training

Some investigators have utilized 'doses' of hypoxia during training to effect a training advantage. Ventura *et al.* (2003) trained athletes for 6 weeks at high intensity with bouts of simulated 3200 m and found no change in performance. Brugniaux *et al.* (2006) had well-trained athletes sleep at simulated altitudes of 1200, 2500, 3000 and 3500 m for 13–18 days and found that 3000 m was safe and induced a degree of ventilatory acclimatization. Truijens *et al.* (2003) trained accomplished swimmers in a flume in an intense interval protocol at either low altitude or while inspiring air consistent with 2500 m altitude for 5 weeks and then measured performance at 100 and 400 m swims and found no difference. In another study, cyclists trained for 4 weeks at either sea level or simulated 2750 m three times per week in 10 intervals at 80% of maximum (Morton and Cable 2005). Without an increase in hemoglobin, the subjects increased their endurance, but not their maximum work intensity, but there was no difference between the hypoxic or sea level-trained athletes. These studies suggest that short-term exposure to hypoxic air during intense training has no discernible benefit for performance.

29.5 LIVING–TRAINING HYPOXIC PARADIGMS

In the late 1990s, a number of elegant studies were undertaken to investigate the various living–training environments in which athletes could realistically be exposed during a period of intense training. In other words, athletes lived high and trained low, lived and trained high, lived low and trained high, and trained and lived low. These studies were designed to take advantage of a number of physiologic responses of acclimatization which might convey an advantage in physical performance.

29.5.1 Training studies

Levine and Stray-Gundersen (1997) suggested that if athletes were acclimatized to a moderate altitude (2500 m) and trained at lower altitude

(1500 m) for 6 weeks, they could get the best of both worlds and improve their performance more than an equivalent control group at sea level or altitude. A 5000 m run time trial was the main measure of performance while they also undertook an additional number of physiologic measurements. The trained runners who 'lived high, trained low' showed an increase above sea level performance. Sea level performance was not improved in those who lived and trained at moderate altitude nor in those who lived and trained at sea level only.

There was, however, considerable individual variation in the response to altitude training, and some do not respond to the 'live high, train low regime' (Chapman *et al.* 1998). The 'responders' had the highest rise in erythropoietin and thus hematocrit, suggesting that the improved endurance was conveyed by the higher oxygen-carrying capacity in that group, but no genetic markers to elucidate this variability could be found (Jedlickova *et al.* 2003). Elite (world championship qualifiers) male and female runners were studied over 4 weeks at 2500 m during continued training; and although there was variability in the results, these already highly trained athletes showed improvement in all variables of performance (Stray-Gundersen *et al.* 2001). Attempts to have similar responses at the same altitude, but for shorter periods of time (5, 10 and 15 days), were unsuccessful in improving exercise performance (Roberts *et al.* 2003). Levine suggests that there is a response threshold such that the response to hypoxia is signaled by hypoxia-inducible factor-1-alpha which can be turned off when the body is not experiencing further stress of hypoxia, thus, gene transcription ceases.

29.5.2 Variations on exposure

In spite of such variable response, athletes have thought hypoxic exposure to be 'worth it.' In attempts to gain a competitive edge, athletes have used tents which allow athletes to sleep in hypoxic conditions at low altitude to mimic the 'live high, train low' construct which some have labeled legal 'blood doping.' To gain advantage with shorter periods of exposure, the concept of 'intermittent hypoxic training' was entertained, and a plethora of studies have emerged to test various doses and time of hypoxic exposure and their effect on exercise performance. Studies were designed based on observations in some animal studies. This approach exposed athletes to short periods (70 min) of hypoxia at rest daily for 4 weeks (Julian *et al.* 2004). There were no changes in any of the hematologic, physiologic or performance variables. Human and animal studies, such as this one, have led to much debate about the 'dose response' of the hypoxic exposure and the subsequent gain or lack thereof in performance (Stray-Gundersen *et al.* 2001; Levine 2005; Levine and Stray-Gundersen 2006).

Using normobaric hypoxia (FiO_2 0.14.5) for 6 weeks, Zoll *et al.* (2006) divided runners into two groups: live low, train low (LLTL) and live low, train high (LLTH). Hey looked at performance ($Vo_{2,max}$, and time to exhaustion) and muscle biopsies to evaluate markers of hypoxic transcription and oxidative phosphorylation. With the LLTH design, they found a modest increase in $Vo_{2,max}$ (5%), a remarkable increase in time to exhaustion (26%) and substantial increase in the transcription factors and markers of oxidative phosphorylation. Gore and colleagues (2006) exposed athletes to a simulated altitude of 4000 to 5500 m for 3 hours per day on 5 days per week for 4 weeks and found an increase in erythropoietin but no increase in markers of red cell production. They also studied swimmers in a similar design and found no improvement in swimming times which led them to conclude that their duration of exposure was not enough.

Not all studies have been negative. Katayama *et al.* (2003) exposed a small group of runners to a simulated altitude of 4500m for 90 minutes per day for 3 weeks. The hypoxic group showed improvement in running time and time to exhaustion, as well as lower Vo_2 levels at submaximal exercise levels with no change in other hematologic variables. One conclusion was that this exposure led to improved exercise efficiency with no mechanism offered.

Different results in similar, well-designed studies are difficult to explain. Robertson *et al.* (2010) exposed highly trained runners to simulate a LHTL (3000 m) and low altitude (600 m) design for 14 hours per day for 3 weeks and measured $Vo_{2,max}$, running economy and hemoglobin mass. They found greater gains in $Vo_{2,max}$ and hemoglobin in the LHTL group and variability in time trial performance. In a double-blind, placebo-controlled study, Siebenmann *et al.* (2012) studied 16 trained cyclists at baseline, during a 2-week lead-in period, and after 3–4 weeks of 16 hours per day of sham or simulated 3000 m altitude exposure and at 2 weeks after the LHTL intervention. After the intervention, $Vo_{2,max}$ at sea level and simulated 2500 m, exercise economy (Vo_2 at 200 watts work), mean power output in a simulated 26.15 km time trial, and hemoglobin were no different in this study designed for the first time to eliminate the placebo effect.

Shorter hypoxic exposure to simulated 3000 m versus low altitude for 3 weeks showed more improvement in all variables in the low altitude group (Roels *et al.*, 2007). Truijens *et al.* (2008) exposed well-trained athletes (runners and swimmers) to higher simulated altitudes (4000–5500 m) for shorter times (3 hours per day, 5 days per week for 4 weeks) or low altitude in a randomized, double-blind design and found no difference in all the measured performance and physiologic variables. In even shorter exposures for 7 days (4 hours per day, 5 days per week), in two studies, Beidleman *et al.* (2008, 2009) showed different results in terms of improved performance.

As one can discern, there is variability in study design and outcomes. It does seem that the studies which imposed longer exposure times to simulated high altitude resulted in some stronger results that were positive for the effect of altitude exposure on aerobic performance. It will, however, be a while before the right dose (degree and duration of exposure) can be recommended to improve exercise performance, and there clearly is heterogeneity in the effect on individuals.

Furthermore, the entire concept of a performance advantage with various constructs of hypoxic exposure has recently incited an intense debate between athletes, investigators and international regulatory agencies which is far from being resolved.

29.6 DETRAINING AND HYPOXIA

It has recently been seen that in elite endurance athletes, $Vo_{2,max}$ can be reduced at altitudes as low as 610 m (Gore *et al.* 1996). This occurred in about 50% of trained subjects with $Vo_{2,max}$ above 65 mL min^{-1} kg^{-1} (Anselme *et al.* 1992), and they appeared to develop a more severe level of arterial hypoxemia during maximal and submaximal exercise than more sedentary controls under hypoxic and normoxic conditions (Lawler *et al.* 1988; Koistenen *et al.* 1995). This might have been due to a detraining effect (Saltin 1967). However, it has also been suggested that intermittent exposure to altitudes between 2300 and 3300 m maximizes the balance between acclimatization and intensity of training (Daniels and Oldridge 1970). It is also possible that the intensity of training at sea level could produce as good a result as intermittent visits to altitude.

29.7 IS ALTITUDE TRAINING WORTH IT?

Is it worthwhile for athletes to train at altitude? At present, there is no clear answer to this question. The relative disadvantages are the minimal risk of acute mountain sickness and high altitude pulmonary and cerebral edema (HACE). The development of HACE would be a remote occurrence at training altitudes. The reduction of $Vo_{2,max}$ and the earlier onset of fatigue means that altitude training is less intense than at sea level. However, living high and training low has shown improved performance in a 5 km time trial.

On the strength of this and other trials, it would seem that for distance events it would be better to live at 2500 m and train at less than 1500 m. Bailey and Davis (1997) reviewed the available evidence for the efficacy of altitude training for sea level events and concluded:

> Scientific evidence to support the claim that either continuous or intermittent hypoxic training will enhance sea level performance remains at present equivocal.

However, many authorities would contest their skepticism and agree that careful modulation of hypoxic exposure and training is beneficial for aerobic exercise performance.

The optimum time of stay at altitude is still not clear, but to increase red cell mass at least 4 weeks at altitude may be necessary, but the associated reduction in training intensity would not be advantageous. To obtain maximum performance after the athlete descends to lower levels, the timing of the event is also not clear: a minimum of 2–3 days with a maximum of 14–21 days has been suggested (Suslov 1994).

29.8 SUSTAINABLE WORK

29.8.1 Mountaineering application

In section 29.2, there were several historic descriptions of elite mountaineers whose feats are clearly athletic. Unlike most low altitude elite athletes from low altitudes whose body build and physiology are somewhat similar in specific sports, there is much more heterogeneity in the physiology and physical stature in the accomplished mountaineer. Two characteristics stand out, however. The first is their ability to perform for long periods of time at a high percentage of their maximal capacity and the other is their ability to move efficiently. In this section, the first characteristic will be discussed.

To climb high peaks, one must have a level of sustainable work that allows them to perform for long periods of time, certainly hours if not days. Physiologically, this level of work is below one's lactate threshold (LT) also referred to as ventilatory or anaerobic threshold. Maintaining work levels above the LT is not possible for more than a few minutes, even in well-trained athletes. Most endurance athletes have a high aerobic capacity ($Vo_{2,max}$) and have LTs that are at a higher percentage of their $Vo_{2,max}$ (~75–90%) than the general population (~55–65%). Functionally, this characteristic translates into physical exertion that optimizes their ability to do well at high altitude.

Of importance to the high altitude climber, is the fact that the muscles involved have great plasticity to adapt to conditions of stress. For instance, in specialized athletes, such as cyclists, muscle mass through repeated training can be progressively recruited such that the oxidative stress is shared (Coyle 1992; Coyle 2005) and rotated to spare the oxidative stress and prolong the LT, increase endurance, delay fatigue, and promote efficiency. Free fatty acids would be the primary fuel and glycolysis which produces more lactate delayed. The onset of fatigue can be induced by a small increment in energy output (Mortensen *et al.* 2005), so it is critical for mountaineers to know this level of exertion to optimize performance and survival. This ability to recognize one's limits is critical for the high altitude mountaineer whether he/she is ascending or trying to escape from danger successfully.

29.8.2 Adaptations

This capability is not impaired by lack of oxygen, but more by perfusion. Cyclists with more endurance have been shown to have a greater capillary density (Coyle 1988; Coyle 2005). Since all of these athletes were well trained, it is not clear whether the ones with greater endurance have an inherently upregulated signal for angiogenesis or not. As described before, at very high altitudes an increase in surface area for perfusion is achieved by the decrease in muscle cell size with a maintenance or even increase in capillary volume.

29.8.3 Lactate threshold

For the mountaineer, it is important to recognize the ability of the muscle to adapt to training in a way so as to increase the level of sustainable work by moving the LT. Since the late 1970s, there have been a number of studies looking at the effect of both aerobic training and mixed intensity training on the LT.

One of the first studies (Davis and Gass 1979) took a group of sedentary men and put them through 9 weeks of aerobic training, 45 minutes per day 4 days per week and found that the LT increased by 44% of its absolute VO_2 and 15% expressed as that of $Vo_{2,max}$. Future studies then began to look at volume versus intensity of work to effect a change in LT. Both aerobic training

and intense or interval training (IT) have been used in varying doses for years, but became the focus of studies to try to answer the question of optimal 'dosing' of these levels of work to achieve a higher level of sustainable work. Three days of intense IT was added to the regimen of trained runners for 8 weeks (Acevedo *et al.* 1989). The results showed no change in $Vo_{2,max}$, but there was improvement in their 10 000 m times, increased time to exhaustion on a treadmill, and lower serum lactate levels at 85–90% of their maximum heart rates. In a less athletic group, a mere six bouts of four to seven 'all-out' Wingate tests over 2 weeks resulted in a 100% increase in endurance time on a cycle ergometer, a 26% increase in muscle glycogen and a 38% increase in citrate synthase, both markers of muscle oxidative capacity (Burgomaster *et al.* 2005). Interestingly, these two studies showed that intense training achieved important gains in the already trained, but clearly much greater gains in the less trained recreational athlete.

Quantity of training apparently is not as important as quality of training to produce beneficial effects of LT. Gibala *et al.* (2006) took 16 men and committed them to either 2.5 or 10.5 hours per week of IT or aerobic training for 2 weeks and found similar improvements in performance, as well as similar changes in markers of oxidative capacity in muscle biopsies. Similar findings emerged from a comparable study (Burgomaster *et al.* 2008). A lower quantity speed IT group maintained similar improvements in aerobic capacity and muscle biopsy capillary density as did a group of high quantity workloads (Iaia *et al.* 2009). How these changes translate into benefits in the high mountains is not known specifically, but carries with it compelling anecdotes from the elite mountaineers whose training regimes are legend.

These studies carry important implications for those individuals who come from busy working lives at low altitude who want to go to the high mountains physically fit so that they can perform efficiently and safely as possible which is critical both for enjoyment, as well as survival and safety. All individuals going on such adventures owe it not only to themselves but also to their fellow trekkers or climbers.

29.9 WORK EFFICIENCY

Mountaineering involves movement over ground which has to be done in the most efficient way, i.e. taking the energy generated by one's aerobic capacity and translating that to effective movement in the most biomechanically and bioenergetically efficient way. Some of these characteristics are inborn. For instance, there are some individuals with prodigious levels of $Vo_{2,max}$ whose biomechanics are not optimal for taking advantage of their 'engine' while by the same token, there are individuals with less than elite levels of $Vo_{2,max}$ who through better biomechanics can cover ground in a most efficient way.

This concept was demonstrated clearly in a study by Ge et al. (1994) who studied 17 Tibetans and 14 recently migrated Han Chinese at 4700 m in Tibet. The Han had higher $Vo_{2,max}$ levels (36 cc/kg/min) than did the Tibetans (30 cc/kg/min), but the Tibetans generated more work at their maximal levels than did the Han (176 versus 150 watts), higher LTs (84 versus 62%) as a percentage of maximum, and lower blood lactate levels. These are remarkable findings as it is well known that the Tibetans are superb performers at high altitude. Of course, the question arises whether these characteristics are inborn or adaptive. If they are the latter, then it would be helpful to know if we can also train efficiency as well as aerobic capacity (see Chapter 4).

There are several studies which have shown that work efficiency can be improved with aerobic, intense and resistive training. In the study by Iaia et al. (2009), IT/aerobic training resulted in 5.7 and 6.6% lower oxygen consumption at preset levels on a treadmill compared with endurance-trained subjects. In another study over 4 weeks in runners comparing IT and aerobic training, there were no changes in $Vo_{2,max}$, but the IT-trained athletes had greater improvement in velocity at maximum levels, suggesting greater running economy (Billat et al. 1999). Similar improvements in running efficiency (5%) at high race speeds were noted in track athletes with intermittent hypoxic training for 3 weeks (Katayama et al. 2003). Part of this improved efficiency may be secondary to a decrease in ventilatory demand which may be modest but potentially important in competitive and stressful environments like high altitude (Franch et al. 1998). Coyle has suggested that continual, intense training can lead to improved efficiency as found in an elite Tour de France rider (Coyle 2005). All of these studies show modest changes in efficiency and do not come close to the findings in the Tibetans, but in environments such as extreme altitude, every small advantage may be crucial.

References

Abassi, Z., Nakhoul, F., Khankin, E. *et al.* (2006) Pulmonary hypertension in chronic dialysis patients with arteriovenous fistula: pathogenesis and therapeutic prospective. *Curr. Opin. Nephrol. Hypertens.* **15**, 353–60.

Abud, E.M., Maylor, J., Undem, C. *et al.* (2012) Digoxin inhibits development of hypoxic pulmonary hypertension in mice. *Proc. Natl. Acad. Sci. USA* **109**, 1239–44.

Abuye, C. Berhane, Y. and Ersumo, T. (2008) The role of changing diet and altitude on goitre prevalence in five regional states in Ethiopia. *East African J. Public Health* **5**, 163–8.

Acevedo, E.O. and Goldfarb, A.H. (1989) Increased training efficiency effects on plasma lactate, ventilatory threshold, and endurance. *Med. Sci. Sports Exer.* **21**, 563–8.

Acosta, I. de (1590) *Historia Natural y Moral de las Indias*, Lib 3, Cap. 9, luan de Leon, Seville. Section of English translation of 1604 (1604), Edward Blount and William Aspley, London. Reprinted in *High Altitude Physiology* (ed. J.B. West), Hutchinson Ross Publishing Company, Stroudsburg, PA, 1981.

Adam, J.M. and Goldsmith, R. (1965) Cold climates, in *Exploration Medicine* (eds. O.G. Edholm and A.L. Bacharach), Wright, Bristol, pp. 245–77.

Adams, W.C., Bernauer, E.M., Dill, D.B., and Bowmar, J.B. Jr (1975) Effects of equivalent sea-level and altitude training on VO_2 max and running performance. *J. Appl. Physiol.* **39**, 262–6.

Adams, W.H. and Strang, L.J. (1975) Haemoglobin levels in persons of Tibetan ancestry living at high altitude. *Proc. Soc. Exp. Biol. Med.* **149**, 1036–9.

Admetlla, J., Leal, C. and Ricart, A. (2001) Management of diabetes at high altitude. *Br. J. Sports Med.* **35**, 282–3.

Adnot, S., Chabrier, P.E., Brun-Buisson, C. *et al.* (1988) Atrial natriuretic factor attenuates the pulmonary pressor response to hypoxia. *J. Appl. Physiol.* **65**, 1975–83.

Adzaku, F., Mohammed, S., Annobil, S. and Addae, S. (1993) Relevant laboratory findings in patients with sickle cell disease living at high altitude. *J. Wilderness Med.* **4**, 374–83.

Aggarwal, S., Negi, S., Jha, P. *et al.* (2010) *EGLN1* involvement in high-altitude adaptation revealed through genetic analysis of extreme constitution types defined in Ayurveda. *Proc. Natl. Acad. Sci.USA* **107**, 18961–6.

Agostoni, P., Cattadori, G., Guazzi, M. *et al.* (2000) Effects of simulated altitude-induced hypoxia on exercise capacity in patients with chronic heart failure. *Am. J. Med.* **109**, 450–5.

Agostoni, P., Contini, M., Magini, A. *et al.* (2006) Carvedilol reduces exercise-induced hyperventilation: a benefit in normoxia and a problem with hypoxia. *Eur. J. Heart Fail.* **8**, 729–35.

Agostini, P., Swenson, E.R., Bussotti, M. *et al.* (2011) High-altitude exposure of three weeks duration increases lung diffusing capacity in humans. *J. Appl. Physiol.* **110**, 1564–71.

Agusti, A.G., Sauleda, J., Miralles, C. *et al.* (2002) Skeletal muscle apoptosis and weight loss in chronic obstructive pulmonary disease. *Am. J. Respir. Crit. Care Med.* **166**, 485–9.

Ahle, N.W., Buroni, J.R., Sharp, M.W. and Hamlet, M.P. (1990) Infrared thermographic measurement of circulatory compromise in trenchfoot-injured Argentine soldiers. *Aviat. Space Environ. Med.* **61**, 247–50.

Ahmad, Y., Shukla, B., Gar, I. *et al.* (2011) Identification of haptoglobin and apolipoprotein A-1 as biomarkers for high altitude pulmonary edema. *Funct. Integr. Genomics* **11**, 407–11.

Aigner, A., Berghold, F. and Muss, N. (1980) Investigations on the cardiovascular system at altitudes up to a height of 7,800 meters. *Z. Kardiol.* **69**, 604–10.

Akero, A., Christensen, C.C., Edvardsen, A. and Skjonsberg, O.H. (2005) Hypoxaemia in chronic obstructive pulmonary disease patients during a commercial flight. *Eur. Respir. J.* **25**, 725–30.

Albrecht, P.H. and Littell, J.K. (1972) Plasma erythropoietin in men and mice during acclimatization to different altitudes. *J. Appl. Physiol.* **32**, 54–8.

Aldashev, A.A., Sarybaev, A.S., Sydykov, A.S. et al. (2002) Characterization of high-altitude pulmonary hypertension in the Kyrgyz: association with angiotensin-converting enzyme genotype. *Am. J. Respir. Crit. Care Med.* **166**, 1396–402.

Aldashev, A.A., Kojonazarov, B.K., Amatov, T.A. et al. (2005) Phosphodiesterase type 5 and high altitude pulmonary hypertension. *Thorax* **60**, 683–7.

Aldenderfer, M. (2011) Peopling the Tibetan plateau: insights from archaeology. *High Alt. Med. Biol.* **12**, 141–7.

Alexander, J. (1994) Coronary heart disease at altitude. *Texas Heart Inst. J.* **21**, 261–6.

Alexander, J. (1995) Age, altitude, and arrhythmia. *Texas Heart Inst. J.* **22**, 308–16.

Alexander, J.K. (1999) Cardiac arrhythmia at high altitude: the progressive effect of aging. *Texas Heart Inst. J.* **26**, 258–63.

Alexander, J.K., Hartley, L.H., Modelski, M. and Grover, R.F. (1967) Reduction of stroke volume during exercise in man following ascent to 3100m altitude. *J. Appl. Physiol.* **23**, 849–58.

Alexander, L. (1945) *The Treatment of Shock from Prolonged Exposure to Cold Especially in Water*, Combined Intelligence Objective Sub-Committee, Item No. **24**, File No. 24–37.

Allegra, L., Cogo, A., Legnani, D. et al. (1995) High altitude exposure reduces bronchial responsiveness to hypo-osmolar aerosol in lowland asthmatics. *Eur. Respir. J.* **8**, 1842–6.

Altman, P.L. and Dittmer, D.S. (1966) Erythrocyte values at altitude; Part 1 Man., in *Environmental Biology* (eds. P.L. Altman and D.S. Dittmer), Fed. Am. Soc. Exper. Biol., Bethesda, pp. 351–5.

American Physiological Society (1995) Standards for the diagnosis and care of patients with chronic obstructive pulmonary disease. *Am. J. Respir. Crit. Care Med.* **152**: S77–120.

Amann, M. and Secher, N.H. (2010) Point: Afferent feedback from fatigued locomotor muscles is an important determinant of endurance exercise performance. *J. Appl. Physiol.* **108**, 452–4.

Amann, M., Eldridge, M.W., Lovering, A.T. et al. (2006a) Arterial oxygenation influences central motor output and exercise performance via effects on peripheral locomotor muscle fatigue in humans. *J. Physiol.* **575**, 937–52.

Amann, M., Romer, L.M., Pegelow, D.F. et al. (2006b) Effects of arterial oxygen content on peripheral locomotor muscle fatigue. *J. Appl. Physiol.* **101**, 119–27.

Amann, M., Romer, L.M., Subudhi, A.W. et al. (2007) Severity of arterial hypoxemia affects the relative contributions of peripheral muscle fatigue to exercise performance in healthy humans. *J. Physiol.* **581**, 389–403.

Anand, A.C., Jha, S.K., Saha, A. et al. (2001) Thrombosis as a complication of extended stay at high altitude. *Natl. Med. J. India* **14**, 197–201.

Anand, A.C., Saha, A., Seth, A.K. et al. (2005) Symptomatic portal system thrombosis in soldiers due to extended stay at extreme altitude. *J. Gastroenterol. Hepatol.* **20**, 777–83.

Anand, I.S. (2001) Letter from the field: letter from Siachen Glacier. *High Alt. Med. Biol.* **2**, 553–7.

Anand, I.S., Harris, E., Ferrari, R. et al. (1986) Pulmonary haemodynamics of the yak, cattle and cross breeds at high altitude. *Thorax* **41**, 696–700.

Anand, I.S., Malhotra, R.M., Chandrashekhar, Y. et al. (1990) Adult subacute mountain sickness – a syndrome of congestive heart failure in man at very high altitude. *Lancet* **335**, 561–5.

Anand, I.S., Chandrashekhar, Y., Rao, S.K. *et al.* (1993) Body fluid compartments, renal blood flow, and hormones at 6000m in normal subjects. *J. Appl. Physiol.* **74**, 1234–9.

Anand, I.S., Prasad, B.A., Chugh, S.S. *et al.* (1998) Effect of inhaled nitric oxide and oxygen in high-altitude pulmonary edema. *Circulation* **98**, 2441–5.

Andersen, P. and Henriksson, J. (1977) Capillary supply of the quadriceps femoris muscle of man: adaptive response to exercise. *J. Physiol. (Lond.)* **270**, 677–90.

Anderson, J.V., Struthers, A.D., Payne, N.N. *et al.* (1986) Atrial natriuretic peptide inhibits the aldosterone response to angiotensin II in man. *Clin. Sci.* **70**, 507–12.

Anderson, P.J., Miller, A.D., O'Malley, K.A. *et al.* (2011) Incidence and symptoms of high altitude illness in South Pole workers: Antarctic Study of Altitude Physiology (ASAP). *Clin. Med. Insights Circ. Respir. Pulm. Med.* **5**, 27–35.

Anderson, S., Herbring, B.G. and Widman, B. (1970) Accidental profound hypothermia (case report). *Br. J. Anaesth.* **42**, 653–5.

Andrew, H.G. (1963) Work in extreme cold. *Trans. Assoc. Indust. Med. Off.* **13**, 16–19.

Anholm, J.D. and Foster, G.P. (2011) Con: Hypoxic pulmonary vasoconstriction is not a limiting factor of exercise at high altitude. *High Alt. Med. Biol.* **12**, 313–17.

Anholm, J.D., Poweles, AC., Downey, R.D. *et al.* (1992) Operation Everest II: arterial oxygen saturation and sleep at extreme simulated altitude. *Am. Rev. Respir. Dis.* **145**, 817–26.

Anholm, J.D., Milne, E.N., Stark, P. *et al.* (1999) Radiographic evidence of interstitial pulmonary edema after exercise at altitude. *J. Appl. Physiol.* **86**, 503–9.

Anonymous (1990) Kiss of life for a cold corpse (Editorial). *Lancet* **335**, 1435.

Anooshiravani, M., Dumont, L., Mardirosoff, C. *et al.* (1999) Brain magnetic resonance imaging (MRI) and neurological changes after a single high altitude climb. *Med. Sci. Sports Exerc.* **31**, 969–72.

Another Ascent of the World's Highest Peak – Qomolangma (1975) Foreign Languages Press, Peking.

Anselme, F., Caillaud, C., Courret, I. and Prefaut, C. (1992) Exercise induced hypoxaemia and histamine excretion in extreme athletes. *Int. J. Sports Med.* **13**, 80–1.

Antezana, A.-M., Richalet, J.-P., Noriega, I. *et al.* (1995) Hormonal changes in normal and polycythemic high-altitude natives. *J. Appl. Physiol.* **79**, 795–800.

Antezana, A.M., Antezana, G., Aparicio, O. *et al.* (1998) Pulmonary hypertension in high altitude chronic hypoxia: response to nifedipine. *Eur. Respir. J.* **12**, 1181–5.

Antezana, G., Leguia, G., Guzman, A.M. *et al.* (1982) Hemodynamic study of high altitude pulmonary edema (12200 ft), in *High Altitude Physiology and Medicine* (eds. W. Brendel and R.A. Zink), Springer-Verlag, New York, pp. 232–41.

Anthony, A., Ackerman, E. and Strother, G.K. (1959) Effects of altitude acclimatization on rat myoglobin. Changes in myoglobin content of skeletal and cardiac muscle. *Am. J. Physiol.* **196**, 512–16.

Aoki, V.S. and Robinson, S.M. (1971) Body hydration and the incidence and severity of acute mountain sickness. *J. Appl. Physiol.* **31**, 363–7.

Appell, H.-J. (1978) Capillary density and patterns in skeletal muscle. III. Changes of the capillary pattern after hypoxia. *Pflügers Arch.* **377**, R53 (abstract).

Appleton, F.M. (1967) Possible influence of altitude on blood pressure. *Circulation* **36** (Suppl. 2), 55.

Araki, T. (1891) Ueber die Bildung von Milchsäure und Glycose im Organismus bei Sauerstoffmangel. *Z. Physiol. Chem.* **15**, 335–70.

Araneda, O.F., Garcia, C., Lagos, N. *et al.* (2005) Lung oxidative stress as related to exercise and altitude. Lipid peroxidation evidence in exhaled breath condensate: a possible predictor of acute mountain sickness. *Eur. J. Appl. Physiol.* **95**, 383–90.

Arbab-Zadeh, A., Levine, B.D., Trost, J.C. *et al.* (2009) The effect of acute hypoxemia on coronary arterial dimensions in patients with coronary artery disease. *Cardiology* **113**, 149–54.

Archer, S.L., Tolins, J.P., Raij, L. and Weir, E.K. (1989) Hypoxic pulmonary vasoconstriction is enhanced by inhibition of the synthesis of an endothelium derived relaxing factor. *Biochem. Biophys. Res. Commun.* **164**, 1198–205.

Arias-Stella, J. (1969) Human carotid body at high altitudes. *Am. J. Pathol.* **55**, 82.

Arias-Stella, J. (1971) Chronic mountain sickness: pathology and definition, in *High Altitude Physiology: Cardiac and Respiratory Aspects*, Ciba Foundation Symposium (eds. R. Porter and J. Knight), Churchill Livingstone, Edinburgh, pp. 31–40.

Arias-Stella, J. and Kruger, H. (1963) Pathology of high altitude pulmonary edema. *Arch. Pathol.* **76**, 147–57.

Arias-Stella, J. and Recavarren, S. (1962) Right ventricular hypertrophy in native children living at high altitude. *Am. J. Pathol.* **41**, 55–64.

Arias-Stella, J. and Saldaña, M. (1962) The muscular arteries in people native to high altitude. *Med. Thorac.* **19**, 55–64.

Arias-Stella, J. and Saldaña, M. (1963) The terminal portion of the pulmonary arterial tree in people native to high altitudes. *Circulation* **28**, 915–25.

Arias-Stella, J. and Topilsky, M. (1971) Anatomy of the coronary circulation at high altitude, in *High Altitude Physiology: Cardiac and Respiratory Aspects* (eds. R. Porter and J. Knight), Churchill Livingstone, London, pp. 149–57.

Arias-Stella, J., Kruger, H. and Recavarren, S. (1973) Pathology of chronic mountain sickness. *Thorax* **28**, 701–8.

Armstrong, L.S. and Maresh, C.M. (1991) The induction and decay of heat acclimatisation in trained athletes. *Sports Med.* **12**, 302–12.

Asano, K., Sub, S., Matsuzaka, A. *et al.* (1986) The influence of simulated high altitude training on work capacity and performance in middle and long distance runners. *Bull. Inst. Health Sports Med.* **9**, 1195–202.

Asano, M., Kaneoka, K., Nomura, T. *et al.* (1998) Increase in serum vascular endothelial growth factor levels during altitude training. *Acta Physiol. Scand.* **162**, 455–9.

Asemu, G., Neckar, J., Szarszoi, O. *et al.* (2003) Decrease in peak rate with acute hypoxia in relation to sea level. *Physiol. Res.* **49**, 597–606.

Ashack, R., Farber, M.O., Weinberger, M.H. *et al.* (1985) Renal and hormonal responses to acute hypoxia in normal individuals. *J. Lab. Clin. Med.* **106**, 12–16.

Ashenden, M.J., Gore, C.J., Martin D,T.*et al.* (1999a) Effects of a 12-day 'live high, train low' camp on reticulocyte production and haemoglobin mass in elite female road cyclists. *Eur. J. Appl. Physiol. Occup. Physiol.* **80**, 472–8.

Ashenden, M.J., Gore, C.J., Dobson, G.P. and Hahn, A.G. (1999b) 'Live high, train low' does not change the total haemoglobin mass of male endurance athletes sleeping at a simulated altitude of 3000m for 23 nights. *Eur. J Appl. Physiol. Occup. Physiol.* **80**, 479–84.

Ashraf, H., Javed, A. and Ashraf, S. (2006) Pulmonary embolism at high altitude and hyperhomocysteinemia. *J. Coll. Physicians Surg. Pak.* **16**, 71–3.

Asmussen, E. and Consolazio, F.C. (1941) The circulation in rest and work on Mount Evans (4,300m). *Am. J. Physiol.* **132**, 555–63.

Aste-Salazar, H. and Hurtado, A. (1944) The affinity of hemoglobin for oxygen at sea level and at high altitudes. *Am. J. Physiol.* **142**, 733–43.

Astrup, P. and Severinghaus, J.W. (1986) *The History of Blood Gases, Acids and Bases*, Munksgaard, Copenhagen.

Atrial natriuretic peptide [editorial]. (1986) *Lancet* **2**, 371–2.

Au, J., Brown, J.E., Lee, M.R. and Boon, N.A. (1990) Effect of cardiac tamponade on atrial natriuretic peptide concentrations: influence of stretch and pressure. *Clin. Sci.* **79**, 377–80.

Auerbach, P.S. (2012) *Wilderness Medicine*, 6th edn. Elsevier Mosby, Philadelphia.

Aughey, R.J., Gore, C.J., Hahn, A.G. *et al.* (2005) Chronic intermittent hypoxia and incremental cycling exercise independently depress muscle in vitro maximal Na+-K+-ATPase activity in well-trained athletes. *J. Appl. Physiol.* **98**, 186–92.

Ayton, J.M. (1993) Polar hands: spontaneous skin fissures closed with cyanoacrylate (Histoacryl Blue) tissue adhesive in Antarctica. *Arctic Med. Res.* **52**, 127–30.

Ayus, J.C., Moritz, M.L. (2008) Exercise-associated hyponatremia masquerading as acute mountain sickness: are we missing the diagnosis? *Clin. J. Sport Med.* **18**, 383–6.

Babcock, M.A., Pegelow, D.F., McClaran, S.R. *et al.* (1995) Contribution of diaphragmatic power output to exercise-induced diaphragm fatigue. *J. Appl. Physiol.* **78**, 1710–19.

Backer, H.D., Shopes, E. and Collins, S.L. (1993) Hyponatemia in recreational hikers in Grand Canyon National Park. *Wilderness. Environ. Med.* **4**, 391–406.

Baddeley, A.D., Cuccaro, W.J., Egstrom, G.H. and Willis, M.A. (1975) Cognitive efficiency of divers working in cold water. *Hum. Factors* **17**, 446–54.

Baertschi, A.J., Hausmaninger, C., Walsh, R.S. *et al.* (1986) Hypoxia-induced release of atrial natriuretic factor (ANF) from isolated rat and rabbit heart. *Biochem. Biophys. Res. Commun.* **140**, 427–33.

Bailey, D.M. and Davies, B. (1997) Physiological implications of altitude training for endurance performance at sea level: a review. *Br. J. Sports Med.* **31**, 183–90.

Bailey, D.M., Davies, B., Romer, L. *et al.* (1998) Implications of moderate altitude training for sea-level endurance in elite distance runners. *Eur. J. Appl. Physiol.* **78**, 360–8.

Bailey, D.M., Davies, B., Young, I.S. *et al.* (2001) A potential role for free radical-mediated skeletal muscle soreness in the pathophysiology of acute mountain sickness. *Aviat. Space Environ. Med.* **72**, 513–21.

Bailey, D.M., Davies, B., Castell, L.M. *et al.* (2003) Symptoms of infection and acute mountain sickness; associated metabolic sequelae and problems in differential diagnosis. *High Alt. Med. Biol.* **4**, 319–31.

Bailey, D.M., Roukens, R., Knauth, M. *et al.* (2005) Free radical-mediated damage to barrier function is not associated with altered brain morphology in high-altitude headache. *J. Cereb. Blood Flow Metab.* **26**, 99–111.

Bailey D.M., Roukens R., Knauth, M. *et al.* (2006) Free radical-mediated damage to barrier function is not associated with altered brain morphology in high-altitude headache. *J. Cereb. Blood Flow Metab.* **26**, 99–111.

Bailey, D.M., Bärtsch, P., Knauth, M. and Baumgartner, R.W. (2009a) Emerging concepts in acute mountain sickness and high-altitude cerebral edema: from the molecular to the morphological. *Cell Mol. Life Sci.* **66**, 3583–94.

Bailey, D.M., Evans, K.A., James, P.E. *et al.* (2009b) Altered free radical metabolism in acute mountain sickness: implications for dynamic cerebral autoregulation and blood-brain barrier function. *J. Physiol.* **587**, 73–85.

Bailey, D.M., Taudorf, S., Berg, R.M. *et al.* (2009c) Increased cerebral output of free radicals during hypoxia: implications for acute mountain sickness? *Am. J. Physiol. Regul. Integr. Comp. Physiol.* **297**, R1283–92.

Bailey, D.M., Dehnert, C., Luks, A.M. *et al.* (2010) High altitude pulmonary hypertension is associated with free radical-mediated reduction and pulmonary nitric oxide bioavailability. *J. Physiol.* **588**, 4837–47.

Bailey, F.M. (1957) *No Passport to Tibet.* Hart Davis, London, p. 261.

Baillie, J.K., Thompson, A.A., Irving, J.B. *et al.* (2009) Oral antioxidant supplementation does not prevent acute mountain sickness: double blind, randomized placebo-controlled trial. *QJM* **102**, 341–8.

Baker, P.T. (1966) Microenvironment cold in a high altitude Peruvian population, in *Human Adaptability and Its Methodology* (eds. H. Yoshimura and J.S. Weiner), Japanese Society for the Promotion of Sciences, Tokyo, pp. 67–77.

Baker, P.T. (1978) *The Biology of High Altitude Peoples.* Cambridge University Press, Cambridge.

Baker, P.T. and Dutt, J.S. (1972) Demographic variables as measures of biological adaptation: a case study of high altitude population, in *The Structure of Human Populations* (eds. G.A. Harrison and A.J. Boyce), Clarendon Press, Oxford, pp. 352–78.

Bakewell, S.E., Hart, N.D., Wilson, C.M. *et al.* (1999) A randomised, double blind placebo controlled trial of the effect of inhaled nedocromil sodium or slameterol xinafoate on the citric acid cough threshold in subjects travelling to high altitude (abstract), in *Hypoxia: Into the Next Millennium* (eds. R.C. Roach, P.D. Wagner and P.H. Hackett), Plenum/Kluwer Academic Publishing, New York, p. 362.

Banchero, N. (1982) Long term adaptation of skeletal muscle capillarity. *Physiologist* **25**, 385–9.

Bandopadhyay, P. and Selvamurthy, W. (2003) Suggested predictive indices for high altitude pulmonary oedema. *J. Assoc. Phys. India* **48**, 290–329.

Bangham, C.R.M. and Hackett, P.H. (1978) Effects of high altitude on endocrine function in the Sherpas of Nepal. *J. Endocrinol.* **79**, 147–8.

Banner, A.S. (1988) Relationship between cough due to hypotonic aerosol and the ventilatory response to CO_2 in normal subjects. *Am. Rev. Respir. Dis.* **137**, 647–50.

Barash, I.A., Beatty, C., Powell, F.L. *et al.* (2001) Nocturnal oxygen enrichment of room air at 3800 meter altitude improves sleep architecture. *High Alt. Med. Biol.* **2**, 525–33.

Barber, S.G. (1978) Drugs and doctoring for trans-Saharan travellers. *BMJ* **2**, 404–6.

Barclay, J.K. (1986) A delivery-independent blood flow effect on skeletal muscle fatigue. *J. Appl. Physiol.* **61**, 1084–90.

Barcroft, J. (1911) The effect of altitude on the dissociation curve of blood. *J. Physiol. (Lond.)* **42**, 44–63.

Barcroft, J. (1925) *The Respiratory Function of the Blood. Part I. Lessons from High Altitudes*, Cambridge University Press, Cambridge.

Barcroft, J. and King, W.O.R. (1909) The effect of temperature on the dissociation curve of blood. *J. Physiol. (Lond.)* **39**, 374–84.

Barcroft, J. and Orbeli, L. (1910) The influence of lactic acid upon the dissociation curve of blood. *J. Physiol. (Lond.)* **41**, 355–67.

Barcroft, J., Camis, M., Mathison, C.G. *et al.* (1914) Report of the Monte Rosa Expedition of 1911. *Philos. Trans. R. Soc. Lond. Ser. B* **206**, 49–102.

Barcroft, J., Cooke, A., Hartridge, H. *et al.* (1920) The flow of oxygen through the pulmonary epithelium. *J. Physiol. (Lond.)* **53**, 450–72.

Barcroft, J., Binger, C.A., Bock, A.V. *et al.* (1923) Observations upon the effect of high altitude on the physiological processes of the human body, carried out in the Peruvian Andes, chiefly at Cerro de Pasco. *Philos. Trans. R. Soc. Lond. Ser. B* **211**, 351–480.

Barer, G.R., Howard, P. and Shaw, J.W. (1970) Stimulus–response curves for the pulmonary vascular bed to hypoxia and hypercapnia. *J. Physiol. (Lond.)* **211**, 139–55.

Barnholt, K.E., Hoffman, A.R., Rock, P.B. *et al.* (2006) Endocrine responses to acute and chronic high-altitude exposure (4,300 meters): modulating effects of caloric restriction. *Am. J. Physiol.* **290**, E1078–88.

Barry, P.W., Mason, N.P. and Collier, D.J. (1995) Sex differences in blood gases during acclimatization, in *Hypoxia and the Brain* (eds. J.R. Sutton, C. S Houston and G. Coates), Queen City Printers, Burlington, VT, p. 314.

Barry, P.W., Mason, N.P., Riordan, M. and O'Callaghan, C. (1997a) Cough frequency and cough receptor sensitivity are increased in man at high altitude. *Clin. Sci.* **93**, 181–6.

Barry, P.W., Mason, N.P., Nicol, A. *et al.* (1997b) Cough receptor sensitivity and dynamic ventilatory response to carbon dioxide in man acclimatized to high altitude (abstract), in *Women at Altitude* (eds. C.S. Houston and G. Coates), Queens City Press, Burlington, VA, p. 303.

Barthelmes, D., Bosch, M.M., Merz, T.M. *et al.* (2011) Delayed appearance of high altitude retinal hemorrhages. *PLoS One* **6**, e11532.

Bartlett, D. Jr and Remmers, J.E. (1971) Effects of high altitude exposure on the lungs of young rats. *Respir. Physiol.* **13**, 116–25.

Bärtsch, P. and Gibbs, J.S. (2007) The effect of altitude on the heart and lungs. *Circulation* **116**, *2191*.

Bärtsch, P., Haeberli, A., Hauser, K. *et al.* (1988) Fibrinogenolysis in the absence of fibrin formation in severe hypobaric hypoxia. *Aviat. Space Environ. Med.* **59**, 428–32.

Bärtsch, P., Shaw, S., Franciolli, M. *et al.* (1988) Atrial natriuretic peptide in acute mountain sickness. *J. Appl. Physiol.* **65**, 1929–37.

Bärtsch, P., Haeberli, A., Franciolli, M. *et al.* (1989) Coagulation and fibrinolysis in acute mountain sickness and beginning pulmonary edema. *J. Appl. Physiol.* **66**, 2136–44.

Bärtsch, P., Lämmle, B., Huber, I. *et al.* (1989) Contact phase of blood coagulation is not activated in edema of high altitude. *J. Appl. Physiol.* **67**, 1336–40.

Bärtsch, P., Pfluger, N., Audetat, M.S. *et al.* (1991a) Effects of slow ascent to 4559m on fluid homeostasis. *Aviat. Space Environ. Med.* **62**, 105–10.

Bärtsch, P., Maggiorini, M., Ritter, M. *et al.* (1991b) Prevention of high-altitude pulmonary edema by nifedipine. *N. Engl. J. Med.* **325**, 1284–9.

Bärtsch, P., Merki, B., Hofsetter, D. *et al.* (1993) Treatment of acute mountain sickness by simulated descent: a randomised controlled trial. *BMJ* **306**, 1098–101.

Bärtsch, P., Grünig, E., Hohenhaus, E. *et al.* (2001) Assessment of high altitude tolerance in healthy individuals. *High Alt. Med. Biol.* **2**, 287–96.

Bärtsch, P., Straub, P.W. and Haeberli, A. (2001) Hypobaric hypoxia. *Lancet* **357**, 955–6.

Bärtsch, P., Swenson, E.R., Paul, A. *et al.* (2002) Hypoxic ventilatory response, ventilation, gas exchange, and fluid balance in acute mountain sickness. *High Alt. Med. Biol.* **3**, 361–76.

Bascom, D.A., Clement, I.D., Cunningham, D.A. *et al.* (1990) Changes in peripheral chemoreceptor sensitivity during sustained isocapnic hypoxia. *Respir. Physiol.* **82**, 161–76.

Basnyat, B. (2001) Isolated facial and hypoglossal nerve palsies at high altitude. *High Alt. Med. Biol.* **2**, 301–3.

Basnyat, B. and Litch, J.A. (1997) Medical problems of porters and trekkers in the Nepal Himalaya. *Wilderness Environ. Med.* **8**, 78–81.

Basnyat, B., Lemaster, J. and Litch, J.A. (1999) Everest or bust: a cross sectional, epidemiological study of acute mountain sickness at 4243 meters in the Himalayas. *Aviat. Space Environ. Med.* **70**, 867–73.

Basnyat, B., Gertsch, J.H., Holck, P.S. *et al.* (2006) Acetazolamide 125mg BD is not significantly different from 375mg BD in the prevention of acute mountain sickness: the prophylactic acetazolamide dosage comparison for efficacy (PACE) trial. *High Alt. Med. Biol.* **7**, 17–27.

Basnyat, B., Holck, P.S., Pun, M. *et al.* (2011) Spironolactone does not prevent acute mountain sickness: a prospective, double-blind, randomized, placebo-controlled trial by SPACE Trial Group (spironolactone and acetazolamide trial in the prevention of acute mountain sickness group). *Wilderness Environ. Med.* **22**, 15–22.

Basnyat, B., Sleggs, J. and Spinger, M. (2000a) Seizures and delirium in a trekker: the consequences of excessive water drinking? *Wilderness. Environ. Med.* **11**, 69–70.

Basnyat, B., Subedi, D., Sleggs, J. *et al.* (2000b) Disoriented and ataxic pilgrims: an epidemiological study of acute mountain sickness and high-altitude cerebral edema at a sacred lake at 4300m in the Nepal Himalayas. *Wilderness. Environ. Med.* **11**, 89–93.

Basnyat, B., Wu, T.Y. and Certsch, J.H. (2004) Neurological conditions at altitude that fall outside the definition of altitude illness. *High Alt. Med. Biol.* **5**, 171–9.

Bates, M.G.D., Thompson, A.A.R., Baillie, K. *et al.* (2011) Sildenafil citrate for the prevention of high altitude hyoxic pulmonary hypertension: double-blind, randomized, placebo-controlled trial. *High Alt. Med. Biol.* **12**, 207–14.

Baumgartner, R.W., Bärtsch, P., Maggiorini, M. *et al.* (1994) Enhanced cerebral blood flow in acute mountain sickness. *Aviat. Space Environ. Med.* **65**, 726–9.

Baumgartner, R.W., Spyridopoulos, I., Bärtsch, P. *et al.* (1999) Acute mountain sickness is not related to cerebral blood flow: a decompression chamber study. *J. Appl. Physiol.* **86**, 1578–82.

Baumgartner, R.W., Siegel, A.M. and Hackett, P.H. (2007) Going high with preexisting neurological conditions. *High Alt. Med. Biol.* **8**, 108–16.

Bayer, A., Yumusak, E., Sahin, O.F. and Uysal, Y. (2004) Intraocular pressure measured at ground level and 10,000 feet. *Aviat. Space Environ. Med.* **75**, 543–5.

Bayliss, R.I.S. (1987) Endocrine manifestations of non-endocrine disease, in *Oxford Textbook of Medicine,* 2nd edn (eds. D.J. Weatherall, J.G.G. Leadingham and D.A. Warrell), Oxford University Press, Oxford, pp. 101–19.

Bazett, H.C. and McGlone, B. (1927) Temperature gradients in the tissues of man. *Am. J. Physiol.* **82**, 415–51.

Beall, C.M. (2000) Tibetan and Andean patterns of adaptation to high-altitude hypoxia. *Hum. Biol.* **72**, 201–28.

Beall, C. (2006) Andean, Tibetan, and Ethiopian patterns of adaptation to high-altitude hypoxia. *Integr. Comp. Biol.* **46**, 18–24.

Beall, C. (2007) Detecting natural selection in high-altitude human populations. *Respir. Physiol. Neurobiol.* **158**, 161–71.

Beall, C.M., Goldstein, M.C. and the Tibetan Academy of Sciences (1987) Hemoglobin concentration of pastoral nomads permanently resident at 4850–5450 meters in Tibet. *Am. J. Phys. Anthropol.* **73**, 433–8.

Beall, C.M., Blangero, J., Williams-Blangero, S. and Goldstein, M.C. (1994) Major gene for percent of oxygen saturation of arterial hemoglobin in Tibetan highlanders. *Am. J. Phys. Anthropol.* **95**, 271–6.

Beall, C.M., Strohl, K.P., Blangero, J. *et al.* (1997a) Ventilation and hypoxic ventilatory response of Tibetan and Aymara high altitude natives. *Am. J. Anthropol.* **104**, 427–47.

Beall, C.M., Strohl, K.P., Blangero, J. *et al.* (1997b) Quantitative genetic analysis of arterial oxygen saturation in Tibetan highlanders. *Hum. Biol.* **69**, 597–604.

Beall, C.M., Brittenham, G.M., Strohl, K.P. *et al.* (1998) Hemoglobin concentration of high-altitude Tibetans and Bolivian Aymara. *Am. J. Anthropol.* **106**, 385–400.

Beall, C.M., Almasy, L.A., Blangero, J. *et al.* (1999) Percent of oxygen saturation of arterial hemoglobin among Bolivian Aymara at 3,990–4,000 m. *Am. J. Phys. Anthropol.* **108**, 41–51.

Beall, C.M., Decker, M.J., Brittenham, G.M. *et al.* (2002) An Ethiopian pattern of human adaptation to high-altitude hypoxia. *Proc. Natl. Acad. Sci. USA* **99**, 17215–8.

Beall, C.M., Song, K., Elston, R.C. and Goldstein, M.C. (2004). Higher offspring survival among Tibetan women with high oxygen saturation genotypes residing at 4,000 m. *PNAS* **101**, 14300–4.

Beall, C.M., Cavalleri, G.L., Deng, L. *et al.* (2010) Natural selection on *EPAS1* (HIF2alpha) associated with low hemoglobin concentration in Tibetan highlanders. *Proc. Natl. Acad. Sci. USA* **107**, 11459–64.

Beall, C.M., Laskowski, D. and Erzurum, S.C. (2012) Nitric oxide in adaptation to altitude. *Free Rad. Biol. Med.* **52**, 1123–34.

Beaumont, M., Goldenberg, F., Lejeune, D. *et al.* (1996) Effect of zolpidem on sleep and ventilatory patterns at simulated altitude of 4,000 meters. *Am. J. Respir. Crit. Care Med.* **153**, 1864–9.

Beaumont, M., Batejat, D., Coste, O. *et al.* (2004) Effects of zolpidem and zaleplon on sleep, respiratory patterns and performance at a simulated altitude of 4,000 m. *Neuropsychobiology* **49**, 154–62.

Beaumont, M., Batejat, D., Pierard, C. *et al.* (2007) Zaleplon and zolpidem objectively alleviate sleep disturbances in mountaineers at a 3,613 meter altitude. *Sleep* **30**, 1527–33.

Becker, P.M., Alcasabas, A., Yu, A.Y. *et al.* (2000) Oxygen-independent upregulation of vascular endothelial growth factor and vascular barrier dysfunction during ventilated pulmonary ischemia in isolated ferret lungs. *Am. J. Respir. Cell. Mol. Biol.* **22**, 272–9.

Beidleman, B.A., Muza, S.R., Rock, P.B. *et al.* (1997) Exercise responses after altitude acclimatization are retained during reintroduction to altitude. *Med. Sci. Sports Exerc.* **29**, 1588–95.

Beidleman, B.A., Rock, P.B., Muza, S.R. *et al.* (1999) Exercise VE and physical performance at altitude are not affected by menstrual cycle phase. *J. Appl. Physiol.* **86**, 1519–26.

Beidleman, B.A., Muza, S.R., Fulco, C.S. *et al.* (2004) Intermittent altitude exposures reduce acute mountain sickness at 4300 m. *Clin. Sci. (Lond)* **106**, 321–8.

Beidleman, B.A., Muza, S.R., Fulco, C.S. *et al.* (2008) Seven intermittent exposures to altitude improves exercise performance at 4300 m. *Med. Sci. Sports Exer.* **40**, 141–8.

Beidleman, B.A., Fulco, C.S., Muza, S.R. *et al.* (2009) Effect of six days of staging on physiologic adjustments and acute mountain sickness during ascent to 4300 meters. *High Alt. Med. Biol.* **10**, 253–60.

Beidleman, B.A., Muza, S.R., Fulco, C.S. *et al.* (2009) Intermittent hypoxic exposure does not improve endurance performance at altitude. *Med. Sci. Sports Exer.* **41**, 1317–25.

Bencowitz, H.Z., Wagner, P.D. and West, J.B. (1982) Effect of change in P_{50} on exercise tolerance at high altitude: a theoretical study. *J. Appl. Physiol.* **53**, 1487–95.

Bender, P.B., DeBehnke, D.J., Swart, G.L. and Hall, K.N. (1995) Serum potassium concentration as a predictor of resuscitation outcome in hypothermic cardiac arrest. *Wilderness Environ. Med.* **6**, 273–82.

Bendz, B., Rostrup, M., Sevre, K. *et al.* (2000) Association between acute hypobaric hypoxia and activation of coagulation in human beings. *Lancet* **356**, 1657–8.

Benesch, R. and Benesch, R.E. (1967) The effect of organic phosphates from the human erythrocyte on the allosteric properties of hemoglobin. *Biochem. Biophys. Res. Commun.* **26**, 162–7.

Benoit, H., Busso, T., Castells, J. *et al.* (2000) Decrease in peak rate with acute hypoxia in relation to sea level $VO_{2,max}$. *Eur. J. Appl. Physiol.* **90**, 514–19.

Benso, A., Broglio, F., Aimaretti, G. *et al.* (2007) Endocrine and metabolic responses to extreme altitude and physical exercise in climbers. *Eur. J. Endocrinol.* **157**, 733–40.

Benson, H., Lehmann, J.W., Malhotra, M.S. *et al.* (1982) Body temperature changes during the practice of g-tum-mo yoga. *Nature* **295**, 234–6.

Berg, B.W., Dillard, T.A., Rajagopal, K.R. and Mehm, W.J. (1992) Oxygen supplementation during air travel in patients with chronic obstructive lung disease. *Chest* **101**, 638–41.

Berg, J.T., Fu, Z., Breen, E.C. *et al.* (1997) High lung inflation increases mRNA levels of ECM components and growth factors in lung parenchyma. *J. Appl. Physiol.* **83**, 120–8.

Berg, J.T., Breen, E.C., Fu, Z. *et al.* (1998) Alveolar hypoxia causes increased gene expression of extracellular matrix proteins and platelet-derived growth factor B in lung parenchyma. *Am. J. Respir. Crit. Care Med.* **158**, 1920–8.

Berger, J., Aguayo, V.M., Tellez, W. *et al.* (1997) Weekly iron supplementation is as effective as 5 day per week iron supplementation in Bolivian school children living at high altitude. *Eur. J. Clin. Nutr.* **51**, 381–6.

Berger, M.M., Dehnert, C., Bailery, D.M. *et al.* (2009) Transpulmonary plasma ET-1 and nitrite differences in high altitude pulmonary hypertension. *High Alt. Med. Biol.* **10**, 17–24.

Berger, M.M., Hesse, C., Dehnert, C. *et al.* (2005) Hypoxia impairs systemic endothelial function in individuals prone to high-altitude pulmonary edema. *Am. J. Respir. Crit. Care. Med.* **172**, 763–7.

Berger, M.M., Rozenval, C.S., Schieber, C. *et al.* (2009) The effect of endothelin-1 on alveolar fluid clearance and pulmonary edema formation in the rat. *Anesth. Analg.* **108**, 225–31.

Berger, M.M., Luks, A.M. and Bailey, D.M. (2011) Transpulmonary plasma catecholamines in acute high-altitude pulmonary hypertension. *Wilderness Environ. Med.* **22**, 37–45.

Bergeron, M., Gidday, J.M., Yu, A.Y. *et al.* (2000) Role of hypoxia-inducible factor-1 in hypoxia-induced ischemic tolerance in neonatal rat brain. *Ann. Neurol.* **48**, 285–96.

Berlin, N.I., Reynafarje, C. and Lawrence, J.H. (1954) Red cell life span in the polycythemia of high altitude. *J. Appl. Physiol.* **7**, 271–2.

Bernardi, L., Road, R.C., Keyl, C. *et al.* (2003) Ventilation, autonomic function, sleep and erythropoietin. Chronic mountain sickness of Andean natives. *Ad. Exper. Med. Biol.* **543**, 161–75.

Bernardi, L., Schneider, A. and Pomidori, L. (2006) Hypoxic ventilatory response in successful extreme altitude climbers. *Eur. Respir. J.* **27**, 165–171.

Bernaudin, M., Nedelec, A.S., Divoux, D. *et al.* (2002) Normobaric hypoxia induces tolerance to focal permanent cerebral ischemia in association with an increased expression of hypoxia-inducible factor-1 and its target genes, erythropoietin and VEGF, in the adult mouse brain. *J. Cereb. Blood Flow Metab.* **22**, 393–403.

Berner, G., Froelicher, V.F. and West, J.B. (1988) Trekking in Nepal: safety after coronary artery bypass. *JAMA* **259**, 3184.

Bernhard, W.N., Schalick, I.M., Delaney, P.A. *et al.* (1998) Acetazolamide plus dexamethasone is better than acetazolamide alone to ameliorate symptoms of acute mountain sickness. *Aviat. Space Environ. Med.* **69**, 883–6.

Bernheim, A.M, Kuencke, A., Fischler, M. *et al.* (2007) Acute changes in pulmonary artery pressures due to exercise and exposure to high altitude do not cause left ventricular diastolic dysfunction. *Chest* **132**, 380–7.

Berssenbrugge, A., Dempsey, J., Iber, C. *et al.* (1983) Mechanisms of hypoxia-induced periodic breathing during sleep in humans. *J. Physiol. (Lond.)* **343**, 507–26.

Bert, P. (1878) *La Pression Barométrique.* Masson, Paris. English translation by M.A. Hitchcock and F.A. Hitchcock, College Book Co., Columbus, OH, 1943.

Berthon-Jones, M. and Sullivan, C.E. (1982) Ventilatory and arousal responses to hypoxia in sleeping humans. *Am. Rev. Respir. Dis.* **125**, 632–9.

Bestle, M.H., Olsen, N.V., Poulsen, T.D. *et al.* (2002) Prolonged hypobaric hypoxemia attenuates vasopressin secretion and renal response to osmostimulation in men. *J. Appl. Physiol.* **92**, 1911–22.

Bhaumik, G., Purkayastha, S.S., Selvamurthy, W. and Banerjee, P.K. (2003) Oxygen saturation response to exercise Vo$_2$ at 2100m and 4350m in women mountaineering trainees. *Indian J. Physiol. Pharmacol.* **47**, 43–51.

Bigard, A.X., Douce, P., Merino, D. *et al.* (1996a) Changes in dietary protein fail to prevent decrease in muscle growth induced by severe hypoxia in rats. *J. Appl. Physiol.* **80**, 208–15.

Bigard, A.X., Lavier, P., Ullman, L. *et al.* (1996b) Branched-chain amino acid supplementation during repeated prolonged skiing exercises at altitude. *Int. J. Sport Nutr.* **6**, 295–306.

Bigham, A., Bauchet, M., Pinto, D. *et al.* (2010) Identifying signatures of natural selection in Tibetan and Andean populations using dense genome scan data. *PLoS Genet.* **6**, e1001116.

Billat, V.L., Flechet, B., Petit, B. *et al.* (1999) Interval training at VO$_{2max}$: effects on aerobic performance and over-training markers. *Med. Sci. Sports Exer.* **31**, 156–63.

Bircher, H.P., Eichenberger, U., Maggiorini, M. *et al.* (1994) Relationship of mountain sickness to physical fitness and exercise intensity during ascent. *J. Wilderness Med.* **5**, 302–11.

Birgegard, G. and Sandhagen, B. (2001) Erythropoetin treatment can increase 2,3-diphosphoglycerate levels in red blood cells. *Scand. J. Clin. Lab. Invest.* **61**, 337–40.

Birukova, A.A. Xing, J. and Fu, P. (2010) Atrial natriuretic peptide attenuates LPS-induced lung vascular leak: role of PAK1. *Am. J. Physiol. Lung Physiol.* **299**, L652–63.

Biscoe, T.J. and Duchen, M.R. (1990) Cellular basis of transduction in carotid body chemoreceptors. *Am. J. Physiol.* **258**, L270–8.

Bishop, R.A., Litch, J.A. and Stanton, J.M. (2000) Ketamine anesthesia at high altitude. *High Alt. Med. Biol.* **1**, 111–14.

Bjurstrom, R.L. and Schoene, R.B. (1986) Ventilatory control in elite synchronized swimmers. *Am. Rev. Respir. Dis.* **133** (Suppl.), A134.

Black, C.P. and Tenney, S.M. (1980) Oxygen transport during progressive hypoxia in high-altitude and sea-level waterfowl. *Respir. Physiol.* **39**, 217–39.

Blauw, G.J., Westerterp, R.G., Srivastava, N. *et al.* (1995) Hypoxia induced arterial endothelin does not influence peripheral vascular tone. *J. Cardiol. Pharm.* **3**, S242–3.

Bledsoe, S.W. and Hornbein, T.F. (1981) Central chemosensors and the regulation of their chemical environment, in *Regulation of Breathing, Part I* (ed. T.F. Hornbein), Marcel Dekker, New York, pp. 347–428.

Bligh, J. and Chauca, D. (1978) The effects of intracerebroventricular injections of carbachol and noradrenaline in cold induced pulmonary artery hypertension in sheep. *J. Physiol.* **284**, 53P.

Bligh, J. and Chauca, D. (1982) Effects of hypoxia, cold exposure and fever on pulmonary artery pressure and their significance for Arctic residents, in *Circum Polar Health 1981* (eds. B. Harvald and J.B. Hart Hansen), Report **32**, Nordic Council for Arctic Medical Research, Copenhagen, pp. 606–7.

Bloch, K.E., Turk, A.J., Maggiorini, M. *et al.* (2009) Effect of ascent protocol on acute mountain sickness and success at Muztagh Ata, 7546 m. *High Alt. Med. Biol.* **10**, 25–32.

Bloch, K.E., Latshang, T.D., Turk, A.J. *et al.* (2010) Nocturnal periodic breathing during acclimatization at very high altitude at Mount Muztagh Ata (7,546 m). *Am. J. Respir. Crit. Care Med.* **182**, 562–8.

Blows from the winter wind (editorial) (1980) *BMJ* **1**, 137–8.

Blume, F.D. (1984) Metabolic and endocrine changes at altitude, in *High Altitude and Man* (eds. J.B. West and S. Lahiri), American Physiological Society, Bethesda, MD, pp. 37–45.

Blume, F.D. and Pace, N. (1967) Effect of translocation to 3800m altitude on glycolysis in mice. *J. Appl. Physiol.* **23**, 75–9.

Blume, F.D. and Pace, N. (1971) The utilisation of ^{14}C-labelled palmitic acid, alanine and aspartic acid at high altitude. *Environ. Physiol.* **1**, 30–6.

Blume, F.D., Boyer, S.J., Braverman, L.E. and Cohen, A. (1984) Impaired osmoregulation at high altitude. *JAMA* **252**, 524–6.

Bocqueraz, O., Koulmann, N., Guigas, B. *et al.* (2004) Fluid-regulatory hormone responses during cycling exercise in acute hypobaric hypoxia. *Med. Sci. Sports Exerc.* **36**, 1730–6.

Bodary, P.F., Pate, R.R., Wu, Q.F. and McMillan, G.S. (1999) Effects of acute exercise on plasma erythropoietin levels in trained runners. *Med. Sci. Sports Exerc.* **31**, 543–6.

Boero, J.A., Ascher, J., Arregui, A. *et al.* (1999) Increased brain capillaries in chronic hypoxia. *J. Appl. Physiol.* **86**, 1211–19.

Boes, D.A., Omura, A.K. and Hennessy, M.J. (2001) Effect of high-altitude exposure on myopic laser *in situ* keratomileusis. *J. Cataract Refract. Surg.* **27**, 1937–41.

Bogaard, H.J., Hopkins, S.R., Yamaya, Y. *et al.* (2002) Role of the autonomic nervous system in the reduced maximal cardiac output at altitude. *J. Appl. Physiol.* **93**, 271–9.

Bohn, D.J. (1987) Treatment of hypothermia in hospital, in *Hypothermia and Cold* (eds. J.R. Sutton, C.S. Houston and G. Coates), Prager, New York, pp. 286–305.

Bohr, C. (1885) *Experimentale Untersuchungen über die Sauerstoffaufnahme des Blutfarbstoffes*, O.C. Olsen, Copenhagen.

Bohr, C. (1891) Über die Lungenatmung. *Skand. Arch. Physiol.* **2**, 236–68. English translation in *Translations in Respiratory Physiology* (ed. J.B. West), Hutchinson Ross, Stroudsburg, PA, 1981.

Bohr, C. (1909) Über die spezifische Tätigkeit der Lungen bei der respiratorischen Gasaufnahmne und ihr Verhalten zu der durch die Alveolarwand stattfindenden Gasdiffusion. *Skand. Arch. Physiol.* **22**, 221–80. English translation in *Translations in Respiratory Physiology* (ed. J.B. West), Hutchinson Ross, Stroudsburg, PA, 1981.

Bohr, C., Hasselbalch, C.B.K. and Krogh, A. (1904) Ueber einen in biologischer Beziehung wichtigen Einfluss, den die Kohlensäurespannuny des Blutes auf dessen Sauerstoffbinding übt. *Skand. Arch. Physiol.* **16**, 402–12.

Bolay, H. and Rapoport, A. (2011) Does low atmospheric pressure independently trigger migraine? *Headache.* **51**, 1355–459.

Bonasoni, P., Laj, P., Angelini, F. *et al.* (2008) The ABC-Pyramid Atmospheric Research Observatory in Himalaya for aerosol, ozone and halocarbon measurements. *Sci. Total Environ.* **391**, 252–61.

Bonelli, J., Waldhausl, W., Magometschnigg, D. *et al.* (1977) Effect of exercise and of prolonged administration of propranolol on haemodynamic variables, plasma renin concentration, plasma aldosterone and c-AMP. *Eur. J. Clin. Invest.* **7**, 337–43.

Boner, A.L., Peroni, D.G., Piacentini, G.L. and Venge, P. (1993) Influence of allergen avoidance at high altitude on serum markers of eosinophil activation in children with allergic asthma. *Clin. Exp. Allergy* **23**, 1021–6.

Boner, A.L., Comis, A., Schiassi, M. *et al.* (1995) Bronchial reactivity in asthmatic children at high and low altitude. Effect of budesonide. *Am. J. Respir. Crit. Care Med.* **151**, 1194–200.

Bonetti, D.L. and Hopkins, W.G. (2009) Sea-level exercise performance following adaptation to hypoxia: a meta-analysis. *Sports Med.* **39**, 107–27.

Bonvalot, G. (1891) *Across Thibet,* Cassell, London.

Borel, C.O., Guy, J., Barcik, U. *et al.* (1998) Effect of hypobaria on ventilatory and CO_2 responses to short-term hypoxic exposure in cats. *Respir. Physiol.* **111**, 45–53.

Borgström, L., Johannsson, H. and Siesjö, B.K. (1975) The relationship between arterial P_{O2} and cerebral blood flow in hypoxic hypoxia. *Acta Physiol. Scand.* **93**, 423–32.

Bosch, M.M., Barthelmes, D., Merz, T.M. *et al.* (2008) High incidence of optic disc swelling at very high altitudes. *Arch. Ophthalmol.* **126**, 644–50.

Bosch, M.M., Barthelmes, D., Merz, T.M. *et al.* (2010) New insights into changes in corneal thickness in healthy mountaineers during a very-high-altitude climb to Mount Muztagh Ata. *Arch. Ophthalmol.* **128**, 184–9.

Bouchama, A. and De Vol, E.B. (2001) Acid–base alterations in heatstroke. *Intensive Care Med.* **27**, 680–5.

Bouchama, A. and Knochel, J.P. (2002) Medical progress: heat stroke. *New Engl. J. Med.* **346**, 1978–88.

Bouissou, P., Peronnet, F., Brisson, C. *et al.* (1986) Metabolic and endocrine responses to graded exercise under acute hypoxia. *Eur. J. Appl. Physiol.* **55**, 290–4.

Bouissou, P., Guezennec, C.Y., Galen, F.X. *et al.* (1988) Dissociated response of aldosterone from plasma renin activity during prolonged exercise under hypoxia. *Horm. Metab. Res.* **20**, 517–21.

Bouissou, P., Richalet, J.-P., Galen, F.X. *et al.* (1989) Effect of β-adrenoreceptor blockade on renin–aldosterone and σ-ANF during exercise at altitude. *J. Appl. Physiol.* **67**, 141–6.

Boulos, P., Kouroukis, C. and Blake, G. (1999) Superior sagittal sinus thrombosis occurring at high altitude associated with protein C deficiency. *Acta Haematol.* **102**, 104–6.

Boussuges, A., Molenat, F., Burnet, H. *et al.* (2000) Operation Everest III (Comex '97): modifications of cardiac function secondary to altitude-induced hypoxia – An echocardiographic and Doppler study. *Am. J. Resp. Crit. Care Med.* **161**, 264–70.

Boutellier, U., Howald, H., di Prampero, P.E. *et al.* (1983) Human muscle adaptations to chronic hypoxia. *Prog. Clin. Biol. Res.* **136**, 273–85.

Boycott, A.E. and Haldane, J.S. (1908) The effects of low atmospheric pressures on respiration. *J. Physiol. (Lond.)* **37**, 355–77.

Boyer, S.J. (1978) Endurance test on Colorado's 14,000 ft peaks. *Summit Magazine* **24**, 30–5.

Boyer, S.J. and Blume, F.D. (1984) Weight loss and changes in body composition at high altitude. *J. Appl. Physiol.* **57**, 1580–5.

Boyle, R. (1660) *New Experiments Physico-Mechanicall, Touching the Spring of the Air, and its Effects.* H. Hall for Tho. Robinson, Oxford.

Boyle, R. (1662) *New Experiments Physico-Mechanical, Touching the Air: Whereunto is Added a Defence of the Authors Explication of the Experiments, Against the Objections of Franciscus Linus, and, Thomas Hobbes.* H. Hall for T. Robinson, Oxford. Relevant pages reprinted in *High Altitude Physiology* (ed. J.B. West), Hutchinson Ross, Stroudsburg, PA, 1981.

Bozzini, C.E., Barcelo, A.C., Conti, M.C. *et al.* (2005) Enhanced erythropoietin production during hypobaric hypoxia in mice under treatments to keep the erythrocyte mass from rising: implication for the adaptive role for polycythemia. *High Alt. Med. Biol.* **6**, 238–46.

Bradwell, A.R., Dykes, P.W., Coote, J.H. *et al.* (1986) Effect of acetazolamide on exercise performance and muscle mass at high altitude. *Lancet* **1**, 1001–5.

Brasher, C. (1986) Wizard of the peaks. *Observer* (London) 29 June.

Brasher, C. (1988) Ascent of superman. *Observer* (London) 26 June.

Braun, B. (1997) Substrate Utilization During Rest and Exercise at High Altitude, in *Women at Altitude* (eds. C.S. Houston and G. Coates), Queen City Printers, Burlington, VT, pp. 20–34.

Braun, B., Butterfield, G.E., Dominick, S.B. *et al.* (1998) Women at altitude: changes in carbohydrate metabolism at 4,300m elevation and across the menstrual cycle. *J. Appl. Physiol.* **85**, 1966–73.

Braun, B., Mawson, J.T., Muza, S.R. *et al.* (2000) Women at altitude: carbohydrate utilization during exercise at 4300m. *J. Appl. Physiol.* **88**, 246–56.

Braun, B., Rock, P.B., Zamudio, S. *et al.* (2001) Women at altitude: Short-term exposure to hypoxia and/or alpha1-adrenergic blockade reduces insulin sensitivity. *J. Appl. Physiol.* **91**, 623–31.

Braun, P. (1985) Pathophysiology and treatment of hypothermia, in *High Altitude Deterioration* (eds. J. Rivolier, P. Cerretelli, J. Foray and P. Segantini), Karger, Basel, pp. 140–8.

Breen, E.C., Johnson, E.C., Wagner, H. *et al.* (1996) Angiogenic growth factor mRNA responses in muscle to a single bout of exercise. *J. Appl. Physiol.* **81**, 355–61.

Brendel, W. (1956) Anpassung von Atmung, Hämoglobin, Körpertemperatur und Kreislauf bei langfristigem Aufenthalt in grossen Höhen (Himalaya). *Pflügers Arch.* **263**, 227–52.

Brennan, P.J., Greenberg, G., Miall, W.E. and Thompson, S.G. (1982) Seasonal variation in arterial blood pressure. *BMJ* **2**, 919–23.

Brenner, I.K.M., Castellani, J.W., Gabaree, C. *et al.* (1999) Immune changes in humans during cold exposure: effects of prior heating and exercise. *J. Appl. Physiol.* **87**, 699–710.

Brent, P. (1974) *Captain Scott and the Antarctic Tragedy,* Weidenfeld and Nicolson, London.

Brinchmann-Hansen, O. and Myhre, K. (1989) Blood pressure, intraocular pressure, and retinal vessels after high altitude mountain exposure. *Aviat. Space Environ. Med.* **60**, 970–6.

Brito, J., Siques, P., Leon-Velard, F. *et al.* (2007) Chronic intermittent hypoxia at high altitude exposure for over 12 years: assessment of hematological, cardiovascular, and renal effects. *High Alt. Med. Biol.* **8**, 236–44.

Brodal, P., Ingjer, F. and Hermansen, L. (1977) Capillary supply of skeletal muscle fibers in untrained and endurance-trained men. *Am. J. Physiol.* **232**, H705–12.

Brookhart, M.A., Schneeweiss, S., Avorn, J. *et al.* (2008) The effect of altitude on dosing and response to erythropoietin in ESRD. *J. Am. Soc. Nephrol.* **19**, 1389–95.

Brooks, G.A., Butterfield, G.E., Wolfe, R.R. *et al.* (1991) Increased dependence on blood glucose after acclimatization to 4300 m. *J. Appl. Physiol.* **70**, 919–27.

Brooks, G.A., Wolfel, E.E., Butterfield, G.E. *et al.* (1998) Poor relationship between arterial [lactate] and leg net release during exercise at 4,300m altitude. *Am. J. Physiol.* **275**, R1192–201.

Broom, J.R., Stoneham, M.D., Beeley, J.M. *et al.* (1994) High altitude headache: treatment with ibuprofen. *Aviat. Space Environ. Med.* **65**, 19–20.

Brown, J.M. and Page, J. (1952) The effect of chronic exposure to cold or temperature and blood flow of the hands. *J. Appl. Physiol.* **5**, 221–7.

Bruce, C.G. (1923) *The Assault on Mt. Everest,* E. Arnold & Co., London.

Brunt, D. (1952) *Physical and Dynamical Meteorology,* 2nd edn, Cambridge University Press, Cambridge, p. 379.

Brutsaert, T.D., Parra, E.J., Shriver, M.D. *et al.* (2003) Spanish genetic admixture is associated with larger V(O2) max decrement from sea level to 4338m in Peruvian Quechua. *J. Appl. Physiol.* **95**, 519–28.

Bucuk, M., Tomic, Z., Tuskan-Mohar, L. *et al.* (2008) Recurrent transient global amnesia at high altitude. *High Alt. Med. Biol.* **9**, 239–40.

Budd, G.M. (1984) Daily fluid balance. International Biomedical Expedition to the Antarctic. *6th International Symposium on Circum Polar Health,* Anchorage, May 1984, pp. 59–60.

Buettner, K.J.K. (1969) The effect of natural sunlight on human skin, in *The Biologic Effects of Ultraviolet Radiation, with Special Emphasis on the Skin* (ed. F. Urbach), Pergamon Press, Oxford, pp. 237–49.

Buguet, A.G.C., Livingstone, S.D. and Reed, L.D. (1979) Skin temperature changes in paradoxical sleep in man in the cold. *Aviat. Space Environ. Med.* **50**, 567–70.

Buick, F., Gledhill, N., Froese, A. *et al.* (1980) Effects of induced erythrocythemia on aerobic work capacity. *J. Appl. Physiol.* **48**, 636–42.

Bulow, K. (1963) Respiration and wakefulness in man. *Acta Physiol. Scand.* **59** (Suppl. 209), 1–110.

Burch, G.E. (1945) Rate of water loss from the respiratory tract of normal subjects in a subtropical climate. *Arch. Int. Med.* **76**, 315–27.

Burchell, H.B., Pruitt, R.D. and Barnes, A.R. (1948) The stress and the electrocardiogram in the induced hypoxemia test for coronary insufficiency. *Am. Heart J.* **36**, 373–89.

Burgess, K.R., Cooper, J., Rice, A. *et al.* (2006) Effect of simulated altitude during sleep on moderate-severity OSA. *Respirology* **11**, 62–9.

Burgess, K.R., Johnson, P.L. and Edwards, N. (2004) Central and obstructive sleep apnoea during ascent to high altitude. *Respirology* **9**, 222–9.

Burgomaster, K.A., Howarth, K.R., Phillips, S.M. *et al.* (2008) Similar metabolic adaptations during exercise after low volume sprint interval and traditional endurance training in humans. *J. Physiol.* **586**: 151–60.

Burgomaster, K.A., Hughes, S.C., Heigenhauser, G.J. *et al.* (2005) Six sessions of sprint interval training increases muscle oxidative potential and cycle endurance capacity in humans. *J. Appl. Physiol.* **98**, 1985–90.

Buroker, N.E., Ning, X.-H., Zhou, Z.-N. *et al.* (2010) Genetic association with mountain sickness in Han and Tibetan residents in the Qinghai-Tibetan plateau. *Clin. Chim. Acta.* **411**, 10–20.

Burr, R.E. (1993) Trench foot. *J. Wilderness Med.* **4**, 348–52.

Burri, P.H. and Weibel, E.R. (1971) Morphometric estimation of pulmonary diffusion capacity. II. Effect of P_{O_2} on the growing lung; adaption of the growing rat lung to hypoxia and hyperoxia. *Respir. Physiol.* **11**, 247–64.

Burton, A.C. and Edholm, O.G. (1955) *Man in a Cold Environment.* Arnold, London.

Burtscher, M., Bachman, O., Hatzl, T. *et al.* (2001) Cardiopulmonary and metabolic responses to healthy elderly humans during a 1 week hiking program at high altitude. *Eur. J. Appl. Physiol.* **84**, 379–86.

Burtscher, M., Brandstätter, E. and Gatterer, H. (2008) Acclimatization in simulated altitudes. *Sleep Breath* **12**, 109–114.

Burtscher, M., Flatz, M. and Faulhaber, M. (2004) Prediction of susceptibility to acute mountain sickness by SaO2 values during short-term exposure to hypoxia. *High Alt. Med. Biol.* **5**, 335–40.

Burtscher, M.B., Likar, R., Nachbauer, W. and Philadelphy, M. (1998) Aspirin for prophylaxis against headache at high altitudes: randomised, double blind, placebo controlled trial. *BMJ* **316**, 1057–8.

Burtscher, M.B., Philadelphy, M., Likar, R. and Nachbauer, W. (1999) Aspirin versus diamox plus aspirin for headache during physical activity at high altitude (abstract), in *Hypoxia: Into the Next Millennium* (eds. R.C. Roach, P.D. Wagner and P.H. Hackett), Plenum/Kluwer, New York, p. 133.

Burtscher, M., Szubski, C. and Faulhaber, M. (2008) Prediction of the susceptibility to AMS in simulated altitude. *Sleep Breath* **12**, 103–8.

Busch, T., Bartsch, P., Pappert, D. *et al.* (2001) Hypoxia decreases exhaled nitric oxide in mountaineers susceptible to high-altitude pulmonary edema. *Am. J. Respir. Crit. Care. Med.* **345**, 107–14.

Buschke, H. (1973) Selective reminding for analysis of memory and learning. *J. Verb. Learn. Verb. Behav.* **13**, 543–50.

Buskirk, E.R. (1977) Temperature regulation with exercise. *Exerc. Sport Sci. Rev.* **5**, 45–88.

Buskirk, E.R. (1978) Work capacity of high-altitude natives, in *The Biology of High Altitude Peoples* (ed. P.T. Baker), Cambridge University Press, Cambridge, pp. 173–87.

Butler, F.K.J. (2007) The eye in the wilderness, *Wilderness Medicine* (ed. P.S. Auerbach), Mosby Elsevier, Philadelphia, pp. 604–24.

Butson, A.R.C. (1949) Acclimatization to cold in Antarctica. *Nature* **163**, 132–3.

Butson, A.R.C. (1975) Effects and prevention of frostbite in wound healing. *Can. J. Surg.* **18**, 145–8.

Butterfield, G.E., Gates, J., Fleming, S. *et al.* (1992) Increased energy intake minimizes weight loss in men at high altitude. *J. Appl. Physiol.* **72**, 1741–8.

Byrne-Quinn, E., Weil, J.V., Sodal, I.E. *et al.* (1971) Ventilatory control in the athlete. *J. Appl. Physiol.* **30**, 91–8.

Cabada, M.M., Maldonado, F., Mozo, K. *et al.* (2010) Pre-travel preparation for Cusco, Peru: a comparison between European and North American travelers. *J. Travel Med.* **17**, 382–6.

Cabanac, M. and LeBlanc, J. (1983) Physiological conflict in humans: fatigue vs. cold discomfort. *Am. J. Physiol.* **244**, R621–8.

Cabrera de Leon, A., Gonzalez, D.A., Mendez, L.I. *et al.* (2004) Leptin and altitude in the cardiovascular diseases. *Obes. Res.* **12**, 1492–8.

Cahoon, R.L. (1972) Simple decision making at high altitude. *Ergonomics* **15**, 157–63.

Cain, S.M. and Dunn, J.E. (1965) Increase of arterial oxygen tension at altitude by carbonic anhydrase inhibition. *J. Appl. Physiol.* **20**, 882–4.

Calbet, J., Radegran, G., Boushel, R. *et al.* (2002) Effect of blood haemoglobin concentration on VO_2max and cardiovascular function in lowlanders acclimatized to 5260 m. *J. Appl. Physiol.* **545**, 715–28.

Calbet, J.A. (2003) Chronic hypoxia increases blood pressure and noradrenalin spillover in healthy subjects. *J. Physiol. (Lond.)* **551**, 379–86.

Calbet, J.A., Radegran, G., Boushel, R. *et al.* (2004) Plasma volume expansion does not increase maximal cardiac ouput or VO_2 max in lowlanders acclimatized to altitude. *Am. J. Physiol Heart Circ. Physiol.* **287**, H1214–24.

Calbet, J.A.L., Radegran, G., Boushel, R. and Saltin, B. (2008a) On the mechanisms that limit oxygen uptake during exercise in acute and chronic hypoxia: role of muscle mass. *J. Physiol.* **587**, 477–90.

Calbet, J.A.L., Robach, P., Lundby, C. and Boushel, R. (2008b) Is pulmonary gas exchange during exercise in hypoxia impaired with an increase in cardiac output? *Appl. Physiol. Nutr. Metab.* **33**, 593–600.

Campbell, R.H.A., Brand, H.L., Cox, J.R. and Howard, P. (1975) Body weight and body water in chronic cor pulmonale. *Clin. Sci. Mol. Med.* **49**, 323–35.

Caplan, C.E. (1999) The big chill: diseases exacerbated by exposure to cold. *Can. Med. Assoc. J.* **160**, 88.

Cargill, R.I., Kiely, D.G., Clark, R.A. and Lipworth, B.J. (1995) Hypoxaemia and release of endothelin-1. *Thorax* **50**, 1308–10.

Carpenter, T.C., Reeves, J.T. and Durmowicz, A.G. (1998) Viral respiratory infection increases susceptibility of young rats to hypoxia-induced pulmonary edema. *J. Appl. Physiol.* **84**, 1048–54.

Carrillo, C. (1996) Pregnancy at high altitude. *Acta Andina* **5**, 67.

Carroll, J.E., Zwillich, C.W. and Weil, J.V. (1977) Ventilatory response in myotonic dystrophy. *Neurology* **27**, 1125–8.

Casa, D.J., McDermott, B.P., Lee, L. *et al.* (2007) Cold water immersion: the gold standard for exertional heatstroke treatment. *Exer. Sports Sci. Rev.* **35**, 141–9.

Cassin, S.R., Gilbert, R.D., Bunnell, C.E. and Johnson, E.M. (1971) Capillary development during exposure to chronic hypoxia. *Am. J. Physiol.* **220**, 448–51.

Castellani, J.W., Young, A.J., Sawka, M.W. *et al.* (1998) Amnesia during cold water immersion. A case report. *Wilderness Environ. Med.* **9**, 153–5.

Castellani, J.W., Young, A.J., Kain, J.E. and Sawka, M.W. (1999a) Thermo regulatory responses to cold water at different times of day. *J. Appl. Physiol.* **87**, 243–6.

Castellani, J.W., Young, A.J., Kain, J.E. *et al.* (1999b) Thermoregulation during cold exposure: effects of prior exercise. *J. Appl. Physiol.* **87**, 247–52.

Castellani, J.W., Muza, S.R., Cheuvront, S.N. *et al.* (2010) Effect of hypohydration and altitude exposure on aerobic exercise performance and acute mountain sickness. *J. Appl. Physiol.* **109**, 1792–800.

Castellini, M.A. and Somero, G.N. (1981) Buffering capacity of vertebrate muscle – correlations with potentials for anaerobic function. *J. Comp. Physiol.* **143**, 191–8.

Castilla, E.E., Lopez-Camelo, J.S. and Campana, H. (1999) Altitude as a risk factor for congenital anomalies. *Am. J. Med. Genet.* **86**, 9–14.

Catron, T.F., Powell, F.L. and West, J.B. (2006) A strategy for determining arterial blood gases on the summit of Mt Everest. *BMC Physiol.* **6**, 3.

Cattermole, T.J. (1999) The epidemiology of cold injury in Antarctica. *Aviat. Space Environ. Med.* **70**, 135–40.

Cauchy, E., Chetaille, E., Marchand, V. and Marsigny, B. (2001) Retrospective study of 70 cases of severe frostbite lesion: a proposed new classification scheme. *Wilderness. Environ. Med.* **12**, 248–55.

Cauchy, E., Chegullaume, B. and Chetalle, E. (2011) A controlled trial of a prostacyclin and rt-PA in the treatment of severe frostbite. *N. Engl. J. Med.* **364**, 189–90.

Cavaletti, G. and Tredici, G. (1993) Long-lasting neuropsychological changes after a single high altitude climb. *Acta Neurol. Scand.* **87**, 103–5.

Cavaletti, G., Moroni, R., Garavaglia, P. and Tredici, G. (1987) Brain damage after high-altitude climbs without oxygen. *Lancet* **1**, 101.

Cerretelli, P. (1976a) Limiting factors to oxygen transport on Mount Everest. *J. Appl. Physiol.* **40**, 658–67.

Cerretelli, P. (1976b) Metabolismo ossidativo ed anaerobico nel soggetto acclimatato all'altitudine. Rilievi sperimentali nel corso della spedizione italiana all'Everest. *Minerva Med.* **67**, 2331–46.

Cerretelli, P. (1980) Gas exchange at high altitude, in *Pulmonary Gas Exchange,* Vol. II (ed. J.B. West), Academic Press, New York, pp. 97–147.

Cerretelli, P. (1987) Extreme hypoxia in air breathers: some problems, in *Comparative Physiology of Environmental Adaptations,* Vol. 2: *Adapatations to Extreme Environments* (ed. P. Dejours), Karger, Basel.

Cerretelli, P. (1992) Energy sources for muscular exercise. *Int. J. Sports Med.* **13**(Suppl. 1), S106–10.

Cerretelli, P. and Hoppeler, H. (1996) Morphologic and metabolic response to chronic hypoxia: the muscle system, in *Handbook of Physiology*, Section 4: *Environmental Physiology*, Vol. II (eds. M.J. Fregly and C.M. Blatteis), American Physiological Society, New York, pp. 1155–81.

Cerretelli, P. and Whipp, B.J. (1980) *Exercise Bioenergetics and Gas Exchange.* Elsevier/North-Holland Biomedical Press, Amsterdam.

Cerretelli, P., Marconi, C., Dériaz, O. and Giezendanner, D. (1984) After effects of chronic hypoxia on cardiac output and muscle blood flow at rest and exercise. *Eur. J. Appl. Physiol.* **53**, 92–6.

Chan, C., Hoar, H., Pattinson, K. *et al.* (2005) Effect of sildenafil and acclimatization on cerebral oxygenation at altitude. *Clin. Sci.* **109**, 319–24.

Chance, B. (1957) Cellular oxygen requirements. *Fed. Proc.* **16**, 671–80.

Chance, B., Cohen, P., Jobsis, F. and Schoener, B. (1962) Intracellular oxidation-reduction states *in vivo. Science* **137**, 499–508.

Chandrashekhar, Y., Anand, I.S., Rao, K.S. and Malhotra, R.M. (1992) Continuous ambulatory electrocardiographic changes after rapid ascent to extreme altitudes. *Indian Heart J.* **44**, 403–5.

Chanutin, A. and Curnish, R.R. (1967) Effect of organic and inorganic phosphates on the oxygen equilibrium of human erythrocytes. *Arch. Biochem. Biophys.* **121**, 96–102.

Chapman, F.S. (1938) *Lhasa. The Holy City,* Chatto and Windus, London, p. 241.

Chapman, J.A., Grant, I.S., Taylor, G. *et al.* (1972) Endemic goitre in the Gilgit Agency, West Pakistan. *Philos. Trans. R. Soc. Lond. Ser. B* **263**, 459–91.

Chapman, K.R. and Cherniack, N.S. (1986) Aging effects on the interaction of hypercapnia and hypoxia as ventilatory stimuli. *Am. Rev. Respir. Dis.* **133**(Suppl. A), 137.

Chapman, R.F., Stray-Gundersen, J. and Levine, B.D. (1998) Individual variation in response to altitude training. *J. Appl. Physiol.* **85**, 1448–56.

Chatterji, J.C., Ohri, V.C., Das, B.K. *et al.* (1982) Platelet count, platelet aggregation and fibrinogen levels following acute induction to high altitude (3200 and 3771 metres). *Thromb. Res.* **26**, 177–82.

Chavez, J.C., Agani, F., Pichiule, P. and LaManna, J.C. (2000) Expression of hypoxia-inducible factor-1alpha in the brain of rats during chronic hypoxia. *J. Appl. Physiol.* **89**, 1937–42.

Chen, Q.H., Ge, R.L., Wang, X.Z. *et al.* (1997) Exercise performance of Tibetan and Han adolescents at altitudes of 3,417 and 4,300 m. *J. Appl. Physiol.* **83**, 661–7.

Chen, Y.C., Wong, L.Z., Mung, Z.H. and Fung, G.Y. (1982) An analysis of 300 cases of high altitude heart disease in adults [in Chinese]. *Zhonghua Xin Xue Guan Bing Za Zhi* **10**, 256–8.

Chen, Y.-F., Feng, J.-A, Li P. *et al.* (2006) Atrial natriuretic peptide-dependent modulation of hypoxia-induced pulmonary vascular remodeling. *Life Sci.* **79**, 1357–65.

Cheng, S., Chng, S.M. and Singh, R. (2009) Cerebral venous infarction during a high altitude expedition. *Sing. Med. J.* **50**, e306–8.

Cherniack, N.S. and Longobardo, G.S. (2006) Mathematical models of periodic breathing and their usefulness in understanding cardiovascular and respiratory disorders. *Exp. Physiol.* **91**, 295–305.

Chernow, B., Lake, C.R., Zaritsky, A. *et al.* (1983) Sympathetic nervous system 'switch off' with severe hypothermia. *Crit. Care Med.* **11**, 677–80.

Chesner, I.M., Small, N.A. and Dykes, P.W. (1987) Intestinal absorption at high altitude. *Postgrad. Med. J.* **63**, 173–5.

Cheyne, J. (1818) A case of apoplexy in which the fleshy part of the heart was converted into fat. *Dublin Hosp. Rep.* **2**, 216–23.

Chiodi, H. (1957) Respiratory adaptations to chronic high altitude hypoxia. *J. Appl. Physiol.* **10**, 81–7.

Choukèr, A., Demetz, F., Martignoni, A. *et al.* (2005) Strenuous physical exercise inhibits granulocyte activation induced by high altitude. *J. Appl. Physiol.* **98**, 640–7.

Chow, T., Browne, V., Heileson, H.L. *et al.* (2005) Ginkgo biloba and acetazolamide prophylaxis for acute mountain sickness: a randomized, placebo-controlled trial. *Arch. Intern. Med.* **165**, 296–301.

Chrenko, F.A. and Pugh, L.G.C.E. (1961) The contribution of solar radiation to the thermal environment of man in Antarctica. *Proc. R. Soc. Lond. Ser. B* **155**, 243–65.

Christensen, C.C., Ryg, M., Refvem, O.K. and Skjonsberg, O.H. (2000) Development of severe hypoxaemia in chronic obstructive pulmonary disease patients at 2,438m (8,000 feet). *Eur. Respir. J.* **15**, 635–9.

Christensen, C.C., Ryg, M.S., Refvem, O.K. and Skjonsberg, O.H. (2002) Effect of hypobaric hypoxia on blood gases in patients with restrictive lung disease. *Eur. Respir. J.* **20**, 300–5.

Christensen, E.H. (1937) Sauerstoffaufnahme und Respiratorische Funktionen in Grossen Höhen. *Skand. Arch. Physiol.* **76**, 88–100.

Christensen, E.H. and Forbes, W.H. (1937) Der Kreislauf in grossen Höhen. *Skand. Arch. Physiol.* **76**, 75–87.

Cibella, F., Cuttitta, G., Romano, S. *et al.* (1999) Respiratory energetics during exercise at high altitude. *J. Appl. Physiol.* **86**, 1785–92.

Clark, C.F., Heaton, R.K. and Wiens, A.N. (1983) Neuropsychological functioning after prolonged high altitude exposure in mountaineering. *Aviat. Space Environ. Med.* **54**, 202–7.

Clark, I.M., Awburn, M.M., Cowden, W.B. and Rockett, K.A. (1999) Can excessive iNOS induction explain much of the illness of acute mountain sickness, in *Hypoxia: Into the Next Millennium* (eds. R.C. Roach, P.D. Wagner and P.H. Hackett), Plenum/Kluwer, New York, p. 373.

Clark, R.T., Criscuolo, D. and Coulson, D.K. (1952) Effects of 20,000 feet simulated altitude on myoglobin content of animals with and without exercise. *Fed. Proc.* **11**, 25.

Clarke, C. and Duff, J. (1976) Mountain sickness, retinal haemorrhages, and acclimatization on Mount Everest in 1975. *BMJ* **2**, 495–7.

Claybaugh, J.R., Wade, C.E., Sato, A.K. *et al.* (1982) Antidiuretic hormone responses to eucapnic and hypocapnic hypoxia in humans. *J. Appl. Physiol. Respir. Environ. Exerc. Physiol.* **53**, 815–23.

Claydon, V.E., Norcliffe, L.J., Moore, J.P. *et al.* (2005) Cardiovascular responses to orthostatic stress in healthy altitude dwellers and altitude residents with chronic mountain sickness. *Exper. Physiol.* **90**, 103–10.

Clegg, E.J. (1978) Fertility and early growth, in *The Biology of High Altitude Peoples* (ed. P.T. Baker), Cambridge University Press, Cambridge, pp. 65–115.

Clini, E., Bianchi, L., Foglio, K. *et al.* (2002) Exhaled nitric oxide and exercise tolerance in severe COPD patients. *Respir. Med.* **96**, 312–16.

Cochand, N.J., Wild, M., Brugniaux, J.V. *et al.* (2011) Sea-level assessment of dynamic cerebral autoregulation predicts susceptibility to acute mountain sickness at high altitude. *Stroke* **42**, 3628–30.

Cochrane, G.M., Prior, J.G. and Wolff, C.B. (1980) Chronic stable asthma and the normal arterial pressure of carbon dioxide in hypoxia. *BMJ* **301**, 705–7.

Cogo, A. and Miserocchi, G. (2011) Pro: most climbers develop subclinical pulmonary interstitial edema. *High Alt. Med. Biol.* **12**, 121–4.

Cogo, A., Basnyat, B., Legnani, D. and Allegra, L. (1997) Bronchial asthma and airway hyperresponsiveness at high altitude. *Respiration* **64**, 444–9.

Cogo, A., Fischer, R. and Schoene, R. (2004) Respiratory diseases and high altitude. *High Alt. Med. Biol.* **5**, 435–44.

Cold hypersensitivity (editorial) (1975) *BMJ* **1**, 643–4.

Colice, C.L. and Ramirez, C. (1986) Aldosterone response to angiotensin II during hypoxemia. *J. Appl. Physiol.* **61**, 150–4.

Collier, D., Wolff, C.B., Nathan, J. *et al.* (1997a) Benzolamide, acidosis and acute mountain sickness, in *Hypoxia: women at altitude* (eds. C.S. Houston and G. Coates), Queen City Printers, Burlington, VT, p. 307.

Collier, D.J., Collier, C.J., Dubowitz, G., and Rosenberg, M. (1997b) Gender and weight loss at altitude (abstract), in *Hypoxia: Women at Altitude* (eds. C.S. Houston and G. Coates), Queen City Printers, Burlington, VT, p. 308.

Collier, D.J., Nickol, A.H., Milledge, J.S. *et al.* (2008) Alveolar PCO_2 oscillations and ventilation at sea level and at high altitude. *J. Appl. Physiol.* **104**, 404–15.

Colquohoun, W.P. (1984) Effects of personality on body temperature and mental efficiency following transmeridian flight. *Aviat. Space Environ. Med.* **55**, 493–6.

Comroe, J.H. (1938) The location and function of the chemoreceptors of the aorta. *Am. J. Physiol.* **127**, 176–91.

Conkin, J. and Wessel, J.H. (2008) Critique of the equivalent air altitude model. *Aviat. Space Environ. Med.* **79**, 975–82.

Conley, K.E., Esselman, P.C., Jubrias, S.A. *et al.* (2000) Ageing, muscle properties and maximal O_2 uptake rate in humans. *J. Physiol.* **526**, 211–17.

Connaughton, J.J., Douglas, N.J., Morgan, A.D. *et al.* (1985) Almitrine improves oxygenation when both awake and asleep in patients with hypoxia and carbon dioxide retention caused by chronic bronchitis and emphysema. *Am. Rev. Respir. Dis.* **132**, 206–10.

Consolazio, C.F., Matoush, L.O., Johnson, H.L. and Daws, T.A. (1968) Protein and water balances of young adults during prolonged exposure to high altitude (4300 m). *Am. J. Clin. Nutr.* **21**, 134–61.

Consolazio, C.F., Matoush, L.O., Johnson, H.L. *et al.* (1969) Effects of high carbohydrate diets on performance and clinical symptomatology after rapid ascent to high altitude. *Fed. Proc.* **28**, 937–43.

Consolazio, C.F., Johnson, H.L., Krzywicki, H.J. and Daws, T.A. (1972) Metabolic aspects of acute altitude exposure (4300 m) in adequately nourished humans. *Am. J. Clin. Nutr.* **25**, 23–9.

Cook, J.D., Boy, E., Flowers, C. and Daroca Mdel, C. (2005) The influence of high-altitude living on body iron. *Blood* **106**, 1441–6.

Coppin, E.G., Livingstone, S.P. and Kuehn, L.A. (1978) Effects on hand grip strength due to arm immersion in a 10°C water bath. *Aviat. Space Environ. Med.* **49**, 1319–26.

Cornolo, J., Brugniaux, J.V., Macarlupu, J.L. *et al.* (2005) Autonomic adaptations in Andean trained participants to a 4220-m altitude marathon. *Med. Sci. Sports Exerc.* **37**, 2148–53.

Cosby, R.L., Sophocles, A.M., Durr, J.A. *et al.* (1988) Elevated plasma atrial natriuretic factor and vasopressin in high-altitude pulmonary edema. *Ann. Intern. Med.* **109**, 796–9.

Costello, M.L., Mathieu-Costello, O. and West, J.B. (1992) Stress failure of alveolar epithelial cells studied by scanning electron microscopy. *Am. Rev. Respir. Dis.* **145**, 1446–55.

Costil, D.L., Coyle, E., Dalsky, G. *et al.* (1977) Effect of elevated plasma FFA and insulin on muscle glycogen usage during exercise. *J. Appl. Physiol.* **43**, 695–9.

Cotes, J.E. (1954) Ventilatory capacity at altitude and its relation to mask design. *Proc. R. Soc. (Lond). Ser. B* **143**, 32–9.

Coward, W.A. (1991) Measurement of energy expenditure: the doubly labelled water method in clinical practice. *Proc. Nutr. Soc.* **50**, 227–37.

Coyle, E.F. (2005) Improved muscle efficiency displayed as Tour de France champion matures. *J. Appl. Physiol.* **98**, 2191–6.

Coyle, E.F., Coggan, A.R., Hopper, M.K. *et al.* (1988) Determinants of endurance in well-trained cyclists. *J. Appl. Physiol.* **64**, 2622–30.

Coyle, E.F., Sidossis, L.S., Horowitz, J.F. *et al.* (1992) Cycling efficiency is related to type 1 muscle fibers. *Med. Sci. Sports Exer.* **24**, 782–8.

Crait, J.R., Prange, H.D., Marshall, N.A. *et al.* (2012) High-altitude diving in river otters: coping with combined hypoxic stresses. *J. Exp. Biol.* **215**, 256–63.

Crawford, J.P. (1979) Endogenous anxiety and circadian rhythms. *BMJ* **1**, 662.

Crawford, R.D. and Severinghaus, J.W. (1978) CSF pH and ventilatory acclimatization to altitude. *J. Appl. Physiol.* **44**, 274–83.

Cremona, G., Asnaghi, R., Baderna, P. *et al.* (2002) Pulmonary extravascular fluid accumulation in recreational climbers: a prospective study. *Lancet* **359**, 303–9.

Crognier, E., Villena, M. and Vargas, E. (2002) Reproduction in high altitude Aymara: physiological stress and fertility planning? *J. Biosoc. Sci.* **34**, 463–73.

Cruden, N.L.M., Newby, D.E., Ross, J.A. *et al.* (1998) Effect of high altitude, cold and exercise on plasma endothelin-1 and markers of endothelial function in man. *Clin. Sci.* **94**, 20.

Cruden, N.L.M., Newby, D.E., Ross, J.A. *et al.* (1999) Effect of cold exposure, exercise and high altitude on plasma endothelin-1 and endothelial cell markers in man. *Scott. Med. J.* **44**, 143–6.

Cruz, J.C., Diaz, C., Marticorena, E. and Hilario, V. (1979) Phlebotomy improves pulmonary gas exchange in chronic mountain polycythemia. *Respiration* **38**, 305–13.

Cruz, J.C., Reeves, J.T., Grover, R.F. *et al.* (1980) Ventilatory acclimatization to high altitude is prevented by CO_2 breathing. *Respiration* **39**, 121–30.

Cudaback, D.M. (1984) Four-km altitude effects on performance and health. *Publ. Astronom. Soc. Pacif.* **96**, 463–77.

Cummings, P. and Lysgaard, M. (1981) Cardiac arrhythmia at high altitude. *West. J. Med.* **135**, 66–8.

Cunningham, D.J.C., Cormack, R.S., O'Riordan, J.L.H. *et al.* (1957) Arrangement for studying the respiratory effect in man of various factors. *Q. J. Exp. Physiol.* **42**, 294–303.

Cunningham, D.J.C., Patrick, J.M. and Lloyd, B.B. (1964) The respiratory response of man to hypoxia, in *Oxygen in the Animal Organism* (eds. F. Dickens and E. Niel), Pergamon, Oxford, pp. 277–93.

Cunningham, W.L., Becker, E.J. and Kreuzer, F. (1965) Catecholamine in plasma and urine at high altitude. *J. Appl. Physiol.* **20**, 607–10.

Curran, L.S., Zhuang, J., Droma, T. and Moore, L.G. (1998) Superior exercise performance in lifelong Tibetan residents of 4,400 m compared with Tibetan residents of 3,658 m. *Am. J. Phys. Anthropol.* **105**, 21–31.

Curran, L.S., Zhuang, J., Droma, T. *et al.* (1995) Hypoxic ventilatory response in Tibetan residents of 4400 m compared with 3658 m. *Respir. Physiol.* **100**, 223–30.

Curran, L.S., Zhuang, J., Sun, S.F. and Moore, L.G. (1997) Ventilation and hypoxic ventilatory responsiveness in Chinese-Tibetan residents at 3,658 m. *J. Appl. Physiol.* **83**, 2098–104.

Dagg, K.D., Thomson, L.J, Clayton, R.A. *et al.* (1997) Effect of acute alterations in inspired oxygen tension on methacholine induced bronchoconstriction. *Thorax* **52**, 453–7.

Dagg, K.D., Thomson, L.J., Clayton, R.A. *et al.* (1997) Effect of acute alterations in inspired oxygen tension on methacholine induced bronchoconstriction in patients with asthma. *Thorax* **52**, 453–7.

Dang, S., Yan, H., Yamamoto, S. *et al.* (2004) Poor nutritional status of younger Tibetan children living at high altitudes. *Eur. J. Clin. Nutr.* **58**, 938–46.

Daniels, J. and Oldridge, N. (1970) The effects of alternate exposure to altitude and sea level on world class middle distance runners. *Med. Sci. Sports Exerc.* **2**, 107–112.

Danzl, D.F., Pozos, R.S. and Hamlet, M.P. (1995) Accidental hypothermia, in *Wilderness Medicine* (ed. P.S. Auerbach), Mosby, St Louis, MO, pp. 51–103.

Das, B.K., Tewari, S.C., Parashar, S.K. *et al.* (1983) Electrocardiographic changes at high altitude. *Indian Heart J.* **35**, 30–3.

Datta, A.K. and Nickol, A. (1995) Dynamic chemoreceptiveness studied in man during moderate exercise breath by breath, in *Modeling and Control of Ventilation* (eds. S.J.G. Semple, L. Adams, and B.J. Whipp), Plenum Press, New York, pp. 235–8.

Davies, A.J., Kalson, N.S., Stokes, S. *et al.* (2009) Determinants of summiting success and acute mountain sickness on Mt Kilimanjaro (5895 m). *Wilderness Environ. Med.* **20**, 311–17.

Davies, R.O., Edwards, M.W. Jr and Lahiri, S. (1982) Halothane depresses the response of carotid body chemoreceptors to hypoxia and hypercapnia in the cat. *Anesthesiology* **57**, 153–9.

Davis, H.A. and Gass, G.C. (1979) Blood lactate concentration during incremental work before and after maximal exercise. *Br. J. Sports Med.* **13**, 165–9.

Dawson, A. (1972) Regional lung function during early acclimatization to 3,100m altitude. *J. Appl. Physiol.* **33**, 218–23.

De Angelis, C., Ferri, C., Urbani, L. and Ferrace, S. (1996) Effect of acute exposure to hypoxia on electrolyes and water metabolism regulatory hormones. *Aviat. Space Environ. Med.* **67**, 746–50.

de Bisschop, C., Martinot, J.-B., Leurquin-Sterk, G. *et al.* (2012) Improvement in lung diffusion by endothelin A receptor blockade at high altitude. *J. Appl. Physiol.* **112**, 20–5.

De Filippi, F. (1912) *Karakoram and Western Himalaya, 1900*, Constable, London.

De Glinsezinski, J., Crampes, F., Harant, I., *et al.* (1999) Decrease in subcutaneous adipose tissue lipolysis after exposure to hypoxia during a simulated ascent of Mt Everest. *Eur. J. Physiol.* **439**, 134–40.

De Jong, G.F. (ed.) (1968) *Demography of High Altitude Populations*, WHO/PAHO/ IBP Meeting of Investigators on Population Biology of Altitude, Pan American Health Organization, WashingtonDC.

de Meer, K., Heymans, H.S. and Zijlstra, W.G. (1995) Physical adaptation of children to life at high altitude. *Eur. J. Ped.* **154**, 263–72.

de Mol, P., Krabbe, H.G., de Vries, S.T. *et al.* (2010) Accuracy of handheld blood glucose meters at high altitude. *PLoS One* **5**, e15485.

de Mol, P., de Vries, S.T., de Koning, E.J. *et al.* (2011) Increased insulin requirements during exercise at very high altitude in type 1 diabetes. *Diabetes Care* **34**, 591–5.

De Pay, A.W. (1982) Medical treatment of hypothermic victims, in *Unterkuhlung im Seenotfall,* 2nd Symposium Deutsche Gesellschaft zur Rettung Schiffbruchiger (eds. P. Koch and M. Kohfahl), Cuxhaven, Germany pp. 146–53.

de Saussure, H.-B. (1786–7) *Voyages Dans Les Alpes*, 4 volumes, Barde, Manget, Geneva.

de Vries, S.T., Kleijn, S.A., van't Hof, A.W. *et al.* (2010) Impact of high altitude on echocardiographically determined cardiac morphology and function in patients with coronary artery disease and healthy controls. *Eur. J. Echocardiogr.* **11**, 446–50.

Debevec, T., Amon, M., Keramidas, M.E. *et al.* (2010) Normoxic and hypoxic performance following four weeks of normobaric hypoxic training. *Aviat. Space Environ. Med.* **81**, 387–93.

Decramer, M., De Benedetto, F., Del Ponte, A. and Marinari, S. (2005) Systemic effects of COPD. *Respir. Med.* **99**(Suppl. B), S3–10.

Deem, S., Hedges, R.G., Kerr, M.E. and Swenson, E.R. (2000) Acetazolamide reduces hypoxic pulmonary vasoconstriction in isolated perfused rabbit lungs. *Respir. Physiol.* **123**, 109–19.

DeGraff, A.C., Jr, Grover, R.F., Johnson, R.L., Jr *et al.* (1970) Diffusing capacity of the lung in Caucasians native to 3,100 m. *J. Appl. Physiol.* **29**, 71–6.

Dehnert, C. and Bärtsch, P. (2010) Can patients with coronary heart disease go to high altitude? *High Alt. Med. Biol.* **11**, 183–8.

Dehnert, C., Weymann, J., Montgomery, H.E. *et al.* (2002a) No association between high-altitude tolerance and the ACE I/D gene polymorphism. *Med. Sci. Sports. Exerc.* **34**, 1928–33.

Dehnert, C., Hutler, M., Liu, Y. *et al.* (2002b) Erythropoiesis and performance after two weeks of living high and training low in well trained triathletes. *Int. J. Sports Med.* **23**, 561–6.

Dehnert, C., Grünig, E., Mereles, D. *et al.* (2005) Identification of individuals susceptible to high-altitude pulmonary oedema at low altitude. *Eur. Resp. J.* **25**, 545–51.

Dehnert, C., Berger, M.M., Maibaurl, H. and Bärtsch, P. (2007) High altitude pulmonary edema: a pressure-induced leak. *Respir. Physiol. Neurobiol.* **158**, 266–73.

Dehnert, C., Luks, A.M., Schendler, G. *et al.* (2010) No evidence for interstitial lung edema by extensive pulmonary function testing at 4559 meters. *Eur. Respir. J.* **35**, 812–20.

Dejours, P., Girard, F., Labrousse, Y. and Teillac, A. (1959) Etude de al régulation de la ventilation de repos chez l'homme en haute altitude. *Rev. Franc. Etudes Clin. et Biol.* **4**, 115–27.

Dellasanta, P., Gaillard, S., Loutan, L. and Kayser, B. (2007) Comparing questionnaires for the assessment of acute mountain sickness. *High Alt. Med. Biol.* **8**, 184–91.

Dempsey, J.A. (1983) Ventilatory regulation in hypoxic sleep: introduction, in *Hypoxia, Exercise, and Altitude* (eds. J.R. Sutton, C.S. Houston and N.L. Jones), Liss, New York, pp. 61–3.

Dempsey, J.A. and Forster, H.V. (1982) Mediation of ventilatory adaptations. *Physiol. Rev.* **62**, 262–346.

Dempsey, J.A., Reddan, W.G., Birnbaum, M.L. *et al.* (1971) Effects of acute through life-long hypoxic exposure on exercise pulmonary gas exchange. *Respir. Physiol.* **13**, 62–89.

Dempsey, J.A., Forster, H.V., Chosy, L.W. *et al.* (1978) Regulation of CSF [$HCO_3{}^2$] during long-term hypoxic hypocapnia in man. *J. Appl. Physiol.* **44**, 175–82.

Dempsey, J.A., Forster, H.V., Bisgard, G.E. *et al.* (1979) Role of cerebrospinal fluid [H^1] in ventilatory deacclimatization from chronic hypoxia. *J. Clin. Invest.* **64**, 199–204.

Dempsey, J.A., Veasey, S.C., Morgan, B.J. and O'Donnell C.P. (2010) Pathophysiology of sleep apnea. *Physiol. Rev.* **90**, 47–112.

Denison, D.M., Ledwith, F. and Poulton, E.C. (1966) Complex reaction times at simulated cabin altitudes of 5,000 feet and 8,000 feet. *Aerosp. Med.* **37**, 1010–13.

Denjean, A., Roux, C., Herve, P. *et al.* (1988) Mild isocapnic hypoxia enhances the bronchial response to methacholine in asthmatic subjects. *Am. Rev. Respir. Dis.* **138**, 789–93.

Desideri, L. (1712–27) Journey across the great desert of Nguari Giongar, and assistance rendered by a Tartar princess and her followers, in *An Account of Tibet* (ed. F. de Filippi), Routledge, London, 1932, p. 87.

Desplanches, D., Hoppeler, H., Linossier, M.T. *et al.* (1993) Effects of training in normoxia and normobaric hypoxia on human muscle structure. *Pflügers Arch.* **425**, 263–7.

Dickinson, J., Heath, D., Gosney, J. and Williams, D. (1983) Altitude-related deaths in seven trekkers in the Himalayas. *Thorax* **38**, 646–56.

Dickinson, J.G. (1979) Severe acute mountain sickness. *Postgrad. Med. J.* **55**, 454–8.

Dickinson, J.G. (1982) Terminology and classification of acute mountain sickness. *BMJ* **285**, 720–1.

Diffey, B.L. (1991) Solar ultraviolet radiation effects on biological systems. *Phys. Med. Biol.* **36**, 299–328.

Dill, D.B., Edwards, H.T., Fölling, A. *et al.* (1931) Adaptations of the organism to changes in oxygen pressure. *J. Physiol. (Lond.)* **71**, 47–63.

Dill, D.B., Talbott, J.H. and Consolazio, W.V. (1937) Blood as a physiochemical system. XII. Man at high altitudes. *J. Biol. Chem.* **118**, 649–66.

Dill, D.B., Robinson, S., Balke, B. and Newton, J.L. (1964) Work tolerance: age and altitude. *J. Appl. Physiol.* **19**, 483–8.

Dillard, T.A. and Ewald Jr, F.W. (2004) The use of pulmonary function testing in piloting, air travel, mountain climbing, and diving. *Clin. Chest Med.* **22**, 795–816.

Dillard, T.A., Berg, B.W., Rajagopal, K.R. *et al.* (1989) Hypoxemia during air travel in patients with chronic obstructive pulmonary disease. *Ann. Intern. Med.* **111**, 362–7.

Dillard, T.A., Beninati, W.A. and Berg, B.W. (1991) Air travel in patients with chronic obstructive pulmonary disease. *Arch. Intern. Med.* **151**, 1793–5.

Dillard, T.A., Rosenberg, A.P. and Berg, B.W. (1993) Hypoxemia during altitude exposure. A meta-analysis of chronic obstructive pulmonary disease. *Chest* **103**, 422–5.

Dillard, T.A., Rajagopal, K.R., Slivka, W.A. *et al.* (1998) Lung function during moderate hypobaric hypoxia in normal subjects and patients with chronic obstructive pulmonary disease. *Aviat. Space Environ. Med.* **69**, 979–85.

Dillard, T.A., Khosla, S., Ewald, F.W. Jr and Kaleem, M.A. (2005) Pulmonary function testing and extreme environments. *Clin. Chest Med.* (S. Ruoss and R.B. Schoene, eds.) **26**, 485–507.

Dimmig, J.W. and Tabin, G. (2003) The ascent of Mount Everest following laser *in situ* keratomileusis. *J. Refract. Surg.* **19**, 48–51.

Dine, C.J. and Kreider, M.E. (2008) Hypoxia altitude simulation test. *Chest* **133**, 1002–5.

Dinmore, A.J., Edwards, J.S.A., Menzies, I.S. and Travis, S.P.L. (1994) Intestinal carbohydrate absorption and permeability at high altitude (5730m). *J. Appl. Physiol.* **76**, 1903–7.

Dombret, M.C., Rouby, J.J., Smeijan, J.M. *et al.* (1987) Pulmonary oedema during pulmonary embolism. *Br. J. Dis. Chest* **81**, 407–10.

Donaldson, G.C., Tchernjavski, V.E., Ermakov, S.P. *et al.* (1998a) Winter mortality and cold stress in Yekaterinburg, Russia: interview survey. *BMJ* **316**, 514–18.

Donaldson, G.C., Ermakov, S.P., Komarov, Y. *et al.* (1998b) Cold related mortalities and protection against cold in Yakutsk, eastern Siberia: observation and interview study. *BMJ* **317**, 978–82.

Donayre, J., Guerra-Garcia, R., Moncloa, F. and Sobrevilla, L.A. (2003) Endocrine studies at high altitude. *J. Reprod. Fertil.* **16**, 55–8.

Donnelly, D.F. and Carroll, J.L. (2005) Mitochondrial function and carotid body transduction. *High Alt. Med. Biol.* **6**, 121–32.

Donnelly, J., Cowan, D.C., Yeoman, D.J. *et al.*(2011) Exhaled nitric oxide and pulmonary artery pressures during graded ascent to high altitude. *Respir. Physiol. Neurobiol.* **177**, 213–17.

Dor, Y., Porat, R. and Keshet, E. (2001) Vascular endothelial growth factor and vascular adjustments to perturbations in oxygen homeostasis. *Am. J. Physiol. Cell Physiol.* **280**, C1367–74.

Doria, C., Toniolo, L., Verratti, V *et al.* (2011) Improved VO2 uptake kinetics and shift in muscle fiber type in high altitude trekkers. *J. Appl. Physiol.* **111**, 1597–605.

Dosman, J.A., Hodgson, W.C. and Cockcroft, D.W. (1991) Effect of cold air on the bronchial response to inhaled histamine in patients with asthma. *Am. Rev. Respir. Dis.* **144**, 45–50.

Doughty, H.A. and Beardmore, C. (1994) Bleeding time at altitude. *J. R. Soc. Med.* **87**, 317–19.

Douglas, C.G. and Haldane, J.S. (1909) The causes of periodic or Cheyne–Stokes breathing. *J. Physiol. (Lond.)* **38**, 401–19.

Douglas, C.G., Haldane, J.S., Henderson, Y. and Schneider, E.C. (1913) Physiological observations made on Pike's Peak, Colorado, with special reference to adaptation to low barometric pressures. *Phil. Trans. R. Soc. (Lond). Ser. B* **203**, 185–381.

Douglas N.J. (2000) Respiratory physiology: control of ventilation, in *Principles and Practice of Sleep Medicine* (eds. M. Kryger, T. Roth and W.C. Dement), W.B. Saunders, Philadelphia, PA, pp. 221–8.

Douglas, N.J., White, D.P., Weil, J.V. *et al.* (1982a) Hypoxic ventilatory response decreases during sleep in normal men. *Am. Rev. Respir. Dis.* **125**, 286–9.

Douglas, N.J., White, D.P., Weil, J.V. *et al.* (1982b) Hypercapnic ventilatory response in sleeping adults. *Am. Rev. Respir. Dis.* **126**, 758–62.

Drinking and drowning (editorial) (1979) *BMJ* **1**, 70–1.

Droma, Y., Hayano, T., Takabayashi, Y. *et al.* (1996a) Endothelin-1 and interleukin-8 in high altitude pulmonary oedema. *Eur. Respir. J.* **9**, 1947–9.

Droma, Y., Ge, R.L., Tanaka, M. *et al.* (1996b) Acute hypoxic pulmonary vascular response does not accompany plasma endothelin-1 elevation in subjects susceptible to high altitude pulmonary edema. *Intern. Med.* **35**, 257–60.

Droma, Y., Hanaoka, M., Ota, M. *et al.* (2002) Positive association of the endothelial nitric oxide synthase gene polymorphisms with high-altitude pulmonary edema. *Circulation* **106**, 826–30.

Droma, Y., Hanaoka, M., Basnyat, B. *et al.* (2008) Adaptation to high altitude in Sherpas: association with the insertion/deletion polymorphism in the angiotensin-converting enzyme gene. *Wilderness Environ. Med.* **19**, 22–9.

Dubas, F. (1980) Aspects de medicaux de l'accident par avalanche. Hypotherme et gelure. *Z. Unfallmed. Berfskr.* **73**, 164–7.

Dubas, F., Henzwlin, R. and Michelet, J. (1991a) Avalanche prevention and rescue, in *A Colour Atlas of Mountain Medicine* (eds. J. Vallotten and F. Dubas), Wolfe, London, pp. 104–12.

Dubas, F., Henzwlin, R. and Michelet, J. (1991b) Rescue in crevasses, in *A Colour Atlas of Mountain Medicine* (eds. J. Vallotten and F. Dubas), Wolfe, London, pp. 112–16.

Dubowitz, D.J., Dyer, E.A., Theilmann, R.J. *et al.* (2009) Early brain swelling in acute hypoxia. *J. Appl. Physiol.* **107**, 244–52.

Dubowitz, G. (1998) Effect of temazepam on oxygen saturation and sleep quality at high altitude: randomised placebo controlled crossover trial. *BMJ* **21**, 587–9.

Dubowitz, G. and Peacock, A.J. (1999) Pulmonary artery pressure variation measured by Doppler echocardiography in healthy subjects at 4250m (abstract), in *Hypoxia: Into the Next Millennium* (eds. R.C. Roach, P.D. Wagner and P.H. Hackett), Plenum/Kluwer, New York, p. 378.

Dubowitz, G., Bickler, P. and Schiller, N. (2004) Patent foramen ovale at high altitude. *High Alt. Med. Biol.* **5**, 482.

Dudley, G.A., Tullson, P.C. and Terjung, R.L. (1987) Influence of mitochondrial content on the sensitivity of respiratory control. *J. Biol. Chem.* **262**, 9109–14.

Duff, J. (1999a) Observations while treating altitude illness. *Wilderness Environ. Med.* **10**, 274.

Duff, J. (1999b) The Tibetan tuck: a dry land cold condition survival position equivalent to that used in cold water. *Wilderness Environ. Med.* **10**, 206–7.

Duffin, J. (2007) Measuring the ventilatory response to hypoxia. *J. Physiol.* **584**, 285–93.

Duke, H.N. (1954) Site of action of anoxia on the pulmonary blood vessels of the cat. *J. Physiol. (Lond.)* **125**, 373–82.

Dumont, L., Mardirosoff, C. and Tramer, M.R. (2000) Efficacy and harm of pharmacological prevention of acute mountain sickness: quantitative systematic review. *BMJ* **321**, 267–72.

Duplain, H., Vollenweider, L., Delabeys, A. *et al.* (1999a) Augmented sympathetic activation during short-term hypoxia and high-altitude exposure in subjects susceptible to high-altitude pulmonary edema. *Circulation* **99**, 1713–18.

Duplain, H., Lepori, M., Sartori, C. *et al.* (1999b) Inflammation does not contribute to high altitude pulmonary edema. *Am. J. Respir. Crit. Care* **159**, A345 (abstract).

Duplain, H., Sartori, C., Lepori, M. *et al.* (2000) Exhaled nitric oxide in high-altitude pulmonary edema: role in the regulation of pulmonary vascular tone and evidence for a role against inflammation. *Am. J. Respir. Crit. Care Med.* **162**, 221–4.

Durand, F., Kippelen, P., Ceugniet, F. *et al.* (2005) Undiagnosed exercise-induced bronchoconstriction in ski-mountaineers. *Int. J. Sports Med.* **26**, 233–7.

Durand, J. and Martineaud, J.P. (1971) Resistance and capacitance vessels of the skin in permanent and temporary residents at high altitude, in *High Altitude Physiology: Cardiac and Respiratory Aspects*, Ciba Foundation (eds. R. Porter and J. Knight), Churchill Livingstone, London, pp. 159–70.

Durand, J. and Raynaud, J. (1987) Limb blood and heat exchange at altitude, in *Hypoxia and Cold* (eds. J.R. Sutton, C.S. Houston and G. Coates), Praeger, New York, pp. 100–13.

Durig, A. (1911) Ergebnisse der Monte Rosa Expedition vom Jahre 1906 von Prof. Dr. A. Durig. Über den Gaswechsel beim Gehen. *Denkschr. d. Mathem.-Naturw. Kl.* **86**, 293–347.

Durmowicz, A.G. (2001) Pulmonary edema in 6 children with Down syndrome during travel to moderate altitudes. *Pediatrics* **108**, 443–7.

Durmowicz, A.G., Noordeweir, E., Nicholas, R. and Reeves, J.T. (1997) Inflammatory processes may predispose children to high altitude pulmonary edema. *J. Pediatr.* **130**, 838–40.

Duteil, L., Queille-Roussel, C., Lorenz, B. *et al.* (2002) A randomized, controlled study of the safety and efficacy of topical corticosteroid treatments of sunburn in healthy volunteers. *Clin. Exp. Dermatol.* **27**, 314–18.

Eady, R.A.J., Bentley-Phillips, C.B., Keahey, T.M. and Greaves, M.W. (1978) Cold urticaria vasculitis. *Br. J. Dermatol.* **99**(Suppl. 16), 9–10.

Eaton, J.W., Skelton, T.D. and Berger, E. (1974) Survival at extreme altitude: protective effect of increased hemoglobin-oxygen affinity. *Science* **183**, 743–4.

Eckardt, K., Boutellier, U., Kurtz, A. *et al.* (1989) Rate of erythropoietin formation in humans in response to acute hypobaric hypoxia. *J. Appl. Physiol.* **66**, 1785–8.

Edwards, H.T. (1936) Lactic acid in rest and work at high altitude. *Am. J. Physiol.* **116**, 367–75.

Edwards, L.M., Murray, A.J., Tyler, D.J. *et al.* (2010) The effect of high-altitude on human skeletal muscle energetics: 31 P-MRS results from the Caudwell Xtreme Everest expedition. *PLoS ONE* **5**, e10681.

Eger, E.I., Kellogg, R.H., Mines, A.H. *et al.* (1968) Influence of CO_2 on ventilatory acclimatization to altitude. *J. Appl. Physiol.* **24**, 607–14.

Egli-Sinclair. (1893) Sur le mal de montagne. *Annals de Observatoire Météorologique, Physique et Glaciaire du Mont Blanc* **1**, 109–30.

Ekblom, B., Goldbarg, A.N. and Gullbring, B. (1972) Response to exercise after blood loss and reinfusion. *J. Appl. Physiol.* **33**, 175–80.

Ekelund, L.G. (1967) Circulatory and respiratory adaptation during prolonged exercise. *Acta Physiol. Scand.* **292**(Suppl.), 1–38.

Eldridge, M.W., Podolsky, A., Richardson, R.S. *et al.* (1996) Pulmonary haemodynamic response to exercise in subjects with prior high-altitude pulmonary edema. *J. Appl. Physiol.* **81**, 911–21.

Eldridge, W.E., Braun, R.K., Yoneda, K.Y. *et al.* (1998) Lung injury after heavy exercise at altitude. *Chest* **114**, 66S–67S.

Ellerton, J.A., Zuljan, I., Agazzi, G. et al. (2009) Eye problems in mountain and remote areas: prevention and onsite treatment—official Recommendations of the International Commission for Mountain Emergency Medicine (ICAR MEDCOM). *Wild. Environ. Med.* **20**, 169–75.

Elliott, A.R., Fu, Z., Tsukimoto, K. *et al.* (1992) Short-term reversibility of ultrastructural changes in pulmonary capillaries caused by stress failure. *J. Appl. Physiol.* **73**, 1150–8.

Elliott, M.E. and Goodfriend, T.L. (1986) Inhibition of aldosterone synthesis by atrial natriuretic factor. *Fed. Proc.* **45**, 2376–81.

Ellsworth, A.J., Larson, E.B. and Strickland, D. (1987) A randomized trial of dexamethasone and acetazolamide for acute mountain sickness prophylaxis. *Am. J. Med.* **83**, 1024–30.

Ellsworth, A.J., Meyer, E.F. and Larson, E.B. (1991) Acetazolamide or dexamethasone use versus placebo to prevent acute mountain sickness on Mount Rainier. *West. J. Med.* **154**, 289–93.

Elterman, L. (1964) *Atmospheric Attenuation Model, 1964, in the Ultraviolet, Visible, and Infrared Regions for Altitudes to 50km*, Environmental Research Papers No. **46**, L.G. Hanscom Field, MA, Air Force Cambridge Research Laboratories, Office of Aerospace Research, AFCRL-64-740.

Enander, A. (1984) Performance and sensory aspects of work in cold environments – a review. *Ergonomics* **27**, 365–78.

Ennemoser, O., Ambach, W. and Flora, G. (1988) Physical assessment of heat insulation of rescue foils. *Int. J. Sports Med.* **9**, 179–82.

Erba, P., Anastasi, S., Senn, O. *et al.* (2004) Acute mountain sickness is related to nocturnal hypoxemia but not to hypoventilation. *Eur. Respir. J.* **24**, 303–8.

Erdman, J., Sun, K.T., Masar, P. and Niederhauser, H. (1998) Effects of exposure to altitude on men with coronary artery disease and impaired left ventricular function. *Am. J. Cardiol.* **81**, 266–70.

Ersanli, D., Yildiz, S., Sonmez, M. *et al.* (2006) Intraocular pressure at a simulated altitude of 9000 m with and without 100% oxygen. *Aviat. Space Environ. Med.* **77**, 704–6.

Erslev, A. (1987) Erythropoietin coming of age. *N. Engl. J. Med.* **316**, 101–3.

Eversman, T., Gottsman, M., Uhlich, E. *et al.* (1978) Increased secretion of growth hormone, prolactin, antidiuretic hormone and cortisol induced by the stress of motion sickness. *Aviat. Space Environ. Med.* **49**, 53–7.

Facco, M., Zilli, C., Siviero, M. *et al.* (2005) Modulation of immune response by the acute and chronic exposure to high altitude. *Med. Sci. Sports Exerc.* **37**, 768–74.

Faeh, D., Gutzwiller, F. and Bopp, M. (2009) Lower mortality from coronary heart disease and stroke at higher altitudes in Switzerland. *Circulation* **120**, 495–501.

Fagan, K.A. and Weil, J.V. (2001) Potential genetic contribution to control of the pulmonary circulation and ventilation at high altitude. *High Alt. Med. Biol.* **2**, 165–71.

Fagenholz, P.J., Gutman, J.A., Murray, A.F. *et al.* (2007) Arterial thrombosis at high altitude resulting in loss of limb. *High Alt. Med. Biol.* **8**, 340–7.

Fagenholz, P.J., Murray, A.F., Gutman, J.A. *et al.* (2007) New-onset anxiety disorders at high altitude. *Wilderness Environ. Med.* **18**, 312–16.

Fagenolz, P.J., Gutman, J.A., Murray, A.F. *et al.* (2007a) Chest ultrasonography for the diagnosis and monitoring of high altitude pulmonary edema. *Chest* **131**, 1013–18.

Fagenholz, P.J., Gutman, J.A., Murray, A.F. *et al.* (2007b) Evidence for increased intracranial pressure and high altitude pulmonary edema. *High Alt. Med. Biol.* **8**, 331–6.

Fagenholz, P.J., Gutman, J.A., Murray, A.F. *et al.* (2009) Optic nerve sheath diameter correlates with the presence and severity of acute mountain sickness: evidence for increased intracranial pressure. *J. Appl. Physiol.* **106**, 1207–11.

Fâ-Hien (399–414) *A Record of Buddhistic Kingdoms, Being an Account by the Chinese Monk Fâ-Hien of his Travels in India and Ceylon (AD 399–414) in Search of the Buddhist Books of Discipline.* Translated and annotated with a Korean recension of the Chinese text by J. Legge, Dover Publications, New York (1965), pp. 40–1 (p. 12 of the Korean text).

Falk, B., Bar-Or, J., Smolander, J. and Frost, G. (1994) Response to rest and exercise in the cold: the effect of age and aerobic fitness. *J. Appl. Physiol.* **76**, 72–8.

Fan, J.-L, Burgess, K.R. Basnyat, R. *et al.* (2010) Influence of high altitude on cerebrovascular and ventilatory responsiveness to CO_2. *J. Physiol.* **588**, 539–49.

Faoro, V., Boldingh, S., Moreels, M. *et al.* (2009) Bosentan decreases pulmonary vascular resistance and improves exercise capacity in acute hypoxia. *Chest* **135**, 1215–22.

Faoro, V., Fink, B., Taudorf, S. *et al.* (2011) Acute in vitro hypoxia and high-altitude (4,559 m) exposure decreases leukocyte oxygen consumption. *Am. J. Physiol. Regul. Integr. Comp. Physiol.* **300**, R32–9.

Faoaro, V., Lamotte, M., Deboeck, G. *et al.* (2007) Effects of sildenafil on exercise capacity in hypoxic normal subjects. *High Alt. Med. Biol.* **8**, 155–63.

Faraci, F.M. (1986) Circulation during hypoxia in birds. *Comp Biochem Physiol A* **85**, 613–20.

Faraci, F.M. and Fedde, M.R. (1986) Regional circulatory responses to hypocapnia and hypercapnia in bar-headed geese. *Am. J. Physiol.* **250**, (3 Pt 2), R499–504.

Farber, M.O., Bright, T.P., Strawbridge, R.A. *et al.* (1975) Impaired water handling in chronic obstructive lung disease. *J. Lab. Clin. Med.* **85**, 41–9.

Fatemian, M., Nieuwenhuijs, D.J., Teppema, L.J. *et al.* (2003) The respiratory response to carbon dioxide in humans with unilateral and bilateral resections of the carotid bodies. *J. Physiol.* **549**, 965–73.

Feddersen, B., Ausserer, H., Haditsch, B. *et al.* (2009) Brain natriuretic peptide at altitude: relationship to diuresis, natriuresis, and mountain sickness. *Aviat. Space Environ. Med.* **80**, 108–11.

Feldman, K.W. and Herndon, S.P. (1977) Positive expiratory pressure for the treatment of high altitude edema. *Lancet* **1**, 1036–7.

Fencl, V., Miller, T.B. and Pappenheimer, J.R. (1966) Studies on the respiratory response to disturbances of acid–base balance, with deductions concerning ionic composition of cerebral interstitial fluid. *Am. J. Physiol.* **210**, 449–72.

Fencl, V., Gabel, R.A. and Wolfe, D. (1979) Composition of cerebral fluids in goats adapted to high altitude. *J. Appl. Physiol.* **47**, 408–13.

Ferrara, N. and Davis-Smyth, T. (1997) The biology of vascular endothelial growth factor. *Endocr. Rev.* **18**, 4–25.

Ferrazzini, G., Maggiorini, M., Kriemler, S. *et al.* (1987) Successful treatment of acute mountain sickness with dexamethasone. *BMJ* **294**, 1380–2.

Ferri, C., Bellini, C., De Angelis, C. *et al.* (1995) Circulating endothelin-1 concentrations in patients with chronic hypoxia. *J. Clin. Pathol.* **48**, 519–24.

Ferrus, L., Guenard, H., Vardon, G. and Varene, P. (1980) Respiratory water loss. *Respir. Physiol.* **39**, 367–81.

Ferrus, L., Commenges, D., Gire, J. and Varene, P. (1984) Respiratory water loss as a function of ventilatory or environmental factors. *Respir. Physiol.* **56**, 11–20.

Fineman, J.R., Heymann, M.A. and Soifer, S.J. (1991) N-nitro-L-arginine attenuates endothelium-dependent pulmonary vasodilation in lambs. *Am. J. Physiol.* **260**, H1299–306.

Finisterer, J. (1999) High altitude illness induced by tooth root infection. *Postgrad. Med. J.* **75**, 227–9.

Fink, K.S., Christensen, D.B. and Ellsworth, A. (2002) Effect of high altitude on blood glucose meter performance. *Diabetes Technol. Ther.* **4**, 627–35.

Fiorenzano, G., Papalia, M.A., Parrivicini, M. *et al.* (1997) Prolonged ECG abnormalities in a subject with high altitude pulmonary edema (HAPE). *J. Sports Med. Phys. Fitness* **37**, 292–6.

Firth, P.G. and Bolay, H. (2004) Transient high altitude neurological dysfunction: an origin in the temporoparietal cortex. *High. Alt. Med. Biol.* **5**, 71–5.

Fischer, A.P., Stumpe, F. and Vallotton, J. (1991) Hypothermia in an avalanche: a case report, in *A Colour Atlas of Mountain Medicine* (eds. J. Vallotton and F. Du Bas), Wolfe, London, pp. 96–7.

Fischer, R., Lang, S.M., Leitl, M. *et al.* (2004) Theophylline and acetazolamide reduce sleep-disordered breathing at high altitude. *Eur. Respir. J.* **23**, 47–52.

Fischer, R., Vollmar, C., Thiere, M. *et al.* (2004) No evidence of cerebral oedema in severe acute mountain sickness. *Cephalalgia* **24**, 66–71.

Fischer, R., Lang, S.M., Bruckner, K. *et al.* (2005) Lung function in adults with cystic fibrosis at altitude: impact on air travel. *Eur. Respir. J.* **25**, 718–24.

Fischer, S., Clauss M., Wiesnet M. *et al.* (1999) Hypoxia induces permeability in brain microvessel endothelial cells via VEGF and NO. *Am. J. Physiol. Cell. Physiol.* **276**, C812–20.

Fischler, M., Maggiorini, M., Dorschner, L. *et al.* (2009) Dexamethasone but not tadalafil improves exercise capacity in adults prone to high altitude pulmonary edema. *Am. J. Respir. Crit. Care Med.* **180**, 346–52.

Fisher, J.W. and Langston, J.W. (1967) The influence of hypoxia and cobalt on erythropoietin production in the isolated perfused dog kidney. *Blood* **29**, 114–25.

Fisher, R., Lang, S.M., Bergner, A. and Huber, R.M. (2005) Monitoring of expiratory flow rates and lung volumes during a high altitude expedition. *Eur. J. Med. Res.* **10**, 469–74.

Fishman, A.P. (1985) Pulmonary circulation, in *Handbook of Physiology*, Section 3: *The Respiratory System*, Vol. 1: *Circulation and Nonrespiratory Functions* (eds. A.P. Fishman and A.B. Fisher), American Physiological Society, Bethesda, MD, pp. 93–165.

Fishman, R.A. (1975) Brain edema. *N. Engl. J. Med.* **293**, 706–11.

Fitch, R.F. (1964) Mountain sickness: a cerebral form. *Ann. Intern. Med.* **60**, 871–6.

Fitzgerald, F.T. and Jessop, C. (1982) Accidental hypothermia. A report of 22 cases and review of the literature. *Adv. Intern. Med.* **27**, 127–50.

FitzGerald, M.P. (1913) The changes in the breathing and the blood at various altitudes.

Philos. Trans. R. Soc. Lond. Ser. B **203**, 351–71.

FitzGerald, M.P. (1914) Further observations on the changes in the breathing and the blood at various high altitudes. *Proc. Roy. Soc. Lond. Ser. B* **88**, 248–58.

Fletcher, E.C., Lesske, J., Behm, R. *et al.* (1992) Carotid chemoreceptors, systemic blood pressure, and chronic episodic hypoxia mimicking sleep apnea. *J. Appl. Physiol.* **72**, 1978–84.

Flora, G. (1985) Secondary treatment of frostbite, in *High Altitude Deterioration* (eds. J. Rivolier, P. Cerretelli, J. Foray and P. Segantini), Karger, Basel, pp. 159–69.

Folsom, A.R., Aleksic, N, Wang, L. *et al.* (2002) Protein C, antithrombin, and venous thromboembolism incidence: a prospective population-based study. *Arterscler. Thromb. Vasc. Biol.* **22**, 1018–22.

Foray, J. and Cahen, C. (1981) Les hypothermies de montagne. *Chirurgie* **107**, 255–310.

Foray, J. and Salon, F. (1985) Casualties with cold injuries: primary treatment, in *High Altitude Deterioration* (eds. J. Rivolier, P. Cerretelli, J. Foray and P. Segantini), Karger, Basel, pp. 149–58.

Forbes, C.B. and Drenick, E.J. (1979) Loss of body nitrogen of fasting. *Am. J. Clin. Nutr.* **32**, 1370–4.

Formenti, F., Constantin-Teodosiub, D., Emmanuela, Y. *et al.* (2010) Regulation of human metabolism by hypoxia-inducible factor. *Proc. Natl. Acad. Sci. USA* **107**, 12722–7.

Forsling, M.L. and Milledge, J.S. (1977) Effect of hypoxia on vasopressin release in man. *J. Physiol.* **267**, 22–23P.

Forsling, M.L. and Milledge, J.S. (1980) The effect of simulated altitude (4000 m) on plasma cortisol and vasopressin concentration in man. *Proc. Int. Union Physiol. Sci.* **14**, 414.

Forster, H.V., Dempsey, J.A. and Chosy, L.W. (1974) Incomplete compensation of CSF [H[1]] in man during acclimatization to high altitude (4300 m). *J. Appl. Physiol.* **38**, 1067–72.

Forster, H.V., Bisgard, G.E. and Klein, J.P. (1981) Effect of peripheral chemoreceptor denervation on acclimatization of goats during hypoxia. *J. Appl. Physiol.* **40**, 392–8.

Forster, P. (1984) Reproducibility of individual response to exposure to high altitude. *BMJ* **289**, 1269.

Forster, P. (1986) Telescopes in high places, in *Aspects of Hypoxia* (ed. D. Heath), Liverpool University Press, Liverpool, pp. 217–33.

Forwand, S.A., Landowne, M., Follansbee, J.N. and Hansen, J.E. (1968) Effect of acetazolamide on acute mountain sickness. *N. Engl. J. Med.* **279**, 839–45.

Fox, V.F. (1967) Human performance in the cold. *Hum. Factors* **9**, 203–90.

Franch, J., Madsen, K., Djurhuus, M.S. *et al.* (1998) Improved running economy following intensified training correlates with reduced ventilatory demands. *Med. Sci. Sports Exer.* **30**, 1250–6.

Francis, T.J.R. and Golden, F. St C. (1985) Non-freezing cold injury: the pathogenesis. *J. R. Nav. Med. Serv.* **71**, 3–8.

Franklin, Q.J. and Compeggie, M. (1999) Splenic syndrome in sickle cell trait: four case presentations and a review of the literature. *Mil. Med.* **164**, 230–3.

Franz, D.R., Berberich, J.J., Blake, S. and Mills, W.J. (1978) Evaluation of fasciotomy and vasodilators for the treatment of frostbite in the dog. *Cryobiology* **15**, 659–69.

Frayser, R., Houston, C.S., Bryan, A.C. *et al.* (1970) Retinal hemorrhage at high altitude. *N. Engl. J. Med.* **282**, 1183–4.

Fred, H.L., Schmidt, A.M., Bates, T. and Hecht, H.H. (1962) Acute pulmonary edema of altitude. Clinical and physiologic observations. *Circulation* **25**, 929–37.

Freeman. K., Shalit. M. and Stroh. G. (2004) Use of the Gamow bag by EMT-basic park rangers for treatment of high-altitude pulmonary edema and high-altitude cerebral edema. *Wilderness. Environ. Med.* **15**, 198–201.

Freer, L. and Imray, C.H.E. (2012) Frostbite, in *Wilderness Medicine*, 6th edn. (ed. P.S. Auerbach), Philadelphia, PA, Mosby, pp. 181–200.

Freitas, J., Costa, O., Carvalho, M.J. and Falcao de Freitas, A. (1996) High altitude-related neurocardiogenic syncope. *Am. J. Cardiol.* **77**, 1021.

Freund, B.J., O'Brien, C. and Young, A.J. (1994) Alcohol ingestion and temperature regulation during cold exposure. *J. Wilderness Med.* **5**, 88–98.

Friedman, N.B. (1945) The pathology of trench foot. *Am. J. Pathol.* **21**, 387–433.

Frisancho, A.R. (1978) Human growth and development among high-altitude populations, in *The Biology of High Altitude Peoples* (ed. P.T. Baker), Cambridge University Press, Cambridge, pp. 117–71.

Frisancho, A.R. (1988) Origins of differences in hemoglobin concentration between Himalayan and Andean populations. *Respir. Physiol.* **72**, 13–18.

Frisancho, A.R. and Baker, P.T. (1970) Altitude and growth: a study of the patterns of physical growth of a high altitude Peruvian Quechua population. *Am. J. Phys. Anthropol.* **32**, 279–92.

Froese, G. and Burton, A.C. (1957) Heat loss from the human head. *J. Appl. Physiol.* **10**, 235–41.

Fromm, R.E., Jr., Varon, J., Lechin, A.E. and Hirshkowitz, M. (1995) CPAP machine performance and altitude. *Chest* **108**, 1577–80.

Frostell, C.G., Blomqvist, H., Hedenstierna, G. *et al.* (1993) Inhaled nitric oxide selectively reverses human hypoxic pulmonary vasoconstriction without causing systemic vasodilation. *Anesthesiology* **78**, 427–35.

Fruehauf, H., Erb, A., Maggiorini, M. *et al.* (2010) Unsedated transnasal esophago-gastroduodenoscopy at 4559m – endoscopic findings in healthy mountaineers after rapid ascent to high altitude. *Swiss Med. Wkly* **140** (Suppl. 183): 5S.

Fu, Z., Costello, M.L., Tsukimoto, K. *et al.* (1992) High lung volume increases stress failure in pulmonary capillaries. *J. Appl. Physiol.* **73**, 123–33.

Fudge, B.W., Westerterp, K.R., Kiplamai, F.K. *et al.* (2006) Evidence of negative energy balance using doubly labelled water in elite Kenyan endurance runners prior to competition. *Br. J. Nutr.* **95**, 59–66.

Fuhrer-Haimendorf, C. von (1964) *The Sherpas of Nepal: Bhuddist Highlanders*, John Murray, London.

Fujimaki, T., Matsutani, M. Asai, A. *et al.* (1986) Cerebral venous thrombosis due to high altitude polycythemia. Case report. *J. Neurosurg.* **64**, 148–50.

Fulco, C.S., Rock, P.B. and Cymerman, A. (1998) Maximal and submaximal exercise performance at altitude. *Aviat. Space Environ. Med.* **69**, 793–801.

Fulco, C.S., Muza, S.R., Beidleman, B.A. *et al.* (2011) Effect of repeated normobaric hypoxia exposures during sleep on acute mountain sickness, exercise performance, and sleep during exposure to terrestrial altitude. *Am. J. Physiol. Regul. Integr. Comp. Physiol.* **300**, R428–36.

Gabry, A.L., Ledoux, X., Mozziconacci, M. and Martin, C. (2003) High-altitude pulmonary edema at moderate altitude (2,400 m; 7,870 feet): a series of 52 patients. *Chest* **123**, 49–53.

Gaillard, S., Dellasanta, P., Loutan, L. and Kayser, B. (2004) Awareness, prevalence, medication use, and risk factors of acute mountain sickness in tourists trekking around the Annapurnas in Nepal: a 12-year follow-up. *High Alt. Med. Biol.* **5**, 410–19.

Gale, G.E., Torre-Bueno, J.R., Moon, R.E. *et al.* (1985) Ventilation–perfusion inequality in normal humans during exercise at sea level and simulated altitude. *J. Appl. Physiol.* **58**, 978–88.

Galeotti, G. (1904) Les variations de l'alcalinité du sang sur le sommet du Mont Rosa. *Arch. Ital. Biol.* **41**, 80–92.

Galileo, G. (1638) *Dialogues Concerning Two New Sciences.* English translation of relevant pages in *High Altitude Physiology* (ed. J.B. West), Hutchinson Ross, Stroudsburg, PA, 1981.

Galton, V.A. (1978) Environmental effects, in *The Thyroid*, 4th edn (eds. S.C. Werner and S.H. Ingbar), Harper Row, New York, pp. 247–52.

Gamboa, A., León-Velarde, F., Rivera-Ch, M. *et al.* (2001) Ventilatory and cardiovascular responses to hypoxia and exercise in Andean natives living at sea level. *High Alt. Med. Biol.* **2**, 341–7.

Gamboa, A., León-Velarde, F., Rivera-Ch, M. *et al.* (2003) Acute and sustained ventilatory responses to hypoxia in high-altitude natives living at sea level. *J. Appl. Physiol.* **94**, 1253–62.

Garcia, N., Hopkins, S.R. and Powell, F.L. (1999) Effects of intermittent vs. continuous hypoxia on the isocapnic ventilatory hypoxic response in man. *Am. J. Crit. Care Respir. Med.* **159**, A44.

Garcia, N., Hopkins, S.R. and Powell, F.L. (2000) Effects of intermittent hypoxia on the isocapnic ventilatory hypoxic response and erythropoiesis in humans. *Respir. Physiol.* **123**, 39–49.

Garcia, N., Hopkins, S.R., Elliott, A.R. *et al.* (2001) Ventilatory response to 2-h sustained hypoxia in humans. *Respir. Physiol.* **124**, 11–22.

Garrido, E., Castello, A., Ventura, J.L. *et al.* (1993) Cortical atrophy and other brain magnetic resonance imaging (MRI) changes after extremely high-altitude climbs without oxygen. *Int. J. Sports Med.* **14**, 232–4.

Garrido, E., Rodas, G., Javierre, C. *et al.* (1997) Cardiorespiratory response to exercise in elite Sherpa climbers transferred to sea level. *Med. Sci. Sports Exerc.* **29**, 937–42.

Garrow, J.S. (1987) Are liquid diets (VLCD) safe or necessary? in *Recent Advances in Obesity Research, V* (eds. E.M. Berry, S.H. Blondheim, H.E. Eliahou and E. Shafrir), Food and Nutrition Press, Westport, CT, pp. 312–16.

Gassmann, M., van Patot, M.T. and Soliz, J. (2009) The neuronal control of hypoxic ventilation, erythropoietin and sexual dimorphism. *Ann. New York Acad. Sci.* **1177**, 151–61.

Gautier, H., Peslin, R., Grassino, A. *et al.* (1982) Mechanical properties of the lungs during acclimatization to altitude. *J. Appl. Physiol.* **52**, 1407–15.

Gautier, H., Bonora, M., Schultz, S.A. and Remmers, J.E. (1987) Hypoxia induced changes in shivering and body temperature. *J. Appl. Physiol.* **62**, 2577–81.

Gautier, J.F., Bigard, A.X., Douce, P. *et al.* (1996) Influence of simulated altitude on the performance of five blood glucose meters. *Diabetes Care* **19**, 1430–3.

Ge, R.L. and Helun, G.W. (2001) Current concept of chronic mountain sickness: pulmonary hypertension-related high-altitude heart disease. *Wilderness. Environ. Med.* **12**, 190–4.

Ge, R.L., Chen, Q.H., Wang, L.H. *et al.* (1994) Higher exercise performance and lower VO2max in Tibetan than Han residents at 4,700m altitude. *J. Appl. Physiol.* **77**, 684–91.

Ge, R.L., Matsuzawa, Y., Takeoka, M. *et al.* (1997) Low pulmonary diffusing capacity in subjects with acute mountain sickness. *Chest* **111**, 58–64.

Ge, R.L., Kubo, K., Kobayashi, T. *et al.* (1998) Blunted hypoxic pulmonary vasoconstrictive response to the rodent *Ochotona curzoniae* (pika) at high altitude. *Am. J. Physiol. Heart Circ. Physiol.* **274**, H1792–9.

Ge, R-L., Shai, H-R., Takaoka, M. *et al.* (2001) Atrial natriuretic peptide and red cell 2,3-diphosphoglyceride in patients with chronic mountain sickness. *Wilderness. Environ. Med.* **12**, 2–7.

Ge, R.L., Stone, J.A., Levine, B.D. and Babb, T.G. (2005) Exaggerated respiratory chemosensitivity and association with SaO2 level at 3568 m in obesity. *Respir. Physiol. Neurobiol.* **146**, 47–54.

Ge, R.-L., Mo, V.Y., Januzzi, J.L. *et al.* (2011) B-type natriuretic peptide, vascular endothelial growth factor, endothelin-1, and nitric oxide synthase in chronic mountain sickness. *Am. J. Physiol. Heart Circ. Physiol.* **300**, H1427–H1433.

Gehr, P., Bachofen, M. and Weibel, E.R. (1978) The normal human lung: ultrastructure and morphometric estimation of diffusion capacity. *Respir. Physiol.* **32**, 121–40.

Geiser, J., Vogt, M., Billeter, R. *et al.* (2001) Training high–living low: changes of aerobic performance and muscle structure with training at simulated altitude. *Int. J. Sports Med.* **22**, 579–85.

GeoNames (2010) GeoNames geographical names. Available from: www.geonames.org.

Gerard, A.B., McElroy, M.D., Taylor M.J. *et al.* (2000) Six percent oxygen enrichment of room air at simulated 5000m altitude improves neuropsychological function. *High Alt. Med. Biol.* **1**, 51–61.

Gertsch, J.H., Seto, T.B., Mor, J. and Onopa, J. (2002) Ginkgo biloba for the prevention of severe acute mountain sickness (AMS) starting one day before rapid ascent. *High Alt. Med. Biol.* **3**, 29–37.

Gertsch, J.H., Basnyat, B., Johnson, E.W. *et al.* (2004) Randomised, double blind, placebo controlled comparison of ginkgo biloba and acetazolamide for prevention of acute mountain sickness among Himalayan trekkers: the prevention of high altitude illness trial (PHAIT). *BMJ* **328**, 797.

Gertsch, J.H., Lipman, G.S., Holck, P.S. *et al.* (2010) Prospective, double-blind, randomized, placebo-controlled comparison of acetazolamide versus ibuprofen for prophylaxis against high altitude headache: the Headache Evaluation at Altitude Trial (HEAT). *Wilderness Environ. Med.* **21**, 236–43.

Ghofrani, H.A., Reichenberger, F., Kohstall, M.G. *et al.* (2004) Sildenafil increased exercise capacity during hypoxia at low altitudes and at Mount Everest base camp: a randomized, double-blind, placebo-controlled crossover trial. *Ann. Intern. Med.* **141**, 169–77.

Gibala, M.J., Little, J.P., van Essen, M. *et al.* (2006) Short-term sprint interval versus traditional endurance training: similar initial adaptations in human skeletal muscle and exercise performance. *J. Physiol.* **575**, 901–11.

Giesbrecht, G.E., Goheen, M.S.L., Johnston, C.E. *et al.* (1997) Inhibition of shivering increases core temperature after drop and attenuates rewarming in hypothermic humans. *J. Appl. Physiol.* **83**, 1630–4.

Gilbert, D.L. (1983) The first documented report of mountain sickness: the China or Headache Mountain story. *Respir. Physiol.* **52**, 315–26.

Gilbert, D.L. (1991) The Pariacaca or Tullujoto story: political realism? *Respir. Physiol.* **86**, 147–57.

Gill, M.B. and Pugh, L.G.C.E. (1964) Basal metabolism and respiration in men living at 5,800 m (19000 ft). *J. Appl. Physiol.* **19**, 949–54.

Gill, M.B., Milledge, J.S., Pugh, L.G.C.E. and West, J.B. (1962) Alveolar gas composition at 21,000 to 25,700 ft (6400–7830 m). *J. Physiol. (Lond.)* **163**, 373–7.

Gill, M.B., Poulton, E.C., Carpenter, A. *et al.* (1964) Falling efficiency at sorting cards during acclimatization at 19,000 ft. *Nature* **203**, 436.

Gillman, P. (1993) *Everest*, Little Brown, Boston.

Glazier, J.B. and Murray, J.F. (1971) Sites of pulmonary vasomotor reactivity in the dog during alveolar hypoxia and serotonin and histamine infusion. *J. Clin. Invest.* **50**, 2550–8.

Glazier, J.B., Hughes, J.M.B., Maloney, J.E. and West, J.B. (1969) Measurements of capillary dimensions and blood volume in rapidly frozen lungs. *J. Appl. Physiol.* **26**, 65–76.

Goedhart, P.T., Khalilzada, M., Bezemer, R. *et al.* (2007). Sidestream Dark Field (SDF) imaging: a novel stroboscopic LED ring-based imaging modality for clinical assessment of the microcirculation. *Opt. Express* **15**, 15101–14.

Goerre, S., Wenk, M., Bärtsch, P. *et al.* (1995) Endothelin-1 in pulmonary hypertension associated with high-altitude exposure. *Circulation* **91**, 359–64.

Golan, Y., Onn, A., Villa, Y. *et al.* (2002) Asthma in adventure travelers: a prospective study evaluating the occurrence and risk factors for acute exacerbations. *Arch. Intern. Med.* **162**, 2421–6.

Golden, F. St C. (1973) Recognition and treatment of immersion hypothermia. *Proc. R. Soc. Med.* **66**, 1058–61.

Golden, F. St C. (1983) Rewarming, in *The Nature and Treatment of Hypothermia* (eds. R.S. Pozos and L.E. Wittmers), Croom Helm, London/University of Minnesota Press, Minneapolis, pp. 194–208.

Golden, F. St C. and Hervey, G.R. (1981) The 'after drop' and death after rescue from immersion in cold water, in *Hypothermia Ashore and Afloat* (ed. J.N. Adams), Aberdeen University Press, Aberdeen, pp. 37–56.

Goldenberg, F., Richalet, J.P., Onnen, I., and Antezana, A.M. (1992) Sleep apneas and high altitude newcomers. *Int. J. Sports Med.* **13**, S34–6.

Goldsmith, R. and Minard, D. (1976) Cold, cold work, in *Occupational Health and Safety*, Vol. 1, International Labour Office, Geneva, pp. 319–20.

Goldstein, M.C. and Beall, C.M. (1989) *Nomads of Western Tibet*, Serindia, London.

Golja, P., Flander, P., Klemenc, M. *et al.* (2008) Carbohydrate ingestion improves oxygen delivery in acute hypoxia. *High Alt. Med. Biol.* **9**, 53–62.

Gollnick, P.D. and Saltin, B. (1982) Significance of skeletal muscle oxidative enzyme enhancement with endurance training. *Clin. Physiol.* **2**, 1–12.

Goñez, C., Villena, A. and Gonzales, G.F. (1993) Serum levels of adrenal androgens up to adrenarche in Peruvian children living at sea level and at high altitude. *J. Endocrinol.* **136**, 517–23.

Gong Jr, H., Tashkin, D.P., Lee, E.Y. and Simmons, M.S. (1984) Hypoxia–altitude simulation test. Evaluation of patients with chronic airway obstruction. *Am. Rev. Respir. Dis.* **130**, 980–6.

Gonzales, G.F. and Salirrosas, A. (2005) Arterial oxygen saturation in healthy newborns delivered at term in Cerro de Pasco (4340 m) and Lima (150 m). *Reprod. Biol. Endocrinol.* **3**, 46.

Gonzales, G.F., Villena, A., Escuderl, F and Coyotupa, J. (1996) Reproduction in the Andes. *Acta Andina* **5**, 68–9.

Gonzales, G.F., Gasco, M., Tapia, V. and Gonzales-Castañeda, C. (2009) High serum testosterone levels are associated with excessive erythrocytosis of chronic mountain sickness in men. *Am. J. Physiol. Endocrinol. Metab.* **296**, E1319–E1325.

Gonzales, G.F., Tapia, V., Gasco, M. *et al.* (2011a) High serum zinc and serum testosterone levels were associated with excessive erythrocytosis in men at high altitudes. *Endocrine* **40**, 472–80.

Gonzales, G.F., Tapia, V., Gasco, M. and Gonzales-Castañeda, C. (2011b) Serum testosterone levels and score of chronic mountain sickness in Peruvian men natives at 4340 m. *Andrologia* **43**, 189–95.

González, A.J., Hernández, D., Vera, A. *et al.* (2006) *ACE* gene polymorphism and erythropoietin in endurance athletes at moderate altitudes. *Med. Sci. Sports Exerc.* **38**, 688–93.

Gonzalez, N.C., Albrecht, T., Sullivan, L.P. and Clancy, R.L. (1990) Compensation of respiratory alkalosis induced after acclimation to simulated altitude. *J. Appl. Physiol.* **69**, 1380–6.

Goodenough, R.D., Royle, G.T., Nadel, E.R. *et al.* (1982) Leucine and urea metabolism in acute human cold exposure. *J. Appl. Physiol.* **53**, 367–72.

Gordon, J.B., Ganz, P., Nabel, E.G. *et al.* (1989) Atherosclerosis influences the vasomotor response of epicardial coronary arteries to exercise. *J. Clin. Invest.* **83**, 1946–52.

Gore, C.J., Hahn, A.G., Watson, D.B. *et al.* (1996) VO$_2$ max and arterial oxygen saturation at sea level and 610m. *Med. Sci. Sports Exerc.* **27**, Abstract 42.

Gore, C., Craig, N., Hahn, A. *et al.* (1998) Altitude training at 2690m does not increase total haemoglobin mass or sea level VO$_2$ max in world champion track cyclists. *J. Sci. Med. Sport.* **1**, 156–70.

Gore, C.J., Rodríguez, F.A., Truijens, M.J. *et al.* (2006) Increased serum erythropoietin but not red cell production after 4 wk of intermittent hypobaric hypoxia (4,000–5,500 m). *J. Appl. Physiol.* **101**, 1386–93.

Gorlin, R. (1966) Physiology of the coronary circulation, in *The Heart* (eds. J.W. Hurst and R.B. Logan), McGraw-Hill, New York, pp. 653–8.

Gosney, J. (1986) Histopathology of the endocrine organs in hypoxia, in *Aspects of Hypoxia* (ed. D. Heath), Liverpool University Press, Liverpool, pp. 131–45.

Gosney, J., Heath, D., Williams, D. and Rios-Dalenz, J. (1991) Morphological changes in the pituitary–adrenocortical axis in natives of La Paz. *Int. J. Biometeorol.* **35**, 1–5.

Graham, J. and Potyk, D. (2005) Age and acute mountain sickness: examining the data. *J. Am. Geriatr. Soc.* **53**, 735.

Graham, L.E. and Basnyat, B. (2001) Cerebral edema in the Himalayas: too high, too fast! *Wilderness. Environ. Med.* **12**, 62.

Graham, W.G.B. and Houston, C.S. (1978) Short-term adaptation to moderate altitude. Patients with chronic obstructive pulmonary disease. *JAMA* **240**, 1491–4.

Grahn, D. and Kratchman, J. (1963) Variations in neonatal death rate and birth weight in the United States and possible relations to environmental radiation, geology and altitude. *Am. J. Hum. Genet.* **15**, 329–52.

Gray, D. (1987) Survival after burial in an avalanche. *BMJ* **294**, 611–12.

Gray, G.W. (1983) High altitude pulmonary edema. *Semin. Respir. Med.* **5**, 141–50.

Gray, G.W., Bryan, A.C., Freedman, M.H. *et al.* (1975) Effect of altitude exposure on platelets. *J. Appl. Physiol.* **39**, 648–52.

Green, H.J., Sutton, J.R., Cymerman, A. *et al.* (1989) Operation Everest II: adaptations in human skeletal muscle. *J. Appl. Physiol.* **66**, 2454–61.

Green, R.L., Huntsman, R.G. and Serjeant, G.R. (1971) The sickle-cell and altitude. *BMJ* **4**, 593–5.

Green, S.P.T. (1992) The 1991 Everest marathon and the Namche Bazaar dental clinic. *J. R. Nav. Med. Serv.* **78**, 165–71.

Greene, R. (1934) Observations on the composition of alveolar air on Mt. Everest. *J. Physiol. (Lond.)* **32**, 481–5.

Greene, R. (1943) The immediate vascular changes in true frostbite. *J. Pathol. Bacteriol.* **55**, 259–68.

Gregory, I.C. (1974) The oxygen and carbon monoxide capacities of foetal and adult blood. *J. Physiol.* **236**, 625–34.

Grissom, C.K. and DeLoughery, T.G. (2007) Chronic diseases and wilderness activities, in *Wilderness Medicine* (ed. P.S. Auerbach), Mosby Elsevier, Philadelphia, PA.

Grissom, C.K., Roach, R.C., Sarnquist, F.H. and Hackett, P.H. (1992) Acetazolamide in the treatment of acute mountain sickness: clinical effect on gas exchange. *Ann. Intern. Med.* **116**, 461–5.

Grissom, C.K., Albertinae, K.H. and Elstsda, M.R. (2000) Alveolar haemorrhage in a case of high altitude pulmonary oedema. *Thorax* **55**, 167–9.

Grissom, C.K., Richer, L.D. and Elstad, M.R. (2005) The effects of a 5-lipoxygenase inhibitor on acute mountain sickness and urinary leukotriene E4 after ascent to high altitude. *Chest* **127**, 565–70.

Grocott, M.P. and Johannson, L. (2007) Ketamine for emergency anaesthesia at very high altitude (4243 m above sea-level). *Anaesthesia* **62**, 959–62.

Grocott, M.P., Martin, D.S., Levett, D.Z. *et al.* (2009) Arterial blood gases and oxygen content in climbers on Mount Everest. *New Engl. J. Med.* **360**, 140–9.

Grocott, M.P., Martin, D.S., Wilson, M.H. *et al.* (2010) Caudwell Xtreme Everest Expedition. *High Alt. Med. Biol.* **11**, 133–7.

Groechenig, E. (1994) Treatment of frostbite with iloprost. *Lancet* **394**, 1152–3.

Grollman, A. (1930) Physiological variations of the cardiac output of man. VII. The effect of high altitude on the cardiac output and its related functions: an account of experiments conducted on the summit of Pikes Peak, Colorado. *Am. J. Physiol.* **93**, 19–40.

Gronbeck, C. (1984) Chronic mountain sickness at an elevation of 2000 metres. *Chest* **85**, 577–8.

Groner, W., Winkelman, J.W., Harris, A.G. *et al.* (1999). Orthogonal polarization spectral imaging: a new method for study of the microcirculation. *Nat. Med.* **5**, 1209–12.

Grootendorst, D.C., Dahlen, S.E., Van Den Bos, J.W. *et al.* (2001) Benefits of high altitude allergen avoidance in atopic adolescents with moderate to severe asthma, over and above treatment with high dose inhaled steroids. *Clin. Exp. Allergy* **31**, 400–8.

Grover, R.F. (1980) Speculations on the pathogenesis of high-altitude pulmonary edema. *Adv. Cardiol.* **27**, 1–5.

Grover, R.F., Lufschanowski, R. and Alexander, J.K. (1970) Decreased coronary blood flow in man following ascent to high altitude. *Adv. Cardiol.* **5**, 72–9.

Groves, B.M., Droma, T., Sutton, J.R. *et al.* (1993) Minimal hypoxic pulmonary hypertension in normal Tibetans at 3,658 m. *J. Appl. Physiol.* **74**, 312–18.

Groves, B.M., Reeves, J.T., Sutton, J.R. *et al.* (1987) Operation Everest II: elevated high-altitude pulmonary resistance unresponsive to oxygen. *J. Appl. Physiol.* **63**, 521–30.

Grunig, E., Mereles, D., Hildebrandt, W. *et al.* (2000) Stress Doppler echocardiography for identification of susceptibility to high altitude pulmonary edema. *J. Am. Coll. Cardiol.* **35**, 980–7.

Guerra-Garcia, R. (1971) Testosterone metabolism in men exposed to high altitude. *Acta Endocrinol. Panama* **2**, 55–9.

Guezennec, C.Y. and Pesquies, P.C. (1985) Biochemical basis for physical exercise fatigue, in *High Altitude Deterioration* (eds. J. Rivolier, P. Cerretelli, J. Foray and P. Segantini), Karger, Basel, pp. 79–89.

Guilleminault, C., Connolly, S., Winkle, R. *et al.* (1984) Cyclical variation of the heart rate in sleep apnoea syndrome. Mechanisms, and usefulness of 24 h electrocardiography as a screening technique. *Lancet* **1**, 126–31.

Guleria, J.S., Pande, J.N. and Khanna, P.K. (1969) Pulmonary function in convalescents of high altitude pulmonary edema. *Dis. Chest* **55**, 434–7.

Guleria, J.S., Pande, J.N., Sethi, P.K. and Roy, S.B. (1971) Pulmonary diffusing capacity at high altitude. *J. Appl. Physiol.* **31**, 536–43.

Gunga, H-C., Kirsch, K., Rocker, L., and Schobersberger, W. (1994) Time course of erythropoietin, triiodothyronine, thyroxin, and thyroid-stimulating hormone at 2315 m. *J. Appl. Physiol.* **76**, 1068–72.

Gupta, M.L., Rao, K.S., Andand, I.S. *et al.* (1992) Lack of smooth muscle in the small pulmonary arteries of the native Ladakhi. *Am. Rev. Respir. Dis.* **145**, 1201–4.

Gustafsson, T., Puntschart, A., Kaijser, L. *et al.* (1999) Exercise-induced expression of angiogenesis-related transcription and growth factors in human skeletal muscle. *Am. J. Physiol. Heart Circ. Physiol.* **276**, 679–85.

Guttman, R. and Gross, M.M. (1956) Relationship between electrical and mechanical changes in muscle caused by cooling. *J. Coll. Comp. Physiol.* **48**, 421–30.

Guyton, A.C., Jones, C.E. and Coleman, T.C. (1973) *Cardiac Output and its Regulation,* 2nd edn, Saunders, Philadelphia, PA, p. 396.

Haab, P., Perret, C. and Piiper, J. (1965) La capacité de diffusion pulmonaire pour l'oxygène chez l'homme normal jeune. *Helv. Physiol. Acta* **23**, C23–5.

Haas, J.D. (1976) Prenatal and infant growth and development, in *Man in the Andes* (eds. P.T. Baker and M.A. Little), Dowden, Hutchinson & Ross, Stroudsburg, PA, pp. 161–78.

Habeler, P. (1979) *Everest: Impossible Victory,* Arlington, London.

Haberman, S., Capildeo, R. and Rose, F. (1981) The seasonal variation in mortality from cerebro-vascular disease. *J. Neurol. Sci.* **52**, 25–36.

Hackett, P. (2001) High altitude and common medical conditions, *High Altitude: An Exploration of Human Adaptation* (eds T.F. Hornbein, R.B. Schoene), Marcel Dekker, New York, pp 839–85.

Hackett, P.H. (2000) Subarachnoid cyst and ascent to high altitude – a problem? *High Alt. Med. Biol.* **1**, 337–9.

Hackett, P.H. (2001) High altitude and common medical conditions, in *High Altitude: an Exploration of Human Adaptation* (eds. T.F. Hornbein and R.B. Schoene), Marcel Decker, New York, pp. 839–85.

Hackett, P.H. (2010) Caffeine at high altitude: java at base camp. *High Alt. Med. Biol.* **11**, 13–17.

Hackett, P.H. and Rennie, D. (1979) Râles, peripheral edema, retinal hemorrhage and acute mountain sickness. *Am. J. Med.* **67**, 214–18.

Hackett, P.H. and Rennie, D. (1982) Cotton wool spots: a new addition to high altitude retinopathy, in *High Altitude Physiology and Medicine* (eds. W. Brendel and R.A. Zink), Springer-Verlag, New York, pp. 215–16.

Hackett, P.H. and Roach, R.C. (2001) Current concepts: high-altitude illness. *N. Engl. J. Med.* **345**, 107–14.

Hackett, P.H., Rennie, D. and Levine, H.D. (1976) The incidence, importance and prophylaxis of acute mountain sickness. *Lancet* **2**, 1149–54.

Hackett, P.H., Forsling, M.L., Milledge, J. and Rennie, D. (1978) Release of vasopressin in man at altitude. *Horm. Metab. Res.* **10**, 571.

Hackett, P.H., Creagh, C.E., Grover, R.F. *et al.* (1980a) High altitude pulmonary edema in persons without the right pulmonary artery. *N. Engl. J. Med.* **302**, 1070–3.

Hackett, P.H., Reeves, J.T., Reeves, C.D. *et al.* (1980b) Control of breathing in Sherpas at low and high altitude. *J. Appl. Physiol.* **49**, 374–9.

Hackett, P.H., Rennie, D., Grover, R.F. and Reeves, J.T. (1981) Acute mountain sickness and the edemas of high altitude: a common pathogenesis? *Respir. Physiol.* **46**, 383–90.

Hackett, P.H., Rennie, D., Hofmeister, S.E. *et al.* (1982) Fluid retention and relative hypoventilation in acute mountain sickness. *Respiration* **43**, 321–9.

Hackett, P.H., Schoene, R.B., Winslow, R.M. *et al.* (1985) Acetazolamide and exercise in sojourners to 6,300m – a preliminary study. *Med, Sci. Sports Exerc.* **17**, 593–7.

Hackett, P.H., Bertman, J. and Rodriguez, G. (1986) Pulmonary edema fluid protein in high-altitude pulmonary edema. *JAMA* **256**, 36.

Hackett, P.H., Roach, R.C., Harrison, C.L. *et al.* (1987a) Respiratory stimulants and sleep periodic breathing at high altitude. Almitrine versus acetazolamide. *Am. Rev. Respir. Dis.* **135**, 896–8.

Hackett, P.H., Hollingshead, K.F., Roach, R.B. *et al.* (1987b) Arterial saturation during ascent predicts subsequent acute mountain sickness (abstract), in *Hypoxia and Cold* (eds. J.R. Sutton, C.S. Houston and G. Coates), Praeger, New York, p. 544.

Hackett, P.H., Hollingshead, K.F., Roach, R.B. *et al.* (1987c) Cortical blindness in high altitude climbers and trekkers – a report of six cases (abstract), in *Hypoxia, and Cold* (eds. J.R. Sutton, C.S. Houston and G. Coates), Praeger, New York, p. 536.

Hackett, P.H., Roach, R.C., Wood, R.A. *et al.* (1988) Dexamethasone for prevention and treatment of acute mountain sickness. *Aviat. Space Environ. Med.* **59**, 950–4.

Hackett, P.H., Roach, R.C., Hartig, G.S. *et al.* (1992) The effect of vasodilators on pulmonary hemodynamics in high altitude pulmonary edema: a comparison. *Int. J. Sports Med.* **13**, S68–S71.

Hackett, P.H., Yarnell, P.R., Hill, R. *et al.* (1998) High-altitude cerebral edema evaluated with magnetic resonance imaging. *JAMA* **280**, 1920–5.

Haddad, G.G. and Jiang, C. (1993) O_2 deprivation in the central nervous system: on mechanisms of neuronal response, differential sensitivity and injury. *Progr. Neurobiol.* **40**, 277–318.

Haditch, B., Roessler, A. and Hinghofer-Szalkay, H.G. (2007) Renal adrenomedullin and high altitude diuresis. *Physiol. Res.* **56**, 779–87.

Hahn, A.G., Gore, C.J., Martin, D.T. *et al.* (2001) An evaluation of the concept of living at moderate altitude and training at sea level. *Comp. Biochem. Physiol. A Mol. Integr. Physiol.* **128**, 777–89.

Haight, J.S.J. and Keatinge, W.R. (1973) Failure of thermoregulation in the cold during hypoglycaemia induced by exercise and ethanol. *J. Physiol. (Lond)* **229**, 87–97.

Hainsworth, R. and Drinkhill, M.J. (2007) Cardiovascular adjustments for life at high altitude. *Respir. Physiol. Neurobiol.* **158**, 204–11.

Haldane, J. and Lorrain Smith, J. (1897) The absorption of oxygen by the lungs. *J. Physiol. (Lond.)* **22**, 231–58.

Haldane, J.S. and Priestley, J.G. (1935) *Respiration*, 2nd edn, Yale University Press, New Haven, CT.

Haldane, J.S., Kellas, A.M., and Kennaway, E.L. (1919) Experiments on acclimatisation to reduced atmospheric pressure. *J. Physiol. (Lond.)* **53**, 181–206.

Hall, C. (2005) NT-ProBNP: the mechanism behind the marker. *J. Cardiac Failure* **11**, S81–S83.

Hall, F.G. (1936) The effect of altitude on the affinity of hemoglobin for oxygen. *J. Biol. Chem.* **115**, 485–90.

Hall, F.G., Dill, D.B. and Guzman-Barron, E.S. (1936) Comparative physiology in high altitudes. *J. Cell. Comp. Physiol.* **8**, 301–13.

Halperin, B.D., Sun, S., Zhuang, J. *et al.* (1998) ECG observations in Tibetan and Han residents of Lhasa. *J. Electrocardiol.* **31**, 237–43.

Hamilton, R.S. and Paton, B.C. (1996) The diagnosis and treatment of hypothermia by mountain rescue teams: a survey. *Wilderness Environ. Med.* **7**, 28–37.

Hamilton, S.J.C. (1980) Hypothermia and unawareness of mental impairment. *BMJ* **1**, 565.

Hamlet, M.P. (1983) Fluid shifts in hypothermia, in *The Nature and Treatment of Hypothermia* (eds. R.S. Pozos and L.E. Wittmers), Croom Helm, London/ University of Minnesota Press, Minneapolis, pp. 94–9.

Hamlet, M.P., Veghte, J., Bowers, W.D. and Boyce, J. (1977) Thermographic evaluation of experimentally produced frostbite of rabbit feet. *Cryobiology* **14**, 197–204.

Hammel, H.T. (1964) Terrestrial animals in the cold. Recent studies in primitive man, in *Handbook of Physiology: Adaptation to the Environment,* American Physiological Society, Washington DC, pp. 413–34.

Hammond, M.D., Gale, G.E., Kapitan, K.S. *et al.* (1986) Pulmonary gas exchange in humans during normobaric hypoxic exercise. *J. Appl. Physiol.* **61**, 1749–57.

Hanaoka, M., Tanaka, M., Ge, R.L. *et al.* (2000) Hypoxia-induced pulmonary blood redistribution in subjects with a history of high-altitude pulmonary edema. *Circulation* **101**, 1418–22.

Hanaoka, M., Droma, Y., Ota, M. *et al.* (2009) Polymorphisms of human vascular endothelial growth factor gene and high altitude pulmonary edema susceptible subjects. *Respirology* **14**, 46–52.

Handley, A.J., Golden, F. St C., Keatinge, W.R. *et al.* (1993) *Report of the Working Party on Out of Hospital Management of Hypothermia,* Medical Commission on Accident Prevention, UK.

Hann, J. von (1901) *Lehrbuch der Meteorologie,* Tauchnitz, Leipzig. English translation by R.D.C. Ward, MacMillan, New York, 1903, p. 222.

Hannon, J. (1966) High altitude acclimatization in women, in *The Effects of Altitude on Physical Performance* (ed. R. Goddard), Athletic Institute, Chicago, pp. 37–44.

Hannon, J. (1978) Comparative adaptability of young men and women, in *Environmental Stress: Individual Human Adaptation* (eds. L. Folinsby, J. Wagner, J. Borgia *et al.*) Academic Press, New York, pp. 335–60.

Hannon J.P. (1967) High altitude acclimatization in women, in *Proceedings of International Symposium on the Effects of Altitude on Physical Performance,* Athletic Institute, Chicago, pp. 37–44.

Hannon, J.P., Shields, J.L. and Harris, C.W. (1969) Effects of altitude acclimatization on blood composition of women. *J. Appl. Physiol.* **26**, 540–7.

Hannon, J.P., Klain, G.J., Sudman, D.M. and Sullivan, F.J. (1976) Nutritional aspects of high-altitude exposure in women. *Am. J. Clin. Nutr.* **29**, 604–13.

Hanoka, M., Kubo, K., Yamazaki, Y. *et al.* (1998) Association of high altitude pulmonary edema with the major histocompatibility complex. *Circulation* **97**, 1124–8.

Hansen, J. and Sander, M. (2003) Sympathetic neural overactivity in healthy humans after prolonged exposure to hypobaric hypoxia. *J. Physiol (Lond.)* **546**, 921–9.

Hanson, J.E., Vogel, J.A., Stelter, G.P. and Consolazio, F. (1967) Oxygen uptake in man during exhaustive work at sea level and high altitude. *J. Appl. Physiol.* **23**, 511–22.

Harber, M.J., Williams, J.D. and Morton, J.J. (1981) Antidiuretic hormone excretion at high altitude. *Aviat. Space Environ. Med.* **52**, 38–40.

Harbinson, M.J. (1999) William Harvey, hypothermia and battle injuries. *BMJ* **319**, 1561.

Harms, C.A., Babcock, M.A., McClaran, S.R. *et al.* (1997) Respiratory muscle work compromises leg blood flow during maximal exercise. *J. Appl. Physiol.* **82**, 1573–83.

Harms, C.A., Wetter, T.J., St. Croix, C.M. *et al.* (2000) Effects of respiratory muscle work on exercise performance. *J. Appl. Physiol.* **89**, 131–8.

Harnett, R.M., Pruitt, J.R. and Sias, F.R. (1983) A review of the literature concerning resuscitation from hypothermia, Part II. Selected rewarming protocols. *Aviat. Space Environ. Med.* **54**, 487–95.

Harper, A.M. and Glass, H.I. (1965) Effect of alterations in the arterial carbon dioxide tension on the blood flow through the cerebral cortex at normal and low arterial blood pressures. *J. Neurol. Neurosurg. Psychiatry* **28**, 449–52.

Harris, N.S., Wenzel, R.P. and Thomas, S.H. (2003) High altitude headache: efficacy of acetaminophen vs. ibuprofen in a randomized, controlled trial. *J. Emerg. Med.* **24**, 383–7.

Harris, P. (1986) Evolution, hypoxia and high altitude, in *Aspects of Hypoxia* (ed. D. Heath), Liverpool University Press, Liverpool, pp. 207–16.

Harris, P., Castillo, Y., Gibson, K. *et al.* (1970) Succinic and lactic dehydrogenase activity in myocardial homogenates from animals at high and low altitude. *J. Mol. Cell. Cardiol.* **1**, 189–93.

Harrison, G.A., Kuchemann, C.F., Moore, M.A.S. *et al.* (1969) The effects of altitudinal variation in Ethiopian populations. *Philos. Trans. R. Soc. Lond. Ser. B* **256**, 147–82.

Harrison, M.H. (1985) Effects of thermal stress and exercise on blood volume in humans. *Physiol. Rev.* **65**, 149–208.

Hartinger, S., Tapia, V., Carrillo, C. *et al.* (2006) Birth weights at high altitudes in Peru. *Intern. J. Gyne. Obs.* **93**, 275–81.

Hartung, G.H., Myhre, L.G., Nunnerly, S.A. and Tucker, D.M. (1984) Plasma substrate response in men and women during marathon running. *Aviat. Space Environ. Med.* **55**, 128–31.

Hashmi, M.A., Bokjari, S.A.H., Rashid, M. *et al.* (1998) Frostbite: epidemiology at high altitude in the Karakoram mountains. *Ann. R. Coll. Surg.* **80**, 91–5.

Hatcher, J.D. (1965) Acute anoxic anoxia, in *The Physiology of Human Survival* (eds. O.G. Edholm and A.L. Bacharach), Academic Press, London, pp. 81–120.

Hathorn, M.K.S. (1971) The influence of hypoxia on iron absorption in the rat. *Gastroenterology,* **60**, 76–81.

Hayward, J.S. (1997) Inhibition of shivering increases core temperature after-drop and attenuates rewarming in hypothermic humans. *J. Appl. Physiol.* **83**, 1030–4.

Hayward, J.S., Eckerson, J.D. and Kemna, D. (1984) Thermal and cardiovascular changes during three methods of resuscitation from mild hypothermia. *Resuscitation* **11**, 21–33.

Hayward, M.G. and Keatinge, W.R. (1979) Progressive symptomless hypothermia in water. Possible cause of diving accidents. *BMJ* **1**, 1222.

Heath, D. (1986) Carotid body hyperplasia, in *Aspects of Hypoxia* (ed. D. Heath), Liverpool University Press, Liverpool, pp. 61–74.

Heath, D. and Williams, D.R. (1995) *High-Altitude Medicine and Pathology.* Oxford University Press, Oxford.

Heath, D., Edwards, C., Winson, M. and Smith, P. (1973) Effects on the right ventricle, pulmonary vasculature, and carotid bodies of the rat of exposure to, and recovery from, simulated high altitude. *Thorax* **28**, 24–8.

Heaton, J.M. (1972) The distribution of brown adipose tissue in the human. *J. Anat.* **112**, 35–9.

Hebbel, R.P., Eaton, J.W., Kronenberg, R.S. *et al.* (1978) Human llamas: adaptation to altitude in subjects with high hemoglobin oxygen affinity. *J. Clin. Invest.* **62**, 593–600.

Hecht, H.H., Lang, R.L., Carnes, W.H. *et al.* (1959) Brisket disease. I. General aspects of pulmonary hypertensive heart disease in cattle. *Trans. Assoc. Am. Physiol.* **72**, 157–72.

Hecht, H.H., Kuida, H., Lange, R.L. *et al.* (1962) Brisket disease. III. Clinical features and hemodynamic observations in altitude-dependent right heart failure of cattle. *Am. J. Med.* **32**, 171–83.

Heffner, J.E. and Sahn, S.A. (1981) High-altitude pulmonary infarction. *Arch. Intern. Med.* **141**, 1721.

Heggers, J.P., Phillips, L.G., McAuley, R.L. and Robson, M.C. (1990) Frostbite: experimental and clinical evaluation of treatment. *J. Wilderness Med.* **1**, 27–32.

Hellems, H.K., Ord, J.W., Talmers, F.N. and Christensen, R.C. (1957) Effects of hypoxia on coronary blood flow and myocardial metabolism in normal human subjects. *Circulation* **16**, 893.

Hemmingsson, T. and Linnarsson, D. (2009) Lower exhaled nitric oxide in hypobaric than in normobapic hypoxia. Resp Physiol Neurobiol. **169**, 74–77

Henderson, A.F., Heaton, R.W., Dunlop, L.S. and Costello, J.F. (1983) Effects of nifedipine on antigen-induced bronchoconstriction. *Am. Rev. Respir. Dis.* **127**, 549–53.

Henderson, Y. (1919) The physiology of the aviator. *Science* **49**, 431–41.

Henderson, Y. (1939) The last thousand feet on Everest. *Nature* **143**, 921–23.

Hepple, R.T., Agey, P.J., Szewczak, J.M. *et al.* (1998) Increased capillarity in leg muscle of finches living at altitude. *J. Appl. Physiol.* **85**, 1871–6.

Hepple, R.T., Hogan, M.C., Stary, C. *et al.* (2000) Structural basis of muscle O_2 diffusing capacity: evidence from muscle function *in situ*. *J. Appl. Physiol.* **88**, 560–6.

Hergistad, M. and Robbins, P.A. (2009) Pulmonary vascular response to air-breathing exercise in humans following an 8-hour exposure to hypoxia. *Respir. Physiol. Neurobiol.* **169**, 11–15.

Herman, J.K., O'Halloran, K.D. and Bisgard, G.E. (2001) Effect of 8-OH DPAT and detanserin on the ventilatory acclimatization to hypoxia in awake goats. *Respir. Physiol.* **124**, 95–104.

Hernandez, M.J. (1983) Cerebral circulation during hypothermia, in *The Nature and Treatment of Hypothermia* (eds. R.S. Pozos and L.E. Wittmers), Croom Helm, London/University of Minnesota, Minneapolis, pp. 61–8.

Herschkowitz, M. (1977) Penile frostbite: an unforeseen hazard of jogging. *N. Engl. J. Med.* **296**, 178.

Hertzman, A.B. (1957) Individual differences in regional sweating patterns. *J. Appl. Physiol.* **10**, 242–8.

Hervey, G.R. (1973) Physiological changes encountered in hypothermia. *Proc. R. Soc. Med.* **66**, 1053–7.

Hervey, G.R. and Tobin, G. (1983) Luxuskonsumption. Diet-induced thermogenesis and brown fat: a critical review. *Clin. Sci.* **64**, 7–22.

Hetzel, B.S. (1989) *The Story of Iodine Deficiency*, Oxford Medical Publications, Oxford.

Heyman, A., Patterson, J.L. and Duke, T.W. (1952) Cerebral circulation and metabolism in sickle cell and other chronic anemias, with observations on the effects of oxygen inhalation. *J. Clin. Invest.* **31**, 824–8.

Heymans, J.-F. and Heymans, C. (1925) Sur le mécanisme de l'apnée réflexe ou pneumogastrique. *Comptes Rendus Soc. Biol.* **92**, 1335–8.

Heymans, J.-F. and Heymans, C. (1927) Sur les modifications directes et sur la regulation reflexe de l'activité du centre respiratoire de la tête isolée du chien. *Arch. Intern. Pharmacodyn.* **33**, 273–370.

Hildebrandt, W., Ottenbacher, A., Schuster, M. *et al.* (2000) Diuretic effect of hypoxia, hypocapnia, and hyperpnea in humans: relation to hormones and O_2 chemosensitivity. *J. Appl. Physiol.* **88**, 599–610.

Hildebrandt, W., Alexander, S., Bärtsch, P. and Draöge, W. (2002) Effect of *N*-acetyl-cysteine on the hypoxic ventilatory response and erythropoietin production: linkage between plasma thiol redox state and O_2 chemosensitivity. *Blood* **99**, 1552–6.

Hill, A.V. (1928) The diffusion of oxygen and lactic acid through tissues. *Proc. R. Soc. Lond. Ser. B* **104**, 39–96.

Hill, L. (1934) Foreword, in *Oxygen and Carbon Dioxide Therapy* (eds A. Campbell and E.P. Poulton), Oxford University Press, London.

Hinchliff, T.W. (1876) *Over the Sea and Far Away*, Longmans Green, London.

Hinson, J.P., Kapas, S. and Smith, D.M. (2000) Adrenomedullin, a multifunctional regulatory peptide. *Endo. Rev.* **21**, 138–67.

Hirata, K., Matsuyama, S. and Saito, A. (1989) Obesity as a risk factor for acute mountain sickness. *Lancet* **2**, 1040–1.

Hirvonen, J. (1982) Accidental hypothermia, in Report 30, Nordic Council for Arctic Medical Research, Copenhagen, pp. 15–19.

Hlatky, M.A., Quertermous, T., Boothroyd, D.B. *et al.* (2007) Polymorphisms in hypoxia inducible factor 1 and the initial clinical presentation of coronary disease. *Am. Heart J.* **154**, 1035–42.

Ho, T.Y., Kao, W.F., Lee, S.M. *et al.* (2011) High-altitude retinopathy after climbing Mount Aconcagua in a group of experienced climbers. *Retina* **31**, 1650–5.

Hochachka, P.W., Clark, C.M., Stanley, C. *et al.* (1996) ^{31}P Magnetic resonance spectroscopy of the Sherpa heart: a phosphocreatine/adenosine defence against hypobaric hypoxia. *Proc. Natl. Acad. Sci. USA* **93**, 1215–20.

Hodges, J.R. and Warlow, C.P. (1990) Syndromes of transient amnesia: towards a classification. A study of 153 cases. *J. Neurol. Neurosurg. Psychiatry* **53**, 834–43.

Hoff, C.J. and Abelson, A.E. (1976) Fertility, in *Man in The Andes, A Multidisciplinary Study of High-Altitude Quechua* (eds. P.T. Baker and M.A. Little), Dowden, Hutchinson & Ross, Stroudsburg, PA, pp. 128–46.

Hoffman, R.C. and Wittmers, L.E. (1990) Cold vasodilatation, pain and acclimatization in Arctic explorers. *J. Wilderness Med.* **1**, 225–34.

Hogan, M.C., Roca, J., Wagner, P.D. and West, J.B. (1988a) Limitation of maximal O_2 uptake and performance by acute hypoxia in dog muscle *in situ*. *J. Appl. Physiol.* **65**, 815–21.

Hogan, M.C., Roca, J., West, J.B., and Wagner, P.D. (1988b) Dissociation of maximal O_2 uptake from O_2 delivery in canine gastrocnemius *in situ*. *J. Appl. Physiol.* **66**, 1219–26.

Hogan, M.C., Bebout, D.E. and Wagner, P.D. (1991) Effect of increased Hb-O_2 affinity on Vo_{2max} at constant O_2 delivery in dog muscle in situ. *J. Appl. Physiol.* **70**, 2656–62.

Hogan, R.P., Kotchen, T.A., Boyd, A.E. and Hartley, L.H. (1973) Effect of altitude on the renin–aldosterone system and metabolism of water and electrolytes. *J. Appl. Physiol.* **35**, 385–90.

Hohenhaus, E., Niroomand, F.G., Goerre, S. *et al.* (1994) Nifedipine does not prevent acute mountain sickness. *Am. J. Respir. Crit. Care* **150**, 857–60.

Hohenhaus, E., Paul, A., McCullough, R.E. *et al.* (1995) Ventilatory and pulmonary vascular response to hypoxia and susceptibility to high altitude pulmonary oedema. *Eur. Respir. J.* **8**, 1825–33.

Höhne, C., Krebs, M.O., Seiferheld, M. *et al.* (2004) Acetazolamide prevents hypoxic pulmonary vasoconstriction in conscious dogs. *J. Appl. Physiol.* **97**, 515–21.

Höhne, C., Pickerodt, P.A., Francis, R.C.E. *et al.* (2006) Pulmonary vasodilation by acetazolamide during acute hypoxia is not related to carbonic anhydrase inhibition. *Am. J. Physiol. Lung Cell Mol. Physiol.* **292**, L178–84.

Hoit, B.D., Dalton, N.D., Erzurum, S.C. *et al.* (2005) Nitric oxide and cardiopulmonary hemodynamics in Tibetan highlanders. *J. Appl. Physiol.* **99**, 1796–801.

Hoit, B.D., Dalton, N.D., Gebremedhin, A. *et al.* (2011) Elevated pulmonary artery pressure among Amhara highlanders in Ethiopia. *Am. J. Hum. Biol.* **23**, 168–76.

Holden, J.E., Stone, C.K., Clark, M. *et al.* (1995) Enhanced cardiac metabolism of plasma glucose in high-altitude natives: adaptation against chronic hypoxia. *J. Appl. Physiol.* **79**, 222–8.

Holditch, T. (1907) *Tibet the Mysterious*, Alston Rivers, London, pp. 242–3.

Holloszy, J.O. and Coyle, E.F. (1984) Adaptations of skeletal muscle to endurance exercise and their metabolic consequences. *J. Appl. Physiol.* **56**, 831–8.

Holloway, C.J., Montgomery, H.E., Murray, A.J. *et al.* (2011) Cardiac response to hypobaric hypoxia: persistent changes in cardiac mass, function, and energy metabolism after a trek to Mt. Everest Base Camp. *FASEB J.* **25**, 792–6.

Holm, P. (1997) Endothelin in the pulmonary circulation with special reference to hypoxic pulmonary vasoconstriction. *Scand. Cardiovasc. J. Suppl.* **46**, 1–40.

Homik, L.A., Bshouty, Z., Light, R.B. and Younes, M. (1988) Effect of alveolar hypoxia on pulmonary fluid filtration in *in-situ* dog lungs. *J. Appl. Physiol.* **65**, 46–52.

Honda, Y., Watanabe, S., Hashizume, I. *et al.* (1979) Hypoxic chemosensitivity in asthmatic patients two decades after carotid body resection. *J. Appl. Physiol.* **46**, 632–8.

Hong, S.I. and Nadel, E.R. (1979) Thermogenic control during exercise in a cold environment. *J. Appl. Physiol.* **47**, 1084–9.

Hong, S.K. (1973) Pattern of cold adaptation in women divers of Korea. *Fed. Proc.* **32**, 1414–22.

Honig, C.R. and Tenney, S.M. (1957) Determinants of the circulatory response to hypoxia and hypercapnia. *Am. Heart J.* **53**, 687–98.

Honig, C.R., Gayeski, T.E.J. and Groebe, K. (1991) Myoglobin and oxygen gradients, in *The Lung: Scientific Foundations* (eds. R.G. Crystal and J.B. West), Raven Press, New York, pp. 1489–96.

Honigman, B., Theis, M.K., Koziol-McLain, J. *et al.* (1993) Acute mountain sickness in a general tourist population at moderate altitudes. *Ann. Intern. Med.* **118**, 587–92.

Hoon, R.S., Sharma, S.C., Balasubramanian, V. and Chadha, K.S. (1977) Urinary catecholamine excretion on induction to high altitude (3658m) by air and road. *J. Appl. Physiol.* **42**, 728–30.

Hopkins, S.R., Garg, J., Bolar, D.S. *et al.* (2005) Pulmonary blood flow heterogeneity during hypoxia and high-altitude pulmonary edema. *Am. J. Resp. Crit. Care Med.* **171**, 83–7.

Hopkins, S.R. (2010a) Point: pulmonary edema does occur in human athletes performing heavy sea level exercise. *J. Appl. Physiol.* **109**, 1270–2.

Hopkins, S.R. (2010b) Stress failure and high altitude pulmonary edema: mechanistic insights from physiology. *Eur. Respir. J.* **35**, 470–2.

Hopkins, S.R., Olfert, I.M. and Wagner, P.D. (2009) Point–counterpoint: Exercise-induced intrapulmonary shunting is imaginary vs. real. *J. Appl. Physiol.* **107**, 993–4.

Hoppeler, H. (1999) Vascular growth in hypoxic skeletal muscle. *Adv. Exp. Med. Biol.* **474**, 277–86.

Hoppeler, H. and Michael Vogt, M. (2001) Muscle tissue adaptations to hypoxia. *J. Exp. Biol.* **204**, 3133–9.

Hoppeler, H., Kayar, S.R., Claassen, H. *et al.* (1987) Adaptive variation in the mammalian respiratory system in relation to energetic demand: III. Skeletal muscles: setting the demand for oxygen. *Respir. Physiol.* **69**, 27–46.

Hoppeler, H., Howald, H. and Cerretelli, P. (1990) Human muscle structure after exposure to extreme altitude. *Experientia* **46**, 1185–7.

Hoppeler, H., Vogt, M., Weibel, R. and Flück, M. (2003) Response of skeletal muscle mitochondria to hypoxia. *Exp. Physiol.* **88**, 109–19.

Horio, T., Kohno, M., Yokokawa, K. *et al.* (1991) Effect of hypoxia on plasma immunoreactive endothelin-1 concentration in anaesthetized rats. *Metabolism* **40**, 999–1001.

Hornbein, T.F., Townes, B.D., Schoene, R.B. *et al.* (1989) The cost to the central nervous system of climbing to extremely high altitude. *N. Engl. J. Med.* **321**, 1714–19.

Horton, B.T. and Brown, G.E. (1929) Systemic histamine like reactions in allergy due to cold. *Am. J. Med. Sci.* **198**, 191–202.

Horvath, S.M. (1981) Exercise in a cold environment. *Exerc Sport Sci. Rev.* **9**, 191–263.

Hossmann, K.A. (1999) The hypoxic brain. Insights from ischemia research. *Adv. Exp. Med. Biol.* **474**, 155–69.

Hotta, J., Hanaoka, M., Droma, Y. *et al.* (2004) Polymorphisms of renin–angiotensin system genes with high-altitude pulmonary edema in Japanese subjects. *Chest* **126**, 825–30.

Houk, V.N. (1959) Transient pulmonary insufficiency caused by cold. *US Armed Forces Med. J.* **10**, 1354–7.

Houston, C.S. (1960) Acute pulmonary edema of high altitude. *N. Engl. J. Med.* **263**, 478–80.

Houston, C.S. (1987) Transient visual disturbance at high altitude (abstract), in *Hypoxia and Cold* (eds. J.R. Sutton, C.S. Houston and G. Coates), Praeger, New York, p. 536.

Houston, C.S. (1988–9) Operation Everest II – 1985. *Alpine J.* **93**, 196–200.

Houston, C.S. and Bates, R. (1979) *K2, The Savage Mountain*, McGraw-Hill, New York, pp. 180–99.

Houston, C.S. and Dickinson, J. (1975) Cerebral form of high-altitude illness. *Lancet* **2**, 758–61.

Houston, C.S. and Riley, R.L. (1947) Respiratory and circulatory change during acclimatization to high altitude. *Am. J. Physiol.* **149**, 565–88.

Houston, C.S., Sutton, J.R., Cymerman, A. and Reeves, J.T. (1987) Operation Everest II: man at extreme altitude. *J. Appl. Physiol.* **63**, 877–82.

Houston, C.S., Cymerman, A. and Sutton, J.R. (1991) *Operation Everest II: Final Days*, US Army Research Institute of Environmental Medicine, Natick, MA, p. 96.

Howald, H. and Hoppeler, H. (2003) Performing at extreme altitude: muscle cellular and subcellular adaptations. *Eur. J. Appl. Physiol.* **90**, 360–4.

Howald, H., Pette, D., Simoneau, J.A. *et al.* (1990) Effect of chronic hypoxia on muscle enzyme activities. *Int. J. Sports Med.* **11**(Suppl. 1), S10–14.

Howard, L.S.G.E. and Robbins, P.A. (1995) Alterations in respiratory control during 8 h of isocapnic and poikilocapnic hypoxia in humans. *J. Appl. Physiol.* **78**, 1089–107.

Howard-Bury, C.K. (1922) *Mt. Everest: The Reconnaissance, 1921*, Arnold, London.

Howarth, M. (1999) High altitude cerebral oedema – a rescue. *ISMM Newsletter* **9**, 15–17.

Hsu, A.R., Barnholt, K.E., Grundmann, N.K. *et al.* (2006) Sildenafil improves cardiac output and exercise performance during acute hypoxia, but not normoxia. *J. Appl. Physiol.* **100**, 2031–40.

Hu, S.T., Huang, W.Y., Chu, S.C. and Pa, C.F. (1982) Chemoreflexive ventilatory response at sea level in subjects with past history of good acclimatization and severe acute mountain sickness, in *High Altitude Physiology and Medicine* (eds. W. Brendel and R.A. Zink), Springer-Verlag, New York, pp. 28–32.

Huang, S.Y., Ning, X.H., Zhou, Z.N. *et al.* (1984) Ventilatory function in adaptation to high altitude: studies in Tibet, in *High Altitude and Man* (eds. J.B. West and S. Lahiri), American Physiological Society, Bethesda, MD, pp. 173–7.

Huang, S.Y., Moore, L.G., McCullough, R.E. *et al.* (1987) Internal carotid and vertebral arterial flow velocity in men at high altitude. *J. Appl. Physiol.* **63**, 395–400.

Huang, S.Y., Tawney, K.W., Bender, P.R. *et al.* (1991) Internal carotid flow velocity with exercise before and after acclimatization to 4300 m. *J. Appl. Physiol.* **71**, 1469–76.

Huang, S.Y., Sun, S., Droma, T. *et al.* (1992) Internal carotid arterial flow velocity during exercise in Tibetan and Han residents of Lhasa (3,658 m). *J. Appl. Physiol.* **73**, 2638–42.

Hubbard, R.W., Gaffin, S.L. and Squire, D.L. (1995) Heat related illness, in *Wilderness Medicine* (ed. P.S. Auerbach), Mosby, St Louis, pp. 167–212.

Huddleston, B., Ataman, E. and Fè de'Ostiane L (2003) Towards a GIS-based analysis of mountain environments and populations. Working paper #10, UN, FAO, Rome. Available on www. fao.org.

Hüfner, C.G. (1890) Uber das Gesetz der Dissociation des Oxyhämoglobins und über einige daran sich knüpfende wichtige Fragen aus der Biologie. *Arch. Pathol. Anat. Physiol.* 1–27.

Huicho, L. and Niermeyer, S. (2006) Cardiopulmonary pathology among children resident at high altitude in Tintaya, Peru: a cross-sectional study. *High Alt. Med. Biol.* **7**, 168–79.

Hultgren, H. and Spickard, W. (1960) Medical experiences in Peru. *Stanford Med. Bull.* **18**, 97–8.

Hultgren, H., Spickard, W. and Lopez, C. (1962) Further studies of high altitude pulmonary edema. *Br. Heart J.* **24**, 95–102.

Hultgren, H.N. (1969) High altitude pulmonary edema, in *Biomedicine Problems of High Terrestrial Altitude* (ed. A.H. Hegnauer), Springer-Verlag, New York, pp. 131–41.

Hultgren, H.N. (1970) Reduction of systemic arterial blood pressure at high altitude. *Adv. Cardiol.* **5**, 49–55.

Hultgren, H.N. (1978) High altitude pulmonary edema, in *Lung Water and Solute Exchange* (ed. N.C. Staub), Dekker, New York, pp. 437–69.

Hultgren, H.N. (1992) Effect of altitude on cardio-vascular diseases. *J. Wilderness Med.* **3**, 301–8.

Hultgren, H.N. (1997) *High Altitude Medicine*, Hultgren Publications, Stanford, CA, p. 12.

Hultgren, H.N., Spickard, W.B., Hellriegel, K. *et al.* (1961) High altitude pulmonary edema. *Medicine (Baltimore)* **40**, 289–313.

Hultgren, H.N., Lopez, C.E., Lundberg, E. and Miller, H. (1964) Physiologic studies of pulmonary edema at high altitude. *Circulation* **29**, 393–408.

Hultgren, H.N., Robison, M.C. and Wuerflein, R.D. (1966) Over perfusion pulmonary edema. *Circulation* **34**(Suppl. 3), 132–3.

Hultgren, H.N., Wilson, R. and Kosek, J.C. (1997) Lung pathology in high-altitude pulmonary edema. *Wilderness. Environ. Med.* **8**, 218–20.

Hunt, J. (1953) *The Ascent of Everest*, Hodder and Stoughton, London.

Hunter, J. (1781) *Original Cases*, Library of Royal College of Surgeons of England, London.

Hunter, J., Kerr, E.H. and Whillans, M.G. (1952) The relation between joint stiffness upon exposure to cold and the characteristics of synovial fluid. *J. Can. Med. Sci.* **39**, 367–77.

Huonker, M., Schmidt-Trucksass, A., Sorichter, S. *et al.* (1997) Highland mountain hiking and coronary artery disease: exercise tolerance and effects on left ventricular function. *Med. Sci. Sports Exerc.* **29**, 1554–60.

Hupperets, M.D., Hopkins, S.R., Pronk, M.G. *et al.* (2004) Increased hypoxic ventilatory responses during 8 weeks at 3800m altitude. *Respir. Physiol. Neurobiol.* **142**, 145–52.

Hurtado, A. (1942) Chronic mountain sickness. *JAMA* **120**, 1278–82.

Hurtado, A. (1964) Animals in high altitudes: resident man, in *Handbook of Physiology, Section IV, Adaptation to the Environment* (ed. D.B. Dill), American Physiological Society, Washington DC, pp. 843–60.

Hurtado, A. (1971) The influence of high altitude on physiology, in *High Altitude Physiology* (eds. R. Porter and J. Knight), Ciba Foundation Symposium, Churchill Livingstone, Edinburgh, pp. 3–13.

Hurtado, A., Rotta, A., Merino, C. and Pons, J. (1937) Studies of myohemoglobin at high altitude. *Am. J. Med. Sci.* **194**, 708–13.

Hurtado, A., Merino, C. and Delgado, E. (1945) Influence of anoxemia on the hemopoietic activity. *Arch. Intern. Med.* **75**, 284–323.

Hussein, M.M., Bakir, N. and Roujouleh, H. (1992) Low-dose recombinant human erythropoietin in dialysis patients living at high altitude. *Nephrol. Dial. Transplant.* **7**, 173–4.

Hutchinson, S.J. and Litch, J.A. (1997) Acute myocardial infarction at high altitude. *JAMA* **278**, 1661–2.

Hyde, R.W., Forster, R.E., Power, G.G. *et al.* (1966) Measurement of O_2 diffusing capacity of the lungs with a stable O_2 isotope. *J. Clin. Invest.* **45**, 1178–93.

Iaia, F.M., Hellsten, Y., Nielsen, J.J. *et al.* (2009) Four weeks of speed endurance training reduces energy expenditure during exercise and maintains muscle oxidative capacity despite a reduction in training volume. *J. Appl. Physiol.* **106**, 73–80.

Ibbertson, H.K., Tair, J.M., Pearl, M. *et al.* (1972) Himalayan cretinism. *Adv. Exp. Med. Biol.* **30**, 51–69.

ICAO (1964) *Manual of the ICAO Standard Atmosphere*, 2nd edn, International Civil Aviation Organization, Montreal, Canada.

Ignarro, L.J., Buga, GM., Wood, K.S. *et al.* (1987) Endothelium-derived relaxing factor produced and released from artery and vein is nitric oxide. *Proc. Natl. Acad. Sci. USA* **84**, 9265–9.

Ikawa, G., Dos Santos, P.A.L., Yamaguchi, K.T. *et al.* (1986) Frostbite and bone scanning: the use of ^{99}m-labelled phosphates in demarcating the line of viability in frostbite victims. *Orthopaedics* **9**, 1257–61.

Iliff, L.D. (1971) Extra-alveolar vessels and edema development in excised dog lungs. *Circ. Res.* **28**, 524–32.

Imray, C.H., Chesner, I., Winterbourn, M. *et al.* (1992) Fat absorption at altitude: a reappraisal. *Int. J. Sports Med.* **13**, 87.

Imray, C.H., Brearey, S., Clarke, T. *et al.* (2000) Cerebral oxygenation at high altitude and the response to carbon dioxide, hyperventilation and oxygen. *Clin. Sci.* **98**, 159–64.

Imray, C.H., Walsh, S., Clarke, T. *et al.* Birmingham Medical Research Expeditionary Society. (2003) Effects of breathing air containing 3% carbon dioxide, 35% oxygen or a mixture of 3% carbon dioxide/35% oxygen on cerebral and peripheral oxygenation at 150 m and 3459 m. *Clin. Sci. (Lond.)* **104**, 203–10.

Imray, C.H.E., Richards, P., Greeves, J. *et al.* (2011) Non-freezing cold injuries. *J. R. Army Med. Corps* **157**, 79–84.

Ind, P.W., Maxwell, D.L., Causon, R.C. *et al.* (1984) Hypoxia and catecholamine secretion in normal man. *Clin. Sci.* **67**, 58–59P.

Ingjer, F. and Brodal, P. (1978) Capillary supply of skeletal muscle fibers in untrained and endurance-trained women. *Eur. J. Appl. Physiol.* **38**, 291–9.

Ingjer, F. and Myhre, K. (1992) Physiological effects of altitude training on elite male cross-country skiers. *J. Sports Sci.* **10**, 37–47.

Insalaco, G., Romano, S., Salvaggio, A. *et al.* (2000) Blood pressure and heart rate during periodic breathing while asleep at high altitude. *J. Appl. Physiol.* **89**, 947–55.

Irwin, B.C., McCord, J.M., Nozik-Grayck, E. *et al.* (2009) A potential role for reactive oxygen species and the HIF-1 Alpha-VEGF pathway hypoxia-induced pulmonary vascular leak. *Free Rad. Biol. Med.* **47**, 55–61.

Irwin, D.C., Subudhi, A.W., Klopp, L. *et al.* (2008) Pulmonary edema induced by cerebral hypoxic insult in a canine model. *Aviat. Environ. Med.* **79**, 472–8.

Irwin, D.C., McCord, J.M., Nozik-Grayek, E. *et al.* (2009) Potential role for reactive oxygen species in the HIF-1 a-DEGF pathway and hypoxia-induced pulmonary vascular leak. *Free Rad. Biol. Med.* **47**, 55–61.

Irwin, M.S., Thorniley, M.S. and Green, C.J. (1994) An investigation into the aetiology of non-freezing cold injury using infrared spectroscopy. *Biochem. Soc. Trans.* **22**, 418S.

Irwin, M.S., Sanders, R., Gren, C.J. and Terenghi, G. (1997) Neuropathy in non-freezing injuries (trench foot). *J. R. Soc. Med.* **90**, 433–8.

Ishizaki, T., Koizumi, T., Ruan, Z. *et al.* (2005) Nitric oxide inhibitor altitude-dependently elevates pulmonary arterial pressure in high-altitude adapted yaks. *Respir. Physiol. Neurobiol.* **146**, 225–30.

ISMM Newsletter (1998) The combined oral contraceptive (COC) at altitude – is it safe? (10 discussants). *ISMM Newsletter* **8**, 11–13.

Itskovitz, J., LaCamma, E.F. and Rudolph, A.M. (1987) Effects of cord compression on fetal blood flow distribution and O_2 delivery. *Am. J. Physiol. (Heart Circ. Physiol.)* **21**, H100–9.

Iwasaki, K., Zhang, R., Zuckerman, J.H. *et al.* (2011) Impaired dynamic cerebral autoregulation at extreme altitude even after acclimatization. *J. Cereb. Blood Flow Metab.* **31**, 283–92.

Jackson, F. and Davies, H. (1960) The electrocardiogram of the mountaineer at high altitude. *Br. Heart J.* **22**, 671–85.

Jackson, F.S. (1968) The heart at high altitude. *Br. Heart J.* **30**, 291–4.

Jackson, F.S., Turner, R.W.D. and Ward, M.P. (1966) *Report on IBP Expedition to North Bhutan,* Royal Society, London.

Jackson, J.A. (1975) Avoidance of cold injury. Outline of basic principles, in *Mountain Medicine and Physiology* (eds. C. Clarke, M.P.

Ward and E.S. Williams), Alpine Club, London, pp. 28–30.

Jafarian, S., Gorouhi, F., Salimi, S. and Lotfi, J. (2007) Sumatriptan for prevention of acute mountain sickness: Randomized clinical trial. *Ann. Neurol.* **62**, 273–7.

Jain, S.C., Singh, M.V., Sharma, V.M. *et al.* (1986) Amelioration of acute mountain sickness: comparative study of acetazolamide and spironolactone. *Int. J. Biometeorol.* **30**, 293–300.

James, M.F., Manson, E.D. and Dennett, J.E. (1982) Nitrous oxide analgesia and altitude. *Anaesthesia* **37**, 285–8.

Jansen, G.F., Krins, A. and Basnyat, B. (1999) Cerebral vasomotor reactivity at high altitude in humans. *J. Appl. Physiol.* **86**, 681–6.

Jansson, E., Sylven, C. and Nordevang, E. (1982) Myoglobin in the quadriceps femoris muscle of competitive cyclists and untrained men. *Acta Physiol. Scand.* **114**, 627–9.

Jean, D. and Moore, L.G. (2012) Travel to high altitude during pregnancy: frequently asked questions and recommendations for clinicians. *High Alt. Med. Biol.* **13**, 73–81.

Jean, D., Leal, C., Kriemler, S. *et al.* (2005) Medical recommendations for women going to altitude. *High Alt. Med. Biol.* **6**, 22–31.

Jedlickova, K., Stockton, D.W., Chen, H. *et al.* (2003) Search for genetic determinants of individual variability of the erythropoietin response to high altitude. *Blood Cells Mol. Dis.* **31**, 175–82.

Jefferson, J.A., Escudero, E., Hertardo, M.E. *et al.* (2002a) Hyperuricemia, hypertension and proteinuria associated with high-altitude polycythemia. *Am. J. Kidney Dis.* **39**, 1135–42.

Jefferson, J.A., Escudero, E., Hurtado, M.-E. *et.al.* (2002b) Excessive erythrocytosis, chronic mountain sickness, and serum cobalt levels. *Lancet* **359**, 407–8.

Jehle, D., Moscati, R., Frye, J. and Reich, N. (1994) The incidence of spontaneous subarachnoid hemorrhage with change in barometric pressure. *Am. J. Emerg. Med.* **12**, 90–1.

Jelkmann, W. and Lundby, C. (2011) Blood doping and its detection. *Blood* **118**, 2395–404.

Jensen, G.M. and Moore, L.G. (1997) The effect of high altitude and other risk factors on birthweight: independent or interactive effect. *Am. J. Public Health* **87**, 1003–7.

Jensen, J.B., Wright, A.D., Lassen, N.A. *et al.* (1990) Cerebral blood flow in acute mountain sickness. *J. Appl. Physiol.* **69**, 430–3.

Jenzer, G. and Bärtsch, P. (1993) Migraine with aura at high altitude: case report. *J. Wilderness. Med.* **4**, 412–15.

Jequier, E., Gygax, P-H., Pittet, P. and Vannotti, A. (1974) Increased thermal body insulation: relationship to the development of obesity. *J. Appl. Physiol.* **36**, 674–8.

Jessen, K. and Hagelstein, J.O. (1978) Peritoneal dialysis in the treatment of profound accidental hypothermia. *Aviat. Space Environ. Med.* **49**, 424–9.

Jha, S.K., Anand, A.C., Sharma, V. *et al.* (2002) Stroke at high altitude: Indian experience. *High Alt. Med. Biol.* **3**, 21–7.

Jiang, C., Liu, F., Luo, Y. *et al.* (2012) Gene expression profiling of high altitude polycythemia in Han Chinese migrating to the Qinghai-Tibetan plateau. *Mol. Med. Rep.* **5**, 287–93.

Jiménez, D. (1995) High altitude intermittent chronic exposure: Andean miners, in *Hypoxia and the Brain* (eds. J.R. Sutton, C.S. Houston and G. Coates), Queen City Printers, Burlington, VT, pp. 284–91.

Joern, A.T., Shurley, J.T., Brooks, R.E. *et al.* (1970) Short-term changes in sleep patterns on arrival at the South Polar Plateau. *Arch. Inern. Med.* **125**, 649–54.

Johnson, B.D., Babcock, M.A., Suman, O.E. and Dempsey, J.A. (1993) Exercise-induced diaphragmatic fatigue in healthy humans. *J. Physiol.* **460**, 385–405.

Johnson, P.L., Popa, D.A., Prisk, G.K. *et al.* (2010) Non-invasive positive pressure ventilation during sleep at 3800 m: Relationship to acute mountain sickness and sleeping oxyhaemoglobin saturation. *Respirology* **15**, 277–82.

Johnson, P.L., Edwards, N., Burgess, K.R. and Sullivan, C.E. (2010a) Sleep architecture changes during a trek from 1400 to 5000 m in the Nepal Himalaya. *J.Sleep Res.* **9**, 148–56.

Johnson, P.L., Popa, D.A., Prisk, G.K. *et al.* (2010b) Non-invasive positive pressure

ventilation during sleep at 3800 m: Relationship to acute mountain sickness and sleeping oxyhaemoglobin saturation. *Respirology* **15**, 277–82.

Johnson, R.L. Jr, Cassidy, S.S., Grover, R.E. *et al.* (1985) Functional capacities of lungs and thorax in beagles after prolonged residence at 3,100 m. *J. Appl. Physiol.* **59**, 1773–82.

Johnson, T.S., Rock, P.B., Fulco, C.S. *et al.* (1984) Prevention of acute mountain sickness by dexamethasone. *N. Engl. J. Med.* **310**, 683–6.

Jones, J.E., Muza, S.R., Fulco, C.S. *et al.* (2008) Intermittent hypoxic exposure does not improve sleep at 4300 m. *High Alt. Med. Biol.* **9**, 281–7.

Jones, N.M. and Bergeron, M. (2001) Hypoxic preconditioning induces changes in HIF-1 target genes in neonatal rat brain. *J. Cereb. Blood Flow. Metab.* **21**, 1105–14.

Jones, R.M., Terhaard, J., Zullo, J. and Tenney, S.M. (1981) Mechanism of reduced water intake in rats at high altitude. *Am. J. Physiol.* **240**, R187–91.

Joseph, V., Soliz, J., Pequignot, J. *et al.* (2000) Gender differentiation of the chemoreflex during growth at high altitude: functional and neurochemical studies. *Am. J. Physiol. Regul. Integr. Comp. Physiol.* **278**, R806–16.

Joseph, V., Pequignot, J.M. and Van Reeth, O. (2002) Neurochemical perspectives on the control of breathing during sleep. *Respir. Physiol. Neurobiol.* **130**, 253–63.

Josephson, M.E. and Wellens, H.J. (eds.) (1984) *Tachycardia: Mechanisms, Diagnosis, Treatment,* Lea and Febiger, Philadelphia, PA.

Jourdanet, D. (1875) *Influence de la Pression de l'Air sur la Vie de l'Homme,* Masson, Paris.

Julian, C.G., Gore, C.J., Wilber, R.L. *et al.* (2004) Intermittent normobaric hypoxia does not alter performance or erythropoietic markers in highly trained distance runners. *J. Appl. Physiol.* **96**, 1800–7.

Julian, C.G., Galan, H.L., Wilson, M.J. *et al.* (2008) Lower uterine artery blood flow and higher endothelin relative to nitric oxide metabolite levels are associated with reductions in birth weight at high altitude.

Am. J. Physiol. Regul. Integr. Comp. Physiol. **295**, R906–15.

Julian, C.G., Subudhi, A.W., Wilson, M.J. *et al.* (2011) Acute mountain sickness, inflammation, and permeability: new insights from a blood biomarker study. *J. Appl. Physiol.* **111**, 392–9.

Juniper, E.F. and Hargreave, F.E. (1986) Airway responsiveness assessed by aerosol inhalation tests: variability in results due to unexpected differences between calibrated nebulizers. *J. Allergy Clin. Immunol.* **78**, 387–91.

Kacimi, R., Richalet, J.-P., Corsin, A. *et al.* (1992) Hypoxia-induced downregulation of β-adrenergic receptors in rat heart. *J. Appl. Physiol.* **73**, 1377–82.

Kallenberg, K., Bailey, D.M., Christ, S. *et al.* (2007) Magnetic resonance imaging evidence of cytotoxic cerebral edema in acute mountain sickness. *J. Cereb. Blood Flow Metab.* **27**, 1064–71.

Kallenberg, K., Dehnert, C., Dorfler, A. *et al.* (2008) Microhemorrhages in non-fatal high-altitude cerebral edema. *J. Cereb. Blood Flow Metab.* **28**, 1635–42.

Kalson, N.S., Davies, A.J., Stokes, S. *et al.* (2007) Climbers with diabetes do well on Mount Kilimanjaro. *Diabet. Med.* **24**, 1496.

Kalson, N.S., Thompson, J., Davie, A.J. *et al.* (2009) The effect of angiotensin-converting enzyme genotype on acute mountain sickness and summit success in trekkers attempting the summit of Mt. Kilimanjaro (5,895 m). *Eur. J. Appl. Physiol.* **105**, 373–9.

Kalson, N.S., Hext, F., Davies, A,J. and Chan, C.W. (2010) Do changes in gastro-intestinal blood flow explain high-altitude anorexia? *Eur. J. Clin. Invest.* **40**, 735–41.

Kamat, S.R. and Banerji, B.C. (1972) Study of cardiopulmonary function on exposure to high altitude. I. Acute acclimatization to an altitude of 3,500 to 4,000 meters in relation to altitude sickness and cardiopulmonary function. *Am. Rev. Respir. Dis.* **106**, 404–13.

Kamin, W., Fleck, B., Rose, D.M. *et al.* (2006) Predicting hypoxia in cystic fibrosis patients during exposure to high altitudes. *J. Cyst. Fibros.* **5**, 223–8.

Kaminsky, D.A., Irvin, C.G., Gurka, D.A. *et al.* (1995) Peripheral airways responsiveness to cool, dry air in normal and asthmatic individuals. *Am. J. Respir. Crit. Care Med.* **152**, 1784–90.

Kapanci, Y., Assimacopoulos, A., Irle, C. *et al.* (1974) 'Contractile interstitial cells' in pulmonary alveolar septa: a possible regulator of ventilation–perfusion ratio? Ultrastructural, immunofluorescence, and in vitro studies. *J. Cell Biol.* **60**, 375–92.

Kaplan, L.A. (1992) Suntan, sunburn and sun protection. *J. Wilderness Med.* **3**, 173–96.

Kapoor, A.K., Kshatriya, G.K. and Kapoor, S. (2003) Fertility and mortality differentials among the population groups of the Himalayas. *Hum Biol.* **75**, 729–47.

Kapoor, S.C. (1984) Changes in electrocardiogram among temporary residents at high altitude. *Defence Sci. J.* **34**, 389–95.

Kappes, B.W. and Mills, W.J. (1984) Thermal biofeedback training with frostbite patients (abstract). *Sixth International Symposium on Circumpolar Health,* 13–18 May, Anchorage, Alaska, p. 100.

Karinen, H., Peltonen, J. and Tikkanen, H. (2008) Prevalence of acute mountain sickness among Finnish trekkers on Mount Kilimanjaro, Tanzania: an observational study. *High Alt. Med. Biol.* **9**, 301–6.

Karinen, H.M., Peltonen, J.E., Kahonen, M. and Tikkanen, H.O. (2010) Prediction of acute mountain sickness by monitoring arterial oxygen saturation during ascent. *High Alt. Med. Biol.* **11**, 325–32.

Karliner, J., Sarnquist, F.H., Graber, D.J. *et al.* (1985) The electrocardiogram at extreme altitude: experience on Mt. Everest. *Am. Heart J.* **109**, 505–13.

Kasch, F.W., Boyer, J.L., Van Camp, S. *et al.* (1995) Cardiovascular changes with age and exercise. A 28-year longitudinal study. *Scan. J. Med. Sci. Sports.* **5**, 147–51.

Katayama, K., Amann, M., Pegelow, D.F. *et al.* (2007) Effect of arterial oxygenation on quadriceps fatiguability during isolated muscle exercise. *Am. J. Physiol. Regul. Integ. Comp. Physiol.* **292**, R1279–R1286.

Katayama, K., Matsuo, H., Ishida, K. *et al.* (2003) Intermittent hypoxia improves endurance performance and submaximal exercise efficiency. *High Alt. Med. Biol.* **4**, 291–304.

Katayama, K., Sato, K. and Hotta, N. (2007) Intermittent hypoxia does not increase exercise ventilation at simulated moderate altitude. *Int. J. Sports Med.* **28**, 480–7.

Kato, M. and Staub, N.C. (1966) Response of small pulmonary arteries to unilobar hypoxia and hypercapnia. *Circ. Res.* **19**, 426–40.

Kaufmann, P.A., Schirlo, C., Pavlicek, V. *et al.* (2001) Increased myocardial blood flow during acute exposure to simulated altitudes. *J. Nucl. Cardiol.* **8**, 158–64.

Kawashima, A., Kubo, K., Matsuwara, Y. *et al.* (1992) Hypoxia-induced ANP secretion in subjects susceptible to high-altitude pulmonary edema. *Respir. Physiol.* **89**, 309–17.

Kay, J.M. and Edwards, F.R. (1973) Ultrastructure of the alveolar-capillary wall in mitral stenosis. *J. Pathol.* **111**, 239–45.

Kay, J.M., Waymire, J.C. and Grover, R.F. (1974) Lung mast cell hyperplasia and pulmonary histamine-forming capacity in hypoxic rats. *Am. J. Physiol.* **226**, 178–84.

Kayser, B. (1991) Acute mountain sickness in Western tourists around the Thorong pass (5400m) in Nepal. *J. Wilderness Med.* **2**, 110–17.

Kayser, B. (1996) Lactate during exercise at high altitude. *Eur. J. Appl Physiol. Occup. Physiol.* **74**, 195–205.

Kayser, B., Hoppeler, H., Desplances, H. and Cerretelli, P. (1991) Muscle ultrastructure and biochemistry of lowland Tibetans. *J. Appl. Physiol.* **70**, 1938–42.

Kayser, B., Acheson, K., Decombaz, J. *et al.* (1992) Protein absorption and energy digestibility at high altitude. *J. Appl. Physiol.* **73**, 2425–31.

Kayser, B., Binzoni, T., Hoppeler, H. *et al.* (1993a) A case of severe frostbite on Mt Blanc: a multi-technique approach. *J. Wilderness Med.* **4**, 167–74.

Kayser, B., Narici, M.V. and Cibella, F. (1993b) Fatigue and performance at high altitude, in *Hypoxia and Molecular Medicine* (eds. J.R. Sutton, C.S. Houston and G. Coates), Queen City Printers, Burlington, VT, pp. 222–34.

Kayser, B., Hoppeler, H., Claassen, C. *et al.* (1996) Muscle structure and performance capacity of Himalayan Sherpas. *J. Appl. Physiol.* **81**, 419–25.

Kayser, B., Hulsebosch, R. and Bosch, F. (2008) Low-dose acetylsalicylic acid analog and acetazolamide for prevention of acute mountain sickness. *High Alt. Med. Biol.* **9**, 15–23.

Kayser, B., Aliverti, A., Pellegrino, R. *et al.* (2010) Comparison of a visual analogue scale and Lake Louise symptom scores for acute mountain sickness. *High Alt. Med. Biol.* **11**, 69–72.

Kayser, B., Dumont, L., Lysakowski, C. *et al.* (2012) Reappraisal of acetazolamide for the prevention of acute mountain sickness: A systematic review and meta-analysis. *High Alt. Med. Biol.* **13**, 82–92.

Kearney, M.S. (1973) Ultrastructural changes in the heart at high altitude. *Pathol. Microbiol.* **39**, 258–65.

Keatinge, W.R. and Cannon, P. (1960) Freezing point of human skin. *Lancet* **1**, 11–14.

Keatinge, W.R., Hayward, M.G. and McIver, N.K.I. (1980) Hypothermia during saturation diving in the North Sea. *BMJ* **1**, 291.

Keatinge, W.R., Coleshaw, S.R.K., Cotter, F. *et al.* (1984) Increases in platelet and red cell counts, blood viscosity and arterial pressure during mild surface cooling: factors in mortality from coronary and cerebral thrombosis in winter. *BMJ* **2**, 1405–8.

Keatinge, W.R., Coleshaw, S.R.K., Millard, C.E. and Axelsson, J. (1986) Exceptional case of survival in cold water. *BMJ* **292**, 171–2.

Keighley, J.H. and Steele, G. (1981) The functional and design requirements of clothing. *Alpine J.* **86**, 138–45.

Kellas, A.M. (1912) The mountains of Northern Sikkim and Garwal. *Alpine J.* **26**, 113–42.

Kellas, A.M. (2001) A consideration of the possibility of ascending Mount Everest. *High Alt. Med. Biol.* **2**, 431–61.

Kellogg, R.H. (1963) The role of CO_2 in altitude acclimatization, in *The Regulation of Human Respiration* (eds. D.J.C. Cunningham and B.B. Lloyd), Blackwell Scientific Publications, Oxford, pp. 379–94.

Kellogg, R.H. (1980) Acid–base balance in high altitude: historical perspective, in *Environmental Physiology: Aging, Heat and*

Altitude (eds. S.M. Horvath and M.K. Yousef), Elsevier, New York, pp. 295–308.

Kelly, K.R., Williamson, D.L., Early, C.E. *et al.* (2010) Acute altitude-induced hypoxia suppresses plasma glucose and leptin in healthy humans. *Metabolism* **57**, 200–5.

Kelly, T.E. and Hackett, P.H. (2010) Acetazolamide and sulfonamide allergy: a not so simple story. *High Alt. Med. Biol.* **11**, 319–23.

Kelman, C.R. (1966a) Digital computer subroutine for the conversion of oxygen tension into saturation. *J. Appl. Physiol.* **21**, 1375–6.

Kelman, C.R. (1966b) Calculation of certain indices of cardio-pulmonary function using a digital computer. *Respir. Physiol.* **1**, 335–43.

Kelman, C.R. (1967) Digital computer procedure for the conversion of Pco_2 into blood CO_2 content. *Respir. Physiol.* **3**, 335–43.

Kennedy, B.C. and Gentle, D.A. (1995) Children in the wilderness, in *Wilderness Medicine* (ed. P.S. Auerbach), Mosby, St Louis, pp. 466–89.

Kennedy, R.S., Dunlap, W.P., Banderet, L.E. *et al.* (1989) Cognitive performance deficits in a simulated climb of Mount Everest: Operation Everest II. *Aviat. Space Environ. Med.* **60**, 99–104.

Kerem, D. and Elsner, R. (1973) Cerebral tolerance to asphyxial hypoxia in the harbor seal. *Respir. Physiol.* **19**, 188–200.

Kerendi, F., Halkos, M.E., Kin, H. *et al.* (2005) Upregulation of hypoxia inducible factor is associated with attenuation of neuronal injury in neonatal piglets undergoing deep hypothermic circulatory arrest. *J. Thorac. Cardiovasc. Surg.* **130**, 1079.

Kety, S.S. (1950) Circulation and metabolism of the human brain in health and disease. *Am. J. Med.* **8**, 205–17.

Keyes, L.E., Armaza, J.F., Niermeyer, S. *et al.* (2003) Intrauterine growth restriction, preeclampsia, and intrauterine mortality at high altitude in Bolivia. *Pediatr. Res.* **54**, 20–5.

Keynes, R.J., Smith, G.W., Slater, J.D.H. *et al.* (1982) Renin and aldosterone at high altitude in man. *J. Endocrinol.* **92**, 131–40.

Keys, A. (1936) The physiology of life at high altitude: the International High Altitude Expedition to Chile 1935. *Sci. Mon.* **43**, 289–312.

Keys, A., Hall, F.G. and Guzman Barron, E.S. (1936) The position of the oxygen dissociation curve of human blood at high altitude. *Am. J. Physiol.* **115**, 292–307.

Keys, A., Stapp, J.P. and Violante, A. (1943) Responses in size, output and efficiency of the human heart to acute alteration in the composition of inspired air. *Am. J. Physiol.* **138**, 763–71.

Khanna, P.K., Dham, S.K. and Hoon, R.S. (1976) Exercise in an hypoxic environment as a screening test for ischaemic heart disease. *Aviat. Space Environ. Med.* **47**, 1114–17.

Khoo, M.C., Anholm, J.D., Ko, S.W. *et al.* (1996) Dynamics of periodic breathing and arousal during sleep at extreme altitude. *Respir. Physiol.* **103**, 33–43.

Khoo, M.C.K., Kronauer, R.E., Strohl, K.P. and Slutsky, A.S. (1982) Factors inducing periodic breathing in humans: a general model. *J. Appl. Physiol.* **53**, 644–59.

Khoury, G.H. and Hawes, C.R. (1963) Primary pulmonary hypertension in children living at high altitude. *J. Pediatrics* **62**, 177–85.

Kim, J.-W., Tchernyshyov, I., Semenza, G.L. *et al.* (2006) HIF-1-mediated expression of pyruvate dehydrogenase kinase: a metabolic switch required for cellular adaptation to hypoxia. *Cell. Metab.* **3**, 177–85.

King, B.R., Goss, P.W., Paterson, M.A. *et al.* (2011) Changes in altitude cause unintended insulin delivery from insulin pumps: mechanisms and implications. *Diabetes Care* **34**, 1932–3.

Klausen, K. (1966) Cardiac output in man in rest and work during and after acclimatization to 3800m. *J. Appl. Physiol.* **21**, 609–16.

Kleger, G.-R., Bärtsch, P., Vock, P. *et al.* (1996) Evidence against an increase in capillary permeability in subjects exposed to high altitude. *J. Appl. Physiol.* **81**, 1917–23.

Kline, D.D., Peng, Y.J., Manalo, J. *et al.* (2002) Defective carotid body function and impaired ventilatory response to chronic hypoxia in mice partially deficient for hypoxia-inducible factor 1α. *Proc. Natl. Acad. Sci. USA* **99**, 821–6.

Klokker, M., Kharazmi, A., Galbo, H. *et al.* (1993) Influence of *in vivo* hypobaric hypoxia on function of lymphocytes, natural killer cells, and cytokines. *J. Appl. Physiol.* **74**, 1100–6.

Klyce, S.D. (1981) Stromal lactate accumulation can account for corneal oedema osmotically following epithelial hypoxia in the rabbit. *J. Physiol.* **321**, 49–64.

Knaupp, W., Khilnani, S., Sherwood, J. *et al.* (1992) Erythropoietin response to acute normobaric hypoxia in humans. *J. Appl. Physiol.* **73**, 837–40.

Knill, R.L. and Celb, A.W. (1978) Ventilatory responses to hypoxia and hypercapnia during halothane sedation and anaesthesia in man. *Anesthesiology* **49**, 244–51.

Knochel, J.P. (1989) Heat stroke and related heat stress disorders. *Dis. Mon.* **35**, 301–77.

Kobrick, J.L. (1972) Effects of hypoxia on voluntary response time to peripheral stimuli during central target monitoring. *Ergonomics* **15**, 147–56.

Kobrick, J.L. (1975) Effects of hypoxia on peripheral visual response to dim stimuli. *Percept. Mot. Skills* **41**, 467–74.

Kobza, R., Duru, F. and Erne, P. (2008) Leisure-time activities of patients with ICDs: findings of a survey with respect to sports activity, high altitude stays, and driving patterns. *Pacing Clin. Electrophysiol.* **31**, 845–9.

Koehle, M.S., Wang, P., Guenette, J.A. and Rupert, J.L. (2006) No association between variants in the ACE and angiotensin II receptor 1 genes and acute mountain sickness in Nepalese pilgrims to the Janai Purnima Festival at 4380 m. *High Alt. Med. Biol.* **7**, 281–9.

Koehle, M.S., Guenette, J.A. and Warburton, D.E. (2010) Oximetry, heart rate variability, and the diagnosis of mild-to-moderate acute mountain sickness. *Eur. J. Emerg. Med.* **17**, 119–22.

Kohlendorfer, U., Kiechl, S. and Sperl. W (1998) Living at high altitude and risk of sudden infant death syndrome. *Arch. Dis. Child.* **79**, 506–9.

Kohler, M., Kriemler, S., Wilhem, E.M. *et al.* (2008) Children at high altitude have less nocturnal periodic breathing than adults. *Eur. Respir. J.* **32**, 189–97.

Koistinen, P., Takala, T., Martikkala, V. and Leppalouto, J. (1995) Aerobic fitness influences the response of maximal oxygen uptake and lactate threshold in acute hypobaric hypoxia. *Int. J. Sports Med.* **26**, 78–81.

Koistinen, P.Q., Rusko, H., Irjala, K. *et al.* (2000) EPO, red cells, and serum transferring receptor in continuous and intermittent hypoxia. *Med. Sci. Sports Exerc.* **32**, 800–4.

Koizumi, T., Kawashima, A., Kubo, K. *et al.* (1994) Radiographic and hemodynamic changes during recovery from high-altitude pulmonary edema. *Intern Med.* **33**, 525–8.

Koizumi, T., Ruan, Z., Sakai, A. *et al.* (2004) Contribution of nitric oxide to adaptation of Tibetan sheep to high altitude. *Respir. Physiol. Neurobiol.* **140**, 189–96.

Kong, F.-Y., Li, Q. and Liu, S.-X. (2011) Poor sleep quality predicts decreased cognitive function independently of chronic mountain sickness score in young soldiers with polycythemia stationed in Tibet. *High Alt. Med. Biol.* **12**, 237–42.

Kontos, H.A. and Lower, R.R. (1963) Role of beta-adrenergic receptors in the circulatory response to high altitude hypoxia. *Am. J. Physiol.* **217**, 756–63.

Kontos, H.A., Levasseur, J.E., Richardson, D.W. *et al.* (1967) Comparative circulatory responses to systemic hypoxia in man and in unanesthetized dog. *J. Appl. Physiol.* **23**, 381–6.

Kosunen, K.J. and Pakarinen, A.J. (1976) Plasma renin, angiotensin II, and plasma and urinary aldosterone in running exercise. *J. Appl. Physiol.* **41**, 26–9.

Kotchen, T.A., Mougey, E.H., Hogan, R.P. *et al.* (1973) Thyroid responses to simulated altitude. *J. Appl. Physiol.* **34**, 145–8.

Koyama, S., Kobayashi, T., Kubo, K. *et al.* (1984) Catecholamine metabolism in patients with high altitude pulmonary edema (HAPE). *Jpn. J. Mount. Med.* **4**, 119.

Krarup, N. and Larsen, J.A. (1972) The effect of slight hypothermia on liver function as measured by the elimination rate of ethanol, the hepatic uptake and excretion of indocyanine green and bile formation. *Acta Physiol. Scand.* **84**, 396–407.

Kreuzer, F. and van Lookeren Campagne, P. (1965) Resting pulmonary diffusing capacity for CO and O_2 at high altitude. *J. Appl. Physiol.* **20**, 519–24.

Kristensen, C., Drenk, N.E. and Jordening, H. (1986) Simple system for central rewarming of hypothermic patients. *Lancet* **2**, 1467–8.

Krogh, A. (1910) On the mechanism of the gas-exchange in the lungs. *Skand. Arch. Physiol.* **23**, 248–78.

Krogh, A. (1919) Number and distribution of capillaries in muscles with calculations of the oxygen pressure head necessary to supplying the tissue. *J. Physiol. (Lond.)* **52**, 409–15.

Krogh, A. (1929) *The Anatomy and Physiology of Capillaries*, Yale University Press, New Haven, CT.

Krogh, A. and Krogh, M. (1910) On the tensions of gases in the arterial blood. *Skand. Archiv. Physiol.* **23**, 179–92.

Krogh, M. (1915) The diffusion of gases through the lungs of man. *J. Physiol. (Lond.)* **49**, 271–96.

Kronenberg, R.S. and Drage, C.W. (1973) Attenuation of the ventilatory and heart rate responses to hypoxia and hypercapnia with ageing in normal men. *J. Clin. Invest.* **52**, 1812–19.

Kronenberg, R.S., Safar, P., Lee, J. *et al.* (1971) Pulmonary artery pressure and alveolar gas exchange in man during acclimatization to 12,470 ft. *J. Clin. Invest.* **50**, 827–37.

Kryger, M., McCullough, R., Doekel, R. *et al.* (1978a) Excessive polycythemia of high altitude: role of ventilatory drive and lung disease. *Am. Rev. Respir. Dis.* **118**, 659–66.

Kryger, M., McCullough, R.E., Collins, D. *et al.* (1978b) Treatment of excessive polycythemia of high altitude with respiratory stimulant drugs. *Am. Rev. Respir. Dis.* **117**, 455–64.

Kubo, K., Hanaoka, M., Hayano, T. *et al.* (1998) Inflammatory cytokines in BAL fluid and pulmonary hemodynamics in high-altitude pulmonary edema. *Respir. Physiol.* **111**, 301–10.

Kuepper, T. Hoefer, M., Gieseler, U. and Netzer, N. (1999) Prevention of acute mountain sickness with theophylline (abstract), in *Hypoxia: Into the Next Millennium* (eds. R.C. Roach, P.D. Wagner and P.H. Hackett), Plenum/Kluwer, New York, p. 400.

Kumar, N., Folger, W.N. and Bolton, C.F. (2004) Dyspnea as the predominant manifestation of bilateral phrenic neuropathy. *Mayo Clin. Proc.* **79**, 1563–5.

Kumar, R., Pasha, Q., Khan, A.P. and Gupta, V. (2004) Renin angiotensin aldosterone system and ACE I/D gene polymorphism in high-altitude pulmonary edema. *Aviat. Space Environ. Med.* **75**, 981–3.

Kumar, V.N. (1982) Intractable foot pain following frostbite. *Arch. Phys. Med. Rehabil.* **63**, 284–5.

Kupper, T.E., Strohl, K.P., Hoefer, M. *et al.* (2008) Low-dose theophylline reduces symptoms of acute mountain sickness. *J. Travel Med.* **15**, 307–14.

Kuwahira, I., Moue, Y., Urano, T. *et al.* (2001) Redistribution of pulmonary blood flow during hypoxic exercise. *Int. J. Sports. Med.* **22**, 393–9.

Lahiri, S. (1972) Dynamic aspects of regulation of ventilation in man during acclimatization to high altitude. *Respir. Physiol.* **16**, 245–58.

Lahiri, S. (1977) Physiological responses and adaptations to high altitude, in *International Review of Physiology Environmental Physiology II, Vol. 14* (ed. D. Robertshaw), University Park Press, Baltimore, MD, pp. 217–51.

Lahiri, S. and Barnard, P. (1983) Role of arterial chemoreflexes in breathing during sleep at high altitude, in *Hypoxia, Exercise and Altitude* (eds. J.S. Sutton, C.S. Houston and N.L. Jones), Liss, New York, pp. 75–85.

Lahiri, S. and Cherniack, N.S. (2001) Cellular and molecular mechanisms of O_2 sensing with special reference to the carotid body, in *High Altitude, Lung Biology in Health and Disease, Vol. 161* (eds. T.F. Hornbein and R.B. Schoene), Marcel Dekker, New York, pp. 101–30.

Lahiri, S. and Delaney, R.G. (1975) Stimulus interaction in the response of carotid body chemoreceptor single afferent fibres. *Respir. Physiol.* **24**, 267–86.

Lahiri, S. and Milledge, J.S. (1967) Acid–base in Sherpa altitude residents and lowlanders at 4880 m. *Respir. Physiol.* **2**, 323–34.

Lahiri, S., Milledge, J.S., Chattopadhyay, H.P. *et al.* (1967) Respiration and heart rate of

Sherpa highlanders during exercise. *J. Appl. Physiol.* **23**, 545–54.

Lahiri, S., Kao, F.F., Velasquez, T. *et al.* (1969) Irreversible blunted sensitivity to hypoxia in high altitude natives. *Respir. Physiol.* **6**, 360–7.

Lahiri, S., Delaney, R.G., Brody, J.S. *et al.* (1976) Relative role of environmental and genetic factors in respiratory adaptation to high altitude. *Nature* **261**, 133–5.

Lahiri, S., Edelman, N.H., Cherniack, N.S. and Fishman, A.P. (1981) Role of carotid chemoreflex in respiratory acclimatization to hypoxemia in goat and sheep. *Respir. Physiol.* **46**, 367–82.

Lahiri, S., Maret, K. and Sherpa, M.G. (1983) Dependence of high altitude sleep apnea on ventilatory sensitivity to hypoxia. *Respir. Physiol.* **52**, 281–301.

Lahiri, S., Maret, K.H., Sherpa, M.G. and Peters, R.M. Jr (1984) Sleep and periodic breathing at high altitude: Sherpa natives versus sojourners, in *High Altitude and Man* (eds. J.B. West and S. Lahiri), American Physiological Society, Bethesda, MD, pp. 73–90.

Lahiri, S., Rozanov, C. and Cherniack, N.S. (2000) Altered structure and function of the carotid body at high altitude and associated chemoreflexes. *High Alt. Med. Biol.* **1**, 63–74.

Lahti, A. (1982) Cutaneous reactions to cold, in Report 30, Nordic Council for Arctic Medical Research, Copenhagen, pp. 32–5.

Lakshminarayan, S. and Pierson, D.J. (1975) Recurrent high altitude pulmonary edema with blunted chemosensitivity. *Am. Rev. Respir. Dis.* **111**, 869–72.

La Manna, J.C., Chavez, J.C. and Pichiule, P. (2004) Structural and functional adaptation to hypoxia in the rat brain. *J. Exp. Biol.* **207**, 3163–9.

Lander, E.S., Linton, L.M., Birren, B. *et al.* (2001) Initial sequencing and analysis of the human genome. *Nature* **409**, 860–921.

Lanfranchi, P.A., Colombo, R., Cremona, G. *et al.* (2005) Autonomic cardiovascular regulation in subjects with acute mountain sickness. *Am. J. Physiol. Heart Circ. Physiol.* **289**, H2364–72.

Lang, S.D.R. and Lang, A. (1971) The Kunde Hospital and a demographic survey of the Upper Khumbu, Nepal. *N.Z. Med. J.* **74**, 1–8.

Laragh, J.H. (1985) Atrial natriuretic hormone, the renin–aldosterone axis, and blood pressure–electrolyte homeostasis. *N. Engl. J. Med.* **313**, 1330–40.

Larsen, E.B., Roach, R.C., Schoene, R.B. and Hornbein, T.F. (1982) Acute mountain sickness and acetazolamide. Clinical efficacy and effect on ventilation. *JAMA* **248**, 328–32.

Larsen, J.J., Hansen, J.M., Olsen, N.V. *et al.* (1997) The effect of altitude hypoxia on glucose homeostasis in men. *J. Physiol.* **504**, 241–9.

Larsson, K., Ohlsen, P., Larsson, L. *et al.* (1993) High prevalence of asthma in cross country skiers. *BMJ* **307**, 1326–9.

Lassvik, C. and Areskog, N.H. (1980) Angina pectoris during inhalation of cold air. Reactions to exercise. *Br. Heart J.* **43**, 661–7.

Laufmann, H. (1951) Profound accidental hypothermia. *JAMA* **147**, 1201–12.

Lawler, J., Powers, S.K., Thompson, D. *et al.* (1988) Linear relationship between VO_2 max and VO_2 maximum decrement during exposure to acute hypoxia. *J. Appl. Physiol.* **64**, 1486–92.

Lawrence, D.L. and Shenker, Y. (1991) Effect of hypoxic exercise on atrial natriuretic factor and aldosterone regulation. *Am. J. Hypertens.* **4**, 341–7.

Lawrence, D.L., Skatrud, J.B. and Shenker, Y. (1990) Effect of hypoxia on atrial natriuretic factor and aldosterone regulation in humans. *Am. J. Physiol.* **258**, E243–8.

Lawrie, R.A. (1953) Effect of enforced exercise on myoglobin concentration in muscle. *Nature* **171**, 1069–70.

Leaf, D.E. and Goldfarb, D.S. (2007) Mechanisms of action of acetazolamide in the prophylaxis and treatment of acute mountain sickness. *J. Appl. Physiol.* **102**, 1313–22.

Leal, C. (2005) Going high with type 1 diabetes. *High Alt. Med. Biol.* **6**, 14–21.

Lechner, A.J., Grimes, M.J., Aquin, L. and Banchero, N. (1982) Adapative lung growth during chronic cold plus hypoxia is age-dependent. *J. Exp. Zool.* **219**, 285–91.

Ledingham, I. McA. (1983) Clinical management of elderly hypothermic patients, in *The Nature and Treatment of Hypothermia* (eds. R.S. Pozos and L.E. Wittmers), Croom Helm, London/University of Minnesota Press, Minneapolis, pp. 165–81.

Ledingham, I. McA. and Mone, J.G. (1980) Treatment of accidental hypothermia: a prospective clinical study. *BMJ* **1**, 1102–5.

Lee, W.C., Chen, J.J., Ho, H.Y. *et al.* (2003) Short-term altitude mountain living improves glycemic control. *High Alt. Med. Biol.* **4**, 81–91.

Lehman, T., Mairbaurl, H., Pleisch, B. *et al.* (2006) Platelet count and function at high altitude and in high-altitude pulmonary edema. *J. Appl. Physiol.* **100**, 690–4.

Lehmann, J.F. (1971) Diathermy, in *Handbook of Physical Medicine and Rehabilitation*, 2nd edn, Saunders, Philadelphia, pp. 1397–442.

Lehmann, T., Mairbaurl, H., Pleisch, B. *et al.* (2006) Platelet count and function at high altitude and in high-altitude pulmonary edema. *J. Appl. Physiol.* **100**, 690–4.

Lehmuskallio, E. (1999) Cold protecting ointment and frostbite: a questionnaire study of 830 conscripts in Finland. *Acta Derm. Venereol.* **79**, 67–70.

Lehmuskallio, E. and Anttonen, H. (1999) Thermal physical effects of ointments in cold: an experimental study with a skin model. *Acta Derm. Venereol.* **79**, 33–6.

Lehmuskallio, E., Linholm, H., Koskenvvo, K. *et al.* (1995) Frostbite of the face and ears: an epidemiological study of risk factors in Finnish conscripts. *BMJ* **311**, 1661–3.

Leiberman, P., Protopapas, A. and Kanki, B.G. (1995) Speech production and cognitive defects on Mt. Everest. *Aviat. Space Environ. Med.* **66**, 857–64.

Leigh-Smith, S. (2004) Blood boosting: a review. *Br. J. Sports Med.* **38**, 99–101.

Leissner, K.B. and Mahmood, F.U. (2009) Physiology and pathophysiology at high altitude: considerations for the anesthesiologist. *J. Anesth.* **23**, 543–53.

Lejeune, P., Brimioulle, S., Leeman, M. *et al.* (1990) Enhancement of hypoxic pulmonary vasoconstriction by metabolic acidosis in dogs. *Anesthesiology* **73**, 256–64.

Lenfant, C. and Sullivan, K. (1971) Adaptation to high altitude. *N. Engl. J. Med.* **284**, 1298–309.

Lenfant, C., Torrance, J., English, E. *et al.* (1968) Effect of altitude on oxygen binding by hemoglobin and on organic phosphate levels. *J. Clin. Invest.* **47**, 2652–6.

Lenfant, C., Ways, P., Aucutt, C. and Cruz, J. (1969) Effect of chronic hypoxic hypoxia on the O_2–Hb dissociation curve and respiratory gas transport in man. *Respir. Physiol.* **7**, 7–29.

Lenfant, C., Torrance, J.D. and Reynafarje, C. (1971) Shift of the O_2–Hb dissociation curve at altitude: mechanism and effect. *J. Appl. Physiol.* **30**, 625–31.

Leonard, W.R., DeWalt, K.M., Stansbury, J.P. and McCaston, M.K. (1995) Growth differences between children of highland and coastal Equador. *Am. J. Phys. Anthropol.* **98**, 47–57.

León-Velarde, F. (1998) First International Group on Chronic Mountain Sickness (CMS) in Matsumoto, in *Progress in Mountain Medicine and High Altitude* (eds. H. Ohno, T. Kobayashi, S. Masuyama and M. Nakashima), Press Committee of the 3rd Congress on Mountain Medicine and High Altitude Physiology, Matsumoto, p. 166.

León-Velarde, F. and Arregui, A. (1993) Hipoxia: Investigacionas Basicas y Clinicias. *Homenajie a Carlos Monge Cassinelli*, Instituto Frances de Estudios Andinos Universidad Peruana Cayetano Heredia, Lima, Peru.

León-Velarde, F. and Richalet, J.P. (2006) Respiratory control in residents at high altitude: physiology and pathophysiology. *High Alt. Med. Biol.* **7**, 125–37.

León-Velarde, F. and Villafuerte, F.C. (2011) High-altitude pulmonary hypertension. *Textbook Pulmon. Vasc. Dis.* **4**, 1211–21.

León-Velarde, F., Monge, C.C., Vidal, A. *et al.* (1991) Serum immunoreactive erythropoietin in high altitude natives with and without excessive erythrocytosis. *Exp. Hematol.* **19**, 257–60.

León-Velarde, F., Arregui, A., Monge C.C. and Ruiz, H. (1993) Ageing at high altitude and the risk of chronic mountain sickness. *J. Wilderness Med.* **4**, 183–8.

León-Velarde, F., Arregui, A., Vargas, M. *et al.* (1994) Chronic mountain sickness and chronic lower respiratory tract disorders. *Chest* **106**, 151–5.

León-Velarde, F., Ramos, M.A., Hermandez, J.A. *et al.* (1997) The role of menopause in the development of chronic mountain sickness. *Am. J. Physiol.* **272**, R90–4.

León-Velarde, F., Gamboa, A., Chuquiza, J.A. *et al.* (2000) Hematological parameters in high altitude residents living at 4,355, 4,660, and 5,500 meters above sea level. *High Alt. Med. Biol.* **1**, 97–104.

León-Velarde, F., Maggiorini, M., Reeves, J.T. *et al.* (2005) Consensus statement on chronic and sub-acute high altitude disease. *High Alt. Med. Biol.* **6**, 147–57.

León-Velarde, F., Villafuerte, F.C. and Richalet, J.-P. (2010) Chronic mountain sickness and the heart. *Prog. Cardiovasc. Dis.* **52**, 540–9.

Lepori, M., Hummler, E., Feihl, F. *et al.* (1999) Amiloride sensitive sodium transport dysfunction augments susceptibility to hypoxia induced lung edema (abstract), in *Hypoxia: Into the Next Millennium* (eds. R.C. Roach, P.D. Wagner and P.H. Hackett), Plenum/Kluwer, New York, p. 403.

Leuthold, E., Hartmann, G., Buhlman, R. *et al.* (1975) Medical and physiological investigations on mountaineers. A field study during a winter climb in the Bernese Oberland, in *Mountain Medicine and Physiology* (eds. C. Clarke, M. Ward and E. Williams), Alpine Club, London, pp. 32–7.

Levett, D.Z, Fernandez, B.O., Riley, H.L. *et al.* (2011) The role of nitrogen oxides in human adaptation to hypoxia. *Sci. Rep.* **1**, 109.

Levett, D.Z., Radford, E.J., Menassa, D.A. *et al.* (2012) Acclimatization of skeletal muscle mitochondria to high-altitude hypoxia during an ascent of Everest. *FASEB J.* **26**, 1431–41.

Levin, E.R. (1995) Endothelins. *N. Engl. J. Med.* **333**, 356–61.

Levine, B.D. (2005) Point: Positive effects of intermittent hypoxia (live high:train low) on exercise performance are mediated primarily by augmented red cell volume. *J. Appl. Physiol.* **99**, 2053–5.

Levine, B.D. and Stray-Gundersen, J. (1992) A practical approach to altitude training: where

to live and train for optimal performance enhancement. *Int. J. Sports Med.* **13**, 5209–12.

Levine, B.D. and Stray-Gundersen, J. (1997) 'Living high–training low': effect of moderate altitude acclimatization with low altitude training on performance. *J. Appl. Physiol.* **83**, 102–12.

Levine, B.D. and Stray-Gundersen, J. (2006) Dose-response of altitude training: how much altitude is enough? *Adv. Exp. Med. Biol.* **588**, 233–47.

Levine, B.D., Yoshimura, K., Kobayashi, T. *et al.* (1989) Dexamethasone in the treatment of acute mountain sickness. *N. Engl. J. Med.* **321**, 1707–13.

Levine, B.D., Zuckerman, J.H. and deFilippi, C.R. (1997) Effect of high-altitude exposure in the elderly: the Tenth Mountain Division study. *Circulation* **96**, 1224–32.

Lewin, S., Brittman, L.R. and Holzman, R.S. (1981) Infections in hypothermic patients. *Arch. Intern. Med.* **141**, 920–5.

Lewis, R.B. and Moen, P.W. (1952) Further studies on the pathogenesis of cold induced muscle necrosis. *Surg. Gynecol. Obstet.* **95**, 543–51.

Lewis, R.F. and Rennick, P.M. (1979) *Manual for the Repeatable Cognitive–Perceptual–Motor Battery*, Axon, Grosse Pointe Park, MI.

Lexow, K. (1991) Severe accidental hypothermia: survival after 6 hrs 30 min of cardio-pulmonary resuscitation. *Arctic Med. Res.* **50**(Suppl. 6), 112–14.

Li, X., Pei, T., Xu, H. *et al.* (2012) Ecological study of community-pevel factors associated with chronic mountain sickness in the young male Chinese immigrant population in Tibet. *J. Epidemiol.* **22**, 136–43.

Li, Y.Z. (1985) The birth weight, distribution of new born (in percentile) in high altitude (abstract), 2nd High Altitude Symposium, Qinghai, China (unpublished proceedings).

Lichty, J.A., Ting, R.Y., Bruns, P.D. and Dyar, E. (1957) Studies of babies born at high altitude. *Am. Med. Assoc. J. Dis. Child.* **93**, 666–7.

Lilja, G.P. (1983) Emergency treatment of hypothermia, in *The Nature and Treatment of Hypothermia* (eds. R.S. Pozos and L.E. Wittmers), Croom Helm, London/ University of Minnesota Press, Minneapolis, pp. 143–51.

Lim, T.P.K. (1960) Central and peripheral control mechanisms of shivering and its effect on respiration. *J. Appl. Physiol.* **15**, 567–74.

Lindgarde, F., Ercilla, M.B., Correa, L.R. and Ahren, B. (2004) Body adiposity, insulin, and leptin in subgroups of Peruvian Amerindians. *High Alt. Med. Biol.* **5**, 27–31.

Lipman, G.S., Kanaan, N.C., Holck, P.S., *et al.* (2012) PAINS Group. Ibuprofen prevents altitude illness: a randomized control trial for prevention of altitude illness with nonsteroidal anti-inflammatories. *Ann Emerg Med.*, Jun; **59**(6): 484–90.

Lippl, F.L., Neubauer, S., Schipfer, S. *et al.* (2010) Hypobaric hypoxia causes body weight reduction in obese subjects. *Obesity* **18**, 675–81.

Litch, J.A. and Bishop, R.A. (1999) Transient global amnesia at high altitude. *N. Engl. J. Med.* **340**, 1444.

Litch, J.A. and Bishop, R.A. (2000) High altitude global amnesia. *Wilderness Exp. Med.* **11**, 25–8.

Liu, L., Cheng, H., Chin, W. *et al.* (1989) Atrial natriuretic peptide lowers pulmonary arterial pressure in patients with high altitude disease. *Am. J. Med. Sci.* **298**, 397–401.

Liu, C., Zhang, L.F., Song, M.L. *et al.* (2009) Highly efficient dissociation of oxygen from hemoglobin in Tibetan chicken embryos compared with lowland chicken embryos incubated in hypoxia. *Poult. Sci.* **88**, 2689–94.

Liu, L.S. (1986) Highlights from the national meeting on hypertension: held by the Chinese Medical Association. *Chin. J. Cardiol.* **14**, 2–3.

Liu, Y., Steinacker, J.M., Dehnert, C. *et al.* (1998) Effect of 'living high-training low' on the cardiac functions at sea level. *Int. J. Sports Med.* **19**, 380–4.

Lloyd, B.B., Jukes, M.G.M. and Cunningham, D.J.C. (1958) The relation of alveolar oxygen pressure and the respiratory response to carbon dioxide in man. *Q. J. Exp. Physiol.* **42**, 214–27.

Lloyd, E.L. (1972) Diagnostic problems and hypothermia. *BMJ* **3**, 417.

Lloyd, E.L. (1973) Accidental hypothermia treated by central re-warming through the airway. *Br. J. Anaesth.* **45**, 41–8.

Lloyd, E.L. (1979) Temperature sensations in veins. *Anaesthesia* **34**, 919.

Lloyd, E.L. (1986) *Hypothermia and Cold Stress*, Croom Helm, London.

Lloyd, E.L. (1996) Accidental hypothermia. *Resuscitation* **32**, 111–24.

Lloyd, E.L. and Mitchell, B. (1974) Factors affecting the onset of ventricular fibrillation in hypothermia: a hypothesis. *Lancet* **2**, 1294–6.

Lloyd, T.C. (1965) Pulmonary vasoconstriction during histotoxic hypoxia. *J. Appl. Physiol.* **20**, 488–90.

Lobenhoffer, H.P., Zink, R.A. and Brendel, W. (1982) High altitude pulmonary edema: analysis of 166 cases, in *High Altitude Physiology and Medicine* (eds. W. Brendel and R.A. Zink), Springer-Verlag, New York, pp. 219–31.

Lockhart, A., Zelter, M., Mensch-Dechene, M. *et al.* (1976) Pressure–flow–volume relationships in pulmonary circulation of normal highlanders. *J. Appl. Physiol.* **41**, 449–56.

Loeppky, J.A., Scotto, P., Charlton, G.C. *et al.* (2001) Ventilation is greater in women than men, but the increase during acute altitude hypoxia is the same. *Respir. Physiol.* **125**, 225–37.

Loeppky, J.A., Icenogle, M.V., Maes, D. *et al.* (2003) Body temperature, autonomic responses and acute mountain sickness. *High Alt. Med. Biol.* **4**, 267–73.

Loeppky, J.A., Icenogle, M.V., Maes, D. *et al.* (2005a) Early fluid retention and severe acute mountain sickness. *J. Appl. Physiol.* **98**, 591–7.

Loeppky, J.A., Roach, R.C., Maes, D. *et al.* (2005b) Role of hypobaria in fluid balance response to hypoxia. *High Alt. Med. Biol.* **6**, 60–71.

Loewy, A. and Gerhartz, H. (1914) Uber de Termperatur de Expirationsluft und der Lungemluft. *Pflüger's Arch. Ges. Physiol.* **155**, 231–44.

Lomax, P., Thinney, R. and Mondino, B.J. (1991) The effects of solar radiation, in *A Colour Atlas of Mountain Medicine* (eds. J. Vallotton and F. Dubas), Wolfe, London, pp. 67–71.

Longmuir, I.S. and Betts, W. (1987) Tissue acclimation to altitude. *Fed. Proc.* **46**, 794.

Lopes, A.A., Bandeira, A.P., Flores, P.C. and Santana, M.V.T. (2010) Pulmonary hypertension in Latin America: pulmonary vascular disease: the global perspective. *Chest* **137**, 78s–84s.

Lorenzo, F., Yang, Y., Simonson, T.S. *et al.* (2009) Genetic adaptation to extreme hypoxia: study at high altitude pulmonary edema in a 3-generation Han Chinese family. *Blood Cell. Mol. Dis.* **43**, 221–5.

Louie, D. and Pare, P.D. (2004) Physiological changes at altitude in nonasthmatic and asthmatic subjects. *Can. Respir. J.* **11**, 197–9.

Lovering, A.T., Eldridge, M.W. and Stickland, M.K. (2009) Counterpoint: Exercise-induced intrapulmonary shunting is real. *J. Appl. Physiol.* **107**, 994–7.

Lovering, A.T., Romer, L.M., Haverkamp, H.C. *et al.* (2008) Intrapulmonary shunting and pulmonary gas exchange during normoxic and hypoxic exercise in healthy subjects. *J. Appl. Physiol.* **104**, 1418–25.

Lugaresi, E., Coccagna, G., Cirignotta, R. *et al.* (1978) Breathing during sleep in man in normal and pathological conditions, in *The Regulation of Respiration during Sleep and Anesthesia* (eds. R.S. Fitzgerald, H. Cautier and S. Lahiri), Plenum, New York, pp. 35–45.

Luks, A.M. (2008) Do we have a 'best practice' for treating high altitude pulmonary edema? *High Alt. Med. Biol.* **9**, 111–14.

Luks, A.M. (2008) Which medications are safe and effective for improving sleep at high altitude? *High Alt. Med. Biol.* **9**, 195–8.

Luks, A.M. (2009a) Do lung disease patients need supplemental oxygen at high altitude? *High Alt. Med. Biol.* **10**, 321–7.

Luks, A.M. (2009b) Should travelers with hypertension adjust their medications when traveling to high altitude? *High Alt. Med. Biol.* **10**, 11–15.

Luks, A.M. and Swenson, E.R. (2007) Travel to high altitude with pre-existing lung disease. *Eur. Respir. J.* **29**, 770–92.

Luks, A.M. and Swenson, E.R. (2008) Medication and dosage considerations in the prophylaxis and treatment of high-altitude illness. *Chest* **133**, 744–55.

Luks, A.M., van Melick, H., Batarse, R. *et al.* (1998) Room oxygen enrichment improves sleep and subsequent day-time performance at high altitude. *Respir. Physiol.* **113**, 247–58.

Luks, A.M., Henderson, W.R. and Swenson, E.R. (2007) Leukotriene receptor blockade does not prevent acute mountain sickness induced by normobaric hypoxia. *High Alt. Med. Biol.* **8**, 131–8.

Luks, A.M., Johnson, R.J. and Swenson, E.R. (2008) Chronic kidney disease at high altitude. *J. Am. Soc. Nephrol.* **19**, 2262–71.

Luks, A.M., Grissom, C.K., Jean, D. and Swenson, E.R. (2009) Can people with Raynaud's phenomenon travel to high altitude? *Wilderness Environ. Med.* **20**, 129–38.

Luks, A.M., McIntosh, S.E., Grissom, C.K. *et al.* (2010) Wilderness Medical Society consensus guidelines for the prevention and treatment of acute altitude illness. *Wilderness Environ. Med.* **21**, 146–55.

Luks, A.M., Stout, K. and Swenson, E.R. (2010) Evaluating the safety of high-altitude travel in patients with adult congenital heart disease. *Congenit Heart Dis* **5**, 220–32.

Lundberg, E. (1952) Edema agudo del pulmon en el soroche. Conferencia sustentada en la ascociacion medica de Yauli, Oroya. (Quoted in Hultgren, H.N., Spickard, W.B., Hellriegel, K. and Houston, C.S. (1961) High altitude pulmonary edema. *Medicine* **40**, 289–313.)

Lundby, C. and Damsgaard, R. (2006) Exercise performance in hypoxia after novel erythropoiesis stimulating protein treatment. *Scand. J. Med. Sci. Sports* **16**, 35–40.

Lundby, C. and van Hall, G. (2001) Peak heart rate at extreme altitudes. *High Alt. Med. Biol.* **2**, 41–5.

Lundby, C and van Hall, G. (2002) Substrate utilization in sea level residents during exercise in acute hypoxia and after 4 weeks acclimatization to 4100 m. *Acta. Physiol. Scand.* **176**, 195–201.

Lundby, C., Boushel, R., Robach, P. *et al.* (2008) During hypoxic exercise some vasoconstriction is needed to match O_2 delivery to O_2 demand at the microcirculatory level. *J. Physiol.* **586**, 123–30.

Lundby, C., Saltin, B. and van Hall, G. (2000) The 'lactate paradox', evidence for a transient change in the course of acclimatization to severe hypoxia in lowlanders. *Acta Physiologica* **170**, 265–9.

Lundby, C., Araoz, M. and van Hall, G. (2001a) Peak heart rate decreases with increasing severity of acute hypoxia. *High Alt. Med. Biol.* **2**, 369–76.

Lundby, C., Moller, P., Kanstrup, I.-L. and Olsen, N.V. (2001b) Heart rate response to hypoxic exercise: role of dopamine D$_2$-receptors and effect of oxygen supplementation. *Clin. Sci. (Lond.)* **101**, 377–83.

Lundby, C., Calber, J.A., van Hall, G. *et al.* (2004a) Pulmonary gas exchange at maximal exercise in Danish lowlanders during 8 weeks of acclimatization to 4,100m and in high-altitude Aymara natives. *Am. J. Physiol.* **287**, R1202–8.

Lundby, C., Pilegaard, H., Andersen, J.L. *et al.* (2004b) Acclimatization to 4100m does not change capillary density or mRNA expression of potential angiogenesis regulatory factors in human skeletal muscle. *J. Exp. Biol.* **207**, 3865–71.

Lundby, C., Nielsen, T.K., Dela, F. and Damsgaard, R. (2005) The influence of intermittent altitude exposure to 4100 m on exercise capacity and blood variables. *Scand. J. Med. Sci. Sports* **15**, 182–7.

Lundby, C., Sander, M., van Hall, G. *et al.* (2006) Determinants of maximal exercise and muscle oxygen extraction in acclimatizing lowlanders and in high altitude natives. *J. Physiol.* **573**, 535–43.

Luo, F.M., Liu, X.J., Li, S.Q. *et al.* (2005) Circulating Ghrelin in patients with chronic obstructive pulmonary disease. *Nutrition* **21**, 793–8.

Lynch, T.F. (1990) Glacial-age man in South America? A critical review. *Am. Antiquity* **55**, 12–36.

Lyons, T.P., Muza, S.R., Rock, P.B. and Cymerman, A. (1995) The effect of altitude pre-acclimatization on acute mountain sickness during reexposure. *Aviat. Space Environ. Med.* **66**, 957–62.

Maa, E.H. (2011) How do you approach seizures in the high altitude traveler? *High Alt. Med. Biol.* **12**, 13–19.

MacDougall, J.D., Green, H., Sutton, J.R. *et al.* (1991) Operation Everest II: structural adaptations in skeletal muscle in response to extreme altitude. *Acta Physiol. Scand.* **142**, 421–7.

Maceluso, A., Young, A., Gibb, K.S. *et al.* (2003) Cycling as a novel approach to resistance training increases muscle strength, power and selected functional abilities in healthy older women. *J. Appl. Physiol.* **95**, 2544–53.

MacInnes, C. (1971) Steroids in mountain rescue. *Lancet* **1**, 599.

MacInnes, C. (1979) Treatment of accidental hypothermia. *BMJ* **1**, 130–1.

MacInnis, M.J., Koehle, M.S., and Rupert, J.L. (2010) Evidence for a genetic basis for altitude illness: 2010 update. *High Alt. Med. Biol.* **11**, 349–68.

MacInnis, M.J., Wang, P., Koehle, M.S. *et al.* (2011) The genetics of altitude tolerance: the evidence for inherited susceptibility to acute mountain sickness. *J. Occup. Environ. Med.* **53**, 159–68.

MacIntyre, B. (1994) Ice-cream comforts girl who survived big freeze. *The Times* (London), 4 March, p. 15.

MacKinnon, P.C.B., Monk-Jones, M.E. and Fotherby, K. (1963) A study of various indices of adrenocortical activity during 23 days at high altitude. *J. Endocrinol.* **26**, 555–6.

MacNeish, R.S. (1971) Early man in the Andes. *Sci. Am.* **224**, 36–46.

Mader, T.H. and Tabin, G. (2003) Going to high altitude with preexisting ocular conditions. *High Alt. Med. Biol.* **4**, 419–30.

Mader, T.H. and White, L.J. (1995) Refractive changes at extreme altitude after radial keratotomy. *Am. J. Ophthalmol.* **119**, 733–7.

Mader, T.H., Blanton, C.L., Gilbert, B.N. *et al.* (1996) Refractive changes during 72-hour exposure to high altitude after refractive surgery. *Ophthalmology* **103**, 1188–95.

Magalhaes, J., Ascensao, A., Viscor, G. *et al.* (2004) Oxidative stress in humans during and after 4 hours of hypoxia at a simulated altitude of 5500 m. *Aviat. Space Environ. Med.* **75**, 16–22.

Maggiorini, M. (2006) High altitude-induced pulmonary oedema. *Cardiovasc. Res.* **72**, 41–50.

Maggiorini, M., Buhler, B., Walter, M. and Oelz, O. (1990) Prevalence of acute mountain sickness in the Swiss Alps. *BMJ* **301**, 853–5.

Maggiorini, M., Bärtsch, P. and Oelz, O. (1997) Association between body temperature and acute mountain sickness: cross sectional study. *BMJ* **315**, 403–4.

Maggiorini, M., Muller, A., Hofstetter, D. *et al.* (1998) Assessment of acute mountain sickness by different score protocols in the Swiss Alps. *Aviat. Space Environ. Med.* **69**, 1186–92.

Maggiorini, M., Melot, C., Pierre, S. *et al.* (2001) High-altitude pulmonary edema is initially caused by an increase in capillary pressure. *Circulation* **103**, 2078–83.

Maggiorini, M., Brunner-La Rocca, H.-P. and Peth, S. *et al.* (2006) Both tadalafil and dexamethasone may reduce the incidence of high-altitude pulmonary edema: a randomized trial. *Ann. Intern. Med.* **145**, 497–506.

Maher, J.T., Jones, L.G. and Hartley, L.H. (1974) Effects of high-altitude exposure on submaximal endurance capacity of men. *J. Appl. Physiol.* **37**, 895–8.

Maher, J.T., Jones, L.G., Hartley, L.H. *et al.* (1975a) Aldosterone dynamics during graded exercise at sea level and high altitude. *J. Appl. Physiol.* **39**, 18–22.

Maher, J.T., Manchanda, S.C., Cymerman, A. *et al.* (1975b) Cardiovascular responsiveness to β-adrenergic stimulation and blockade in chronic hypoxia. *Am. J. Physiol.* **228**, 477–81.

Maher, J.T., Cymerman, A., Reeves, J.T. *et al.* (1975c) Acute mountain sickness: increased severity in eucapnic hypoxia. *Aviat. Space Environ. Med.* **46**, 826–9.

Maher, J.T., Denniston, J.C., Wolfe, D.L. and Cymerman, A. (1978) Mechanism of the attenuated cardiac response to β-adrenergic stimulation in chronic hypoxia. *J. Appl. Physiol. Respir. Environ. Exerc. Physiol.* **44**, 647–51.

Maher, J.T., Levine, P.H. and Cymerman, A. (1976) Human coagulation abnormalities during acute exposure to hypobaric hypoxia. *J. Appl. Physiol.* **41**, 702–7.

Mahfouz, AA., El-Aid, R.M.M., Alakija, W. and Al-Erian, R.A.G. (1994) Altitude and socio-biological determinants of pregnancy-associated hypertension. *Int. J. Obstet. Gynecol.* **44**, 135–8.

Mahony, B.S. and Githens, J.H. (1979) Sickling crises and altitude. Occurrence in the Colorado patient population. *Clin Pediatr (Phila)* **18**, 431–8.

Maignan, M., Rivera-Ch, M., Privat, C. *et al.* (2009) Pulmonary pressure and cardiac function in chronic mountain sickness patients. *Chest* **135**, 499–504.

Mairbaurl, H. (2006) Role of alveolar epithelial sodium transport in high altitude pulmonary edema (HAPE). *Respir. Physiol. Neurobiol.* **151**, 178–91.

Mairbaurl, H., Schobersberger, W., Hasibeder, W. *et al.* (1989a) Increase in Hb-O2-affinity at moderate altitude (2000 m) in patients on maintenance hemodialysis. *Clin. Nephrol.* **31**, 198–203.

Mairbaurl, H., Schobersberger, W., Hasibeder, W. *et al.* (1989b) Exercise performance of hemodialysis patients during short-term and prolonged exposure to altitude. *Clin. Nephrol.* **32**, 31–9.

Mairbaurl, H., Schwobel, F., Hoschele, S. *et al.* (2003) Altered ion transporter expression in bronchial epithelium in mountaineers with high-altitude pulmonary edema. *J. Appl. Physiol.* **95**, 1843–50.

Malconian, M.K., Rock, P.B., Hultgren, H.N. *et al.* (1990) The electrocardiogram at rest and exercise during a simulated ascent of Mt. Everest (Operation Everest II). *Am. J. Cardiol.* **65**, 1475–80.

Malconian, M.K., Rock, P.B., Reeves, J.T. and Houston, C.S. (1993) Operation Everest II: gas tensions in expired air and arterial blood at extreme altitude. *Aviat. Space Environ. Med.* **64**, 37–42.

Malik, M.T., Peng, Y.J., Kline, D.D. *et al.* (2005) Impaired ventilatory acclimatization to hypoxia in mice lacking the immediate early gene fos B. *Respir. Physiol. Neurobiol.* **145**, 23–31.

Malik, R.A., Masson, E.A., Sharma, A.K. *et al.* (1990) Hypoxic neuropathy: relevance to human diabetic neuropathy. *Diabetologia* **33**, 311–18.

Maloiy, G.M.O., Heglund, G.M., Prager, N.C. et al. (1986) Energetic cost of carrying loads: have African women discovered an economic way? *Nature* **319**, 668–9.

Manier, C., Guenard, H., Castaing, Y. et al. (1988) Pulmonary gas exchange in Andean natives with excessive polycythemia – effect of hemodilution. *J. Appl. Physiol.* **65**, 2107–17.

Mannucci, P.M., Gringeri, A., Peyvandi, F. et al. (2002) Short-term exposure to high altitude cause coagulation activation and inhibits fibrinolysis. *Thromb. Haemost.* **87**, 342–3.

Mansell, A., Powles, A. and Sutton, J. (1980) Changes in pulmonary PV characteristics of human subjects at an altitude of 5366m. *J. Appl. Physiol.* **49**, 79–83.

Marciniuk, D., McKim, D., Sanii, R. and Younes, M. (1994) Role of central respiratory muscle fatigue in endurance exercise in normal subjects. *J. Appl. Physiol.* **76**, 236–41.

Marconi, C., Marzorati, M., Grassi, B. et al. (2004) Second generation Tibetan lowlanders acclimatize to high altitude more quickly than Caucasians. *J. Physiol.* **556**, 661–71.

Marconi, C., Marzorati, M., Sciuto, D. et al. (2005) Economy of locomotion in high-altitude Tibetan migrants exposed to normoxia. *J. Physiol.* **569**, 667–75.

Marconi, C., Marzorati, M. and Cerretelli, P. (2006) Work capacity of permanent residents of high altitude. *High Alt. Med. Biol.* **7**, 105–15.

Marcora, S. (2010) Counterpoint: Afferent feedback from fatigued locomotor muscles is not an important determinant of endurance exercise performance. *J. Appl. Physiol.* **108**, 454–6.

Marcus, P. (1979) The treatment of acute accidental hypothermia. Proceedings of a Symposium held at the RAF Institute of Aviation Medicine. *Aviat. Space Environ. Med.* **50**, 834–43.

Maresh, C.M., Kreamer, W.J., Judelson, A. et al. (2004) Effects of high altitude and water deprivation on arginine vasopressin release in man. *Am. J. Physiol Endocrinol. Metab.* **286**, E20–4.

Maret, K.H., Billups, J.O., Peters, R.M. and West, J.B. (1984) Automatic mechanical alveolar gas sampler for multiple sample collection in the field. *J. Appl. Physiol.* **56**, 1435–8.

Margaria, R. (1957) The contribution of hemoglobin to acid-base equilibrium of the blood in health and disease. *Clin. Chem.* **3**, 306–18.

Margaria, R. (ed.) (1967) *Exercise at Altitude*, Excerpta Medica Foundation, Amsterdam.

Marine, D. and Kimball, O.P. (1920) Prevention of simple goiter in man. *Arch. Intern. Med.* **25**, 661–72.

Marinelli, M., Roi, G.S., Giacometti, M. et al. (1994) Cortisol, testosterone and free testosterone in athletes performing a marathon at 4,000m altitude. *Horm. Res.* **41**, 225–9.

Marsh, A.R. (1983) A short but distant war: the Falklands Campaign. *J. R. Soc. Med.* **76**, 972–82.

Marshall, H.C. and Goldman, R.F. (1976) Electrical response of nerve to freezing injury, in *Circumpolar Health* (eds. R.J. Shephard and S. Itoh), University Press, Toronto, p. 77.

Marsigny, B. (1998) Mountain frostbite. *ISSM Newsletter* **8**, 8–10.

Marti, H.J.H., Bernaudin, M., Bellail, M. et al. (2000) Hypoxia-induced vascular endothelial growth factor expression precedes neovascularization after cerebral ischemia. *Am. J. Pathol.* **156**, 965–76.

Marticorena, E., Severino, J., Peñaloza, A.D. and Neuriegel, K. (1959) Influencia de las grandes alturas en la determinacion de la persistencia del canal arterial. Observaciones realizadas en 3500 escolares de altura a 4300 m. Sombre el niuel dez mar. Primeros resultados operatorios. *Rev. Asoc. Med. Prov. Yauli* Nos 1–2, La Oroya.

Marticorena, E., Tapia, F.A., Dyer, J. et al. (1964) Pulmonary edema by ascending to high altitudes. *Dis. Chest* **45**, 273–83.

Marticorena, E., Ruiz, L., Severino, J. et al. (1969) Systemic blood pressure in white men born at sea level: changes after long residence in high altitudes. *Am. J. Cardiol.* **23**, 364–8.

Martin, B.J., Wiel, J.V., Sparks, K.E. et al. (1978) Exercise ventilation corresponds positively with ventilatory chemoresponsiveness. *J. Appl. Physiol.* **44**, 447–84.

Martin, D. and Pyne, D. (1998) Altitude training at 2690m does not increase total haemoglobin mass or sea level VO$_2$max in world champion track cyclists. *J. Sci. Med. Sport* **1**, 156–70.

Martin, D.S., Ince, C., Goedhart, P. *et al.* (2009) Abnormal blood flow in the sublingual microcirculation at high altitude. *Eur. J. Appl. Physiol.* **106**, 473–8.

Martin, D.S., Goedhart, P., Vercueil, A. *et al.* (2010) Changes in sublingual microcirculatory flow index and vessel density on ascent to altitude. *Exp. Physiol.* **95**, 880–91.

Martin, D.S., Levett, D.Z.H., Grocott, M.P.W. and Montgomery, H.E. (2010) Variation of human performance in the hypoxic mountain environment. *Exp. Physiol.* **95**, 463–70.

Mason, N.P. and Barry, P.W. (2007) Altitude-related cough. *Pulm. Pharmacol. Ther.* **20**, 388–95.

Mason, N.P., Barry, P.W., Despiau, G. *et al.* (1999) Cough frequency and cough receptor sensitivity to citric acid challenge during a simulated ascent to extreme altitude. *Eur. Respir. J.* **13**, 508–13.

Mason, N.P., Petersen, M., Melot, C. *et al.* (2003) Serial changes in nasal potential difference and lung electrical impedance tomography at high altitude. *J. Appl. Physiol.* **94**, 2043–50.

Mason, N.P., Petersen, M., Melot, C. *et al.* (2009) Changes in plasma bradykinin concentration and citric acid cough threshold at high altitude. *Wilderness Environ. Med.* **20**, 353–8.

Masuda, A., Kobayashi, T., Honda, Y. *et al.* (1992) Effect of high altitude on respiratory chemosensitivity. *Jpn. J. Mount. Med.* **12**, 177–81.

Mathew, J., Basheeruddin, K. and Prabhakar, S. (2001) Differences in frequency of the deletion polymorphism of the angiotensin-converting enzyme gene in different ethnic groups. *Angiology* **52**, 375–9.

Mathews, C.E. (1898) *Annals of Mont Blanc,* T. Fisher Unwin, London, p. 82.

Mathieu-Costello, O. (1987) Capillary tortuosity and degree of contraction or extension of skeletal muscle. *Microvasc. Res.* **33**, 98–117.

Mathieu-Costello, O. (1989) Muscle capillary tortuosity in high altitude mice depends on sarcomere length. *Respir. Physiol.* **76**, 289–302.

Mathieu-Costello, O. (2001) Muscle adaptation to altitude: tissue capillarity and capacity for aerobic metabolism. *High Alt. Med. Biol.* **2**, 413–25.

Mathieu-Costello, O., Agey, P.J., Wu, L. *et al.* (1998) Increased fiber capillarization in flight muscle of finch at altitude. *Respir. Physiol.* **111**, 189–99.

Matsuyama, S., Kimura, H., Sugita, T. *et al.* (1986) Control of ventilation in extreme altitude climbers. *J. Appl. Physiol.* **61**, 400–6.

Matsuyama, S., Kohchiyama, S., Shinozaki, T. *et al.* (1989) Periodic breathing at high altitude and ventilatory responses to O_2 and CO_2. *Jpn. J. Physiol.* **39**, 523–35.

Matsuzawa, Y., Fujimoto, K., Kobayashi, T. *et al.* (1989) Blunted hypoxic ventilatory drive in subjects susceptible to high-altitude pulmonary edema. *J. Appl. Physiol.* **66**, 1152–7.

Matthews, B. (1954) Discussion on physiology of man at high altitudes; limiting factors at high altitude. *Proc. R. Soc. Lond. Ser. B* **143**, 1–4.

Matthews, B.H.C. (1932) Loss of heat at high altitudes. *J. Physiol. (Lond.)* **77**, 28-9P (Abstr.).

Maugham, R.J. (1984) Temperature regulation during marathon competition. *Br. J. Sports Med.* **22**, 257–60.

Mawson, J.T., Braun, B., Rock, P.B. *et al.* (2000) Women at altitude: energy requirement at 4,300 m. *J. Appl. Physiol.* **88**, 272–81.

Mayhew, T. (1986) Morphometric diffusing capacity for oxygen of the human term placenta at high altitude, in *Aspects of Hypoxia* (ed. D. Heath), Liverpool University Press, Liverpool, pp. 181–90.

Mayhew, T.M. (1991) Scaling placental oxygen diffusion to birthweight: studies on placentae from low- and high-altitude pregnancies. *J. Anat.* **175**, 187–94.

Mayhew, T.M. (2003) Changes in fetal capillaries during preplacental hypoxia: growth, shape remodelling and villous capillarization in placentae from high-altitude pregnancies. *Placenta* **24**, 191–8.

Mazzeo, R.S. (2005) Altitude, exercise and immune function. *Exerc. Immunol. Rev.* **11**, 6–16.

Mazzeo, R.S. and Reeves, J.T. (2003) Adrenergic contribution during acclimatization to high altitude: perspectives from Pikes Peak. *Exerc Sport Sci. Rev.* **31**, 13–18.

Mazzeo, R.S., Bender, P.R., Brooks, G.A. *et al.* (1991) Arterial catecholamine responses during exercise with acute and chronic high-altitude exposure. *Am. J. Physiol.* **261**, E419–24.

Mazzeo, R.S., Child, A., Butterfield, G.E. *et al.* (1998) Catecholamine response during 12 days of high-altitude exposure (4,300 m) in women. *J. Appl. Physiol.* **84**, 1151–7.

Mazzeo, R.S., Carroll, J.D., Butterfield, G.E. *et al.* (2001) Catecholamine responses to alpha-adrenergic blockade during exercise in women acutely exposed to altitude. *J. Appl. Physiol.* **90**, 121–6.

Mazzeo, R.S., Dubay, A., Kirsch, J. *et al.* (2003) Influence of α-adrenergic blockade on the catecholamine response to exercise at 4,300 meters. *Metabolism* **52**, 1471–7.

McAuliffe, F., Kameta, N., Ratterty, G.F. *et al.* (2003) Pulmonary diffusing capacity in pregnancy at sea level and at high altitude. *Respir. Physiol. Neurobiol.* **134**, 85–92.

McCarrison, R. (1908) Observations on endemic cretinism in the Chitral and Gilgit valleys. *Lancet* **2**, 1275–80.

McCarrison, R. (1913) *The Pathology of Endemic Goitre (Milroy Lectures 1913)*, Bale Sons and Danielson, London.

McCauley, R.C., Smith, D.J., Robson, M.C. and Heggers, J.P. (1995) Frostbite and other cold related injuries, in *Wilderness Medicine* (ed. P.S. Auerbach), Mosby, St Louis, MO, pp. 129–40.

McClung, J.P. (1969) *Effects of High Altitude on Human Birth,* Harvard University Press, Cambridge, MA.

McCormack, P.D., Thomas, J., Malik, M. and Staschen, C. (1998) Cold stress, reverse T3 and lymphocyte function. *Alaska Med.* **40**, 55–62.

McDonough, P., Merrill Dane, D., Hsia, C.C.W. *et al.* (2006) Long-term enhancement of pulmonary gas exchange after high-altitude residence during maturation. *J. Appl. Physiol.* **100**, 474–81.

McElroy, M.K., Gerard, A., Powell, F.L. *et al.* (2000) Nocturnal O_2 enrichment of room air at high altitude increases daytime O_2 saturation without changing control of ventilation. *High Alt. Med. Biol.* **1**, 197–206.

McFadden, D.M., Houston, C.S., Sutton, J.R. *et al.* (1981) High-altitude retinopathy. *J. Am Med. Assoc.* **245**, 581–6.

McFarland, R.A. (1937a) Psycho-physiological studies at high altitude in the Andes. I. The effects of rapid ascents by aeroplane and train. *Comp. Psychol.* **23**, 191–225.

McFarland, R.A. (1937b) Psycho-physiological studies at high altitude. II. Sensory and motor responses during acclimatization. *Comp. Psychol.* **23**, 227–58.

McFarland, R.A. (1938a) Psycho-physiological studies at high altitude in the Andes. III. Mental and psycho-somatic responses during gradual adaptation. *Comp. Psychol.* **24**, 147–88.

McFarland, R.A. (1938b) Psycho-physiological studies at high altitude. IV. Sensory and circulatory responses of the Andean residents at 17500 feet. *Comp. Psychol.* **24**, 189–220.

McIntyre, L. (1987) The high Andes. *Natl. Geogr.* **171**, 422–59.

McKendry, R.J.R. (1981) Frostbite arthritis. *Can. Med. Assoc. J.* **125**, 1128–30.

Mecham, R.P., Whitehouse, L.A., Wrenn, D.S. *et al.* (1987) Smooth muscle-mediated connective tissue remodeling in pulmonary hypertension. *Science* **237**, 423–6.

Meehan, R., Duncan, U., Neal, L. *et al.* (1988) Operation Everest II: alterations in the immune system at high altitudes. *J. Clin. Immunol.* **8**, 397–406.

Meehan, R.T. (1987) Immune suppression at high altitude. *Ann. Emerg. Med.* **16**, 974–9.

Meerson, F.Z., Ustinova, E.E. and Orlova, E.H. (1987) Prevention and elimination of heart arrhythmias by adaptation to intermittent high altitude hypoxia. *Clin. Cardiol.* **10**, 783–9.

Megirian, D.A., Ryan, A.T. and Sherrey, J.H. (1980) An electrophysiological analysis of sleep and respiration of rats breathing different gas mixtures: diaphragmatic muscle function. *Electroencephalogr. Clin. Neurophysiol.* **50**, 303–13.

Meir, J.U. and Ponganis, P.J. (2009) High-affinity hemoglobin and blood oxygen saturation in diving emperor penguins. *J. Exp. Biol.* **212**, 3330–8.

Mejia, O.M., Prchal, J.T., León-Velarde, F. *et al.* (2005) Genetic association analysis of chronic mountain sickness in an Andean high-altitude population. *Haematologica* **90**, 13–19.

Melin, A., Fauchier, L., Dubuis, E. *et al.* (2003) Heart rate variability in rats acclimatized to high altitude. *High Alt. Med. Biol.* **4**, 375–87.

Menon, N.D. (1965) High altitude pulmonary edema: a clinical study. *N. Engl. J. Med.* **273**, 66–73.

Menzies, I.S. (1984) Transmucosal passage of inert molecules in health and disease, in *Intestinal Absorption and Secretion*, Falk Symposium 36 (eds. E. Skadhauge and K. Heintze), MTP Press, Lancaster, pp. 527–43.

Mercker, H. and Schneider, M. (1949) Uber capillarveranderungen des gehirns bei hohenanpassung. *Pflügers Arch.* **251**, 49–55.

Merino, C.F. (1950) Studies on blood formation and destruction in the polycythaemia of high altitude. *Blood* **5**, 1–31.

Messner, R. (1979) The mountain, in *Everest: Expedition to the Ultimate*, Kaye & Ward, London, pp. 47–217.

Messner, R. (1981) At my limit. *Natl. Geogr.* **160**, 553–66.

Meyrick, B. and Reid, L. (1978) The effect of continued hypoxia on rat pulmonary arterial circulation. An ultrastructural study. *Lab. Invest.* **38**, 188–200.

Meyrick, B. and Reid, L. (1980) Hypoxia-induced structural changes in the media and adventitia of the rat hilar pulmonary artery and their regression. *Am. J. Pathol.* **100**, 151–78.

Michel, C.C. and Milledge, J.S. (1963) Respiratory regulation in man during acclimatization to high altitude. *J. Physiol.* **168**, 631–43.

Milledge, J.S. (1963) Electrocardiographic changes at high altitude. *Br. Heart J.* **25**, 291–8.

Milledge, J.S. (1968) The control of breathing at high altitude, MD thesis, University of Birmingham.

Milledge, J.S. (1972) Arterial oxygen desaturation and intestinal absorption of xylose. *BMJ* **2**, 557–8.

Milledge, J.S. (1992) Respiratory water loss at altitude. *ISMM Newsletter* **2**, 5–7.

Milledge, J.S. and Catley, D.M. (1982) Renin, aldosterone and converting enzyme during exercise and acute hypoxia in humans. *J. Appl. Physiol.* **52**, 320–3.

Milledge, J.S. and Catley, D.M. (1987) Angiotensin converting enzyme activity and hypoxia. *Clin. Sci.* **72**, 149.

Milledge, J.S. and Cotes, P.M. (1985) Serum erythropoietin in humans at high altitude and its relation to plasma renin. *J. Appl. Physiol.* **59**, 360–4.

Milledge, J.S. and Lahiri, S. (1967) Respiratory control in lowlanders and Sherpa highlanders at altitude. *Respir. Physiol.* **2**, 310–22.

Milledge, J.S. and Sorensen, S.C. (1972) Cerebral arteriovenous oxygen difference in man native to high altitude. *J. Appl. Physiol.* **32**, 687–9.

Milledge, J.S. and Stott, F.D. (1977) Inductive plethysmography – a new respiratory transducer. *J. Physiol. (Lond)* **267**, 4p–5p.

Milledge, J.S., Iliff, L.D. and Severinghaus, J.W. (1968) The site of vascular leakage in hypoxic pulmonary edema, in *Proceedings of the International Union of Physiological Sciences, Abstracts*, vol. 44, *International Congress*, p. 883.

Milledge, J.S., Halliday, D., Pope, C. *et al.* (1977) The effects of hypoxia on muscle glycogen resynthesis in man. *Q. J. Exp. Physiol.* **62**, 237–45.

Milledge, J.S., Catley, D.M., Ward, M.P. *et al.* (1983a) Renin–aldosterone and angiotensin-converting enzyme during prolonged altitude exposure. *J. Appl. Physiol.* **55**, 699–702.

Milledge, J.S., Catley, D.M., Blume, F.D. and West, J.B. (1983b) Renin, angiotensin-converting enzyme, and aldosterone in humans on Mount Everest. *J. Appl. Physiol.* **55**, 1109–12.

Milledge, J.S., Ward, M.P., Williams, E.S. and Clarke, C.R. (1983c) Cardiorespiratory response to exercise in men repeatedly exposed to extreme altitude. *J. Appl. Physiol.* **55**, 1379–85.

Milledge, J.S., Catley, D.M., Williams, E.S. *et al.* (1983d) Effect of prolonged exercise at altitude on the renin–aldosterone system. *J. Appl. Physiol.* **55**, 413–18.

Milledge, J.S., Thomas, P.S., Beeley, J.M. and English, J.S.C. (1988) Hypoxic ventilatory response and acute mountain sickness. *Eur. Respir. J.* **1**, 948–51.

Milledge, J.S., Beeley, J.M., McArthur, S. and Morice, A.H. (1989) Atrial natriuretic peptide, altitude and acute mountain sickness. *Clin. Sci.* **77**, 509–14.

Milledge, J.S., Beeley, J.M., Broom, J. *et al.* (1991a) Acute mountain sickness susceptibility, fitness and hypoxic ventilatory response. *Eur. Respir. J.* **4**, 1000–3.

Milledge, J.S., McArthur, S., Morice, A. *et al.* (1991b) Atrial natriuretic peptide and exercise-induced fluid retention in man. *J. Wilderness Med.* **2**, 94–101.

Miller, D. (1999) Menstrual cycle abnormalities and the oral contraceptive pill at high altitude (abstract), in *Hypoxia: Into the Next Millennium* (eds. R.C. Roach, P.D. Wagner and P.H. Hackett), Plenum/Kluwer, New York, p. 412.

Mills, W.J. (1973a) Frostbite and hypothermia. Current concepts. *Alaska Med.* **15**, 26–59.

Mills, W.J. (1973b) Frostbite. A discussion of the problem and a review of an Alaskan experience. *Alaska Med.* **15**, 27–47.

Mills, W.J. (1983a) General hypothermia. *Alaska Med.* **25**, 29–32.

Mills, W.J. (1983b) Frostbite. *Alaska Med.* **25**, 33–8.

Mills, W.J. and Rau, D. (1983) University of Alaska, Anchorage. Section of high latitude study, and the Mount McKinley Project. *Alaska Med.* **25**, 21–8.

Mines, A.H. (1981) *Respiratory Physiology*, Raven Press, New York.

Minetti, A.E., Formenti, F. and Ardigo, L.A. (2006) Himalayan porter's specialization: metabolic power, economy and skill. *Proc. Roy. Soc. Ser. B* **273**, 2791–7.

Mirrakhimov, M.M. (1978) Biological and physiological characteristics of high altitude natives of Tien Shan and the Pamirs, in *The Biology of High Altitude Peoples* (ed. P.T. Baker), Cambridge University Press, Cambridge, p. 313.

Mirrakhimov, M.M. and Meimanaliev, T.S. (1981) Heart rhythm disturbances in the inhabitants of mountainous regions. *Cor. Vasa.* **23**, 359–65.

Misset, B., De Jonghe, B., Bastuji-Garin, S. *et al.* Mortality in patients with heatstroke admitted to intensive care units during the 2003 heat wave in France: a national multiple-center risk-factor study. *Crit. Care Med.* **34**, 1087–92.

Mitchell, I.R. and Rodway, G.W. (2011) *Prelude to Everest*. Luath Press, Edinburgh.

Mitchell, R.A. (1963) The role of the medullary chemoreceptors in acclimatization to high altitude, in *Proceedings: International Symposium Cardiovascular Respiration*, Karger, Basel, pp. 124–44.

Miyamoto, O. and Auer, R.N. (2000) Hypoxia, hyperoxia, ischemia, and brain necrosis. *Neurology* **54**, 362–71.

Mizuno, M., Savard, G., Areskog, N.-H. *et al.* (2008) Skeletal muscle adaptations to prolonged exposure to extreme altitude: a role of physical activity? *High Alt. Med. Biol.* **9**, 311–17.

Modesti, P.A., Vanni, S., Morabito, M. *et al.* (2006) Role of endothelin-1 in exposure to high altitude: Acute Mountain Sickness and Endothelin-1 (ACME-1 Study). *Circulation* **114**, 1410–16.

Møller, K., Strauss, G.I., Thomsen, G. *et al.* (2002) Cerebral blood flow, oxidative metabolism and cerebrovascular carbon dioxide reactivity in patients with acute bacterial meningitis. *Acta Anaes. Scand.* **46**, 567.

Molnar, G.W., Hughes, A.L., Wilson, O. and Goldman, R.F. (1973) Effect of wetting skin on finger cooling and freezing. *J. Appl. Physiol.* **35**, 205–7.

Moncada, S.R., Palmer, M.J. and Higgs, E.A. (1991) Nitric oxide physiology, pathophysiology, and pharmacology. *Pharmacol. Rev.* **43**, 109–42.

Moncloa, F., Donayre, J., Sobrevilla, L.A. and Guerra-Garcia, R. (1965) Endocrine studies at high altitude: I. Adrenal cortical function in sea level natives exposed to high altitudes (4300 m) for two weeks. *J. Clin. Endocrinol. Metab.* **25**, 1640–2.

Monge, C.C. and Whittembury, J. (1976) Chronic mountain sickness. *Johns Hopkins Med. J.* **139**, 87–9.

Monge, C.C., Bonavia, D., León-Velarde, F. and Arregui, A. (1990) High altitude populations in Nepal and the Andes, in *Hypoxia: the Adaptations* (eds. J.R. Sutton, G. Coates and J.E. Remmers), Decker, Toronto, pp. 53–8.

Monge, M.C. (1925) Sobre el primer caso del policitemia encontrado en el Peru. *Bull. Acad. Méd. Lima*.

Monge, M.C. (1928) *La Enfermedad de los Andes*, Imp. Americana, Lima.

Monge, M.C. (1948) *Acclimatization in the Andes: Historical Confirmations of 'Climatic Aggression' in the Development of Andean Man*, Johns Hopkins University Press, Baltimore, MD.

Montgomery, H., Clarkson, P., Barnard, M. *et al.* (1999) Angiotensin-converting-enzyme gene insertion/deletion polymorphism and response to physical training. *Lancet* **253**, 1884–5.

Montgomery, H.E., Marshal, R., Hemingway, S. *et al.* (1998) Human gene for physical performance. *Nature* **393**, 221.

Mooi, W., Smith, P. and Heath, D. (1978) The ultrastructural effects of acute decompression on the lung of rats: the influence of frusemide. *J. Pathol.* **126**, 189–96.

Moore, G.W.K. and Semple J.L. (2011) Freezing and frostbite on Mount Everest: new insights into wind chill and freezing times at extreme altitude. *High Alt. Med. Biol.* **12**, 271–5.

Moore, K., Vizzard, N., Coleman, C. *et al.* (2001) Extreme altitude mountaineering and Type 1 diabetes; the Diabetes Federation of Ireland Kilimanjaro Expedition. *Diabet. Med.* **18**, 749–55.

Moore, L.G. (2000) Comparative human ventilatory adaptation to high altitude. *Respir. Physiol.* **121**, 257–76.

Moore, L.G. (2001) Human genetic adaptation to high altitude. *High Alt. Med. Biol.* **2**, 257–79.

Moore, L.G., Cymerman, A., Huang, S.Y. *et al.* (1987) Propranolol blocks the metabolic rate increase but not ventilatory acclimatization to 4300 m. *Respir. Physiol.* **70**, 195–204.

Moore, L.G., Niermeyer, S. and Zamudio, S. (1998a) Human adaptation to high altitude: regional and life cycle perspectives. *Am. J. Physical. Anthropol. Ybk.* **41**, 25–64.

Moore, L.G., Asmus, I. and Curran, L. (1998b) Chronic mountain sickness: gender and geographical variation, in *Progress in Mountain Medicine and High Altitude* (eds. H. Ohno, T. Kobayashi, S. Masuyama and M. Nakashima), Press Committee of the 3rd Congress on Mountain Medicine and High Altitude Physiology, Matsumoto, pp. 114–19.

Moore, L.G., Young, D., McCullough, R.E. *et al.* (2001a) Tibetan protection from intrauterine growth restriction (IUGR) and reproductive loss at high altitude. *Am. J. Hum. Biol.* **13**, 635–44.

Moore, L.G., Zamudio, S., Zhuang, J. *et al.* (2001b) Oxygen transport in Tibetan women during pregnancy at 3,658 m. *Am. J. Phys. Anthropol.* **114**, 42–53.

Moore, L.G., Zamudio, S., Zhuang, J. *et al.* (2002) Analysis of the myoglobin gene in Tibetans living at high altitude. *High. Alt. Med. Biol.* **3**, 39–47.

Moore, L.G., Shriver, M., Bemis, L. *et al.* (2004) Maternal adaptation to high-altitude pregnancy: an experiment of nature–a review. *Placenta* **25**(Suppl. A), S60–71.

Moore, L.G., Niermeyer, S. and Vargas, E. (2007) Does chronic mountain sickness (CMS) have perinatal origins? *Respir. Physiol. Neurobiol.* **158**, 180–9.

Moraga, F.A., Flores, A., Serra, J. *et al.* (2007) Ginkgo biloba decreases acute mountain sickness in people ascending to high altitude at Ollague (3696 m) in northern Chile. *Wilderness Environ. Med.* **18**, 251–7.

Mordes, J.P., Blume, F.D., Boyer, S. *et al.* (1983) High-altitude pituitary–thyroid dysfunction on Mount Everest. *N. Engl. J. Med.* **308**, 1135–8.

Moret, P.R. (1971) Coronary blood flow and myocardial metabolism in man at high altitude, in *High Altitude Physiology: Cardiac and Respiratory Aspects* (eds. R. Porter and J. Knight), Churchill Livingstone, Edinburgh, pp. 131–44.

Morgan, J., Wright, A., Hoar, H. *et al.* (1999) Near-infrared spectroscopy to assess cerebral oxygenation at high altitude (abstract), in *Hypoxia: Into the Next Millennium* (eds. R.C. Roach, P.D. Wagner and P.H. Hackett), Plenum/Kluwer, New York, p. 413.

Morganti, A., Giussani, M., Sala, C. *et al.* (1995) Effects of exposure to high altitude on plasma endothelin-1 levels in normal subjects. *J. Hyperten.* **13**, 859–65.

Morice, A., Pepke-Zaba, J., Loysen, E. *et al.* (1988) Low dose infusion of atrial natriuretic peptide causes salt and water excretion in normal man. *Clin. Sci.* **74**, 359–63.

Morocz, I.A., Zientara, G.P., Gudbjartsson, H. *et al.* (2001) Volumetric quantification of brain swelling after hypobaric hypoxia exposure. *Exp. Neurol.* **168**, 96–104.

Morote-Garcia, J.C., Rosenberger, P., Kuhlicke, J. et al. (2008) HIF-1-dependent repression of adenosine kinase attenuates hypoxia-induced vascular leak. *Blood* **111**, 5571–80.

Morpurgo, G., Arese, P., Bosia, A. et al. (1976) Sherpas living permanently at high altitude: a new pattern of adaptation. *Proc. Natl. Acad. Sci. USA* **73**, 747–51.

Morrell, N.W., Sarybaev, A.S., Alikhan, A. et al. (1999) ACE genotype and risk of high altitude pulmonary hypertension in Kyrghyz highlanders. *Lancet* **353**, 814.

Morris, D.S., Somner, J.E., Scott, K.M. et al. (2007) Corneal thickness at high altitude. *Cornea* **26**, 308–11.

Mortensen, S.P., Dawson, E.A., Yoshiga, S.C. et al. (2005) Limitations to systemic and locomotor limb muscle oxygen delivery and uptake during maximal exercise in adults. *J. Physiol.* **566**, 273–85.

Mortola, J.P., Rezzonico, R., Fisher, J.T. et al. (1990) Compliance of the respiratory system in infants born at high altitude. *Am. Rev. Respir. Dis.* **142**, 43–8.

Morton, J.P. and Cable, N.T. (2005) Effects of intermittent hypoxic training on aerobic and anaerobic performance. *Ergonomics* **48**, 1535–46.

Mosso, A. (1897) *Fisiologia Dell'uomo Sulle Alpi: Studii Fatti Sul Monte Rosa*, Treves, Milan.

Mosso, A. (1898) *Life of Man on the High Alps*. T. Fisher Unwin, London.

Motley, H.L., Cournand, A., Werko, L. et al. (1947) Influence of short periods of induced acute anoxia upon pulmonary artery pressure in man. *Am. J. Physiol.* **150**, 315–20.

Moudgil, R., Michelakis, E.D. and Archer, S.L. (2005) Hypoxic pulmonary vasoconstriction. *J. Appl. Physiol.* **98**, 390–403.

Mounier, R., Amonchot, A., Caillot, N. et al. (2011) Pulmonary arterial systolic pressure and susceptibility to high altitude pulmonary edema. *Respir. Physiol. Neurobiol.* **179**, 294–9.

Muelleman, R.L., Grandstaff, P.M. and Robinson, W.A. (1997) The use of pegorgotein in the treatment of frostbite. *Wilderness Environ. Med.* **8**, 17–19.

Mulligan, E., Lahiri, S. and Storey, B.T. (1981) Carotid body O_2 chemoreception and mitochondrial oxidative phosphorylation. *J. Appl. Physiol.* **51**, 438–46.

Murata, T., Hori, M., Sakamoto, K. et al. (2004) Dexamethasone blocks hypoxia-induced endothelial dysfunction in organ-cultured pulmonary arteries. *Am. J. Respir. Crit. Care. Med.* **170**, 647–55.

Murdoch, D. (1995a) Altitude illness among tourists flying to 3740 meters elevation in the Nepal Himalayas. *J. Travel Med.* **2**, 255–6.

Murdoch, D.R. (1994) Lateral rectus palsy at high altitude. *J. Wilderness Med.* **5**, 179–81.

Murdoch, D.R. (1995) Focal neurological deficits and migraine at high altitude. *J. Neurol. Neurosurg. Psychiatry* **58**, 637.

Murdoch, D.R. (1995) Symptoms of infection and altitude illness among hikers in the Mount Everest region of Nepal. *Aviat. Space Environ. Med.* **66**, 148–51.

Murdoch, D.R. (1995b) Focal neurological defects and migraine at high altitude. *J. Neurol. Neurosurg. Psychiatry* **58**, 637.

Murdoch, D.R. (1996) Focal neurological deficits associated with high altitude. *Wilderness Environ. Med.* **7**, 79–82.

Murdoch, D.R. (1999) How fast is too fast? Attempts to define a recommended ascent rate to prevent acute mountain sickness. *ISMM Newsletter* **9**, 3–6.

Mustafa, S., Thulesius, O. and Ismael, H.N. (2003) Hyperthermia-induced vasoconstriction of the carotid artery, a possible causative factor of heatstroke. *J. Appl. Physiol.* **96**, 1875–8.

Muza, S.R., Rock, P.B., Fulco, C.S. et al. (2001) Women at altitude: ventilatory acclimatization at 4,300 m. *J. Appl. Physiol.* **91**, 1791–9.

Muza, S.R., Kaminsky, D., Fulco, C.S. et al. (2004) Cysteinyl leukotriene blockade does not prevent acute mountain sickness. *Aviat. Space Environ. Med.* **75**, 413–19.

Muza, S.R., Beidleman, B.A. and Fulco, C.S. (2010) Altitude preexposure recommendations for inducing acclimatization. *High Alt. Med.Biol.* **11**, 87–92.

Myerson, S., Hemingway, H., Budget, R. et al. (1999) Human angiotensin I-converting enzyme gene and endurance performance. *J. Appl. Physiol.* **87**, 1313–16.

Myres, J.E., Malan, M., Shumway, J.B. *et al.* (2000) Haplogroup-associated differences in neonatal death and incidence of low birth weight at elevation: a preliminary assessment. *Am. J. Obstet. Gynecol.* **182**, 1599–605.

Naeije, R. (2010) Physiological adaptation of the cardiovascular system to high altitude. *Prog. Cardiovasc. Dis.* **52**, 456–66.

Naeije, R. (2011) Pro: Hypoxic pulmonary vasoconstriction is a limiting factor of exercise at high altitude. *High Alt. Med.Biol.* **12**, 309–12.

Naeije, R., De Backer, D., Vachiery, J.L. and De Vuyst, P. (1996) High-altitude pulmonary edema with primary pulmonary hypertension. *Chest* **110**, 286–9.

Naeije, R., Huez, S., Lamotte, M. et al. (2010) Pulmonary artery pressure limits exercise capacity at high altitude. *Eur. Resp. J.* **36**, 1049–55.

Nahum, G.G. and Stanislaw, H. (2004) Hemoglobin, altitude and birth weight: does maternal anemia during pregnancy influence fetal growth? *J. Reprod. Med.* **49**, 297–305.

Nair, C.S., Malhotra, M.S. and Gopinarth, P.M. (1971) Effect of altitude and cold acclimatization on the basal metabolism in man. *Aerosp. Med.* **42**, 1056–9.

Nakagawa, S., Kubo, K., Koizumi, T. *et al.* (1993) High-altitude pulmonary edema with pulmonary thromboembolism. *Chest* **103**, 948–50.

Nakashima, M. (1983) High altitude medical research in Japan. *Jpn. J. Mount. Med.* **3**, 19–27.

Nanduri, J., Wang, N., Yuan, G. *et al.* (2009) Intermittent hypoxia degrades HIF-2α via calpains resulting in oxidative stress: implications for recurrent apnea-induced morbidities. *Proc. Natl. Acad. Sci. USA* **106**, 1199–1204.

National Fire Protection Association (1993) *Standard for Hypobaric Facilities*, Quincy, MA, NFPA Code 99B.

National Oceanic and Atmospheric Administration (1976) *US Standard Atmosphere*, 1976, NOAA, Washington, DC.

Nattie, E.E. (2002) Central chemosensitivity, sleep and wakefulness. *Respir. Physiol.* **129**, 257–68.

Nayak, N.C., Roy, S. and Narayanan, T.K. (1964) Pathologic features of altitude sickness. *Am. J. Pathol.* **45**, 381–7.

Newhouse, M.T., Becklake, M.R., Macklem, P.T. and McGregor, M. (1964) Effect of alterations in end-tidal CO_2 tension on flow resistance. *J. Appl. Physiol.* **19**, 745–9.

NHS (1974) *Accidental Hypothermia.* NHS Memorandum No. 1974 (Gen.) 7, Scottish Home and Health Department.

Niazi, S.A. and Lewis, F.J. (1958) Profound hypothermia in man: report of a case. *Ann. Surg.* **147**, 254–6.

Nicholas, M., Thullier-Lestienne, F., Bouquet, C. *et al.* (2000) A study of mood changes and personality during a 31-day period of chronic hypoxia in a hypobaric chamber (Everest-Comex '97). *Psychol. Reports* **86**, 119–26.

Nicholas, R., O'Meara P.D. and Calonge, N. (1992) Is syncope related to moderate altitude exposure? *JAMA* **268**, 904–6.

Nickol, A.H., Leverment, J., Richards, P. *et al.* (2006) Temazepam at high altitude reduces periodic breathing without impairing next-day performance: a randomized cross-over double-blind study. *J. Sleep Res.* **15**, 445–54.

Niermeyer, S. (2003) Cardiopulmonary transition in the high altitude infant. *High Alt. Med. Biol.* **4**, 225–39.

Niermeyer, S. (2007) Going to high altitude with a newborn infant. *High Alt. Med. Biol.* **8**, 117–23.

Niermeyer, S., Yang, P., Shanmina, D. *et al.* (1995) Arterial oxygen saturation in Tibetan and Han infants born in Lhasa, Tibet. *N. Engl. J. Med.* **333**, 1248–52.

Noda, M., Suzuki, S., Tsubochi, H. *et al.* (2003) Single dexamethasone injection increases alveolar fluid clearance in adult rats. *Crit. Care Med.* **4**, 1183–9.

Norboo, T., Saiyed, H.N., Angchuk, P.T. *et al.* (2004) Mini review of high altitude health problems in Ladakh. *Biomed. Pharmacother.* **58**, 220–5.

Norese, M.F., Lezon, C.E., Alippi, R.M. *et al.* (2002) Failure of polycythemia-induced increase in arterial oxygen content to suppress the anorexic effect of simulated high altitude in the adult rat. *High Alt. Med. Biol.* **3**, 49–57.

Normand, H., Barragan, M., Benoit, O. et al. (1990) Periodic breathing and O_2 saturation in relation to sleep stages in normal subjects. Am. J. Respir. Crit. Care Med. **149**, 229–35.

Norton, E.F. (1925) Norton and Somervell's attempt, in The Fight for Everest (ed. E.F. Norton), Arnold, London, pp. 90–119.

Nugent, S.K. and Rogers, M.C. (1980) Resuscitation and intensive care monitoring following immersion hypothermia. J. Trauma **20**, 814–15.

Nukada, H., Pollock, M. and Allpress, S. (1981) Experimental cold injury to nerve. Brain **104**, 779–813.

Nummela, A. and Rusko, H. (2000) Acclimatization to altitude and normoxic training improve 400-m running performance at sea level. J. Sports Sci. **18**, 411–19.

Nussbaumer-Ochsner, Y., Schuepfer, N., Ulrich, S. and Bloch, K.E. (2010) Exacerbation of sleep apnoea by frequent central events in patients with the obstructive sleep apnoea syndrome at altitude: a randomised trial. Thorax **65**, 429–35.

Nussbaumer-Ochsner, Y., Latshang, T.D., Ulrich, S. et al. (2012a) Patients with obstructive sleep apnea syndrome benefit from acetazolamide during an altitude sojourn: a randomized, placebo-controlled, double-blind trial. Chest **141**, 131–8.

Nussbaumer-Ochsner, Y., Ursprung, J., Siebenmann, C. et al. (2012b) Effect of short-term acclimatization to high altitude on sleep and nocturnal breathing. Sleep **35**, 419–23.

Nusshag, W. (1954) Hygiene der Haustiere, Hirzel, Leipzig, p. 86.

Nygaard, E. and Nielsen, E. (1978) Skeletal muscle fibre capillarization with extreme endurance training in man, in Swimming Medicine IV (eds. B. Eriksson and B. Furberg), University Park Press, Baltimore, MD.

O'Brien, C., Young, A.J. and Sawka, M.N. (1998) Hypothermia and thermoregulation in cold air. J. Appl. Physiol. **83**, 185–9.

O'Brodovich, H., Andrew, M., Gray, G.W. and Coates, G. (1984) Hypoxia alters blood coagulation during acute decompression in humans. J Appl Physiol **56**, 666–70.

O'Connor, T., Dubowitz, G. and Bickler, P.E. (2004) Pulse oximetry in the diagnosis of acute mountain sickness. High Alt. Med. Biol. **5**, 341–8.

O'Donnell, W.J., Rosenberg, M., Niven, R.W. et al. (1992) Acetazolamide and furosemide attenuate asthma induced by hyperventilation of cold, dry air. Am. Rev. Respir. Dis. **146**, 1518–23.

Oades, P.J., Buchdahl, R.M. and Bush, A. (1994) Prediction of hypoxaemia at high altitude in children with cystic fibrosis. BMJ **308**, 15–18.

Oberg, D. and Ostenson, C.G. (2005) Performance of glucose dehydrogenase- and glucose oxidase-based blood glucose meters at high altitude and low temperature. Diabetes Care **28**, 1261.

Oelz, O., Howald, H., di Prampero, P.E. et al. (1986) Physiological profile of world-class high-altitude climbers. J. Appl. Physiol. **60**, 1734–42.

Oelz, O., Maggiorini, M., Ritter, M. et al. (1989) Nifedipine for high altitude pulmonary oedema. Lancet **2**, 1241–4.

Ogilvie, J. (1977) Exhaustion and exposure. Climber Rambler Sept., 34–9; Oct., 52–5.

Ohkuda, K., Nakahara, K., Weidner, W.J. et al. (1978) Lung fluid exchange after uneven pulmonary artery obstruction in sheep. Circ. Res. **43**, 152–61.

Okumura, A., Fuse, H., Kawauchi, Y. et al. (2003) Changes in male reproductive function after high altitude mountaineering. High Alt. Med. Biol. **4**, 349–53.

Olfert, I.M., Breen, E.C., Mathieu-Costello, O. and Wagner, P.D. (2001) Chronic hypoxia attenuates resting and exercise-induced VEGF, flt-1, and flk-1 mRNA levels in skeletal muscle. J. Appl. Physiol. **90**, 1532–8.

Oliver, S.J., Golija, P. and Macdonald, J.H. (2012) Carbohydrate supplementation and exercise performance at high altitude: a randomized controlled trial. High Alt. Med. Biol. **13**, 22–31.

Olsen, N.V., Hansen, J.-M., Kanstrup, I. et al. (1993) Renal hemodynamics, tubular function, and the response to low-dose dopamine during acute hypoxia in humans. J. Appl. Physiol. **74**, 2166–73.

Omura, A., Roy, R. and Jennings, T. (2000) Inhaled nitric oxide improves survival in the rat model of high-altitude pulmonary edema. *Wilderness Environ. Med.* **11**, 251–6.

Onywera, V.O., Kiplamai, F.K., Boit, M.K. and Pitsiladis, Y.P. (2004) Food and macronutrient intake of elite Kenyan distance runners. *Int. J. Sport Nutr. Exerc. Metab.* **14**, 709–19.

Oort, A.H. and Rasmusson, E.M. (1971) *Atmospheric Circulation Statistics*, US Department of Commerce, NOAA, Rockville, MD, pp. 84–5.

Opitz, E. (1951) Increased vascularization of the tissue due to acclimatization to high altitude and its significance of oxygen transport. *Exp. Med. Surg.* **9**, 389–403.

Orem, J. and Kubin, L. (2000) Respiratory physiology: central neural control, in *Principles and Practice of Sleep Medicine* (eds. M. Kryger, T. Roth and W.C. Dement), W.B. Saunders, Philadelphia, PA, pp. 205–20.

Orr, K.D. and Fainer, D.C. (1951) *Cold Injuries in Korea During Winter 1950–51*, Army Medical Research Laboratory, Fort Knox, KY.

Osborne, J.J. (1953) Experimental hypothermia: respiratory and blood pH changes in relation to cardiac function. *Am. J. Physiol.* **175**, 389–98.

Ou, L.C. and Tenney, S.M. (1970) Properties of mitochondria from hearts of cattle acclimatized to high altitude. *Respir. Physiol.* **8**, 151–9.

Pace, N., Griswold, R.L. and Grunbaum, B.W. (1964) Increase in urinary norepinephrine excretion during 14 days sojourn at 3800m elevation. *Fed. Proc.* **23**, 521.

Palatini, P., Businaro, R., Berton, G. *et al.* (1989) Effects of low altitude exposure on 24-hour blood pressure and adrenergic activity. *Am. J. Cardiol.* **64**, 1379–82.

Palmer, S.K., Moore, L.G., Young, D. *et al.* (1999) Altered blood pressure course during normal pregnancy and increased preeclampsia at high altitude (3100 meters) in Colorado. *Am. J. Obstet. Gynecol.* **180**, 1161–8.

Pandolf, K.B., Young, A.J., Sawka, M.N. *et al.* (1998) Does erythrocyte infusion improve 3.2km run performance at high altitude? *Eur. J. Appl. Physiol.* **79**, 1–6.

Pappenheimer, J. (1988) Physiological regulation of transepithelial impedance in the intestinal mucosa of rats and hamsters. *J. Membr. Biol.* **100**, 137–48.

Pappenheimer, J.R. (1977) Sleep and respiration of rats during hypoxia. *J. Physiol. (Lond.)* **266**, 191–207.

Pappenheimer, J.R., Fencl, V., Heisey, S.R. and Held, D. (1964) Role of cerebral fluids in control of respiration as studied in unanesthetized goats. *Am. J. Physiol.* **208**, 436–40.

Parker, J.C., Breen, E.C. and West, J.B. (1997) High vascular and airway pressures increase interstitial protein mRNA expression in isolated rat lungs. *J. Appl. Physiol.* **83**, 1697–705.

Parkins, K.J., Poets, C.F., O'Brien, L.M. *et al.* (1998) Effect of exposure to 15% oxygen on breathing patterns and oxygen saturation in infants: interventional study. *BMJ* **316**, 887–91.

Pascal, B. (1648) *Story of the Great Experiment on the Equilibrium of Fluids*. English translation of relevant pages in *High Altitude Physiology* (ed. J.B. West), Hutchinson Ross, Stroudsburg, PA, 1981.

Paschen, W. (1996) Disturbances of calcium homeostasis within the endoplasmic reticulum may contribute to the development of ischemic cell damage. *Med. Hypotheses* **47**, 283–8.

Pasha, Q. and Gassmann, M. (2010) Taskforce: pulmonary hypertension associated with high altitude and hypoxia – annual report 2009. *PVRI Rev.* **2**, 36–41.

Passino, C., Bernardi, L., Spadacini, G. *et al.* (1996) Autonomic regulation of heart rate and peripheral circulation: comparison of high altitude and sea level residents. *Clin. Sci.* **91**, 81–3.

Patel, S., Woods, D.R., Macleod, N.J. *et al.* (2003) Angiotensin-converting enzyme genotype and the ventilatory response to exertional hypoxia. *Eur. Resp. J.* **22**, 755–60.

Paton, B.C. (1983) Accidental hypothermia. *Pharmacol. Ther.* **22**, 331–77.

Paton, B.C. (1987) Pathophysiology of frostbite, in *Hypoxia and Cold* (eds. J.R. Sutton, C.S. Houston and G. Coates), Praeger, New York, pp. 329–39.

Paton, B.C. (1991) Hypothermia, in *A Colour Atlas of Mountain Medicine* (eds. J. Vallotton and F. Dubas), Wolfe, London, pp. 92–6.

Pattengale, P.K. and Holloszy, J.O. (1967) Augmentation of skeletal muscle myoglobin by a program of treadmill running. *Am. J. Physiol.* **213**, 783–5.

Pattinson, K., Myers, S. and Gardner-Thorpe, C. (2004) Problems with capnography at high altitude. *Anaesthesia* **59**, 69–72.

Patton, J.F. and Doolittle, W.H. (1972) Core rewarming by peritoneal dialysis following induced hypothermia in the dog. *J. Appl. Physiol.* **33**, 800–4.

Patz, D.S., Swihart, B. and White, D.P. (2010) CPAP pressure requirements for obstructive sleep apnea patients at varying altitudes. *Sleep* **33**, 715–18.

Paul, M.A. and Fraser, W.D. (1994) Performance during mild acute hypoxia. *Aviat. Space. Environ. Med.* **65**, 891–9.

Pavan, P., Sarto, P., Merlo, L. *et al.* (2003) Extreme altitude mountaineering and type 1 diabetes: the Cho Oyu alpinisti in Alta Quota expedition. *Diabetes Care* **26**, 3196–7.

Pavan, P., Sarto, P., Merlo, L. *et al.* (2004) Metabolic and cardiovascular parameters in type 1 diabetics at extreme altitude. *Med. Sci. Sports Exerc.* **36**, 1283–9.

Pawson, I.G. (1977) Growth characteristics of populations of Tibetan origin in Nepal. *Am. J. Phys. Anthropol.* **47**, 473–82.

Peacock, A.J. and Jones, P.L. (1997) Gas exchange at extreme altitude: results from the British 40th Anniversary Everest Expedition. *Eur. Respir. J.* **10**, 1439–44.

Pearn, J.H. (1982) Cold injury complicating trauma in sub-zero environments. *Med. J. Aust.* **1**, 505–7.

Pecchio, O., Maule, S., Migliardi, M. *et al.* (2000) Effects of exposure at an altitude of 3,000 m on performance of glucose meters. *Diabetes Care* **23**, 129–31.

Pedlar, C., Whyte, G., Emegbo, S. *et al.* (2005) Acute sleep responses in a normobaric hypoxic tent. *Med. Sci. Sports Exerc.* **37**, 1075–9.

Pei, S.X., Chen, X.J., Si Ren, B.Z. *et al.* (1989) Chronic mountain sickness in Tibet. *Q. J. Med.* **71**, 555–74.

Peñaloza, D. (1971) Discussion, in *High Altitude Physiology: Cardiac and Respiratory Aspects* (eds. R. Porter and J. Knight), Churchill Livingstone, Edinburgh, p. 169.

Peñaloza, D. (2007) High altitude pulmonary hypertension. Reappraisal of the Consensus Statement on Chronic and Subacute High Altitude Diseases, *Problems of High Altitude Medicine and Biology* (eds A. Aldashev and R. Naeije). Actas del Taller en Investigaciones Avanzadas Sobre Medicina y Biología Aplicada a la Altura, Organizada por la OTAN. Springer, Berlin, 2007, 11–37.

Peñaloza, D. and Arias-Stella, J. (2007) The heart and pulmonary circulation at high altitudes healthy highlanders and chronic mountain sickness. *Circulation* **115**: 1132–46.

Peñaloza, D. and Echevarria, M. (1957) Electrocardiographic observations on ten subjects at sea level and during one year of residence at high altitudes. *Am. Heart J.* **54**, 811–22.

Peñaloza, D. and Sime, F. (1969) Circulatory dynamics during high altitude pulmonary edema. *Am. J. Cardiol.* **23**, 369–78.

Peñaloza, D. and Sime, F. (1971) Chronic cor pulmonale due to loss of altitude acclimatization (chronic mountain sickness). *Am. J. Med.* **50**, 728–43.

Peñaloza, D., Sime, F., Banchero, N. and Gamboa, R. (1962) Pulmonary hypertension in healthy man born and living at high altitudes. *Med. Thorac.* **19**, 449–60.

Peñaloza, D., Sime, F., Banchero, N. *et al.* (1963) Pulmonary hypertension in healthy men born and living at high altitudes. *Am. J. Cardiol.* **11**, 150–7.

Peñaloza, D., Arias-Stella, J., Sime, F. *et al.* (1964) The heart and pulmonary circulation in children at high altitudes: physiological, anatomical, and clinical observations. *Pediatrics* **34**, 568–82.

Peñaloza, D., Sime, F., Ruiz. L. (2008) Pulmonary hemodynamics and children living at high altitudes. *High Alt. Med. Biol.* **9**, 199–207.

Peng, Y.-J., Yuan, G., Ramakrishnan, D. *et al.* (2006) Heterozygous HIF-1α deficiency impairs carotid body-mediated systemic responses and reactive oxygen species generation in mice exposed to intermittent hypoxia. *J. Physiol.* **577**, 705–16.

Peng, Y., Yang, Z., Zhang, H. et al. (2011) Genetic variations in Tibetan populations and high altitude adaptation at the Himalayas. Mol. Biol. Evol. 28, 1075–81.

Perez-Pinzon, M.A., Chan, C.Y., Rosenthal, M. and Sick, T.J. (1992) Membrane and synaptic activity during anoxia in the isolated turtle cerebellum. Am. J. Physiol. 263, R1057–63.

Peroni, D.G., Boner, A.L., Vallone, G. et al. (1994) Effective allergen avoidance at high altitude reduces allergen-induced bronchial hyperresponsiveness. Am. J. Respir. Crit. Care Med. 149, 1441–6.

Perrill, C.V. (1993) High-altitude sycope: history repeats itself. JAMA 269, 587.

Pesce, C., Leal, C., Pinto, H. et al. (2005) Determinants of acute mountain sickness and success on Mount Aconcagua (6962 m). High Alt. Med. Biol. 6, 158–66.

Petetin, D. (1991) Eye protection at high altitude, in A Colour Atlas of Mountain Medicine (eds. J. Vallotton and F. Dubas), Wolfe, London, pp. 71–2.

Petit, J.M., Milic-Emili, J. and Troquet, J. (1963) Travail dynamique pulmonaire et altitude. Rev. Med. Aerosp. 2, 276–9.

Peyronnard, J.M., Pednault, M. and Aquayo, A.J. (1977) Neuropathies due to cold. Quantitative studies of structural changes in human and animal nerves, in Proceedings of the 11th World Congress of Neurology, Amsterdam, pp. 308–29.

Pham, I., Uchida, T., Planes, C. et al. (2002) Hypoxia upregulates VEGF expression in alveolar epithelial cells in vitro and in vivo. Am. J. Physiol., Lung Cell. Mol. Physiol. 283, L1133–42.

Pham, I., Wuerzner, G., Richaler, J.-P. et al. (2010) Endothelin receptors blockade blunts hypoxia-induced increase in PAP in humans. Eur. J. Clin. 40, 195–202.

Phillipson, E.A., Sullivan, C.E., Read, D.J.C. et al. (1978) Ventilatory and waking responses to hypoxia in sleeping dogs. J. Appl. Physiol. Respir. Environ. Exerc. Physiol. 44, 512–20.

Pialoux, V., Hanly, P.J. and Foster, G.E. (2009) Effects of exposure to intermittent hypoxia on oxidative stress and acute hypoxic ventilatory response in humans. Am. J. Respir. Crit. Care Med. 180, 1002–9.

Pichiule, P. and LaManna, J.C. (2002) Angiopoietin-2 and rat brain capillary remodeling during adaptation and deadaptation to prolonged mild hypoxia. J. Appl. Physiol. 93, 1131–9.

Pickering, B.G., Bristow, G.K. and Craig, D.B. (1977) Core rewarming by peritoneal irrigation in accidental hypothermia. Anesth. Analg. 56, 574–7.

Picon-Reategui, E. (1961) Basal metabolic rate and body composition at high altitudes. J. Appl. Physiol. 16, 431–4.

Pierre, B. and Aulard, C. (1985) Escalades et Randonnés du Hoggar et dans les Tassilis, Arthaud, Paris, p. 153.

Piiper, J. and Scheid, P. (1980) Blood–gas equilibration in lungs, in Pulmonary Gas Exchange, vol. 1, Ventilation, Blood Flow, and Diffusion (ed. J.B. West), Academic Press, New York, pp. 131–71.

Piiper, J. and Scheid, P. (1986) Cross-sectional P_{O_2} distributions in Krogh cylinder and solid cylinder models. Respir. Physiol. 64, 241–51.

Pines, A. (1978) High altitude acclimatization and proteinuria in East Africa. Br. J. Dis. Chest 72, 196–8.

Pines, A., Slater, J.D.H. and Jowett, T.P. (1977) The kidney and aldosterone in acclimatization at altitude. Br. J. Dis. Chest 71, 203–7.

Pison, U., López, F.A., Heidelmeyer, C.F. et al. (1993) Inhaled nitric oxide reverses hypoxic pulmonary vasoconstriction without impairing gas exchange. J. Appl. Physiol. 74, 1287–92.

Pitsiou, G., Kyriazis, G., Hatzizisi, O. et al. (2002) Tumor necrosis factor-alpha serum levels, weight loss and tissue oxygenation in chronic obstructive pulmonary disease. Respir. Med. 96, 594–8.

Pitt, P. (1970) Surgeon in Nepal, Murray, London, p. 135.

Planes, C., Escoubet, B., Blot-Chabaud, M. et al. (1997) Hypoxia downregulates expression and activity of epithelial sodium channels in rat alveolar epithelial cells. Am. J. Respir. Cell. Mol. Biol. 17, 508–18.

Plata, R., Cornejo, A., Arratia, C. et al. (2002) Angiotensin-converting-enzyme inhibition therapy in altitude polycythemia: a prospective randomized trial. *Lancet* **359**, 663–6.

Plutarch (46–120) Alexander and Caesar. *Loeb Classics,* vol. 7. (1971) Heinemann, London, p. 389.

Podolsky, A., Eldridge, M.W., Richardson, R.S. *et al.* (1996) Exercise-induced VA/Q inequality in subjects with prior high-altitude pulmonary edema. *J. Appl. Physiol.* **81**, 922–32.

Pohjantahti, H., Laitinen, J. and Parkkari, J. (2005) Exercise-induced bronchospasm among healthy elite cross country skiers and non-athletic students. *Scand. J. Med. Sci. Sports* **15**, 324–8.

Poiani, G.J., Tozzi, C.A., Yohn, S.E. *et al.* (1990) Collagen and elastin metabolism in hypertensive pulmonary arteries of rats. *Circ. Res.* **66**, 968–78.

Pollard, A.J. and Murdoch, D.R. (1997) Children at altitude, in *The High Altitude Medicine Handbook*, 2nd edn, Radcliffe Medical Press, Oxford, pp. 39–49.

Pollard, A.J., Mason, N.P., Barry, P.W. *et al.* (1996) Effect of altitude on spirometric parameters and the performance of peak flow meters. *Thorax* **51**, 175–8.

Pollard, A.J., Murdoch, D.R. and Bärtsch, P. (1998) Children at altitude. *BMJ* **316**, 874–5.

Pollard, A.J., Niermeyer, S., Barry, P. *et al.* (2001) Children at altitude: an international consensus statement by an *ad hoc* committee of the International Society for Mountain Medicine. *High Alt. Med. Biol.* **2**, 389–403.

Poole, D.C. and Mathieu-Costello, O. (1990) Effects of hypoxia on capillary orientation in anterior tibialis muscle of highly active mice. *Respir. Physiol.* **82**, 1–10.

Porter, M.M., Vandervoort, A.A. and Lexell, J. (1995) Aging of the human muscle: structure, function and adaptability. *Scan. J. Med. Sci. Sports.* **5**, 127–8.

Potter, R.F. and Groom, A.C. (1983) Capillary diameter and geometry in cardiac and skeletal muscle studied by means of corrosion casts. *Microvasc. Res.* **25**, 68–84.

Poulin, M.J., Cunningham, D.A., Paterson, D.H. *et al.* (1993) Ventilatory sensitivity to CO_2 in hyperoxia and hypoxia in older humans. *J. Appl. Physiol.* **75**, 2209–16.

Poulsen, T.D., Klausen, T., Richalet, J.P. *et al.* (1998) Plasma volume in acute hypoxia: comparison of a carbon monoxide rebreathing method and dye dilution with Evans' blue. *Eur. J. Appl. Physiol.* **77**, 457–61.

Povea, C., Schmitt, L., Brugniaux, J. *et al.* (2005) Effects of intermittent hypoxia on heart rate variability during rest and exercise. *High Alt. Med. Biol.* **6**, 215–25.

Powell, F.L. and Garcia, N. (2000) Physiological effects of intermittent hypoxia. *High Alt. Med. Biol.* **1**, 125–36.

Prabhakar, H.R. (2000) Oxygen sensing by the carotid body chemoreceptors. *J. Appl. Physiol.* **88**, 2287–95.

Prabhakar, H.R. and Jacono, F.J. (2005) Cellular and molecular mechanisms associated with carotid body adaptations to chronic hypoxia. *High Alt. Med. Biol.* **6**, 112–120.

Prabhakar, H.R. and Overholt, J.L. (2000) Cellular mechanisms of oxygen sensing at the carotid body: haem and ion channels. *Respir. Physiol.* **122**, 209–21.

Pradhan, S., Yadav, S., Neupane, P. and Subedi, P. (2009) Acute mountain sickness in children at 4380 meters in the Himalayas. *Wilderness Environ. Med.* **20**, 359–63.

Pratali, L., Cavana, M., Sicarir, R. and Picano, E. (2010) Frequent subclinical high-altitude pulmonary edema detected by chest sonography as ultrasound lung comets in recreational climbers. *Crit. Care Med.* **38**, 1818–23.

Pratali, L., Rimoldi, S.F., Rexhaj, E. *et al.* (2012) Exercise induces rapid interstitial lung water accumulation in patients with chronic mountain sickness. *Chest* **141**, 953–8.

Pretorius, H.A. (1970) Effect of oxygen on night vision. *Aerospace Med.* **41**, 560–2.

Prisk, G.K., Elliott, A.R. and West J.B. (2000) Sustained microgravity reduces the human ventilatory response to hypoxia but not to hypercapnia. *J. Appl. Physiol.* **88**, 1421–30.

Pritchard, J.S. and Lane, D.J. (1974) Intestinal absorption studied in patients with chronic obstructive airways disease. *Thorax* **29**, 609.

Pugh, L.G.C.E. (1950) Physiological studies on HMS *Vengeance*: Royal Navy cold weather cruise 1994, *MRC Royal Naval Personnel Research Committee RNP 49/561.*

Pugh, L.G.C.E. (1955) Report on Cho Oyu 1952 and Everest 1953 expeditions. (Unpublished archival material held in the Archival Collection in High Altitude Medicine and Physiology at University of California, San Diego, USA.)

Pugh, L.G.C.E. (1957) Resting ventilation and alveolar air on Mount Everest: with remarks on the relation of barometric pressure to altitude in mountains. *J. Physiol. (Lond.)* **135**, 590–610.

Pugh, L.G.C.E. (1958) Muscular exercise on Mt. Everest. *J. Physiol. (Lond.)* **141**, 233–61.

Pugh, L.G.C.E. (1959) Carbon monoxide hazard in Antarctica. *BMJ* **1**, 192–6.

Pugh, L.G.C.E. (1962a) Physiological and medical aspects of the Himalayan Scientific and Mountaineering Expedition, 1960–61. *BMJ* **2**, 621–33.

Pugh, L.G.C.E. (1962b) Solar heat gain by man in the high Himalaya: UNESCO Symposium on Environmental Physiology and Psychology, Lucknow, India, pp. 325–9.

Pugh, L.G.C.E. (1963) Tolerance to extreme cold at altitude in a Nepalese pilgrim. *J. Appl. Physiol.* **18**, 1234–8.

Pugh, L.G.C.E. (1964a) Man at high altitude. *Scientific Basis of Medicine, Annual Review* 32–54.

Pugh, L.G.C.E. (1964b) Blood volume and haemoglobin concentration at altitudes above 18000 ft (5500 m). *J. Physiol.* **170**, 344–54.

Pugh, L.G.C.E. (1964c) Animals in high altitudes: man above 5000 m mountain exploration, in *Handbook of Physiology, Adaptation to the Environment,* section 4 (eds. D.B. Dill, E.F. Adolph and C.C. Wilber), Washington, DC, pp. 861–8.

Pugh, L.G.C.E. (1964d) Cardiac output in muscular exercise at 5800 m (19,000 ft). *J. Appl. Physiol.* **19**, 441–7.

Pugh, L.G.C.E. (1965) Altitude and athletic performance. *Nature* **207**, 1397–8.

Pugh, L.G.C.E. (1966) Clothing insulation and accidental hypothermia in youth. *Nature* **209**, 1281–6.

Pugh, L.G.C.E. (1967) Cold stress and muscular exercise with special reference to accidental hypothermia. *BMJ* **2**, 333–7.

Pugh, L.G.C.E. (1969) Blood volume changes in outdoor exercise of 8–10 h duration. *J. Physiol. (Lond.)* **200**, 345–51.

Pugh, L.G.C.E. and Band, G. (1953) Appendix VI: Diet, in *The Ascent of Everest* (ed. J. Hunt), Hodder and Stoughton, London, pp. 263–9.

Pugh, L.G.C.E. and Ward, M.P. (1956) Some effects of high altitude on man. *Lancet* **2**, 1115–21.

Pugh, L.G.C.E., Gill, M.B., Lahiri, S. *et al.* (1964) Muscular exercise at great altitudes. *J. Appl. Physiol.* **19**, 431–40.

Pulfery, S.M. and Jones, P.L. (1996) Energy expenditure and requirement while climbing above 6,000 m. *J. Appl. Physiol.* **81**, 1306–11.

Puri, G.D., Jayant, A., Dorje, M. and Tashi, M. (2008) Propofol-fentanyl anaesthesia at high altitude: anaesthetic requirements and haemodynamic variations when compared with anaesthesia at low altitude. *Acta Anaesthesiol. Scand.* **52**, 427–31.

Purkayastha, S.S., Bhaumik, G., Sharma, R.P. *et al.* (2000) Effects of mountaineering training at high altitude (4,350 m) on physical work performance of women. *Aviat. Space Environ. Med.* **71**, 685–91.

Puthucheary, Z., Skipworth, J.R.A., Rawal, J. *et al.* (2011) The *ACE* gene and human performance: 12 years on. *Sports Med.* **41**, 433–48.

Pyne, D.B., Gleeson, M., McDonald, W.A. *et al.* (2000) Training strategies to maintain immunocompetence in athletes. *Int. J. Sports Med.* **21**(Suppl. 1), S51–60.

Qi, Y., Niu, W., Zhu, T. *et al.* (2008) Synergistic effect of the genetic polymorphisms of the renin-angiotensin, aldosterone system on high altitude pulmonary edema. A study from Qinghai–Tibet altitude. *Eur. J. Epidemiol.* **22**, 143–52.

Qi, Y., Niu, W., Zhu, T. *et al.* (2009) Genetic interaction of Hsp70 family genes polymorphisms with high altitude pulmonary edema among Chinese railway constructors at altitudes exceedingly 4000 meters. *Clin. Chim. Acta* **405**, 17–22.

Qi, Y., Sun, J., Zhu, T. *et al.* (2011) Association of angiotensin-converting enzyme gene insertion/deletion polymorphism with high altitude pulmonary edema: meta-analysis. *J. Renin-Angiotensin-Aldosterone Syst.* **12**, 617–23

Quick, J., Eichenberger, A. and Binswanger, U. (1992) Stimulation of erythropoietin in renal insufficiency by hypobaric hypoxia. *Nephrol. Dial. Transplant.* **7**, 1002–6.

Radomski, M.N. and Boutelier, C. (1982) Hormone response of normal and intermittent cold pre-adapted humans to continuous cold. *J. Appl. Physiol.* **53**, 610–16.

Raff, H. and Kohandarvish, S. (1990) The effect of oxygen on aldosterone release from bovine adrenocortical cells *in vitro*. *Endocrinology* **127**, 682–7.

Raff, H., Jankowski, B.M., Engeland, W.C. and Oaks, M.K. (1996) Hypoxia *in vivo* inhibits aldosterone and aldosterone synthase mRNA in rats. *J. Appl. Physiol.* **81**, 604–10.

Raguso, C.A., Guinot, S.L., Janssens, J-P. *et al.* (2004) Chronic hypoxia: common traits between chronic obstructive pulmonary disease and altitude. *Curr. Opin. Clin. Nutr. Metab. Care* **7**, 411–17.

Rahn, H. and Fenn, W.O. (1955) *A Graphical Analysis of the Respiratory Gas Exchange*, American Physiological Society, Washington, DC.

Rahn, H. and Otis, A.B. (1949) Man's respiratory response during and after acclimatization to high altitude. *Am. J. Physiol.* **157**, 445–62.

Rai, R.M., Malhotra, M.S., Dimri, G.P. and Sampathkumar, T. (1975) Utilization of different quantities of fat at high altitude. *Am. J. Clin. Nutr.* **28**, 242–5.

Raichle, M.E. and Hornbein, T.F. (2001) The high-altitude brain, in *High Altitude: An Exploration of Human Adaptation* (eds. T.F. Hornbein and R.B. Schoen), Marcel Dekker, New York, pp. 377–423.

Raifman, M.A., Berant, M. and Levarsky, C. (1978) Cold weather and rhabdomyolysis. *J. Paediatr.* **93**, 970–1.

Raja, K.B., Pippard, M.J., Simpson, R.J. and Peters, T.J. (1986) Relationship between erythropoiesis and the enhanced intestinal uptake of ferric iron in hypoxia in the mouse. *Br. J. Haematol.* **64**, 587–93.

Ramanathan, V., Li, F., Ramana, M.V. *et al.* (2007) Atmospheric brown clouds: Hemispherical and regional variations in long-range transport, absorption, and radiative forcing. *J. Geophys. Res.* **112**, D22S21, 26 PP.

Ramirez, G., Bittle, P.A., Hammond, M. *et al.* (1988) Regulation of aldosterone secretion during hypoxemia at sea level and moderately high altitude. *J. Clin. Endocrinol. Metab.* **67**, 1162–5.

Ramirez, G., Hammon, M., Agousti, S.J. *et al.* (1992) Effects of hypoxemia at sea level and high altitude on sodium excretion and hormonal levels. *Aviat. Space Environ. Med.* **63**, 891–8.

Ramirez, G., Herrera, R., Pineda, D. *et al.* (1995) The effects of high altitude on hypothalamic–pituitary secretory dynamics in men. *Clin. Endocrinol.* **43**, 11–18.

Ramirez, G., Pineda, D., Bittle, P.A. *et al.* (1998) Partial renal resistance to arginine vasopressin as an adaptation to high altitude living. *Aviat. Space Environ. Med.* **69**, 58–65.

Ramos, D.A., Kruger, H., Muro, M. and Arias-Stella, J. (1967) Patologica del hombre nativo de las grande alturas: investigacion de las causes de muerte en 300 autopsias. *Bon. Sanit. Panam.* **62**, 497–507.

Rankinen, T., Pérusse, L., Gagnon, J. *et al.* (2000a) Angiotensin-converting enzyme ID polymorphism and fitness phenotype in the HERITAGE Family Study. *J. Appl. Physiol.* **88**, 1029–35.

Rankinen, T., Wolfarth, B., Simoneau, J.-A. *et al.* (2000b) No association between the angiotensin-converting enzyme ID polymorphism and elite endurance athlete status. *J. Appl. Physiol.* **88**, 1571–5.

Rassler, B., Marx, G., Reissig, C. *et al.* (2007) Time course of hypoxia-induced lung injury in rats. *Respir. Physiol. Neurobiol.* **159**, 45–54.

Rastogi, C.K., Malholtra, M.S., Srivastava, M.C. *et al.* (1977) Study of the pituitary–thyroid functions at high altitude in man. *J. Clin. Endocrinol. Metab.* **44**, 447–52.

Ratan, R.R., Siddiq, A., Aminova, L. *et al.* (2004) Translation of ischemic preconditioning to the patient: prolyl hydroxylase inhibition and hypoxia inducible factor-1 as novel targets for stroke therapy. *Stroke* **35**, 2687.

Rathat, C., Richalet, J.-P., Herry, J.-P. and Largmighat, P. (1992) Detection of high-risk subjects for high altitude diseases. *Int. J. Sports Med.* **13**, S76–8.

Ravenhill, T.H. (1913) Some experience of mountain sickness in the Andes. *J. Trop. Med. Hyg.* **16**, 313–20.

Raynaud, J., Drouet. L., Martineaud, J.P. *et al.* (1981) Time course of plasma growth hormone during exercise in humans at altitude. *J. Appl. Physiol.* **50**, 229–33.

RCP (1966) *Report of Committee on Accidental Hypothermia,* Royal College of Physicians, London.

Read, J. and Fowler, K.T. (1964) Effect of exercise on zonal distribution of pulmonary blood flow. *J. Appl. Physiol.* **19**, 672–8.

Rebuck, A.S. and Campbell, E.J.M. (1974) A clinical method for assessing the ventilatory response to hypoxia. *Am. Rev. Respir. Dis.* **109**, 345–50.

Recavarren, S. and Arias-Stella, J. (1964) Right ventricular hypertrophy in people born and living at high altitudes. *Br. Heart J.* **26**, 806–12.

Reed, D.J.C. (1967) A clinical method of assessing the ventilatory response to carbon dioxide. *Australas. Ann. Med.* **16**, 20–32.

Reeves, J.A. (2004) Is increased hematopoiesis needed at altitude? *J. Appl. Physiol.* **96**, 1579–80.

Reeves, J.T. and Grover, R.F. (1975) High-altitude pulmonary hypertension and pulmonary edema. *Prog. Cardiol.* **4**, 99–118.

Reeves, J.T. and Grover, R.F. (2005) Insights by Peruvian scientists into the pathogenesis of human chronic hypoxic pulmonary hypertension. *J. Appl. Physiol.* **98**, 384–9.

Reeves, J.T. and Weil, J.V. (2001) Chronic mountain sickness. A view from the crows nest. *Ad. Exper. Med. Biol.* **542**, 419–37.

Reeves, J.T., Moore, L.G., McCullough, R.E. *et al.* (1985) Headache at high altitude is not related to internal carotid arterial blood velocity. *J. Appl. Physiol.* **59**, 909–15.

Reeves, J.T., Groves, B.M., Sutton, J.T. *et al.* (1987) Operation Everest II: preservation of cardiac function at extreme altitude. *J. Appl. Physiol.* **63**, 531–9.

Reeves, J.T., Wagner, J., Zafren, K. *et al.* (1994) Seasonal variation in barometric pressure and temperature: effect on altitude illness, in

Hypoxia and Molecular Medicine (eds. J.R. Sutton, C.S. Houston and G. Coates), Queen City Printers, Burlington, VT, pp. 275–81.

Regard, M., Oelz, O., Brugger, P. and Landis, T. (1989) Persistent cognitive impairment in climbers after repeated exposure to extreme altitude. *Neurology* **39**, 210–13.

Reichl, M. (1987) Neuropathy of the feet due to running on cold surfaces. *BMJ* **294**, 348–9.

Reinhart, W.H., Kayser, B., Singh, A. *et al.* (1991) Blood rheology and acute mountain sickness and high-altitude pulmonary edema. *J. Appl. Physiol.* **71**, 934–8.

Reitan, R.M. and Davison, L.A. (eds.) (1974) *Clinical Neuropsychology: Current Status and Applications,* Winston, Washington DC.

Reite, M., Jackson, D., Cahoon, R.L. and Weil, J.V. (1975) Sleep physiology at high altitude. *Electroencephalogr. Clin. Neurophysiol.* **38**, 463–71.

Remillard, C.V. and Yuan, J.X. (2005) High altitude pulmonary hypertension: role of K^+ and Ca^{2+} channels. *High Alt. Med. Biol.* **6**, 133–46.

Remmers, J.E. and Mithoefer, J.C. (1969) The carbon monoxide diffusing capacity in permanent residents at high altitudes. *Respir. Physiol.* **6**, 233–44.

Ren, Y., Fu, Z., Shen, W. *et al.* (2010). Incidence of high altitude illnesses among unacclimatized persons who acutely ascended to Tibet. *High Alt. Med. Biol.* **11**, 39–42.

Rennie, D. (1973) Field studies in hypoxia and the kidney, in *Cornell Seminars in Nephrology* (ed. E.L. Becker), Wiley, New York, pp. 193–206.

Rennie, D. (1989) Will mountain trekkers have heart attacks? *JAMA* **261**, 1045–6.

Rennie, D. and Morrissey, J. (1975) Retinal changes in Himalayan climbers. *Arch. Ophthalmol.* **93**, 395–400.

Rennie, D. and Wilson, R. (1982) Who should not go high, in *Hypoxia: Man at Altitude* (eds. J.R. Sutton, N.L. Jones, and C.S. Houston), Thieme-Stratton, New York, pp. 186–90.

Rennie, D., Lozano, R., Monge, C. *et al.* (1971a). Renal oxygenation in male Peruvian natives living permanently at high altitude. *J. Appl. Physiol.* **30**, 450–6.

Rennie, D., Marticorena, E., Monge, C. and Sirotzky, L. (1971b) Urinary protein excretion in high altitude residents. *J. Appl. Physiol.* **31**, 257–9.

Rennie, D., Frayser, R., Gray, G. and Houston, C. (1972) Urine and plasma proteins in men at 5,400 m. *J. Appl. Physiol.* **32**, 369–73.

Rennie, I.D.B. and Joseph, B.L. (1970) Urinary protein excretion in climbers at high altitude. *Lancet* **1**, 1247–51.

Rennie, M.J., Babij, P., Sutton, J.R. *et al.* (1983) Effects of acute hypoxia on forearm leucine metabolism, in *Hypoxia, Exercise and Altitude* (eds. J.R. Sutton, C.S. Houston and N.L. Jones), Liss, New York, pp. 317–24.

Resar, J.R., Roguin, A., Voner, J. *et al.* (2005) Hypoxia-inducible factor 1alpha polymorphism and coronary collaterals in patients with ischemic heart disease. *Chest* **128**, 787–91.

Reshetnikova, O.S., Burton, G.J. and Milovanov, A.P. (1994) Effects of hypobaric hypoxia on the fetoplacental unit: the morphometric diffusing capacity of the villous membrane at high altitude. *Am. J. Obstet. Gynecol.* **171**, 1560–5.

Rexhaj, E., Garcin, S., Rimoldi, S.F. *et al.* (2011) Reproducibility of acute mountain sickness in children and adults: a prospective study. *Pediatrics* **127**, e1145–8.

Reynafarje, B. (1962) Myoglobin content and enzymatic activity of muscle and altitude adaptation. *J. Appl. Physiol.* **17**, 301–5.

Reynolds, R.D., Lickteig, J.A., Deuster, P.A. *et al.* (1999) Energy metabolism increases and regional body fat decreases while regional muscle mass is spared in humans climbing Mt. Everest. *J. Nutr.* **129**, 1307–14.

Rhodes, J. (2005) Comparative physiology of hypoxic pulmonary hypertension: historical clues from brisket disease. *J. Appl. Physiol.* **98**, 1092–100.

Ricart, A., Maristany, J., Fort, N. *et al.* (2005) Effects of sildenafil on the human response to acute hypoxia and exercise. *High Alt. Med. Biol.* **6**, 43–9.

Rice, L., Ruiz, W., Driscoll, T. *et al.* (2001) Neocytolysis on descent from altitude: a newly recognised mechanism for the control of red cell mass. *Ann. Intern. Med.* **134**, 652–6.

Richalet, J.-P. (1990) The heart and adrenergic system, in *Hypoxia: the Adaptations* (eds. J.R.

Sutton, G. Coates and J.E. Remmers), Dekker, Philadelphia, pp. 231–40.

Richalet, J.-P. (2010) Operation Everest III: COMEX '97. *High Alt. Med. Biol.* **11**, 121–32.

Richalet, J.-P., Keromes, A., Dersch, B. *et al.* (1988) Caractéristiques physiologiques des alpinistes de haute altitude. *Sci. Sports* **3**, 89–108.

Richalet, J.-P., Rutgers, V., Bouchet, P. *et al.* (1989) Diurnal variation of acute mountain sickness, colour vision, and plasma cortisol and ACTH at high altitude. *Aviat. Space Environ. Med.* **60**, 105–11.

Richalet, J.-P., Hornych, A., Rathat, C. *et al.* (1991) Plasma prostaglandins, leukotrienes and thromboxane in acute high altitude hypoxia. *Respir. Physiol.* **85**, 205–15.

Richalet, J.-P., Bittel, J. and Herry, J.P. (1992) Use of a hypobaric chamber for preacclimatization before climbing Mount Everest. *Int. J. Sports Med.* **13**(Suppl. 1), 216–20.

Richalet, J.-P., Souberbielle, J.C., Antezana, A.M. *et al.* (1994) Control of erythropoiesis in humans during prolonged exposure to the altitude of 6542 m. *Am. J. Physiol.* **266**, R756–64.

Richalet, J.-P., Dechaux, M., Bienvenu, A. *et al.* (1995) Erythropoiesis and renal function at the altitude of 6,542 m. *Jpn. J. Mount. Med.* **15**, 135–50.

Richalet, J.-P., Vargas Donoso M., Jiménez D. *et al.* (2002) Chilean miners commuting from sea level to 4500m: a prospective study. *High Alt. Med. Biol.* **3**, 159–66.

Richalet, J.-P., Gratadour, P., Robach, P. *et al.* (2005a) Sildenafil inhibits altitude-induced hypoxemia and pulmonary hypertension. *Am. J. Respir. Crit. Care Med.* **171**, 275–81.

Richalet, J.-P., Rivera, M., Bouchet, P. *et al.* (2005b) Acetazolamide: a treatment for chronic mountain sickness. *Am. J. Resp. Crit. Care Med.* **172**, 1427–33.

Richalet, J.-P., Rivera, M., Maignan, M. *et al.* (2008) Acetazolamide for Monge's disease: efficiency and tolerance of 6-month treatment. *Am. J. Respir. Crit. Care Med.* **177**, 1370–6.

Richalet, J.-P., Rivera, M., Maignan, M. *et al.* (2009) Pulmonary hypertension and Monge's disease. *PVRI Rev.* **1**, 114–9.

Richalet, J.-P., Letournel, M. and Souberbielle, J.-C. (2010) Effects of high-altitude hypoxia on the hormonal response to hypothalamic factors. *Am. J. Physiol. Regul. Integr. Comp. Physiol.* **299**, R1685–92.

Richalet, J.-P., Larmignat, P., Poitrine, E. *et al.* (2011) Physiological risk factors of severe high altitude illness: a prospective cohort study. *Am. J. Respir. Crit. Care Med.* **185**, 192–8.

Richalet, J.-P., Letournel, M. and Salama, J. (2011) Holmes-AD syndrome associated with high altitude pulmonary edema and low chemo-responsiveness to hypoxia. *Clin. Auton. Res.* **21**, 55–6.

Richalet, J.-P., Larmignat, P., Poitrine, E. *et al.* (2012) Physiological risk factors for severe high-altitude illness: a prospective cohort study. *Am. J. Respir. Crit. Care Med.* **185,** 192–8.

Richardson, A., Watt, P. and Maxwell, N. (2009) Hydration and the physiological responses to acute normobaric hypoxia. *Wilderness Environ. Med.* **20**, 212–20.

Richardson, R.S., Noyszewski, E.A., Kendrick, K.F. *et al.* (1995) Myoglobin O_2 desaturation during exercise. Evidence of limited O_2 transport. *J. Clin. Invest.* **96**, 1916–26.

Richardson, R.S., Tagore, K., Haseler, L.J. *et al.* (1998) Increased $\dot{V}O_{2,max}$ with right-shifted Hb–O_2 dissociation curve at a constant O_2 delivery in dog muscle in situ. *J. Appl. Physiol.* **84**, 995–1002.

Richardson, R.S., Newcomer, S.C. and Noyszewski, E.A. (2001) Skeletal muscle intracellular P_{O_2} assessed by myoglobin desaturation: response to graded exercise. *J. Appl. Physiol.* **91**, 2679–85.

Richardson, T.Q. and Guyton, A.C. (1959) Effects of polycythemia and anemia on cardiac output and other circulatory factors. *Am. J. Physiol.* **197**, 1167–79.

Riley, D.J. (1991) Vascular remodeling, in *The Lung: Scientific Foundations* (eds. R.C. Crystal and J.B. West), Raven Press, New York, pp. 1189–98.

Riley, R.L. and Houston, C.S. (1951) Composition of alveolar air and volume of pulmonary ventilation during long exposure to high altitude. *J. Appl. Physiol.* **3**, 526–34.

Riley, R.L., Shephard, R.H., Cohn, J.E. *et al.* (1954) Maximal diffusing capacity of the lungs. *J. Appl. Physiol.* **6**, 573–87.

Ri-Li, G., Chase, P.J., Witkowski, S. *et al.* (2003) Obesity: associations with acute mountain sickness. *Ann Intern Med* **139**, 253–7 (first author, Ge R.L.)

Rios, B., Driscoll, D.J. and McNamara, D.G. (1985) High-altitude pulmonary edema with absent right pulmonary artery. *Pediatrics* **75**, 314–17.

Rios, E.J., Fallon, M., Wang, J. *et al.* (2005) Chronic hypoxia elevates intracellular pH and activates Na^+/H^+ exchange in pulmonary arterial smooth muscle cells. *Am. J. Physiol. Lung Cell. Mol. Physiol.* **289**, L867–74.

Risso, A., Turello, M., Biffoni, F. and Antonutto, G. (2007) Red blood cell senescence and neocytolysis in humans after high altitude acclimatization. *Blood Cells Mol. Dis.* **38**, 83–92.

Rivera, M., Huicho, L., Bouchet, P. *et al.* (2008) Effect of acetazolamide on ventilatory response in subjects with chronic mountain sickness. *Respir. Physiol. Neurobiol.* **162**, 184–9.

Roach, R.C. and Hackett, P.H. (1992) Hyperbaria and high altitude illness, in *Hypoxia and Mountain Medicine* (eds. J.R. Sutton, C.S. Houston and G. Coates), Queen City Printers, Burlington, VT, pp. 266–73.

Roach, R.C. and Hackett, P.H. (2001) Frontiers of hypoxia research: acute mountain sickness. *J. Exp. Biol.* **204**, 3161–70.

Roach, R.C., Bärtsch, P., Hackett, P.H. and Oelz, O. (1993) The Lake Louise acute mountain sickness scoring system, in *Hypoxia and Mountain Medicine* (eds. J.R. Sutton, C.S. Houston and G. Coates), Queen City Printers, Burlington, VT, pp. 272–4.

Roach, R.C., Houston, C.S., Hogigman, B. *et al.* (1995) How do older persons tolerate moderate altitude? *West. J. Med.* **162**, 32–6.

Roach, R.C., Loeppky, J.A. and Icenogle, M.V. (1996) Acute mountain sickness: Increased severity during simulated altitude compared with normobaric hypoxia. *J. Appl. Physiol.* **81**, 1908–10.

Roach, R.C., Greene, E.R., Schoene, R.B. and Hackett, P.H. (1998) Arterial oxygen saturation for prediction of acute mountain sickness. *Aviat. Space Environ. Med.* **69**, 1182–5.

Roach, R.C., Maes, D., Sandoval, D. et al. (2000) Exercise exacerbates acute mountain sickness at simulated high altitude. *J. Appl. Physiol.* **88**, 581–5.

Roach, R.C, Kayser, B. and Hackett, P. (2011) Pro: Headache should be a required symptom for the diagnosis of acute mountain sickness. *High Alt. Med. Biol.* **12**, 21–2; discussion 29.

Robach, P., Déchaux, M., Jarrot, S. et al. (2000) Operation Everest III: role of plasma volume expansion on VO$_2$max during prolonged high-altitude exposure. *J. Appl. Physiol.* **89**, 29–37.

Robach, P., Lafforgue, E., Olsen, N.V. et al. (2002) Recovery of plasma volume after 1 week of exposure at 4,350 m. *Pflügers Arch.* **444**, 821–8.

Robach, P., Schmitt, L., Brugniaux, J.V. et al. (2006) 'Living high–training low': Effect on erythropoiesis and aerobic performance in highly-trained swimmers. *Eur. J. Appl. Physiol.* **96**, 423–33.

Robach, P., Schmitt, L., Brugniaux, J.V. et al. (2006) Living high-training low: effect on erythropoiesis and maximal aerobic performance in elite Nordic skiers. *Eur. J. Appl. Physiol.* **97**, 695–705.

Roberovsky, V. (1896) The Central Asian Expedition of Capt. Roberovsky and Lt. Kozloff. *Geogr. J.* **8**, 161.

Roberts, A.C., Butterfield, G.E., Cymerman, A. et al. (1996) Acclimatization to 4,300m altitude decreases reliance on fat as a substrate. *J. Appl. Physiol.* **81**, 1762–71.

Roberts, A.D., Clark, S.A., Townsend, N.E. et al. (2003) Changes in performance, maximal oxygen uptake and maximal accumulated oxygen deficit after 5, 10 and 15 days of live high:train low altitude exposure. *Eur. J. Appl. Physiol.* **88**, 390–5.

Roberts, D., Smith, D.J., Donnelly, S. and Simard, S. (2000) Plasma-volume contraction and exercise-induced hypoxaemia modulate erythropoietin production in healthy humans. *Clin. Sci.* **98**, 39–45.

Robertson, E., Saunders, P.U., Pyne, D.B. et al. (2010) Effectiveness in intermittent training in hypoxia combined with live high/train low. *Eur. J. Appl. Physiol.* **110**, 379–87.

Robertson, J.A. and Shlim, D.R. (1991) Treatment of moderate acute mountain sickness with pressurization in a portable hyperbaric (Gamow) bag. *J. Wilderness Med.* **2**, 268–73.

Robin, E.D. and Gardner, F.H. (1953) Cerebral metabolism and hemodynamics in pernicious anemia. *J. Clin. Invest.* **32**, 598.

Roca, J.M., Hogan, M.C., Storey, D. et al. (1989) Evidence for tissue limitation of VO$_{2,max}$ in normal man. *J. Appl. Physiol.* **67**, 291–9.

Rock, P.B., Johnson, T.S., Larsen, R.F. et al. (1989) Dexamethasone prophylaxis for acute mountain sickness. Effect of dose level. *Chest* **95**, 568–73.

Röggla, G., Röggla, M., Wagner, A. and Laggner, A.N. (1995) Poor ventilatory response to mild hypoxia may inhibit acclimatization at moderate altitude in elderly patients after carotid surgery. *Br. J. Sports Med.* **29**, 110–12.

Röggla, G., Röggla, M., Podolsky, A. et al. (1996) How can acute mountain sickness be quantified at moderate altitude? *J. R. Soc. Med.* **89**, 141–3.

Roels, B., Bentley, D.J., Coste, O. et al. (2007) Effects of intermittent hypoxic training on cycling peformance in well-trained athletes. *Eur. J. Appl. Physiol.* **101**, 359–68.

Rogers, T.A. (1971) The clinical course of survival in the Arctic. *Hawaii Med. J.* **30**, 31–4.

Röggla, G. and Moser, B. (2006) The function of metered dose inhalers at moderate altitude. *J. Travel Med.* **13**, 248; author reply 248–9.

Röggla, G., Röggla, M., Wagner, A. et al. (1994) Effect of low dose sedation with diazepam on ventilatory response at moderate altitude. *Wien Klin. Wochenschr.* **106**, 649–51.

Röggla, G., Röggla, M., Podolsky, A. et al. (1996) How can acute mountain sickness be quantified at moderate altitude? *J. R. Soc. Med.* **89**, 141–3.

Röggla, G., Moser, B. and Röggla, M. (2000) Effect of temazepam on ventilatory response at moderate altitude. *BMJ* **320**, 56.

Roi, G.S., Giacometti, M. and Von Duvillard, S.P. (1999) Marathons in altitude. *Med. Sci. Sports Exerc.* **31**, 723–8.

Romer, L.M., Haverkamp, H.C., Amann, M. et al. (2007) Effect of acute severe hypoxia on peripheral fatigue and endurance capacity in healthy humans. *Am. J. Physiol: Reg. Integ. Comp. Physiol.* **292**, R598–R606.

Roncin, J.P., Schwartz, F. and D'Arbigny, P. (1996) EGb 761 in control of acute mountain sickness and vascular reactivity to cold exposure. *Aviat. Space Environ. Med.* **67**, 445–52.

Roscoe, C., Baker, E., Johnston, E. *et al.* (2008) Carbon monoxide exposure on Denali: comparing the 2004 and 2005 climbing seasons. *Wilderness Environ. Med.* **19**, 15–21.

Rose, D.M., Fleck, B., Thews, O. and Kamin, W.E. (2000) Blood gas-analyses in patients with cystic fibrosis to estimate hypoxemia during exposure to high altitude. *Eur. J. Med. Res.* **26**, 9–12.

Rose, M.S., Houston, C.S., Fulco, C.S. *et al.* (1988) Operation Everest II: nutrition and body composition. *J. Appl. Physiol.* **65**, 2545–51.

Roskamm, F., Londry, F.K., Samek, L.L. *et al.* (1969) Effects of standardised ergometer training produced at three different altitudes. *J. Appl. Physiol.* **27**, 840–7.

Ross, J.H. and Attwood, E.C. (1984) Severe repetitive exercise and haematological status. *Postgrad. Med. J.* **60**, 454–7.

Ross, R.T. (1985) The random nature of cerebral mountain sickness. *Lancet* **1**, 990–1.

Rossis, C.G., Yiacoumettis, A.M. and Elemenoglou, J. (1982) Squamous cell carcinoma of the heel developing at site of previous frostbite. *J. R. Soc. Med.* **75**, 715–18.

Roth, W.T., Gomolla, A., Meuret, A.E. *et al.* (2002) High altitudes, anxiety, and panic attacks: is there a relationship? *Depress. Anxiety* **16**, 51–8.

Rothwell, N.J. and Stock, M.J. (1983) Luxuskonsumption. Diet-induced thermogenesis and brown fat: the case in favour. *Clin. Sci.* **64**, 19–23.

Rotta, A., Canepa, A., Hurtado, A. *et al.* (1956) Pulmonary circulation at sea level and at high altitudes. *J. Appl. Physiol.* **9**, 328–36.

Roughton, F.J. (1945) Average time spent by blood in human lung capillary and its relation to the rates of CO uptake and elimination in man. *Am. J. Physiol.* **143**, 621–33.

Roughton, F.J.W. (1964) Transport of oxygen and carbon dioxide, in *Handbook of Physiology*, Section 3, *Respiration*, Vol. 1 (eds. W.O. Fenn and H. Rahn), American Physiological Society, Washington, DC, pp. 767–825.

Roughton, F.J.W. and Forster, R.E. (1957) Relative importance of diffusion and chemical reaction rates in determining rate of exchange of gases in the human lung, with special reference to true diffusing capacity of pulmonary membrane and volume of blood in the lung capillaries. *J. Appl. Physiol.* **11**, 291–302.

Roussel, B., Dittmar, A., Delhomm, C. *et al.* (1982) Normal and pathological aspects of skin blood flow measurements by thermal clearance method, in *Biomedical Thermology* (eds. M. Guthrie, E. Albert and R. Alar), Liss, New York, pp. 421–9.

Rowell, G. (1982) High altitude pulmonary oedema during rapid ascent, in *Hypoxia: Man at High Altitude* (eds. J.R. Sutton, N.L. Jones and C.S. Houston), Thieme Stratton, New York, pp. 168–71.

Roy, S.B., Guleria, J.S., Khanna, P.K. *et al.* (1969) Haemodynamic studies in high altitude pulmonary oedema. *Br. Heart J.* **31**, 52–8.

Ruiz, L. and Peñaloza, D. (1977) Altitude and hypertension. *Mayo Clin. Proc.* **52**, 442–5.

Rupert, J.L. and Koehle, M.S. (2006) The evidence for a genetic basis for altitude-related illness. *High Alt. Med. Biol.* **7**, 150–67.

Russell, E. (1975) A multiple scoring method for the assessment of complex memory functions. *J. Consult. Clin. Psychol.* **43**, 800–9.

Ruttledge, H. (1937) *Everest: the Unfinished Adventure*, Hodder and Stoughton, London, p. 212.

Ruttman, E., Weissenbacher, A., Ulmar, U. *et al.* (2007) Prolonged extracorporeal membrane oxygenation-assisted support provides improved survival in hypothermic patients with cardiocirculatory arrest. *J. Thorac. Cardiovasc. Surg.* **134**, 594–600.

Ryn, Z. (1970) Mental disorders in alpinists under conditions of stress at high altitudes, Doctoral thesis, University of Cracow, Poland.

Ryn, Z. (1971) Psychopathology in alpinism. *Acta Med. Pol.* **12**, 453–67.

Ryujin, D.T., Mannebach, S.C., Samuelson, W.M. and Marshall, B.C.(2001) Oxygen saturation in adult cystic fibrosis patients during exercise at high altitude. *Pediatr. Pulmonol.* **32**, 437–41.

Sadikali, F. and Owor, R. (1974) Hypothermia in the tropics. A review of 24 cases. *Trop. Geogr. Med.* **26**, 265–70.

Sahn, S.A., Lakshminarayan, S., Pierson, D.J. and Weil, J.V. (1974) Effect of ethanol on the ventilatory responses to oxygen and carbon dioxide in man. *Clin. Sci. Mol. Med.* **49**, 33–8.

Saito, S., Tobe, K., Harada, N. *et al.* (2002) Physical condition among middle altitude trekkers in an ageing society. *Am. J. Emerg. Med.* **20**, 291–4.

Sakaguchi, E. and Yurugi, R. (1983) Retinal haemorrhages at simulated high altitude. *Jpn. J. Mount. Med.* **3**, 107–8.

Saldana, M. and Arias-Stella, J. (1963a) Studies on the structure of the pulmonary trunk. I. Normal changes in the elastic configuration of the human pulmonary trunk at different ages. *Circulation* **27**, 1086–93.

Saldana, M. and Arias-Stella, J. (1963b) Studies on the structure of the pulmonary trunk. II. The evolution of the elastic configuration of the pulmonary trunk in people native to high altitudes. *Circulation* **27**, 1094–100.

Saldana, M. and Arias-Stella, J. (1963c) Studies on the structure of the pulmonary trunk. III. The thickness of the media of the pulmonary trunk and ascending aorta in high altitude natives. *Circulation* **27**, 1101–4.

Saldana, M.J., Salem, L.E. and Travezan, R. (1973) High altitude hypoxia and chemodectoma. *Hum. Pathol.* **4**, 251–63.

Saldeen, T. (1976) The microembolism syndrome. *Microvasc. Res.* **11**, 187–259.

Salimi, Z. (1985) Assessment of tissue viability by scintigraphy. *Postgrad. Med.* **17**, 133–4.

Salisbury, R. and Hawley, E. (2007) The Himalaya by the Numbers: A Statistical Analysis of Mountaineering in the Nepal Himalaya. Available from: www.himalayandatabase.com/downloads/HimalayaByNbrs.pdf.

Saltin, B. (1967) Aerobic and anaerobic work capacity at 2300 m. *Med. Thorac.* **24**, 205–10.

Saltin, B. and Gollnick, P.D. (1983) Skeletal muscle adaptability: significance for metabolism and performance, in *Handbook*

of Physiology, Section 10 (ed. L.D. Peachey), American Physiological Society, Bethesda, MD, pp. 555–631.

Salvaggio, A., Insalaco, G., Marrone, O. *et al.* (1998) Effects of high-altitude periodic breathing on sleep and arterial oxyhaemoglobin saturation. *Eur. Respir. J.* **12**, 408–13.

Samaja, M., Veicsteinas, A. and Cerretelli, P. (1979) Oxygen affinity of blood in altitude Sherpas. *J. Appl. Physiol.* **47**, 337–41.

Samaja, M., Mariani, C., Prestini, A. and Cerretelli, P. (1997) Acid–base balance and O_2 transport at high altitude. *Acta Physiol. Scand.* **159**, 249–56.

Samaja, M., Crespi, T., Guazzi, M. and Vandergriff, K.D. (2003) Oxygen transport in blood at high altitude: role of the hemoglobin–oxygen affinity and impact of the phenomena related to hemoglobin allosterism and red cell function. *Eur. J. Appl. Physiol.* **90**, 351–9.

Sampson, J.B., Cymerman, A., Burse, R.J. *et al.* (1983) Procedures for the measurement of acute mountain sickness. *Aviat. Space Environ. Med.* **54**, 1063–73.

San Miguel, J.L., Spielvogel, H., Berger, J. *et al.* (2002) Effect of high altitude on protein metabolism in Bolivian children. *High Alt. Med. Biol.* **3**, 377–86.

Sanchez, C., Merino, C. and Figallo, M. (1970) Simultaneous measurement of plasma volume and cell mass in polycythemia of high altitude. *J. Appl. Physiol.* **30**, 775–8.

Sandham, J.D., Shaw, D.T. and Guenter, C.A. (1977) Acute supine respiratory failure due to bilateral diaphragmatic paralysis. *Chest* **72**, 96–8.

Santolaya, R.B., Lahiri, S., Alfaro, R.T. and Schoene, R.B. (1989) Respiratory adaptation in the highest inhabitants and highest Sherpa mountaineers. *Respir. Physiol.* **77**, 253–62.

Santos, J.L., Perez-Bravo, F., Carrasco, E. *et al.* (2001) Low prevalence of type 2 diabetes despite a high average body mass index in the Aymara natives from Chile. *Nutrition* **17**, 305–9.

Sarnquist, F.H., Schoene, R.B., Hackett, P.H. and Townes, B.D. (1986) Hemodilution of polycythemic mountaineers: effect on exercise and mental function. *Aviat. Space Environ. Med.* **57**, 313–17.

Sartori, C., Allemann, Y., Trueb, L. *et al.* (1999a) Augmented vaso-reactivity in adult life associated with perinatal vascular insult. *Lancet* **353**, 2205–7.

Sartori, C., Vollenweider, L., Löffler, B-M. *et al.* (1999b) Exaggerated endothelin release in high-altitude pulmonary edema. *Circulation* **99**, 2665–8.

Sartori, C., Allemann, Y., Duplain, H. *et al.* (2002) Salmeterol for the prevention of high-altitude pulmonary edema. *N. Engl. J. Med.* **346**, 1631–6.

Sartori, C., Duplain, H., Lepori, M. *et al.* (2004) High altitude impairs nasal transepithelial sodium transport in HAPE-prone subjects. *Eur. Respir. J.* **23**, 916–20.

Sato, M., Severinghaus, J.W., Powel, F.L. *et al.* (1992) Augmented hypoxic ventilatory response in men at altitude. *J. Appl. Physiol.* **73**, 101–7.

Sato, M., Severinghaus, J.W. and Bickler, P. (1994) Time course of augmentation and depression of hypoxic ventilatory response at altitude. *J. Appl. Physiol.* **77**, 313–16.

Saunders, P.U., Telford, R.D., Pyne, D.B. *et al.* (2004) Improved running economy in elite runners after 20 days of simulated moderate-altitude exposure. *J. Appl. Physiol.* **96**, 931–7.

Saunders, R. (1789) Some account of the vegetable and mineral productions of Boutan and Tibet. *Philos. Trans. R. Soc.* **79**, 79–111.

Savard, G.K., Cooper, K.E., Veal, W.L. and Malkinson, T.J. (1985) Peripheral blood flow during rewarming from mild hypothermia in humans. *J. Appl. Physiol.* **58**, 4–13.

Savonitto, S., Cardellino, G., Doveri, G. *et al.* (1992) Effects of acute exposure to altitude (3460 m) on blood pressure response to dynamic and isometric exercise in men with systemic hypertension. *Am. J. Cardiol.* **70**, 1493–7.

Savourey, B., Launay, J.-C., Besnard, Y. *et al.* (2003) Normo- and hypobaric hypoxia: are there any physiological differences? *Eur. J. Appl. Physiol.* **89**, 122–6.

Savourey, G., Moirant, C., Eterradossi, J. and Bittel, J. (1995) Acute mountain sickness relates to sea-level partial pressure of oxygen. *Eur. J. Appl. Physiol.* **70**, 469–76.

Savourey, G., Garcia, N., Caravel, C. *et al.* (1998) Pre-adaptation, adaptation and de-adaptation to high altitude in humans: hormonal and biochemical changes at sea level. *Eur. J. Appl. Physiol.* **77**, 37–43.

Sawhney, R.C. and Malhotra, A.S. (1991) Thyroid function in sojourners and acclimatized low landers at high altitude in man. *Horm. Metab. Res.* **23**, 81–4.

Sawhney, R.C., Chabra, P.C., Malhotra, A.S. *et al.* (1985) Hormone profiles at high altitude in man. *Andrologia* **17**, 178–84.

Sawhney, R.C., Malhotra, A.S., Singh, T. *et al.* (1986) Insulin secretion at high altitude in man. *Int. J. Biometeorol.* **30**, 23–8.

Saxena, S., Kumar, R., Madan, T. *et al.* (2005) Association of polymorphisms in pulmonary surfactant protein A1 and A2 genes with high-altitude pulmonary edema. *Chest* **128**, 1611–19.

Schaefer, O., Eaton, R.D.P., Timmermans, F.J.W. and Hildes, J.A. (1980) Respiratory function impairment and cardiopulmonary consequences in long term residents of the Canadian Arctic. *Can. Med. Assoc. J.* **119**, 997–1004.

Scheinfeldt, L.B., Soi, S., Thompson, S. *et al.* (2012) Genetic adaptation to high altitude in the Ethiopian highlands. *Genome Biol.* **13**, R1.

Scherrer, U., Vollenweider, L., Delabays, A. *et al.* (1996) Inhaled nitric oxide for high-altitude pulmonary edema. *N. Engl. J. Med.* **334**, 624–9.

Scheult, R.D., Ruh, K., Dada, L. *et al.* (2009) Endothelin does not improve exercise capacity or lower pulmonary artery systolic pressure at high altitude. *Respir. Physiol. Neurobiol.* **165**, 123–30.

Schirlo, C., Pavlicek, V., Jacomet, A. *et al.* (2002) Characteristics of the ventilatory response in subjects susceptible to high altitude pulmonary edema during acute and prolonged hypoxia. *High Alt. Med. Biol.* **3**, 267–76.

Schmid, J.P., Noveanu, M., Gaillet, R. *et al.* (2006) Safety and exercise tolerance of acute high altitude exposure (3454m) among patients with coronary artery disease. *Heart* **92**, 921–5.

Schmid-Schonbein, H. and Neumann, F.J. (1985) Pathophysiology of cutaneous frost injury: disturbed microcirculation as a consequence of abnormal flow behaviour of the blood. Application of new concepts of blood rheology, in *High Altitude Deterioration* (eds. J. Rivolier, P. Cerretelli, J. Foray and P. Segantini), Karger, Basel, pp. 20–38.

Schmidt, W. (2002) Effects of intermittent exposure to high altitude on blood volume and erythropoietic activity. *High Alt. Med. Biol.* **3**, 167–76.

Schmidt, W., Brabant, C., Kröger, C. *et al.* (1990) Atrial natriuretic peptide during and after maximal and submaximal exercise under normoxic and hypoxic conditions. *Eur. J. Appl. Phsyiol.* **61**, 398–407.

Schmidt, W., Eckhart, K.U., Hilgendorf, A. *et al.* (1991) Effects of maximal and submaximal exercise under normoxic and hypoxic condition on serum erythropoietin level. *Int. J. Sports Med.* **12**, 457–61.

Schmidt, W., Heinicke, K., Rojas, J. *et al.* (2002) Blood volume and hemoglobin mass in endurance athletes from moderate altitude. *Med. Sci. Sports Exerc.* **34**, 1934–40.

Schneider, M., Bernasch, D., Weymann, J. *et al.* (2002) Acute mountain sickness: influence of susceptibility, preexposure, and ascent rate. *Med. Sci. Sports Exerc.* **34**, 1886–91.

Schoch, H.J., Fischer, S. and Marti, H.H. (2002) Hypoxia-induced vascular endothelial growth factor expression causes vascular leakage in the brain. *Brain* **125**, 2549–57.

Schoeller, D.A. and Van Santen, E. (1982) Measurement of energy expenditure in humans by doubly labelled water method. *J. Appl. Physiol.* **53**, 955–9.

Schoene, R.B. (1982) Control of ventilation in climbers to extreme altitude. *J. Appl. Physiol.* **43**, 886–90.

Schoene, R.B. (2001) Limits of human lung function at high altitude. *J. Exp. Biol.* **204**, 3121–7.

Schoene, R.B., Lahiri, S., Hackett, P.H. *et al.* (1984) Relationship of hypoxic ventilatory response to exercise performance on Mount Everest. *J. Appl. Physiol.* **56**, 1478–83.

Schoene, R.B., Roach, R.C., Hackett, P.H. *et al.* (1985) High altitude pulmonary edema and exercise at 4400m on Mount McKinley. Effect of expiratory positive airway pressure. *Chest* **87**, 330–3.

Schoene, R.B., Hackett, P.H. and Roach, R.C. (1987) Blunted hypoxic chemosensitivity at altitude and sea level in an elite high altitude climber, in *Hypoxia and Cold* (eds. J.R. Sutton, C.S. Houston and G. Coates), Praeger, New York, p. 532.

Schoene, R.B., Robertson, H.T., Pierson, D.J. and Peterson, A.P. (2001) Respiratory drives and exercise in menstrual cycles of athletic and nonathletic women. *J. Appl. Physiol.* **50**, 1300–5.

Scholander, P. (1960) Oxygen transport through hemoglobin solution. *Science* **131**, 585–90.

Schoonman, G.G., Sandor, P.S., Nirkko, A.C. *et al.* (2008) Hypoxia-induced acute mountain sickness is associated with intracellular cerebral edema: a 3 T magnetic resonance imaging study. *J. Cereb. Blood Flow Metab.* **28**, 198–206.

Schuler, B., Thomsen, J.J., Gassman, M. and Lundby, C. (2007) Timing the arrival at 2340 m altitude for aerobic performance. *Scand. J. Med. Sci. Sports.* **17**, 588–94.

Schwandt, H-J., Heyduck, B., Gunga, H-C. and Röcker, L. (1991) Influence of prolonged physical exercise on the erythropoietin concentration in blood. *Eur. J Appl. Physiol.* **63**, 463–6.

Schwarcz, T.H., Hogan, L.A., Endean, E.D. *et al.* (1993) Thromboembolic complications of polycythemia: polycythemia vera versus smokers' polycythemia. *J. Vasc. Surg.* **17**, 518–22; discussion 522–3.

Scoggin, C.H., Hyers, T.M., Reeves, J.T. and Grover, R.F. (1977) High-altitude pulmonary edema in the children and young adults of Leadville, Colorado. *N. Engl. J. Med.* **297**, 1269–72.

Scott, G.R., Schulte, P.M., Eddington, S. *et al.* (2011) Molecular evolution of cytochrome C oxidase underlies high-altitude adaptation in the bar-headed goose. *Mol. Biol. Evol.* **28**, 351–63.

Scrase, E., Laverty, A., Gavlak, J.C.D. *et al.* (2009) The Young Everest Study: Effects of hypoxia at high altitude on cardiorespiratory function and general well-being in healthy children. *Arch. Dis. Child.* **94**, 621–6.

Seccombe, L.M., Kelly, P.T., Wong, C.K. *et al.* (2004) Effect of simulated commercial flight on oxygenation in patients with interstitial lung disease and chronic obstructive pulmonary disease. *Thorax* **59**, 966–70.

Sediame, S., Zerah-Lancner, F., d'Ortho, M.P. *et al.* (1999) Accuracy of the i-STAT bedside gas analyzer. *Eur. Respir. J.* **14**, 214–17.

Seheult, R.D., Ruh, K., Foster, G.P. and Anholm, J.D. (2009) Prophylactic bosentan does not improve exercise capacity or lower pulmonary artery systolic pressure at high altitude. *Respir. Physiol. Neurobiol.* **165**, 123–30.

Selkon, J. and Gould, J.C. (1966) Bacteriology, in *Report on IBP Expedition to North Bhutan* (eds. F.S. Jackson, R.W.D. Turner and M.P. Ward), Royal Society, London, pp. 88–98.

Sellassie, S.H. (1972) *Ancient and Medieval Ethiopian History to 1270,* United Printers, Addis Ababa, Ethiopia.

Semenza, G.L. (2000) Surviving ischemia: adaptive responses mediated by hypoxia-inducible factor 1. *J. Clin. Invest.* **106**, 809–12.

Semenza, G.L. (2009) Involvement of oxygen-sensing pathways in physiologic and pathologic erythropoiesis. *Blood* **114**, 2015–19.

Semenza, G.L. (2012) Hypoxia-inducible factors in physiology and medicine. *Cell* **143**, 399–408.

Semenza, G.L. and Wang, G.L. (1992) A nuclear factor induced by hypoxia via de novo protein synthesis binds to the human erythropoietin gene enhancer at a site required for transcriptional activation. *Mol. Cell. Biol.* **12**, 5447–54.

Semenza, G.L., Agani, F., Iyer, N. *et al.* (1998) Hypoxia-inducible factor-1: from molecular biology to cardiopulmonary physiology. *Chest* **114**, 40S–45S.

Semple, J.L. and Moore, G.W.K. (2008) First observations of surface ozone concentration from the summit region of Mount Everest. *Geophys. Res. Lett.* **35**, L20818, 5PP.

Semple, J.L. and Moore, G.W.K (2009) Ozone exposure and mortality. *N. Eng. J. Med.* **360**, 2786–9.

Semple, P. d'A. (1986) The clinical endocrinology of hypoxia, in *Aspects of Hypoxia* (ed. D. Heath), Liverpool University Press, Liverpool, pp. 147–61.

Serebrovskaya, T., Karaban, I., Monskovskaya, I. *et al.* (1998) Hypoxic ventilatory responses and gas exchange in patient with Parkinson's disease. *Respiration* **65**, 28–33.

Serebrovskaya, T.V. and Ivashkevich, A.A. (1992) Effects of a 1-yr stay at altitude on ventilation, metabolism and work capacity. *J. Appl. Physiol.* **73**, 1749–55.

Serebrovskaya, T.V., Karaban, I.N., Kolesnikova, T.M. *et al.* (1999) Human hypoxic ventilatory response with blood dopamine content under intermittent hypoxic training. *Can. J. Physiol. Pharmcol. Rev.* **77**, 967–73.

Serebrovskaya, T.V., Karaban, I.N., Kolesnikova, E.E. *et al.* (2000) Geriatric men at altitude: hypoxic sensitivity and blood dopamine changes. *Respiration* **67**, 253–60.

Sergeyeva, A., Gordeuk, V.R., Tokarev, Y.N. *et al.* (1997) Congenital polycythemia in Chuvashia. *Blood* **89**, 2148–54.

Severinghaus, J.W. (1977) Pulmonary vascular function. *Am. Rev. Respir. Dis.* **115**(Suppl.), 149–58.

Severinghaus, J.W. (1995) Hypothetical roles of angiogenesis, osmotic swelling, and ischemia in high-altitude cerebral edema. *J. Appl. Physiol.* **79**, 375–9.

Severinghaus, J.W. (2008) History of measuring O_2 and CO_2 responses. *Adv. Exp. Med. Biol.* **605**, 3–8.

Severinghaus, J.W. and Carcelen, A. (1964) Cerebrospinal fluid in man native to high altitude. *J. Appl. Physiol.* **19**, 319–21.

Severinghaus, J.W., Mitchell, R.A., Richardson, B.W. and Singer, M.M. (1963) Respiratory control at high altitude suggesting active transport regulation of CSF pH. *J. Appl. Physiol.* **18**, 1155–66.

Severinghaus, J.W., Bainton, C.K. and Carcelen, A. (1966a) Respiratory insensitivity to hypoxia in chronically hypoxic man. *Respir. Physiol.* **1**, 308–34.

Severinghaus, J.W., Chiodi, H., Eger, E.I. *et al.* (1966b) Cerebral blood flow in man at high altitude. *Circ. Res.* **19**, 274–302.

Shapiro, C.M., Goll, C.C., Cohen, G.R. and Oswald, I. (1984) Heat production during sleep. *J. Appl. Physiol.* **56**, 671–7.

Sharma, S.C. (1980) Platelet count in temporary residents of high altitude. *J. Appl. Physiol.* **49**, 1047–8.

Sharma, S.C. (1980) Platelet count on acute induction to high altitude. *Thromb. Haemost.* **43**, 24.

Sharma, S.C., Balasubramanian, V. and Chadha, K.S. (1980) Platelet adhesiveness in permanent residents of high altitude. *Thromb. Haemost.* **42**, 1508–12.

Sharma, V.M. and Malhotra, M.S. (1976) Ethnic variations in psychological performance under altitude stress. *Aviat. Space Environ. Med.* **47**, 248–51.

Sharma, V.M., Malhotra, M.S. and Baskaran, A.S. (1975) Variations in psychomotor efficiency during prolonged stay at high altitude. *Ergonomics* **18**, 511–16.

Sharp, C.R. (1978) Hypoxia and hyperventilation, in *Aviation Medicine Physiology and Human Factors* (ed. J. Ernsting), Tir-Med Books, London, p. 78.

Sharp, F.R., Bergeron, M. and Bernaudin, M. (2001) Hypoxia-inducible factor in brain. *Adv. Exp. Med. Biol.* **502**, 273–91.

Shepard, R.H., Varnauskas, E., Martin, H.B. *et al.* (1958) Relationship between cardiac output and apparent diffusing capacity of the lung in normal men during treadmill exercise. *J. Appl. Physiol.* **13**, 205–10.

Shephard, R.J. (1985) Adaptation to exercise in the cold. *Sports Med.* **2**, 59–71.

Sheridan, R.L., Goldstein, M.A., Stoddard, F.J. and Walker, T.G. (2009) Case 41-2009: a 16-year-old boy with hypothermia and frostbite. *N Engl. J. Med.* **361**, 2645–62.

Sherrer, U. and Sciler, C. (2006) High altitude pulmonary edema and patent foramen ovale. *JAMA* **296**, 2954–58.

Shi, Z.Y., Ning, X.H., Huang, P.G. *et al.* (1979) Comparison of physiological responses to hypoxia at high altitudes between highlanders and lowlanders. *Sci. Sin.* **22**, 1446–69.

Shigeoka, J.W., Colice, G.L. and Ramirez, G. (1985) Effect of normoxemic and hypoxemic exercise on renin and aldosterone. *J. Appl. Physiol.* **59**, 142–8.

Shih, W.J., Riley, C., Magoun, S. and Ryo, U.Y. (1988) Intense bone imaging agent uptake in the soft tissues of the lower legs and feet relating to ischemia and cold exposure. *Eur. J. Nucl. Med.* **14**, 419–21.

Shimoda, L.A. and Semenza, G.L. (2011) HIF and the lung: role of hypoxia-inducible factors in pulmonary development and disease. *Am.J Respir.Crit. Care Med.* **183**, 152–6.

Shimoda, L.A., Manalo, D.J., Sham, J.S.K. *et al.* (2001) Partial HIF-1α deficiency impairs pulmonary arterial myocyte electrophysiological responses to hypoxia. *Am. J. Physiol. Lung Cell. Mol. Physiol.* **281**, L202–8.

Shipton, E. (1938) *Blank on the Map,* Hodder and Stoughton, London, p. 265.

Shlim, D.R. and Papenfus, K. (1995) Pulmonary embolism presenting as high-altitude pulmonary edema. *Wilderness Environ. Med.* **6**, 220–4.

Shlim, D.R., Nepal, K. and Meijer, H.J. (1991) Suddenly symptomatic brain tumors at altitude. *Ann. Emerg. Med.* **20**, 315–16.

Shlim, D.R., Hackett, P., Houston, C. *et al.* (1995) Diplopia at high altitude. *Wilderness Environ. Med.* **6**, 341.

Shrestha, P., Basnyat, B., Kupper, T. and van der Giet, S. (2012) Cerebral venous sinus thrombosis at high altitude. *High Alt. Med. Biol.* **13**, 60–2.

Shukitt-Hale, B., Banderet, L.E. and Lieberman, H.R. (1991) Relationships between symptoms, moods, performance, and acute mountain sickness at 4700 meters. *Aviat. Space Environ. Med.* **62**, 865–9.

Shukla, D., Saxena, S., Purushothman, J. *et al.* (2011) Hypoxic preconditioning with cobalt ameliorates hypobaric hypoxia-induced pulmonary edema in rats. *Eur. J. Pharmacol.* **656**, 101–9.

Shukla, V., Singh, S.N., Vats, P. *et al.* (2005) Ghrelin and leptin levels of sojourners and acclimatized lowlanders at high altitude. *Nutr. Neurosci.* **8**, 161–5.

Shults, W.T. and Swan, K.C. (1975) High altitude retinopathy in mountain climbers. *Arch. Ophthalmol.* **93**, 404–8.

Siebenmann, C., Bloch, K.E., Lundby, C. *et al.* (2010) Dexamethasone improves maximum exercise capacity of individuals susceptible to high altitude pulmonary edema at 4559 m. *High Alt. Med. Biol.* **12**, 169–77.

Siebenmann, C., Robach, P., Jacobs, R.A. *et al.* (2012) 'Live high–train low' using normobaric hypoxia: a double-blind, placebo-controlled study. *J. Appl. Physiol.* **112**, 106–17.

Siebkhe, H., Breivik, H., Rod, T. and Lind, B. (1975) Survival after 40 minutes' submersion without cerebral sequelae. *Lancet* **1**, 1275–9.

Sierra-Johnson, J., Romero-Corral, A., Vierend, K.S. and Johnson, B.D. (2008) Viewpoint: Effect of altitude on leptin levels, does it go up or down? *J. Appl. Physiol.* **105**, 1684–5.

Siesjo, B.K. (1992a) Pathophysiology and treatment of focal cerebral ischemia. Part I. Pathophysiology. *J. Neurosurg.* **77**, 169–84.

Siesjo, B.K. (1992b) Pathophysiology and treatment of focal cerebral ischemia. Part II. Mechanisms of damage and treatment. *J. Neurosurg.* **77**, 337–54.

Siesjo, B.K. and Kjallquist, A. (1969) A new theory for the regulation of extra-cellular pH in the brain. *Scand. J. Clin. Lab. Invest.* **24**, 1–9.

Silber, E., Sonnenberg, P., Collier, D.J *et al.* (2003) Clinical features of headache at altitude: a prospective study. *Neurology* **60**, 1167–71.

Sime, F., Peñaloza, D., Ruiz, L. *et al.* (1974) Hypoxemia, pulmonary hypertension, and low cardiac output in newcomers at low altitude. *J. Appl. Physiol.* **36**, 561–65.

Simonson, T.S., Yang, Y., Huff, C.D. *et al.* (2010) Genetic evidence for high-altitude adaptation in Tibet. *Science* **329**, 72–5.

Singh, I., Kapila, C.C., Khanna, P.K. *et al.* (1965) High-altitude pulmonary oedema. *Lancet* **1**, 229–34.

Singh, I., Khanna, P.K., Srivastava, M.C. *et al.* (1969) Acute mountain sickness. *N. Engl. J. Med.* **280**, 175–84.

Singh, I., Malhotra, M.S., Khanna, P.K. *et al.* (1974) Changes in plasma cortisol, blood antidiuretic hormone and urinary catecholamine in high altitude pulmonary oedema. *Int. J. Biometeorol.* **18**, 211–21.

Sirén, A.-L., Fratelli, M., Brines, M. *et al.* (2001) Erythropoietin prevents neuronal apoptosis after cerebral ischemia and metabolic stress. *Proc. Natl Acad. Sci. USA* **98**, 4044–9.

Siri, W.E., Van Dyke, D.C., Winchell, H.S. *et al.* (1966) Early erythropoietin, blood, and physiological responses to severe hypoxia in man. *J. Appl. Physiol.* **21**, 73–80.

Siri, W.E., Cleveland, A.S. and Blanche, P. (1969) Adrenal gland activity in Mount Everest climbers. *Fed. Proc.* **28**, 1251–6.

Slater, J.D.H., Tuffley, R.E., Williams, E.S. *et al.* (1969) Control of aldosterone secretion during acclimatization to hypoxia in man. *Clin. Sci.* **37**, 327–41.

Slutsky, A.S. and Strohl, K.P. (1980) Quantification of oxygen saturation during episodic hypoxemia. *Am. Rev. Respir. Dis.* **121**, 893–5.

Smith, C. (1999) Blood pressures of Sherpa men in modernizing Nepal. *Am. J. Hum. Biol.* **11**, 469–79.

Smith, C.A., Bisgard, G.E., Nielsen, A.M. *et al.* (1986) Carotid bodies are required for ventilatory acclimatization to chronic hypoxia. *J. Appl. Physiol.* **60**, 1003–10.

Smith, C.A., Dempsey, J.A. and Hornbein, T.F. (2001) Control of breathing at high altitude, in *High Altitude* (eds. T.F. Hornbein and R.B. Schoene), Lung Biology in Health and Disease, vol 161, Marcel Dekker, New York, pp. 140–8.

Smith, J.D., Cianflone, K., Martin, J. *et al.* (2011) Plasma adipokine and hormone changes in mountaineers on ascent to 5300 meters. *Wilderness Environ. Med.* **22**, 107–14.

Smith, T.G., Brooks, J.T., Balanos, G.M. *et al.* (2006) Mutation of von Hippel–Lindau tumour suppressor and human cardiopulmonary physiology. *PLoS Med.* **3**, e290.

Smith, T.G., Talbot, N.P., Privat, C. *et al.* (2009) Effects of iron supplementation and depletion on hypoxic pulmonary hypertension. Two randomized controlled trials. *JAMA* **302**, 1444–50.

Smyth, R. (1988) Alpine runners racing danger. *Observer* (London), 7 August.

Snellgrove, D. (1961) *Himalayan Pilgrimage*, Cassirer, Oxford.

Snodgrass, A.M. (1993) The early history of the Alps. *Alpine J.* **98**, 213–22.

Snyder, L.R.G., Born, S. and Lechner, A.L. (1982) Blood oxygen affinity in high- and low-altitude populations of the deer mouse. *Respir. Physiol.* **48**, 89–105.

Sobrevilla, L.A., Romero, L., Moncloa, F. *et al.* (1967) Endocrine studies of high altitude. III. Urinary gonadotrophins in subjects native to and living at 14000 feet and during acute exposure of men living at sea level to high altitude. *Acta Endocrinol.* **56**, 369–75.

Somers, V.K., Anderson, J.V., Conway, J. *et al.* (1986) Atrial natriuretic peptide is released by dynamic exercise in man. *Horm. Metab. Res.* **18**, 871–2.

Somers, V.K., Mark, A.L. and Abboud, F.M. (1991) Interaction of baroreceptor and chemoreceptor reflex control of sympathetic nerve activity in normal humans. *J. Clin. Invest.* **87**, 1953–7.

Somervell, T.H. (1925) Note on the composition of alveolar air at extreme heights. *J. Physiol. (Lond.)* **60**, 282–5.

Somervell, T.H. (1936) *After Everest,* Hodder and Stoughton, London, p. 132.

Somner, J.E., Morris, D.S., Scott, K.M. *et al.* (2007) What happens to intraocular pressure at high altitude? *Invest. Ophthalmol. Vis. Sci.* **48**, 1622–6.

Song, S.Y., Asaji, T., Tanizaki, Y. *et al.* (1986) Cerebral thrombosis at altitude. Its pathogenesis and the problems of prevention and treatment. *Aviat. Space Environ. Med.* **57**, 71–6.

Sorensen, S.C. (1970) Ventilatory acclimatization to hypoxia in rabbits after denervation of peripheral chemoreceptors. *J. Appl. Physiol.* **28**, 836–9.

Sorensen, S.C. and Milledge, J.S. (1971) Cerebrospinal fluid acid–base composition at high altitude. *J. Appl. Physiol.* **31**, 28–30.

Sorensen, S.C. and Mines, A.H. (1970) Ventilatory responses to acute and chronic hypoxia in goats after sinus nerve section. *J. Appl. Physiol.* **28**, 832–4.

Sorensen, S.C. and Severinghaus, J.W. (1968) Respiratory sensitivity to acute hypoxia in man at sea level and at high altitude. *J. Appl. Physiol.* **24**, 211–16.

Southard, A., Niermeyer, S. and Yaron, M. (2007) Language used in Lake Louise Scoring System underestimates symptoms of acute mountain sickness in 4- to 11-year-old children. *High Alt. Med. Biol.* **8**, 124–30.

Specht, H. and Fruhmann, G. (1972) Incidence of periodic breathing in 2000 subjects without pulmonary or neurological disease. *Bull. Physio-Pathol. Respir.* **98**, 1075–83.

Speechley-Dick, M.E., Rimmer, S.J. and Hodson, M.E. (1992) Exacerbations of cystic fibrosis after holidays at high altitude – a cautionary tale. *Respir. Med.* **86**, 55–6.

Spicuzza, L., Casiraghi, N., Gamboa, A. *et al.* (2004) Sleep-related hypoxaemia and excessive erythrocytosis in Andean high-altitude natives. *Eur. Resp. J.* **23**, 41–6.

Spieksma, F.T., Zuidema, P. and Leupen, M.J. (1971) High altitude and house-dust mites. *BMJ* **1**, 82–4.

Spriet, L.L., Cledhill, N., Froese, A.B. and Wilkes, D.L. (1986) Effect of graded erythrocythemia on cardiovascular and metabolic responses to exercise. *J. Appl. Physiol.* **61**, 1942–8.

Stathokostas, L., Jacob-Johnson, S., Petrella, R.J. and Paterson, D.H. (2004) Longitudinal changes in aerobic power in older men and women. *J. Appl. Physiol.* **97**, 781–9.

Steele, P. (1971) Medicine on Mount Everest. *Lancet* **ii**, 32–9.

Stefano, F., Rimoldi, M.D., Rexhaj, E. *et al.* (2012) Systemic vascular dysfunction in patients with chronic mountain sickness. *Chest* **141**, 139–46.

Stein, R.A. (1972) *Tibetan Civilization,* Faber, London, pp. 26–37.

Steinacker, J.M., Liu, Y., Boning, D. *et al.* (1996) Lung diffusion capacity, oxygen uptake, cardiac output and oxygen transport during exercise before and after a Himalayan expedition. *Eur. J. Appl. Physiol. Occup. Physiol.* **74**, 187–93.

Steinacker, J.M., Tobias, P., Menold, E. *et al.* (1998) Lung diffusing capacity and exercise in subjects with previous high altitude pulmonary edema. *Eur. Respir. J.* **11**, 643–50.

Steinbrook, R.A., Donovan, J.C., Gabel, R.A. *et al.* (1983) Acclimatization to high altitude in goats with ablated carotid bodies. *J. Appl. Physiol.* **44**, 16–21.

Stelzner, T.J., O'Brien, R.F., Sato, K. and Weil, J.V. (1988) Hypoxia-induced increases in pulmonary transvascular protein escape in rats. Modulation by glucocorticoids. *J. Clin. Invest.* **82**, 1840–7.

Stephens, D.H. (1982) Sleeping snugly in damp bedrooms. *J. R. Soc. Health* **6**, 272–5.

Stewart, A.G., Bardsley, P.A., Baudouin, S.V. *et al.* (1991a) Changes in atrial natriuretic peptide concentrations during intravenous saline infusion in hypoxic cor pulmonale. *Thorax* **46**, 829–34.

Stewart, A.G., Thompson, J.S., Rogers, T.K. and Morice, A.H. (1991b) Atrial natriuretic peptide-induced relaxation of pre-constricted isolated rat perfused lungs: a comparison in control and hypoxia-adapted animals. *Clin. Sci.* **81**, 201–8.

Stock, M.J., Norgan, N.G., Ferro-Luzzi, A. and Evans, E. (1978a) Effect of altitude on dietary-induced thermogenesis at rest and during light exercise in man. *J. Appl. Physiol. Respir. Environ. Exerc. Physiol.* **45**, 345–9.

Stock, M.J., Chapman, C., Stirling, J.L. and Campbell, I.T. (1978b) Effects of exercise, altitude, and food on blood hormone and metabolite levels. *J. Appl. Physiol: Respir. Environ. Exerc. Physiol.* **45**, 350–4.

Stohl, A., Spichtinger-Rakowsky, N., Bonasoni, P. *et al.* (2000) The influence of stratospheric intrusions on alpine ozone concentrations. *Atmos. Environ.* **34**, 1323–54.

Stokes, S., Kalson, N., Earl, M. *et al.* (2008) Bronchial asthma on Mount Kilimanjaro is not a disadvantage. *Thorax* **63**, 936–7.

Stokes, S., Kalson, N.S., Earl, M. *et al.* (2010) Age is no barrier to success at very high altitudes. *Age. Ageing* **39**, 262–5.

Stokes, W. (1854) *The Diseases of the Heart and Aorta*, Hodges and Smith, Dublin, p. 320.

Stoneham, M.D. (1995) Anaesthesia and resuscitation at altitude. *Eur. J. Anaesthesiol.* **12**, 249–57.

Storz, J.F., Natarajan, C., Cheviron, Z.A. *et al.* (2012) Altitudinal variation at duplicated β-globin genes in deer mice: effects of selection, recombination, and gene conversion. *Genetics.* **190**, 203–216.

Strauss, R.H., McFadden, E.R., Ingram, R.H. *et al.* (1978) Influence of heat and humidity on the airway obstruction induced by exercise in asthma. *J. Clin. Invest.* **61**, 433–40.

Stray-Gundersen, J., Chapman, R.F. and Levine, B.D. (2001) 'Living high–training low' altitude training improves sea level performance in male and female elite runners. *J. Appl. Physiol.* **91**, 1113–20.

Stream, J.O., Luks, A.M. and Grissom, C.K. (2009) Lung disease at high altitude. *Exp. Rev. Respir. Med.* **3**, 635–50.

Strong, L.H., Gin, G.K. and Goldman, R.F. (1985) Metabolic and vasomotor insulative responses occurring on immersion in cold water. *J. Appl. Physiol.* **58**, 964–77.

Stuber, T., Sartori, C., Schwab, M. *et al.* (2010) Exaggerated pulmonary hypertension during mild exercise I chronic mountain sickness. *Chest* **137**, 388–92.

Sturdy, S.W. (1988) Biology as a social theory: John Scott Haldane and physiological regulation. *Br. J. Hist. Sci.* **21**, 315–40.

Suarez, J., Alexander, J.K. and Houston, C.S. (1987) Enhanced left ventricular systolic performance at high altitude during Operation Everest II. *Am. J. Cardiol.* **60**, 137–42.

Subedi, B.H., Pokharel, J., Goodman, T.L. *et al.* (2010) Complications of steroid use on Mt. Everest. *Wilderness Environ. Med.* **21**, 345–8.

Subudhi, A.W., Dimmen, A.C., Julian, C.G. *et al.* (2011) Effects of acetazolamide and dexamethasone on cerebral hemodynamics in hypoxia. *J. Appl. Physiol.* **110**, 1219–25.

Sui, G.J., Lui, Y.H., Cheng, X.S. *et al.* (1988) Subacute infantile mountain sickness. *J. Pathol.* **155**, 161–70.

Sumner, D.S., Boswick, J.A. and Doolittle, W.H. (1971) Prediction of tissue loss in human frostbite with xenon-133. *Surgery* **69**, 899–903.

Sumner, D.S., Criblez, T. and Doolittle, W. (1974) Host factors in human frostbite. *Mil. Med.* **139**, 454–61.

Sun, J.H., Lin, Z.P. and Hu, X.L. (1985) An observation on the development of normal children age between 7–17 years at three elevations (abstract), 2nd High Altitude

Symposium, Qinghai, China (unpublished proceedings).

Sun, S.F. (1985) Epidemiology of hypertension on the Tibetan plateau (abstract), 2nd High Altitude Symposium, Qinghai, China (unpublished proceedings).

Sun, S.F., Droma, T.S., Zhang, J.G. *et al.* (1990) Greater maximal O_2 uptake and vital capacities in Tibetan than Han residents of Lhasa. *Respir. Physiol.* **79**, 151–62.

Sun, Y., Fang, M., Uniu, W. *et al.* (2010) Endothelial nitric oxide synthase gene polymorphisms associated with susceptibility to high altitude pulmonary edema in Chinese railway construction workers at Qinjhai–Tibet over 4500 meters above sea level. *Chin. Med. Sci. J.* **25**, 215–21.

Suri, M.L., Vijayan, G.P., Puri, H.C. *et al.* (1978) Neurological manifestations of frostbite. *Indian J. Med. Res.* **67**, 292–9.

Surks, M.I. (1966) Elevated PBI, free thyroxine, and plasma protein concentration in man at high altitude. *J. Appl. Physiol.* **21**, 1185–90.

Suslov, F.P. (1994) Basic principles of training at high altitude. *New Studies in Athletes IAAF Quart. Mag.* **2**, 45–9.

Sutton, J.R. (1977) Effect of acute hypoxia on the hormonal response to exercise. *J. Appl. Physiol. Respir. Environ. Exerc. Physiol.* **42**, 587–92.

Sutton, J.R. (1987) Energy substrates and hypoglycaemia, in *Hypoxia and Cold* (eds. J.R. Sutton, C.S. Houston and G. Coates), Prager, New York, pp. 487–92.

Sutton, J.R., Bryan, A.C., Gray, G.W. *et al.* (1976) Pulmonary gas exchange in acute mountain sickness. *Aviat. Space Environ. Med.* **47**, 1032–7.

Sutton, J.R., Viol, G.W., Gray, G.W. *et al.* (1977) Renin, aldosterone, electrolyte, and cortisol responses to hypoxic decompression. *J. Appl. Physiol. Respir. Environ. Exerc. Physiol.* **43**, 421–4.

Sutton, J.R., Houston, C.S. and Jones, N.L. (1983) *Hypoxia, Exercise, and Altitude*, Liss, New York.

Sutton, J.R., Houston, C.S. and Coates, G. (1987) *Hypoxia: the Tolerable Limits*, Benchmark Press, Indianapolis, IN.

Sutton, J.R., Reeves, J.T., Wagner, P.D. *et al.* (1988) Operation Everest II: oxygen transport during exercise at extreme simulated altitude. *J. Appl. Physiol.* **64**, 1309–21.

Svedenhag, J., Henriksson, J. and Sylven, C. (1983) Dissociation of training effects on skeletal muscle mitochondrial enzymes and myoglobin in man. *Acta Physiol. Scand.* **117**, 213–18.

Swenson, E.R. (1998) Carbonic anhydrase inhibitors and ventilation: a complex interplay of stimulation and suppression. *Eur. Respir. J.* **12**, 1242–7.

Swenson, E.R. (2001) Renal function and fluid homeostasis, in *High Altitude: An Exploration of Human Adaptation* (eds. T.F. Hornbein and R.B. Schoene), Marcel Dekker, New York, pp. 525–68.

Swenson, E.R. (2006) Carbonic anhydrase inhibitors and hypoxic pulmonary vasoconstriction. *Respir. Physiol. Neurobiol.* **151**, 209–16.

Swenson, E.R. (2011a) Con: most climbers do not develop subclinical interstitial pulmonary edema. *High Alt. Med. Biol.* **12**, 125–8.

Swenson, E.R. (2011b) Con: rebuttal. *High Alt. Med. Biol.* **12**, 131–2.

Swenson, E.R. and Teppema, L.J. (2007) Prevention of acute mountain sickness by acetazolamide: as yet an unfinished story. *J. Appl. Physiol.* **102**, 1305–7.

Swenson, E.R., Leatham, K.L., Roach, R.C. *et al.* (1991) Renal carbonic anhydrase inhibition reduces high altitude sleep periodic breathing. *Respir. Physiol.* **86**, 333–43.

Swenson, E.R., MacDonald, A., Vatheuer, M. *et al.* (1997) Acute mountain sickness is not altered by a high carbohydrate diet nor associated with elevated circulating cytokines. *Aviat. Space Environ. Med.* **68**, 499–503.

Swenson, E.R., Mongovin, S., Gibbs, S. *et al.* (2000) Stress failure in high altitude pulmonary edema (HAPE). *Am. J. Respir. Crit. Care Med.* **161**, A418.

Swenson, E.R., Maggiorini, M., Mongovin, S. *et al.* (2002) Pathogenesis of high-altitude pulmonary edema: inflammation is not an etiologic factor. *JAMA* **287**, 2228–35.

Taber, R. (1994) A child in the pressure bag: a case. *ISMM Newsletter* **4**, 4–5.

Takeno, Y., Kamijo, Y.I. and Nose, H. (2001) Thermoregulatory and aerobic changes after endurance training in a hypobaric hypoxic and warm environment. *J. Appl. Physiol.* **91**, 1520–8.

Talbott, J.H. and Dill, D.B. (1936) Clinical observations at high altitude. *Am. J. Med. Sci.* **192**, 626–39.

Tannheimer, M., Thomas, A. and Gerngross, H. (2002) Oxygen saturation course and altitude symptomatology during an expedition to broad peak (8047 m). *Int. J. Sports Med.* **23**, 329–35.

Tannheimer, M., Albertini, N., Ulmer, H.V. *et al.* (2009) Testing individual risk of acute mountain sickness at greater altitudes. *Mil. Med.* **174**, 363–9.

Tansey, W.A. (1973) Medical aspects of cold water immersion: a review. *US Navy Submarine Medical Research Laboratory Report* NSMRL, 763, NTIS Document AD-775–687.

Tansley, J.G., Fatmian, M., Howard, L.S.G.E. *et al.* (1998) Changes in respiratory control during and after 48h of isocapnic and poikilocapnic hypoxia in humans. *J. Appl. Physiol.* **85**, 2125–34.

Tappan, D.V. and Reynafarje, B.D. (1957) Tissue pigment manifestation of adaptation to high altitude. *Am. J. Physiol.* **190**, 99–103.

Tasker, J. (1981) *Everest the Cruel Way*, Eyre Methuen, London.

Tatsumi, K., Pickett, C.K. and Weil, J.V. (1991) Attenuated carotid body hypoxic sensitivity after prolonged hypoxic exposure. *J. Appl. Physiol.* **70**, 748–55.

Taylor, M.S. (1999) Lumbar sympathectomy for frostbite injuries of the foot. *Mil. Med.* **164**, 566–7.

Tek, D. and Mackey, S. (1993) Non-freezing cold injury in a marine infantry battalion. *J. Wilderness Med.* **4**, 353–7.

Tenney, S.M. and Ou, L.C. (1970) Physiological evidence for increased tissue capillarity in rats acclimatized to high altitude. *Respir. Physiol.* **8**, 137–50.

Tenney, S.M. and Ou, L.C. (1977) Ventilatory response of decorticate and decerebrate

cats to hypoxia and CO_2. *Respir. Physiol.* **29**, 81–2.

Teppema, L.J. and Dahan, A. (2010) The ventilatory response to hypoxia in mammals: mechanisms, measurement, and analysis. *Physiol. Rev.* **90**, 675–754.

Tewari, S.C., Jayaswal, R., Kasturi, A.S. *et al.* (1991) Excessive polycythaemia of high altitude. Pulmonary function studies including carbon monoxide diffusion capacity. *J. Assoc. Physicians India* **39**, 453–5.

The Times (1999) Queen Victoria's Gurkha was a trailblazer extraordinary, 8 July, p. 50.

Theis, M.K., Honigman, B., Yip, R. *et al.* (1993) Acute mountain sickness in children at 2835 metres. *Am. J. Dis. Child.* **147**, 143–5.

Thews, O., Fleck, B., Kamin, W.E.S. and Rose, D.-M. (2004) Respiratory function and blood gas variables in cystic fibrosis patients during reduced environmental pressure. *Eur. J. Appl. Physiol.* **92**, 493–7.

Thomas, D.J., Marshall, J., Ross Russell, R.W. *et al.* (1977) Cerebral blood-flow in polycythaemia. *Lancet* **2**, 161–3.

Thomas, P.K., King, R.H.M., Feng, S.F. *et al.* (2000) Neurological manifestations in chronic mountain sickness: the burning feet-burning hands syndrome. *J. Neurol. Neurosurg. Psychiatry* **69**, 447–52.

Thomas, P.S., Harding, R.M. and Milledge, J.S. (1990) Peak expiratory flow at altitude. *Thorax* **45**, 620–2.

Thomas, P.W. (1894) Rocky Mountain sickness. *Alpine J.* **17**, 140–9.

Thompson, A.A., Baillie, J.K., Bates, M.G. *et al.* (2009) The citric acid cough threshold and the ventilatory response to carbon dioxide on ascent to high altitude. *Respir. Med.* **103**, 1182–8.

Thompson, A.A.R., Baillie, J.K., Sutherland, A.I. *et al.* (2011) Sildenafil citrate for the prevention of high altitude hypoxic pulmonary hypertension: double blind, randomized, placebo-controlled trial. *High Alt. Med. Biol.* **12**, 207–14.

Thompson, D.G., Richelson, E. and Malagelada, J.R. (1983) A perturbation of upper gastro-intestinal function by cold stress. *Gut* **24**, 277–83.

Thompson, J., Raitt, J., Hutchings, L. *et al.* (2007) Angiotensin-converting enzyme genotype and successful ascent to extreme high altitude. *High Alt. Med. Biol.* **8**, 278–85.

Thompson, R.L. and Hayward, J.S. (1996) Wet cold exposure and hypothermia: thermal and metabolic responses to prolonged exercise in rain. *J. Appl. Physiol.* **81**, 1128–37.

Thompson, W.O., Thompson, P.K. and Dailey, M.M. (1928) The effect of posture on the composition and volume of the blood in man. *J. Clin. Invest.* **5**, 573–604.

Tierman, C.J. (1999) Splenic crisis at high altitude in two white men with sickle cell trait. *Ann. Emerg. Med.* **33**, 230–3.

Tikusis, P., Ducharme, M.B., Moroz, D. and Jacobs, I. (1999) Physiological responses on exercise fatigued individuals exposed to wet cold conditions. *J. Appl. Physiol.* **86**, 1319–25.

Tilman, H.W. (1948) *Mount Everest 1938,* Cambridge University Press, Cambridge, pp. 93–4.

Tilman, H.W. (1952) *Nepal Himalaya*, Cambridge University Press, Cambridge.

Tilman, H.W. (1975) Practical problems of nutrition, in *Mountain Medicine and Physiology* (eds. C. Clarke, M. Ward and E. Williams), Alpine Club, London, pp. 62–6.

Timmons, B.A., Ararujo, J. and Thomas, T.R. (1985) Fat utilization in a cold environment. *Med. Sci. Sports Exerc.* **17**, 673–8.

Ting, S. (1984) Cold induced urticaria in infancy. *Pediatrics* **73**, 105–6.

Tiollier, E., Schmitt, L., Burnat, P. *et al.* (2005) Living high–training low altitude training: effects on mucosal immunity. *Eur. J. Appl. Physiol.* **94**, 298–304.

Tissandier, G. (1875) Le voyage à grande hauteur du ballon 'Le Zenith'. *La Nature Paris* **3**, 337–44.

Tissot van Patot, M., Grill, A., Chapman, P. *et al.* (2003) Remodelling of uteroplacental arteries is decreased in high altitude placentae. *Placenta* **24**, 326–30.

Tissot van Patot, M.C., Leadbetter, G., Keyes, L.E. *et al.* (2005) Greater free plasma VEGF and lower soluble VEGF receptor-1 in acute mountain sickness. *J. Appl. Physiol.* **98**, 1626–9.

Toepfer, M., Hartmann, G., Schlosshauer, M. *et al.* (1998) Adrenomedullin: a player at high altitude? *Chest* **113**, 1428.

Toff, N.J. (1993) Hazards of air travel for the obese: Miss Pickwick and the Boeing 747. *J. R. Coll. Phys. Lond.* **27**, 375–6.

Tolman, K.G. and Cohen, A. (1970) Accidental hypothermia. *Can. Med. Assoc. J.* **103**, 1357–61.

Tomashefski, J.F., Feeley, D.R. and Shillito, F.H. (1966) Effects of altitude on emphysematous blebs and bullae. *Aerosp. Med.* **37**, 1158–62.

Tomiyama, Y., Brian Jr., J.E. and Tod, M.M. (2000) Plasma viscosity and cerebral blood flow. *Am. J. Physiol. Heart Circ. Physiol.* **279**, H1949–54.

Torgovicky, R., Azaria, B., Grossman, A. *et al.* (2005) Sinus vein thrombosis following exposure to simulated high altitude. *Aviat. Space Environ. Med.* **76**, 144–6.

Torrington, K.G. (1989) Recurrent high-altitude illness associated with right pulmonary artery occlusion from granulomatous mediastinitis. *Chest* **96**, 1422–4.

Toshner, M.R., Thompson, A.A.R., Irving, J.B. *et al.* (2008) NT-proBNP does not rise on acute ascent to high altitude. *High Alt. Med. Biol.* **9**, 307–310.

Townes, B.D., Hornbein, T.F., Schoene, R.B. *et al.* (1984) Human cerebral function at extreme altitude, in *High Altitude and Man* (eds. J.B. West and S. Lahiri), American Physiological Society, Bethesda, MD, pp. 32–6.

Townsend, N.E., Gore, C.J., Hahn, A.G. *et al.* (2002) Living high–training low: increased hypoxic ventilatory response of well-trained endurance athletes. *J. Appl. Physiol.* **93**, 1498–505.

Townsend, N.E., Gore, C.J., Hahn, A.G. *et al.* (2004) Hypoxic ventilatory response is correlated with increased submaximal exercise ventilation after live high, train low. *Eur. J. Appl. Physiol.* **94**, 207–15.

Tozzi, C.A., Poiani, G.J., Harangozo, A.M. *et al.* (1989) Pressure-induced connective tissue synthesis in pulmonary artery segments is dependent on intact endothelium. *J. Clin. Invest.* **84**, 1005–12.

Travis, S.P.L. and Menzies, I.S. (1992) Intestinal permeability: functional assessment and significance. *Clin. Sci.* **82**, 471–88.

Travis, S.P.L., A'Court, C., Menzies, I.S. *et al.* (1993) Intestinal function at altitudes above 5000m. *Gut* **34**, T165.

Treating accidental hypothermia (editorial). (1978) *BMJ* **2**, 1383–4.

Tripathy, V. and Gupta, R. (2005) Birth weight among Tibetans at different altitudes in India: are Tibetans better protected from IUGR? *Am. J. Hum. Biol.* **17**, 442–50.

Truijens, M.J., Toussaint, H.M., Dow, J. and Levine, B.D. (2003) Effect of high-intensity hypoxic training on sea-level swimming performances. J. Appl. Physiol. **94**, 733–43.

Truijens, M.J., Rodriquez, F.A., Townsend, N.E. *et al.* (2008) The effect of intermittent hypoxic exposure and sea level training on submaximal economy in well-trained swimmers and runners. *J. Appl. Physiol.* **104**, 328–37.

Tsianos, G., Eleftheriou, K.I., Hawe, E. *et al.* (2005) Performance at altitude and angiotensin I-converting enzyme genotype. *Eur. J. Appl. Physiol.* **93**, 630–5.

Tsukimoto, K., Mathieu-Costello, O., Prediletto, R. *et al.* (1991) Ultrastructural appearances of pulmonary capillaries at high transmural pressures. *J. Appl. Physiol.* **71**, 573–82.

Tsukimoto, K., Yoshimura, N., Ichioka, M. *et al.* (1994) Protein, cell, and leukotriene B4 concentrations of lung edema fluid produced by high capillary transmural pressures in rabbit. *J. Appl. Physiol.* **76**, 321–67.

Tucker, A. and Rhodes, J. (2001) Role of vascular smooth muscle in the development of high altitude pulmonary hypertension: an interspecies evaluation. *High Alt. Med. Biol.* **2**, 349–60.

Tuffley, R.E., Rubenstein, D., Slater, J.D.H. and Williams, E.S. (1970) Serum renin activity during exposure to hypoxia. *J. Endocrinol.* **48**, 497–510.

Turek, Z., Kreuzer, F. and Hoofd, L.J.C. (1973) Advantage or disadvantage of a decrease of blood oxygen affinity for tissue oxygen supply at hypoxia; a theoretical study comparing man and rat. *Pflügers Arch.* **342**, 185–97.

Turek, Z., Kreuzer, F. and Ringnalda, B.E.M. (1978) Blood gases at several levels of oxygenation in rats with a left shifted blood oxygen dissociation curve. *Pflügers Arch.* **376**, 7–13.

Turino, C.M., Bergofsky, E.H., Goldring, R.M. and Fishman, A.P. (1963) Effect of exercise on pulmonary diffusing capacity. *J. Appl. Physiol.* **18**, 447–56.

Unger, C., Weiser, J.K., McCullough, R.E. *et al.* (1988) Altitude, low birth weight, and infant mortality in Colorado. *JAMA* **259**, 3427–32.

Ungley, G.G., Channell, G.D. and Richards, R.L. (1945) The immersion foot syndrome. *Br. J. Surg.* **33**, 17–31.

Vachiery, J.L., McDonald, T., Moraine, J.J. *et al.* (1995) Doppler assessment of hypoxic pulmonary vasoconstriction and susceptibility to high altitude pulmonary oedema. *Thorax* **50**, 22–7.

Valdivia, E. (1958) Total capillary bed in striated muscle of guinea pigs native to the Peruvian mountains. *Am. J. Physiol.* **194**, 585–9.

Valletta, E.A., Comis, A., Del Col, G. *et al.* (1995) Peak expiratory flow variation and bronchial hyperresponsiveness in asthmatic children during periods of antigen avoidance and reexposure. *Allergy* **50**, 366–9.

Valletta, E.A., Piacentini, G.L., Del Col, G. and Boner, A.L. (1997) FEF25-75 as a marker of airway obstruction in asthmatic children during reduced mite exposure at high altitude. *J. Asthma.* **34**, 127–31.

van den Elshout, F.J., van Herwaarden, C.L. and Folgering, H.T. (1991) Effects of hypercapnia and hypocapnia on respiratory resistance in normal and asthmatic subjects. *Thorax* **46**, 28–32.

van Hall, G. (2007) Counterpoint: The lactate paradox does not occur during exercise at high altitude. *J. Appl. Physiol.* **102**, 2399–401.

Van Osta, A., Moraine, J.J., Melot, C. *et al.* (2005) Effects of high altitude exposure on cerebral hemodynamics in normal subjects. *Stroke* **36**, 557–60.

Van Patot, M.C., Hill, A.E., Dingmann, C. *et al.* (2006) Risk of impaired coagulation in warfarin patients ascending to altitude (>2400 m). *High Alt. Med. Biol.* **7**, 39–46.

van Patot, M.C., Leadbetter, G., 3rd, Keyes, L.E. *et al.* (2008) Prophylactic low-dose acetazolamide reduces the incidence and severity of acute mountain sickness. *High Alt. Med. Biol.* **9**, 289–93.

Van Ruiten, H.J.A. and Daanen, H.A.M. (1999) Cold induced vasodilatation at altitude (abstract), in *Hypoxia: Into the Next Millennium* (eds. R.C. Roach, P.D. Wagner and P.H. Hackett), Plenum/Kluwer, New York, p. 436.

van Velzen, E., van den Bos, J.W., Benckhuijsen, J.A. *et al.* (1996) Effect of allergen avoidance at high altitude on direct and indirect bronchial hyperresponsiveness and markers of inflammation in children with allergic asthma. *Thorax* **51**, 582–4.

Vardy, J., Vardy, J. and Judge, K. (2005) Can knowledge protect against acute mountain sickness? *J. Public Health (Oxford)* **27**, 366–70.

Vargas, M., León-Velarde, F., Monge, C.C. *et al.* (1998) Similar hypoxic ventilatory response in sea-level natives and Andean natives living at sea level. *J. Appl. Physiol.* **84**, 1024–9.

Vargas, M., Vargas, E., Julian, C.G. *et al.* (2007) Determinants of blood oxygenation during pregnancy in Andean and European residents of high altitude. *Am. J. Physiol. Regul. Physiol.* **293**, R1303–12.

Vasquez, R. and Villena, M. (2001) Normal hematological values for healthy persons living at 4000 meters in Bolivia. *High Alt. Med .Biol.* **2**, 361–7.

Vats, P., Singh, S.N., Shyam, R. *et al.* (2004) Leptin may not be responsible for high altitude anorexia. *High Alt. Med. Biol.* **5**, 90–2.

Vaughan, B.E. and Pace, N. (1956) Changes in myoglobin content of the high altitude acclimatized rat. *Am. J. Physiol.* **185**, 549–56.

Vaughn, P.B. (1942) Local cold injury – menace to military operations. A review. *Mil. Med.* **145**, 305–11.

Velásquez, M.T. (1956) *Maximal Diffusing Capacity of the Lungs at High Altitudes.* Report 56–108, USAF School of Aviation Medicine, Randolph Air Force Base, TX.

Velasquez, T. (1976) Pulmonary function and oxygen transport, in *Man in the Andes: a Multidisciplinary Study of High-altitude Quechua* (eds. P.T. Baker and M.A. Little), Dowden, Hutchinson & Ross, Stroudsburg, PA, pp. 237–60.

Vella, M.A., Jenner, C., Betteridge, D.J. and Jowett, N.I. (1988) Hypothermia induced thrombocytopenia. *J. R. Soc. Med.* **81**, 228–9.

Venter, J.C., Adams, M.D., Myers, E.W. *et al.* (2001) The sequence of the human genome. *Science* **291**, 1304–51.

Ventura, N., Hoppeler, H., Seiler, R. *et al.* (2003) The response of trained athletes to six weeks of endurance training in hypoxia or normoxia. *Int. J. Sports Med.* **24**, 166–72.

Verratti, V., Berardinelli, F. and Di Giulio, C. (2008) Evidence that chronic hypoxia causes reversible impairment on male fertility. *Asian J. Androl.* **10**, 602–6.

Viault, F. (1890) Sur l'augmentation considerable de nombre des globules rouges dans le sang chez les habitants des haut plateaux de l'Amérique du Sud. *Comptes Rendus, Hebdomaire Des Seances de l'Academie Des Sciences (Paris)*, **III**, 917–18. English translation (1981) in *High Altitude Physiology* (ed. J.B. West), Hutchinson Ross, Stroudsburg, PA, 1981, pp. 333–4.

Viault, F. (1891) Sur la quantité d'oxygène contenue dans le sang des animaux des hauts plateaux de l'Amérique du Sud. *C. R. Acad. Sci. (Paris)* **112**, 295–8.

Vij, A.G. (2009). Effect of prolonged stay at high altitude on platelet aggregation and fibrinogen levels. *Platelets* **20**, 421–7.

Villafuerte, F.C., Cardenas, R., and Monge-C.C. (2004) Optimal hemoglobin concentration and high altitude: a theoretical approach for Andean men at rest. *J. Appl. Physiol.* **96**, 1579–8.

Vinnikov, D., Brimlulov, N., Redding-Jones, R. and Jumabaeva, K. (2010) Exhaled nitric oxide is reduced upon chronic intermittent hypoxia exposure in well-acclimatized mine workers. *Respir. Physiol. Neurobiol.* **175**, 261–4.

Virmani, S.K. and Swamy, A.S. (1993) Cranial nerve palsy at high altitude. *J. Assoc. Physicians India* **41**, 460.

Virokannas, H. and Anttonen, H. (1993) Risk of frostbite in vibration-induced finger cases. *Arctic Med. Res.* **52**, 69–72.

Viswanathan, R., Subramanian, S. and Radha, T.C. (1979) Effect of hypoxia on regional lung perfusion, by scanning. *Respiration* **37**, 142–7.

Vitzthum, V.J. (2001) The home team advantage: reproduction in women indigenous to high altitude. *J. Exp. Biol.* **204(Pt 18)**, 3141–50.

Vitzthum, V.J. and Wiley, A.S. (2003) The proximate determinants of fertility in populations exposed to chronic hypoxia. *High Alt. Med. Biol.* **4**, 125–39.

Vitzthum, V.J., Ellison, P.T., Sukalich, S. *et al.* (2000a) Does hypoxia impair ovarian function in Bolivian women indigenous to high altitude? *High Alt. Med. Biol.* **1**, 39–49.

Vitzthum, V.J., Spielvogel, H., Caceres, E. and Gaines, J. (2000b) Menstrual patterns and fecundity among non-lactating and lactating cycling women in rural highland Bolivia: implications for contraceptive choice. *Contraception* **62**, 181–7.

Vitzthum, V.J., Bentley, G.R., Spielvogel, H. *et al.* (2002) Salivary progesterone levels and rate of ovulation are significantly lower in poorer than in better-off urban-dwelling Bolivian women. *Hum. Reprod.* **17**, 1906–13.

Vivona, M.L., Matthay, M., Chabaud, M.B. *et al.* (2001) Hypoxia reduces alveolar epithelial sodium and fluid transport in rats: reversal by beta-adrenergic agonist treatment. *Am. J. Respir. Cell. Mol. Biol.* **25**, 554–61.

Vock, P., Fretz, C., Franciolli, M. and Bärtsch, P. (1989) High-altitude pulmonary edema: findings at high-altitude chest radiography and physical examination. *Radiology* **170**, 661–6.

Vock, P., Brutsche, M.H., Nanzer, A. and Bärtsch, P. (1991) Variable radiomorphologic data of high altitude pulmonary edema. Features from 60 patients. *Chest* **100**, 1306–11.

Voelkel, N.F., Hegstrand, L., Reeves, J.T. *et al.* (1981) Effects of hypoxia on density of β-adrenergic receptors. *J. Appl. Physiol.* **50**, 363–6.

Vogel, J.A. and Harris, C.W. (1967) Cardiopulmonary responses of resting man during early exposure to high altitude. *J. Appl. Physiol.* **22**, 1124–8.

Vogel, J.A., Hansen, J.E. and Harris, C.W. (1967) Cardiovascular responses in man during exhaustive work at sea level and high altitude. *J. Appl. Physiol.* **23**, 531–9.

Vogel, J.A., Hartley, L.H. and Cruz, J.C. (1974) Cardiac output during exercise in altitude natives at sea level and high altitude. *J. Appl. Physiol.* **36**, 173–6.

Vogt, M., Puntschart, A., Geiser, J. *et al.* (2001) Molecular adaptations in human skeletal muscle to endurance training under simulated hypoxic conditions. *J. Appl. Physiol.* **91**, 173–82.

Von Euler, U.S. and Liljestrand, G. (1946) Observations on the pulmonary arterial blood pressure in the cat. *Acta Physiol.* **22**, 1115–23.

Vonmoos, S., Nussberger, J., Waeber, J. *et al.* (1990) Effect of metoclopramide on angiotensin, aldosterone and atrial peptide during hypoxia. *J. Appl. Physiol.* **69**, 2072–9.

Vovk, A., Smith, W.D.F., Paterson, N.D. *et al.* (2004) Peripheral chemoreceptor control of ventilation following sustained hypoxia in young and older adult humans. *Exp. Physiol.* **86**, 647–56.

Vuolteenaho, O., Koistinen, P., Martikkala, V. *et al.* (1992) Effect of physical exercise in hypobaric conditions on atrial natriuretic peptide secretion. *Am. J. Physiol.* **263**, R647–52.

Wagenvoort, C.A. and Wagenvoort, N. (1973) Hypoxic pulmonary vascular lesions in man at high altitude and in patients with chronic respiratory disease. *Pathol. Microbiol.* **39**, 276–82.

Wagenvoort, C.A. and Wagenvoort, N. (1976) Pulmonary venous changes in chronic hypoxia. *Virchows Arch. [A]* **372**, 51–6.

Waggener, T.B., Brusil, P.J., Kronauer, R.E. *et al.* (1984) Strength and cycle time of high-altitude ventilatory patterns in unacclimatized humans. *J. Appl. Physiol.* **56**, 576–81.

Wagner, D.R., Fargo, J.D., Parker, D. *et al.* (2006) Variables contributing to acute mountain sickness on the summit of Mt Whitney. *Wilderness Environ. Med.* **17**, 221–8.

Wagner, D.R., Tatsugawa, K., Parker, D. and Young, T.A. (2007) Reliability and utility of a visual analog scale for the assessment of acute mountain sickness. *High Alt. Med. Biol.* **8**, 27–31.

Wagner, P.D. (1988) An integrated view of the determinants of maximum oxygen uptake, in *Oxygen Transfer from Atmosphere to Tissues*, vol. 227 (eds. N.C. Gonzalez and M.R. Fedde), Plenum, New York, pp. 246–56.

Wagner, P.D. (1996) A theoretical analysis of factors determining $V_{O_2,max}$ at sea level and altitude. *Respir. Physiol.* **106**, 329–43.

Wagner, P.D. and West, J.B. (1972) Effects of diffusion impairment of O_2 and CO_2 time courses in pulmonary capillaries. *J. Appl. Physiol.* **33**, 62–71.

Wagner, P.D., Saltzman, H.A. and West, J.B. (1974) Measurement of continuous distributions of ventilation–perfusion ratios: theory. *J. Appl. Physiol.* **36**, 588–99.

Wagner, P.D., Sutton, J.R., Reeves, J.T. *et al.* (1987) Operation Everest II. Pulmonary gas exchange during a simulated ascent of Mt. Everest. *J. Appl. Physiol.* **63**, 2348–59.

Wagner, P.D., Hedenstierna, G. and Rodriguez-Roisin, R. (1996) Gas exchange, expiratory flow obstruction and the clinical spectrum of asthma. *Eur. Respir. J.* **9**, 1278–82.

Wagner, P.D., Araoz, M., Boushel, R. *et al.* (2002) Pulmonary gas exchange and acid-base status at 5,260m in high-altitude Bolivians and acclimatized lowlanders. *J. Appl. Physiol.* **92**, 1393–400.

Waller, D. (1990) *The Pundits: British Exploration of Tibet and Central Asia*, University Press of Kentucky, Lexington, KY.

Walter, R., Maggiorini, M., Scherrer, U. *et al.* (2001) Effects of high-altitude exposure on vascular endothelial growth factor levels in man. *Eur. J. Appl. Physiol.* **85**, 113–17.

Wanderer, A.A. (1979) An 'allergy' to cold. *Hosp. Pract.* **14**, 136–7.

Wang, J., Weigand, L., Lu, W. *et al.* (2006) Hypoxia inducible factor 1 mediates hypoxia-induced TRPC expression and elevated intracellular Ca^{2+} in pulmonary arterial smooth muscle cells. *Circ. Res.* **98**, 1528–37.

Wang, L.C.H. (1978) Factors limiting maximum cold induced heat production. *Life Sci.* **23**, 2089–98.

Wang, P., Koehle, M.S. and Rupert, J.L. (2010) No association between alleles of the bradykinin receptor-B2 gene and acute mountain sickness. *Exp. Biol. Med.* **235**, 737–40.

Ward, M.P. (1954) High altitude deterioration, in: A discussion on the physiology of man at high altitude. *Proc. R. Soc., Series B, London* **143**, 40–2.

Ward, M.P. (1968) Diseases occurring at altitudes exceeding 17500 ft. MD thesis, University of Cambridge, pp. 66–9.

Ward, M.P. (1973) Periodic respiration. *Am. R. Coll. Surg. Engl.* **52**, 330–4.

Ward, M.P. (1974) Frostbite. *BMJ* **1**, 67–70.

Ward, M.P. (1975) *Mountain Medicine, a Clinical Study of Cold and High Altitude*, Crosby Lockwood Staples, London.

Ward, M.P. (1987) Cold, hypoxia and dehydration, in *Hypoxia and Cold* (eds. J.R. Sutton, C.S. Houston and G. Coates), Prager, New York, pp. 475–86.

Ward, M.P. (1990) Tibet: human and medical geography. *J. Wilderness Med.* **1**, 36–46.

Ward, M.P. (1991) Medicine in Tibet. *J. Wilderness Med.* **2**, 198–205.

Ward, M.P. (1993) The first ascent of Mount Everest, 1953: the solution of the problem of the 'last thousand feet'. *J. Wilderness Med.* **4**, 312–18.

Ward, M.P. and Jackson, F.S. (1965) Medicine in Bhutan. *Lancet* **1**, 811–13.

Warren, C.B.M. (1939) Alveolar air on Mount Everest. *J. Physiol. (Lond.)* **96**, 34–5.

Washburn, B. (1962) Frostbite. What it is – and how to prevent it – emergency treatment. *N. Engl. J. Med.* **266**, 974–89.

Watson, J.D. and Crick, F.H. (1953) Molecular structure of nucleic acids; a structure for deoxyribose nucleic acid. *Nature* **171**, 737–38.

Waypa, G.B. and Schumacker, P.T. (2008) Oxygen sensing in hypoxic pulmonary vasoconstriction: using new tools to answer an age-old question. *Exp. Physiol.* **93**, 133–8.

Webb, P. (1951) Air temperature in respiratory tracts of resting subjects in cold. *J. Appl. Physiol.* **4**, 378–82.

Webb, P. (1986) After drop of body temperature during re-warming – an alternative explanation. *J. Appl. Physiol.* **60**, 385–90.

Weber, R.E. (2007) High-altitude adaptations in vertebrate hemoglobins. *Respir. Physiol. Neurobiol.* **158**, 132–42.

Wedin, B., Vanggaard, L. and Hirvonen, J. (1979) 'Paradoxical undressing' in fatal hypothermia. *J. Forensic Sci.* **24**, 543–53.

Wedzicha, J.A., Cotes, P.M., Empey, D.W. *et al.* (1985) Serum immunoreactive erythropoietin in hypoxic lung disease with and without polycythaemia. *Clin. Sci.* **69**, 413–22.

Weeke, J. and Gundersen, H.J.G. (1983) The effect of heating and cold cooling on serum TSH, GH and norepinephrine in resting normal man. *Acta Physiol. Scand.* **47**, 33–9.

Wehrlin, J.P. and Hallen, J. (2006) Linear decrease in VO2 max and performance with increasing altitude in endurance athletes. *Eur. J. Appl. Physiol.* **96**, 404–12.

Wehrlin, J.P. and Marti, B. (2006) Live high–train low associated with increased haemoglobin mass as preparation for the 2003 World Championships in two native European world class runners. *Br. J. Sports Med.* **40**, e3; discussion e3.

Wehrlin, J.P., Zuest, P., Hallen, J. and Marti, B. (2006) Live high - train low for 24 days increases hemoglobin mass and red cell volume in elite endurance athletes. *J. Appl. Physiol.* **100**, 1938–45.

Weibel, E.R. (1970) Morphometric estimation of pulmonary diffusion capacity. *Respir. Physiol.* **11**, 54–75.

Weil, J.V. (2004) Sleep at high altitude. *High Alt. Med. Biol.* **5**, 180–9.

Weil, J.V. and White, D.P. (2001) Sleep, in *High Altitude* (eds. T.F. Hornbein and R.B. Schoene), Marcel Dekker, New York, pp. 707–76.

Weil, J.V., Byrne-Quinn, E., Sodal, I.E. *et al.* (1970) Hypoxic ventilatory drive in normal man. *J. Clin. Invest.* **49**, 1061–72.

Weil, J.V., Byrne-Quinn, E., Ingvar, E. *et al.* (1971) Acquired attenuation of chemoreceptor function in chronically hypoxic man at high altitude. *J. Clin. Invest.* **50**, 186–95.

Weil, J.V., Kryger, M.H. and Scoggin, C.H. (1978) Sleep and breathing at high altitude, in *Sleep Apnea Syndromes* (eds. C. Guilleminault and W. Dement), Liss, New York, pp. 119–36.

Weilenmann, D., Duru, F., Schonbeck, M. *et al.* (2000) Influence of acute exposure to high altitude and hypoxemia on ventricular stimulation thresholds in pacemaker patients. *Pacing Clin. Electrophysiol.* **23**, 512–15.

Weiss, E.A. (1991) Environmental heat illness, in *Proceedings of the First World Congress on Wilderness Medicine,* Wilderness Medical Society, Point Reyes Station, CA, pp. 347–57.

Weiss, R.G., Bottomley, P.A., Hardy, C.J. and Gerstenblith, G. (1990) Regional myocardial metabolism of high-energy phosphates during isometric exercise in patients with coronary artery disease. *N. Engl. J. Med.* **323,** 1593–1600.

Weisse, A.B., Moschos, C.B., Frank, M.L. *et al.* (1975) Haemodynamic effects of staged haematocrit reduction in patients with stable cor pulmonale and severely elevated haematocrit. *Am. J. Med.* **58**, 92–8.

Weitz, C.A. and Garruto, R.M. (2004) Growth of Han migrants at high altitude in central Asia. *Am. J. Hum. Biol.* **16**, 405–19.

Weller, A.S., Millard, C.E., Stroud, M.A. *et al.* (1997) Physiological responses to a cold, wet and windy environment during prolonged intermittent walking. *Am. J. Physiol.* **272**, R226–33.

Welsh, C.H., Wagner, P.D., Reeves, J.T. *et al.* (1993) Operation Everest II: spirometric and radiographic changes in acclimatized humans at simulated high altitudes. *Am. Rev. Respir. Dis.* **147**, 1239–44.

Wen, T.C., Sadamoto, Y., Tanaka, J. *et al.* (2002) Erythropoietin protects neurons against chemical hypoxia and cerebral ischemic injury by up-regulating Bcl-xL expression. *J. Neurosci. Res.* **67**, 795–803.

West, J.B. (1962a) Diffusing capacity of the lung for carbon monoxide at high altitude. *J. Appl. Physiol.* **17**, 421–6.

West, J.B. (1962b) Regional differences in gas exchange in the lung of erect man. *J. Appl. Physiol.* **17**, 893–8.

West, J.B. (1981) *High Altitude Physiology: Benchmark Papers in Physiology,* vol. 15,

Hutchinson Ross, Stroudsburg, PA, p. 328.

West, J.B. (1982) Diffusion at high altitude. *Fed. Proc.* **41**, 2128–30.

West, J.B. (1983) Climbing Mt. Everest without oxygen: an analysis of maximal exercise during extreme hypoxia. *Respir. Physiol.* **52**, 265–79.

West, J.B. (ed.) (1985b) *Best and Taylor's Physiological Basis of Medical Practice*, 11th edn, Williams and Wilkins, Baltimore, MD.

West, J.B. (1986a) Highest inhabitants in the world. *Nature* **324**, 517.

West, J.B. (1986b) Lactate during exercise at extreme altitude. *Fed. Proc.* **45**, 2953–7.

West, J.B. (1987) Alexander M. Kellas and the physiological challenge of Mount Everest. *J. Appl. Physiol.* **63**, 3–11.

West, J.B. (1988a) Rate of ventilatory acclimatization to extreme altitude. *Respir. Physiol.* **74**, 323–33.

West, J.B. (1988b) Tolerable limits to hypoxia on high mountains, in *Hypoxia: the Tolerable Limits* (eds. J.R. Sutton, C.S. Houston and G. Coates), Benchmark Press, Indianapolis, IN, pp. 353–62.

West, J.B. (1988c) *High Life: A History of High-altitude Physiology and Medicine*. Oxford University Press, Oxford, pp. 358–63.

West, J.B. (1990) *Ventilation/Blood Flow and Gas Exchange*, 5th edn, Blackwell Scientific, Oxford.

West, J.B. (1993a) Acclimatization and tolerance to extreme altitude. *J. Wilderness Med.* **4**, 17–26.

West, J.B. (1993b) The Silver Hut expedition, high-altitude field expeditions, and low-pressure chamber simulations, in *Hypoxia and Molecular Medicine* (eds. J.R. Sutton, C.S. Houston and G. Coates), Queen City Printers, Burlington, VT, pp. 190–202.

West, J.B. (1995) Oxygen enrichment of room air to relieve the hypoxia of high altitude. *Respir. Physiol.* **99**, 225–32.

West, J.B. (1996a) Prediction of barometric pressures at high altitudes with the use of model atmospheres. *J. Appl. Physiol.* **81**, 1850–4.

West, J.B. (1996b) T.H. Ravenhill and his contributions to mountain sickness. *J. Appl. Physiol.* **80**, 715–24.

West, J.B. (1997) Fire hazard in oxygen-enriched atmospheres at low barometric pressures. *Aviat. Space Envir. Med.* **68**, 159–62.

West, J.B. (1998) *High Life: A History of High-Altitude Physiology and Medicine*, Oxford University Press, New York.

West, J.B. (1999a) Barometric pressures on Mt. Everest: new data and physiological significance. *J. Appl. Physiol.* **86**, 1062–6.

West, J.B. (1999b) The original presentation of Boyle's law. *J. Appl. Physiol.* **87**, 1543–5.

West J.B. (2001) Safe upper limits for oxygen enrichment of room air at high altitude. *High Alt Med Biol* **2**, 47–51.

West, J.B. (2002a) Highest permanent human habitation. *High Alt. Med. Biol.* **3**, 401–7.

West, J.B. (2002b) Potential use of oxygen enrichment of room air in mountain resorts. *High Alt. Med. Biol.* **3**, 59–64.

West, J.B. (2004a) Gulmuf–Lhasa rail link: an enormous challenge in high altitude medicine. *High Alt. Med. Biol.* **5**, 3.

West, J.B. (2004b) The physiologic basis of high-altitude disease. *Ann. Intern. Med.* **141**, 789–800.

West, J.B. (2005a) *Respiratory Physiology – The Essentials,* 7th edn, Williams & Wilkins, Baltimore, MD.

West J.B. (2005b) Robert-Boyle's landmark book of 1660 with the first experiments on rarified air. *J. Appl. Physiol.* **98**, 31–9.

West, J.B. (2007) Point: The lactate paradox does occur during exercise at high altitude. *J. Appl. Physiol.* **102**, 2398–9.

West, J.B. (2009) Arterial blood measurements in climbers on Mount Everest. *Lancet* **373**, 1589–90.

West, J.B. (2011) Con: Headache should not be a required symptom for the diagnosis of acute mountain sickness. *High Alt. Med. Biol.* **12**, 23–5; discussion 27.

West, J.B. and Mathieu-Costello, O. (1992a) High altitude pulmonary edema is caused by stress failure of pulmonary capillaries. *Intl. J. Sports Med.* **13**(Suppl. 1), S54–8.

West, J.B. and Mathieu-Costello, O. (1992b) Strength of the pulmonary blood–gas barrier. *Respir. Physiol.* **88**, 141–8.

West, J.B. and Mathieu-Costello, O. (1992c) Stress failure of pulmonary capillaries: role in lung and heart disease. *Lancet* **340**, 762–7.

West, J.B. and Readhead, A. (2004) Working at high altitude: medical problems, misconceptions, and solutions. *Observatory* **124**, 1–14.

West, J.B. and Wagner, P.D. (1977) Pulmonary gas exchange, in *Bioengineering Aspects of the Lung* (ed. J.B. West), Dekker, New York, pp. 361–457.

West, J.B. and Wagner, P.D. (1980) Predicted gas exchange on the summit of Mt Everest. *Respir. Physiol.* **42**, 1–16.

West, J.B., Lahiri, S., Gill, M.B. *et al.* (1962) Arterial oxygen saturation during exercise at high altitude. *J. Appl. Physiol.* **17**, 617–21.

West, J.B., Lahiri, S., Maret, K.H. *et al.* (1983a) Barometric pressures at extreme altitudes on Mt. Everest: physiological significance. *J. Appl. Physiol.* **54**, 1188–94.

West, J.B., Hackett, P.H., Maret, K.H. *et al.* (1983b) Pulmonary gas exchange on the summit of Mount Everest. *J. Appl. Physiol.* **55**, 678–87.

West, J.B., Boyer, S.J., Graber, D.J. *et al.* (1983c) Maximal exercise at extreme altitudes on Mount Everest. *J. Appl. Physiol.* **55**, 688–98.

West, J.B., Peters, R.M., Aksnes, G. *et al.* (1986) Nocturnal periodic breathing at altitudes of 6300 and 8050 m. *J. Appl. Physiol.* **61**, 280–7.

West, J.B., Tsukimoto, K., Mathieu-Costello, O. and Prediletto, R. (1991) Stress failure in pulmonary capillaries. *J. Appl. Physiol.* **70**, 1731–42.

West, J.B., Mathieu-Costello, O., Jones, J.H. *et al.* (1993) Stress failure of pulmonary capillaries in racehorses with exercise-induced pulmonary hemorrhage. *J. Appl. Physiol.* **75**, 1097–109.

West, J.B., Colice, G.L., Lee, Y.-J. *et al.* (1995) Pathogenesis of high-altitude pulmonary edema: direct evidence of stress failure of pulmonary capillaries. *Eur. Respir. J.* **8**, 523–9.

West, J.P. (1985a) *Everest – the Testing Place.* McGraw-Hill, New York.

Westendorp, R.G., Blauw, G.J., Frolich, M. and Simons, R. (1997) Hypoxic syncope. *Aviat. Space Environ. Med.* **68**, 410–4.

Westendorp, R.G.J., Frölich, M. and Meinders, A.E. (1993) What to tell steroid substituted patients about the effects of high altitude? *Lancet* **342**, 310–11.

Westerterp, K.R. (2001) Limits to sustainable human metabolic rate. *J. Exp. Biol.* **204**, 3183–7.

Westerterp, K.R., Kayser, B., Brouns, F. *et al.* (1992) Energy expenditure climbing Mt. Everest. *J. Appl. Physiol.* **73**, 1815–19.

Westerterp, K.R., Kayser, B., Wouters, L. *et al.* (1994) Energy balance at high altitude of 6,542 m. *J. Appl. Physiol.* **77**, 862–6.

Westerterp, K.R., Meijer, E.P., Rubbens, M. *et al.* (2000) Operation Everest III: energy and water balance. *Eur. J. Physiol.* **439**, 483–8.

Westerterp-Plantegna, M.S., Westerterp, K.R., Rubbens, M. *et al.* (1999) Appetite at high altitude [(Operation Everest III Comex-97)]: A simulated ascent of Mount Everest. *J. Appl. Physiol.* **87**, 391–9.

Weston, A.R., Karamizrak, O., Smith, A. *et. al* (1999) African runners who lived at sea level exhibited greater fatigue resistance, lower lactate accumulation and higher oxidative activity. *J. Appl. Physiol.* **86**, 915–23.

Wetter, T.J., Harms, C.A., Nelson, W.B. *et al.* (1999) Influence of respiratory muscle work on V_{O_2} and leg blood flow during submaximal exercise. *J. Appl. Physiol.* **87**, 643–51.

Whayne, T.F. and Severinghaus, J.W. (1968) Experimental hypoxic pulmonary edema in the rat. *J. Appl. Physiol.* **25**, 729–32.

White, D.P., Gleeson, K., Pickett, C.K. *et al.* (1987) Altitude acclimatization: influence on periodic breathing and chemoresponsiveness during sleep. *J. Appl. Physiol.* **63**, 401–12.

Whittembury, J., Lozano, R. and Monge, C.C. (1968) Influence of cell concentration in the electrometric determination of blood pH. *Acta Physiol. Lat. Am.* **18**, 263–5.

Whymper, E. (1891–1892) *Travels among the Great Andes of the Equator.* John Murray, London.

Wickramasinghe, H. and Anholm, J.D. (1999) Sleep and breathing at high altitude. *Sleep Breath.* **3**, 89–102.

Wickwire, J. (1982) Pulmonary embolus and/or pneumonia on K2, in *Hypoxia, Man at Altitude* (eds. J.R. Sutton, N.L. Jones and C.S. Houston), Thieme Stratton, New York, pp. 173–6.

Wiedman, M. and Tabin, G.C. (1999) High-altitude retinopathy and altitude illness. *Ophthalmology* **106**, 1924–6.

Wielicki, K. (1985) Broad peak climbed in one day. *Alpine J.* **90**, 61–3.

Wilber, R.L., Holm, P.L., Morris, D.M. *et al.* (2003) Effect of F(I)O(2) on physiological responses and cycling performance at moderate altitude. *Med. Sci. Sports Exerc.* **35**, 1153–9.

Wiles, P.G., Grant, P.J., Jones, R.G. *et al.* (1986) Lowered skin blood flow at exhaustion. *Lancet* **2**, 295.

Wilkerson, J.A., Bangs, C.C. and Hayward, J.S. (1986) *Hypothermia, Frostbite and Other Cold Injuries*, The Mountaineers, Seattle, p. 45.

Wilkins, D.C. (1973) Acclimation to heat in the Antarctic, in *Polar Human Biology* (eds. O.G. Edholm and E.K.E. Gunderson), Heinemann Medical, London, pp. 171–81.

Wilkinson, R., Milledge, J.S. and Landon, M.J. (1993) Microalbuminuria in chronic obstructive lung disease. *BMJ* **307**, 239–40.

Will, D.H., McMurty, I.F., Reeves, T.J. *et al.* (1978) Cold-induced pulmonary hypertension in cattle. *J. Appl. Physiol.* **45**, 469–73.

Williams, E.S. (1961) Salivary electrolyte composition at high altitude. *Clin. Sci.* **21**, 37–42.

Williams, E.S. (1975) Mountaineering and the endocrine system, in *Mountain Medicine and Physiology* (eds. C. Clarke, M. Ward and E. Williams), Proceedings of a Symposium for Mountaineers, Expedition Doctors and Physiologists, Alpine Club, London, pp. 38–44.

Willison, J.R., Thomas, D.J., DuBoulay, G.H. *et al.* (1980) Effects of high haematocrit on alertness. *Lancet* **1**, 846–8.

Wilson, D.F., Erecińska, M., Drown, C. and Silver, I.A. (1977) Effect of oxygen tension on cellular energetics. *Am. J. Physiol.* **233**, C135–40.

Wilson, D.F., Roy, A. and Lahiri, S. (2005) Immediate and long-term responses of the carotid body to high altitude. *High Alt. Med. Biol.* **6**, 97–111.

Wilson, M.H. and Milledge, J. (2008) Direct measurement of intracranial pressure at high altitude and correlation of ventricular size with acute mountain sickness: Brian Cummins' results from the 1985 Kishtwar expedition. *Neurosurgery* **63**, 970–4; discussion 974–5.

Wilson, M.H., Levett, D.Z., Dhillon, S. *et al.* (2010) Stroke at high altitude diagnosed in the field using portable ultrasound. *Wilderness Environ. Med.* **22**, 54–7.

Wilson, M.H., Imray, C.H.E. and Hargens, A.R. (2011) The headache of high altitude and microgravity – similarities with clinical syndromes of cerebral venous hypertension. *High Alt. Med. Biol.* **12**, 379–86.

Wilson, M.J., Lopez, M., Vargas, M. *et al.* (2007) Greater uterine artery blood flow during pregnancy in multigenerational (Andean) than shorter-term (European) high-altitude residents. *Am. J. Physiol. Regul. Physiol.* **293**, R1313–24.

Winkle, R.K., Mader, T.H., Parmley, V.C. *et al.* (1998) The etiology of refractive changes at high altitude following radial keratotomy: hypoxia versus hypobaria. *Ophthalmology* **105**, 282–6.

Winslow, R.M. and Monge, C.C. (1987) *Hypoxia, Polycythemia, and Chronic Mountain Sickness*, Johns Hopkins University Press, Baltimore, MD, pp. 182–4 and 64–74.

Winslow, R.M., Monge, C.C., Statham, N.J. *et al.* (1981) Variability of oxygen affinity of blood: human subjects native to high altitude. *J. Appl. Physiol.* **51**, 1411–16.

Winslow, R.M., Samaja, M. and West, J.B. (1984) Red cell function at extreme altitude on Mount Everest. *J. Appl. Physiol.* **56**, 109–16.

Winslow, R.M., Monge, C.C., Brown, E.G. *et al.* (1985) Effects of hemodilution on O_2 transport in high-altitude polycythemia. *J. Appl. Physiol.* **59**, 1495–502.

Winslow, R.M., Chapman, K.W., Gibson, C.C. *et al.* (1989) Different haematologic response to hypoxia in Sherpas and Quechua Indians. *J. Appl. Physiol.* **66**, 1561–9.

Winter, R.J.D., Melaegros, L., Pervez, S. et al. (1987a) Plasma atrial natriuretic factor and ultrastructure of atrial specific granules following chronic hypoxia in rats. Clin. Sci. **72**, 26P.

Winter, R.J.D., Davidson, A.C., Treacher, D.F. et al. (1987b) Plasma atrial natriuretic factor in chronically hypoxaemic patients with pulmonary hypertension. Clin. Sci. **73**, 51P.

Winter, R.J.D., Melaegros, L., Pervez, S. et al. (1989) Atrial natriuretic peptide levels in plasma and in cardiac tissues after chronic hypoxia in rats. Clin. Sci. **76**, 95–101.

Winterstein, H. (1911) Die Regulierung der Atmung durch das Blut. Pflügers Arch. Ges. Physiol. **138**, 167–84.

Winterstein, H. (1915) Neue Untersuchungen über die physikalisch-chemische Regulierung der Atmung. Biochem. Z. **70**, 45–73.

Withey, W.R., Milledge, J.S., Williams, E.S. et al. (1983) Fluid and electrolyte homeostasis during prolonged exercise at altitude. J. Appl. Physiol. **55**, 409–12.

Wittenberg, J.B. (1959) Oxygen transport: a new function proposed for myoglobin. Biol. Bull. **117**, 402–3.

Wohns, R.N. (1986) Transient ischemic attacks at high altitude. Crit. Care Med. **14**, 517–18.

Wohns, R.N.W. (1987) Transient ischemic attacks at high altitude, in Hypoxia and Cold (eds. J.R. Sutton, C.S. Houston and G. Coates), Praeger, New York, p. 536.

Wolde-Gebriel, Z., Demeke, T., West, C.E. and Van der Haar, F. (1993) Goitre in Ethiopia. Br. J. Nutr. **69**, 257–68.

Wolfel, E.E., Groves, B.M., Brooks, G.A. et al. (1991) Oxygen transport during steady state submaximal exercise in chronic hypoxia. J. Appl. Physiol. **70**, 1129–36.

Wolfel, E.E., Selland, M.A., Mazzeo, R.S. and Reeves, J.T. (1994) Systemic hypertension at 4,300m is related to sympathoadrenal activity. J. Appl. Physiol. **76**, 1643–50.

Wolff, C.B. (1980) Normal ventilation in chronic hypoxia. J. Physiol. **308**, 118–19P.

Wolff, C.B. (2000) Cerebral blood flow and oxygen delivery at high altitude. High Alt. Med. Biol. **1**, 33–8.

Wood, S., Norboo, T., Lilly, M. et al. (2003) Cardiopulmonary function in high altitude residents of Ladakh. High Alt. Med. Biol. **4**, 445–54.

Woods, D., Hickman, M., Jamshidi,Y. et al. (2001) Elite swimmers and the D allele of the ACE I/D polymorphism. Hum. Genet. **108**, 230–2.

Woods, D., Hooper, T., Hodkinson, P. et al. (2011) Effect of altitude exposure on brain natriuretic peptide in humans. Eur. J. Appl. Physiol. **111**, 2687–93.

Woods, D.R., Brull, D. and Montgomery, H.E. (2000) Endurance and the ACE gene. Sci. Prog. **83**, 317–36.

Woods, D.R. and Montgomery, H.E. (2001) Angiotensin-converting enzyme and genetics at high altitude. High Alt. Med. Biol. **2**, 201–10.

Woods, D.R., Pollard, A.J., Collier, D.J. et al. (2002) Insertion/deletion polymorphism of the angiotensin I-converting enzyme gene and arterial oxygen saturation at high altitude. Am. J. Respir. Crit. Care Med. **166**, 362–6.

Woods, D.R., Allen, S., Betts, T.R. et al. (2008) High altitude arrhythmias. Cardiology **111**, 239–46.

Woods, D.R., Begley, J., Stacey, M. et al. (2012a) Severe acute mountain sickness, brain natriuretic peptide and NT–proBNF in humans. Acta Physiol. **205**, 349–55.

Woods, D.R., Davidson, A., Stacey, M. et al. (2012b) The cortisol response to hypobaric hypoxia at rest and post-exercise. Horm. Metab. Res. **44**, 1–4.

Woolcott, O.O., Castillo, O.A., Torres, J. et al. (2002) Serum leptin levels in dwellers from high altitude lands. High Alt. Med. Biol. **3**, 245–6.

World Health Organization. 2. Introduction to mountain regions, WHO Publication Available from: www.searo.who.int/LinkFiles/Publications_and_Documents_healthImapctsC2.pdf

Wren, A.M., Seal, L.J., Cohen, M.A. et al. (2001) Ghrelin enhances appetite and increases food intake in humans J. Clin. Endocrinol. Metabol. **86**, 5992–5.

Wright, A.D., Imray, C.H., Morrissey, M.S. et al. (1995) Intracranial pressure at high altitude and acute mountain sickness. *Clin. Sci. (Lond)* **89**, 201–4.

Wu, T. (1994b) Children on the Tibetan plateau. *ISMM Newsletter* **4**, 5–6.

Wu, T., Li, S., and Ward, M.P. (2005) Tibetans at extreme altitude. *Wilderness Environ. Med.* **16**, 47–54.

Wu, T., Wang, X., Wei, C. *et al.* (2005) Hemoglobin levels in Qinghai-Tibet: different effects of gender for Tibetans versus Han. *J. Appl. Physiol.* **98**, 598–604.

Wu, T.Y. (1994a) Low prevalence of systemic hypertension in Tibetan native highlanders. *ISMM Newsletter* **4**, 5–7.

Wu, T.Y. (2000) Take note of altitude gastrointestinal bleeding. *ISMM Newsletter* **10**, 9–10.

Wu, T.Y. (2005) Chronic mountain sickness on the Qinghai–Tibetan plateau. *Chin. Med. J.* **118**, 161–8.

Wu, T.Y., Ding, S.Q., Liu, J.L. *et al.* (2007a) High-altitude gastrointestinal bleeding: an observation in Qinghai–Tibetan railroad construction workers on Mountain Tanggula. *World J. Gastroenterol.* **13**, 774–80.

Wu, T.Y., Ding, S.Q., Liu, J.L. *et al.* (2007b) Who should not go high: chronic disease and work at altitude during construction of the Qinghai–Tibet railroad. *High Alt. Med. Biol.* **8**, 88–107.

Wu, T.Y., Ding, S.Q., Liu, J.L. *et al.* (2009) Reduced incidence and severity of acute mountain sickness in Qinghai–Tibet railroad construction workers after repeated 7-month exposures despite 5-month low altitude periods. *High Alt. Med. Biol.* **10**, 221–32.

Wu, T.Y., Ding, S.Q., Zhang, S.L. *et al.* (2010) Altitude illness in Qinghai–Tibet railroad passengers. *High Alt. Med. Biol.* **11**, 189–98.

Wu, T-Y. and Liu, Y.R. (1995) High altitude heart disease. *Chin. J. Pediatr.* **6**, 348–50.

Wu, T-Y., Zhang, Q., Jin, B. *et al.* (1992) Chronic mountain sickness (Monge's disease): an observation in Quinghai–Tibet plateau, in *High Altitude Medicine* (eds. G. Ueda, J.T. Reeves and M. Sekiguchi), Sinshu University Press, Matsumoto, pp. 314–24.

Wyss, C.A., Koepfli, P., Fretz, G. *et al.* (2003) Influence of altitude exposure on coronary flow reserve. *Circulation* **108**, 1202–7.

Xing, G., Qualls, C., Huicho, L. *et al.* (2008) Adaptation and maladaptation to ambient hypoxia: Andean, Ethiopian, and Himalayan patterns. *PLoS* **3**, e2342.

Xu, F. and Severinghaus, J.W. (1998) Rat brain VEGF expression in alveolar hypoxia: possible role in high-altitude cerebral edema. *J. Appl. Physiol.* **85**, 53–7.

Xu, K. and Lamanna, J.C. (2006) Chronic hypoxia and the cerebral circulation. *J. Appl. Physiol.* **100**, 725–30.

Xu, S., Li, S., Yang, Y. *et al.* (2011) A genome-wide search for signals of high altitude adaptation in Tibetans. *Mol. Biol. Evol.* **28**, 1003–11.

Xu, X.-Q. and Jing, Z.-C. (2009) High-altitude pulmonary hypertension. *Eur. Respir. Rev.* **18**, 13–17.

Yagi, H., Yamada, H., Kobayashi, T. and Sekiguchi, M. (1990) Doppler assessment of pulmonary hypertension induced by hypoxic breathing in subjects susceptible to high altitude pulmonary edema. *Am. Rev. Respir. Dis.* **142**, 796–801.

Yamaguchi, S., Matsuzawa, S., Yoshikawa, S. *et al.* (1991) Effect of acclimatization and deacclimatization on hypoxic ventilatory response. *Jpn. J. Mount. Med.* **11**, 77–84.

Yamamoto, W.S. and Edwards, M.W. (1960) Homeostasis of carbon dioxide during intravenous infusion of carbon dioxide. *J. Appl. Physiol.* **15**, 807–18.

Yanagidaira, Y., Sakai, A., Kashimura, O. *et al.* (1994) The effects of prolonged exposure to cold on hypoxic pulmonary hypertension in rats. *J. Wilderness Med.* **5**, 11–19.

Yanda, R.L. and Herschensohn, H.L. (1964) Changes in lung volumes of emphysema patients upon short exposures to simulated altitude of 18,000 feet. *Aerosp. Med.* **35**, 1201–3.

Yang, S.P., Bergo, G.W., Krasney, E. and Krasney, J.A. (1994) Cerebral pressure-flow and metabolic responses to sustained hypoxia: effect of CO2. *J. Appl. Physiol.* **76**, 303–13.

Yarnell, P.R., Heit, J. and Hackett, P.H. (2000) High-altitude cerebral edema (HACE): the Denver/Front Range experience. *Semin. Neurol.* **20**, 209–17.

Yaron, M. and Niermeyer, S. (2008) Travel to high altitude with young children: an approach for clinicians. *High Alt. Med. Biol.* **9**, 265–9.

Yaron, M., Waldman, N., Niermeyer, S. *et al.* (1998) The diagnosis of acute mountain sickness in preverbal children. *Arch. Pediatr. Adolesc. Med.* **152**, 683–7.

Yaron, M., Niermeyer, S., Lindgren, K.N. and Honigman, B. (2002) Evaluation of diagnostic criteria and incidence of acute mountain sickness in preverbal children. *Wilderness Environ. Med.* **13**, 21–6.

Yaron, M., Niermeyer, S., Lindgren, K.N. *et al.* (2003) Physiologic response to moderate altitude exposure among infants and young children. *High Alt. Med. Biol.* **4**, 53–9.

Yaron, M., Lindgren, K.N., Halbower, A.C. *et al.* (2004) Sleep disturbance after rapid ascent to moderate altitude among infants and preverbal young children. *High Alt. Med. Biol.* **5**, 314–20.

Yi, X., Liang, Y., Huerta-Sanchez, E. *et al.* (2010). Sequencing of 50 human exomes reveals adaptation to high altitude. *Science* **329**, 75–8.

Yoneda, I. and Watanabe, Y. (1997) Comparison of altitude tolerance and hypoxia symptoms between non-smokers and habitual smokers. *Aviat. Space Environ. Med.* **68**, 807–11.

Young, A.J., Muza, S.R., Sawka, M.N. *et al.* (1986) Human thermo-regulatory responses to cold air are altered by repeated cold water immersion. *J. Appl. Physiol.* **60**, 1542–8.

Young, A.J., Sawka, M.N., Muza, S.R. *et al.* (1996) Effects of erythrocyte infusion on Vo_{2max} at high altitude. *J. Appl. Physiol.* **81**, 252–9.

Young, A.J., Castellani, J.W., O'Brian, C. *et al.* (1998) Exertional fatigue, sleeplessness and negative energy balance increases susceptibility to hypothermia. *J. Appl. Physiol.* **85**, 1210–17.

Young, P.M., Rose, M.S., Sutton, J.R. *et al.* (1989) Operation Everest II: plasma lipid and hormonal responses during a simulated ascent of Mt Everest. *J. Appl. Physiol.* **66**, 1430–5.

Zacarian, S.A. (1985) Cryogenics: the cryolesions and the pathogenesis of cryonecrosis, in *Cryosurgery for Skin and Cutaneous Diseases* (ed. S.A. Zacarian), Mosby, St Louis, MO.

Zaccaria, M., Rocco, S., Noventa, D. *et al.* (1998) Sodium regulating hormones at high altitude: basal and post-exercise levels. *J. Clin. Endocrinol. Metab.* **83**, 570–4.

Zaccaria, M., Ermolao, A., Bonvicini, P. *et al.* (2004) Decreased serum leptin levels during prolonged high altitude exposure. *Eur. J. Appl. Physiol.* **92**, 249–53.

Zafren, K. (1998) Hyponatremia in a cold environment. *Wilderness Environ. Med.* **9**, 54–5.

Zafren, K., Reeves, J.T. and Schoene, R. (1996) Treatment of high-altitude pulmonary edema by bed rest and supplemental oxygen. *Wilderness Environ. Med.* **7**, 127–32.

Zafren, K., Feldman, J., Becker, R.J. *et al.* (2011) D-dimer is not elevated in asymptomatic high altitude climbers after descent to 5340 m: the Mount Everest Deep Venous Thrombosis Study (Ev-DVT). *High Alt. Med. Biol.* **12**, 223–7.

Zamudio, S. (2003) The placenta at high altitude. *High Alt. Med. Biol.* **4**, 171–91.

Zamudio, S. (2007) High-altitude hypoxia and preeclampsia. *Front. Biosci.* **12**, 2967–77.

Zamudio, S., Baumann, M.U. and Illsley, N.P. (2006) Effects of chronic hypoxia in vivo on the expression of human placental glucose transporters. *Placenta* **27**, 49–55.

Zhai, Z., Wang, J., Zhao, L. *et al.* (2010) Pulmonary hypertension in China: pulmonary vascular disease: the global perspective. *Chest* **137**, 69s–77s.

Zhang, E.G., Burton, G.J., Smith, S.K. and Charnock-Jones, D.S. (2002) Placental vessel adaptation during gestation and to high altitude: changes in diameter and perivascular cell coverage. *Placenta* **23**, 751–62.

Zhang, H., Wu, C.X., Chamba, Y., and Ling, Y. (2007) Blood characteristics for high altitude adaptation in Tibetan chickens. *Poult. Sci.* **86**, 1384–9.

Zhang, Y.B. (1985) *An Introduction to Medical Research in Qinghai*, High Altitude Medical Research Institute, Qinghai, China.

Zhao, L., Mason, N.A., Morrell, N.W. *et al.* (2001) Sildenafil inhibits hypoxia-induced pulmonary hypertension. *Circulation* **104**, 424–8.

Zhao, X., Li, S., He, F. *et al.* (2012) Prevalence, awareness, treatment, and control of hypertension among herdsmen living at 4,300 m in Tibet. *Am. J. Hypertens.* **5**, 583–9.

Zhongyuan, S., Xuehan, N., Shoucheng, Z. *et al.* (1980) Electrocardiogram made on ascending the mount Qomolangma from 50 m A.S.L. *Sci. Sin.* **23**, 1316–25.

Zhongyuan, S., Deming, Z., Changming, L. and Miaoshen, Q. (1983) Changes of electroencephalogram under acute hypoxia and relationship between tolerant ability to hypoxia and adaptation ability to high altitudes. *Sci. Sin.* **26**, 58–69.

Zhou, Q., Tan, X., Wang, J. *et al.* (2011) Increased permeability of the blood–brain barrier caused by inflammatory mediators is involved in high-altitude cerebral edema. *Sci. Res. Essays.* **6**, 607–15.

Zhu, T., Lin, W., Song, Y. *et al.* (2006) Downward transport of ozone-rich air near Mt. Everest. *Geophys. Res. Lett.* **33**, L23809, 4PP.

Zhuang, J., Droma, T., Sun, S. *et al.* (1993) Hypoxic ventilatory responsiveness in Tibetan compared with Han residents of 3,658 m. *J. Appl. Physiol.* **74**, 303–11.

Zielinski J., Koziej, M., Mankowski, M. *et al.* (2000) The quality of sleep and periodic breathing in healthy subjects at an altitude of 3200 metres: sleep at high altitude. *High Alt. Med. Biol.* **1**, 331–6.

Zimmerman, G.A. and Crapo, R.O. (1980) Adult respiratory distress syndrome secondary to high altitude pulmonary edema. *West. J. Med.* **133**, 335–7.

Zoll, J., Ponsot, F., Dufour, S. *et al.* (2006) Exercise training in normobaric hypoxia in endurance runners: muscular adjustments of selected gene transcripts. *J. Appl. Physiol.* **100**, 1258–66.

Zuntz, N., Loewy, A., Müller, F. and Caspari, W. (1906) *Höhenklima und Bergwanderungen in ihrer Wirkung auf den Menschen*, Bong, Berlin. An English translation of the relevant passages can be found in *High Altitude Physiology* (ed. J.B. West), Hutchinson Ross, Stroudsburg, PA, 1981.

Index